HANDBOOK OF
CRYOGENIC ENGINEERING

HANDBOOK OF CRYOGENIC ENGINEERING

Edited by

J. G. Weisend II

Deutsches Elektronen-Synchrotron (DESY)
Hamburg, Germany

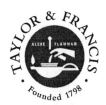

USA	Publishing Office	Taylor & Francis 325 Chestnut St., #800 Philadelphia, PA 19106 Tel: (215) 625-8900 Fax: (215) 625-2940
	Distribution Center	Taylor & Francis 1900 Frost Road, Suite 101 Bristol, PA 19007-1598 Tel: (215) 785-5800 Fax: (215) 785-5515
UK		Taylor & Francis Ltd. 1 Gunpowder Square London EC4A 3DE Tel: 0171 583 0490 Fax: 0171 583 0581

HANDBOOK OF CRYOGENIC ENGINEERING

1 2 3 4 5 6 7 8 9 0   E B E B   9 0 9 8

A CIP catalog record for this book is available from the British Library.
⊗ The paper in this publication meets the requirements of the ANSI Standard Z39.48-1984 (Permanence of Paper)

Library of Congress Cataloging-in-Publication Data

Handbook of cryogenic engineering / edited by John G. Weisend II.
     p.   cm.
   Includes bibliographical references.
   ISBN 1-56032-332-9 (case : alk. paper)
   1. Low temperature engineering.   I. Weisend, J. G.
TP482.H36   1998
621.5′9—dc21   97-48881
                                       CIP

ISBN 1-56032-332-9

CONTENTS

Preface   xiii
List of Contributors   xvii

1   PROPERTIES OF CRYOGENIC FLUIDS
       V. Arp and J. G. Weisend II   1

1-1   Introduction   1
1-2   Thermophysical Properties of Fluids   1
       1-2-1   Fluid State Properties   2
       1-2-2   Thermal Conductivity and Viscosity   18
       1-2-3   Computer Programs for Fluid Properties   21
1-3   Tabular Data for Particular Fluids   21
1-4   Sources for Fluid Property Computer Programs   71
       References   71

2   PROPERTIES OF CRYOGENIC MATERIALS
       T. H. K. Frederking, R. Flükiger, J. L. Hall, J. A. Barclay, X. Y. Liu,
       G. Hartwig, and V. L. Morris   73

2-1   Friction Coefficients and Related Phenomena
       T. H. K. Frederking   73
       2-1-1   Introduction   73
       2-1-2   Phenomena of Static and Dynamic Friction   74
       2-1-3   Experimental Methods   78
       2-1-4   Friction Data   80
       2-1-5   Magnet Tribology and Related Parameters   83

	Acknowledgments		89
	Nomenclature		90
	References		90
2-2	Composite Materials		
	V. L. Morris		92
	2-2-1	Introduction	92
	2-2-2	Composite Materials	92
	2-2-3	Structural Design	96
	2-2-4	Composite Structure Uses	98
	Nomenclature		101
	References		102
2-3	Critical Current-Density in Bi,Pb(2223) Tapes		
	R. Flükiger		103
	2-3-1	Introduction	103
	2-3-2	Fabrication of Bi-2223 Tapes	103
	2-3-3	Variation of $j_c(B)$ for Multifilamentary Bi-2223 Tapes	108
	2-3-4	Conclusion	110
	References		111
2-4	Magnetic Materials for Cryogenic Refrigeration		
	J. L. Hall, J. A. Barclay, and X. Y. Liu		112
	2-4-1	Introduction	112
	2-4-2	Classification of Magnetic Refrigerant Materials	114
	2-4-3	Representative Magnetic Refrigerant Data	115
	2-4-4	Passive Magnetic Regenerator Materials	115
	Nomenclature		118
	References		119
2-5	Cryogenic Properties of Polymers		
	G. Hartwig		121
	2-5-1	Introduction	121
	2-5-2	Accuracy of Data	122
	2-5-3	Sample Treatments and Their Influence on Cryogenic Properties	123
	2-5-4	Cryogenic Applications of Polymers	123
	2-5-5	Scientific Aspects of Low-Temperature Polymer Investigations	124
	2-5-6	Glass Transitions and Properties	127
	2-5-7	Damping Behavior	127
	2-5-8	Deformation Behavior	130
	2-5-9	Dielectric Permittivity	134
	2-5-10	Fracture Behavior	135
	2-5-11	Fatigue Behavior	137
	2-5-12	Thermal Vibrations of Polymers	138
	2-5-13	Specific Heat	139
	2-5-14	Thermal Expansion	141
	2-5-15	Thermal Conductivity	145
	2-5-16	Gas Permeability	147
	2-5-17	Radiation Damage	151
	Nomenclature		156
	References		156
	Bibliography		157
	Appendix		158

3 CRYOGENIC HEAT TRANSFER
P. Kittel, T. Nast, L. J. Salerno, M. Shiotsu, and J. G. Weisend II 163

3-1 Introduction 163
3-2 Conduction Heat Transfer 163
   3-2-1 Thermal Conductivity Integrals
     J. G. Weisend II 163
   3-2-2 Thermal Contact Conductance
     L. J. Salerno and P. Kittel 164
   Nomenclature 178
3-3 Convection Heat Transfer 178
   3-3-1 Correlations for Forced Convection Heat Transfer
     J. G. Weisend II 178
   Nomenclature 180
   3-3-2 Predicting the Critical Heat Flux for a Horizontal
     Cylinder in Saturated Liquid He I
     M. Shiotsu 181
   Nomenclature 185
3-4 Radiation Heat Transfer 186
   3-4-1 Multilayer Insulation Systems
     T. Nast 186
   Nomenclature 200
   Acknowledgments 200
   References 200

4 CRYOGENIC INSTRUMENTATION
D. S. Holmes and S. S. Courts 203

4-1 Measurement Systems 203
   4-1-1 Balanced Design of a Measurement System 203
   4-1-2 Defining the Measurement 204
   4-1-3 Selecting a Sensor 205
   4-1-4 Measurement Uncertainty 206
   4-1-5 Sources of Measurement Uncertainty 207
   4-1-6 Other Measurement System Considerations 211
4-2 Temperature Measurement 216
   4-2-1 Metallic Resistors 219
   4-2-2 Semiconducting Resistors 222
   4-2-3 Semiconductor Diodes 227
   4-2-4 Capacitors 228
   4-2-5 Thermocouples 229
   4-2-6 Self-Heating of Temperature Sensors 231
   4-2-7 Temperature Sensor Calibration 234
4-3 Strain Measurement 234
4-4 Pressure Measurement 236
   4-4-1 Piezoresistive or Strain Gauge Pressure Sensors 237
   4-4-2 Capacitance Pressure Sensors 241
   4-4-3 Variable Reluctance Pressure Sensors 241
   4-4-4 Piezoelectric Pressure Sensors 241

4-5	Flow Measurement	242
	4-5-1 Mass Flowmeters	242
	4-5-2 Volumetric Flowmeters	243
	4-5-3 Differential Pressure Flowmeters	245
4-6	Liquid Level Measurement	247
4-7	Magnetic Measurements	248
	4-7-1 Hall Effect	248
	4-7-2 Induction Coils	249
	4-7-3 Magnetoresistance	249
	4-7-4 NMR	249
	4-7-5 SQUIDs	250
4-8	Others Measurements	250
	References for Section 4-8	251
4-9	Commercial Sources	252
	Nomenclature	253
	References	253

5 CRYOSTAT DESIGN
G. McIntosh 259

5-1	Introduction	259
5-2	Materials	260
	5-2-1 Austenitic Stainless Steels: Types 304, 304L, 304N, 316, 316L, and 321	260
	5-2-2 Nickel Steels: Primarily 9% Nickel Steel	260
	5-2-3 Aluminum Alloys: Alloys 1100, 3003, 6061, 6063, and 5083	261
	5-2-4 Copper: Commercial Alloys CDA 101 (OFHC), 110 (ETP), and 120 (Phosphorous Deoxidized)	261
	5-2-5 Fiber–Epoxy Composites: NEMA Grades G-10-CR, G-11-CR, and Others	261
	5-2-6 Other Structural Materials: Titanium, Invar, Maraging Steels, Hastelloy Alloys	262
5-3	Cold Seals	263
5-4	Cryostat and Dewar Supports	267
5-5	Helium Cryostat and Dewar Design with Vapor-Cooled Shields	268
5-6	Vacuum-Jacketed Transfer Line Design	269
	References	278

6 REFRIGERANTS FOR NORMAL REFRIGERATION
W. E. Kraus and M. Kauschke 279

6-1	Introduction	279
6-2	Classification of Refrigerants	279
	6-2-1 General	279
	6-2-2 Isomers	280
	6-2-3 R4XX: Refrigerant Mixtures (Blends)	280
	6-2-4 R5XX: Azeotropic Refrigerant Mixtures	282
	6-2-5 Butane Compounds	282
	6-2-6 R7XX: Inorganic Compounds	282

6-3   Environmental Impact of Refrigerants   283
6-4   Selection of Refrigerants   284
       References   285

7   SMALL CRYOCOOLERS
       L. Duband and A. Ravex   287

7-1   Introduction   287
7-2   Thermodynamic Considerations of Cryocoolers   288
       7-2-1   Theoretical Reversible Cycles   288
       7-2-2   Joule–Thomson Expansion   293
7-3   Inefficiencies and Parasitic Losses in Real Cryocoolers   295
       7-3-1   Piston Motion   296
       7-3-2   Dead Volumes   297
       7-3-3   Pressure Drop   297
       7-3-4   Nonisothermal Operation   297
       7-3-5   Regenerator or Counterflow Heat Exchanger Inefficiency   297
       7-3-6   Thermal Losses   298
       7-3-7   Conclusion   298
7-4   Cryocoolers: Applications and State of the Art   299
       7-4-1   Joule–Thomson Expansion Cryocoolers   299
       7-4-2   Gifford–McMahon Cryocoolers   302
       7-4-3   Compound Gifford–McMahon and Joule–Thomson Cryocoolers   306
       7-4-4   Stirling Cryocoolers   308
7-5   Future Trends in Cryocooler Development   311
       7-5-1   Magnetic Materials for Regenerators   312
       7-5-2   Gas Mixtures for Joule–Thomson Expansion Coolers   313
       7-5-3   Pulse-Tube Refrigerators   314
       7-5-4   Adsorption Coolers   318
7-6   Choosing a Cryocooler   319
       Nomenclature   319
       References   320

8   SUPERCONDUCTING MAGNET TECHNOLOGY
       A. Devred, H. Desportes, F. Kircher, C. Lesmond, C. Meuris, J. M. Rey,
       and J. L. Duchateau   321

8-1   Introduction   321
8-2   General Properties of Superconductors   322
       8-2-1   Critical Parameters   322
       8-2-2   Different Types of Superconductors   323
8-3   Practical Superconducting Materials   325
       8-3-1   Niobium Titanium   325
       8-3-2   Niobium Tin and Niobium Aluminum   326
       8-3-3   Conductor Assembly   329
8-4   Conceptual Design of Superconducting Magnets   330
       8-4-1   User's Specifications   330
       8-4-2   First Design Approach   331

		8-4-3	Conceptual Choices	331
		8-4-4	Complete Design	333
	8-5	AC Losses		334
		8-5-1	Superconducting Magnetization	334
		8-5-2	Coupling Current Losses in Composites and Cables	337
	8-6	Thermal Stability		340
		8-6-1	General Stability Concepts	341
		8-6-2	Stability Criteria of Windings Cooled by Helium Channels	342
		8-6-3	Stability of Internally Cooled Conductors	344
	8-7	Electrical Insulation		346
		8-7-1	Specification	346
		8-7-2	The Different Insulation Materials	346
		8-7-3	Temperature Dependence of the Insulation Material Properties	347
		8-7-4	Influence of the Cooling Technique on the Insulation	348
		8-7-5	Impregnated Superconducting Coils	348
	8-8	Quench Protection		349
		8-8-1	Quench Mechanism	349
		8-8-2	Maximum Temperature and Voltage	350
		8-8-3	Protection Techniques	353
	8-9	Some Applications		356
		Nomenclature		361
		References		363
		Bibliography		364

9 CRYOGENIC EQUIPMENT
D. E. Daney, J. E. Dillard, and M. D. Forsha   365

	9-1	Cryogenic Transfer Systems		365
		9-1-1	Introduction	365
		9-1-2	Pressure Drop	369
	9-2	Pumps		380
		9-2-1	Introduction	380
		9-2-2	Centrifugal Pumps	381
		9-2-3	Positive Displacement Pumps	392
	9-3	Cold Compressors		393
		9-3-1	Introduction	393
		9-3-2	Turbo Compressors	395
		9-3-3	Ejectors	398
	9-4	Current Leads		399
		9-4-1	Introduction	399
		9-4-2	Conduction-Cooled Current Leads	403
		9-4-3	Gas-Cooled Current Leads	404
		9-4-4	Hybrid Current Leads	408
	9-5	Heat Exchangers		413
		9-5-1	Introduction	413
		9-5-2	Types of Heat Exchangers	415
		9-5-3	Heat Exchanger Design	423
		9-5-4	Regenerator Design	429

9-5-5   Heat Transfer Coefficients and Pressure Drop   430
Nomenclature   436
References   438

10   He II (SUPERFLUID HELIUM)
         S. W. Van Sciver   443

10-1   Introduction   443
10-2   Properties of He II   444
       10-2-1   Phase Diagram   444
       10-2-2   State Properties   445
       10-2-3   Transport Properties   450
       10-2-4   Surface Heat Transfer   460
10-3   Technology of He II Applications   463
       10-3-1   Refrigeration Techniques   463
       10-3-2   Heat Exchangers   466
       10-3-3   Pumping Methods   470
       10-3-4   He II Flowmetering Techniques   475
10-4   Summary   478
       Nomenclature   478
       References   479

11   SAFETY
         F. J. Edeskuty and M. Daugherty   481

11-1   Introduction   481
11-2   Sources of Hazards   481
11-3   Physiological Hazards   481
       11-3-1   Cold Damage to Living Tissue   482
       11-3-2   Asphyxiation   483
       11-3-3   Toxicity   484
11-4   Physical (or Mechanical) Hazards   484
       11-4-1   Embrittlement   484
       11-4-2   Buildup of Pressure   486
       11-4-3   Condensation of Atmospheric Gases and Higher-Boiling Substances   491
       11-4-4   Stresses Caused by Thermal Contraction   492
11-5   Combustion Hazards   494
       11-5-1   Fuels (Hydrogen and LNG)   495
       11-5-2   Oxidizers   495
11-6   Regulations, Standards, and Guidelines   496
11-7   Conclusions   497
       References   498

INDEX   499

PREFACE

Cryogenics is the science and technology of very low temperatures. Traditionally, the field of cryogenics is taken to start at temperatures below 120 K. Although cryogenics may seem like an esoteric field, it plays a major role in modern industry and science. Large-scale air separation plants use cryogenics to break down air into its component elements for industrial and medical uses. The resulting products are frequently transported and stored as cryogenic fluids for efficiency. Magnetic resonance imaging (MRI) systems that use superconducting magnets cooled by liquid helium have become a common feature in modern hospitals. In space technology, cryogenics is found in the liquid hydrogen and oxygen fuels used in rocket engines and in applications such as the Cosmic Background explorer (COBE) satellite, whose superfluid (He II) cooled sensors have detected remnants of the Big Bang. The Large Hadron Collider, currently under construction, will use thousands of superconducting magnets cooled to 1.8 K to study the fundamental laws of matter. At a smaller scale, cryocoolers are used to provide cooling for night-vision systems.

The study of cryogenics* started back in the nineteenth century as scientists and engineers raced each other to liquefy gases and reach ever lower temperatures. This process started in 1887 with the announcement of the liquefaction of oxygen (Pictet and Cailletet). In 1898, James Dewar first liquefied hydrogen. Dewar also developed the vacuum-insulated flask with reflective walls for containing cryogenic liquids. His design is still at the heart of cryogenic containers today, which in tribute are frequently called Dewars. The last and most difficult gas to be liquified was helium. This gas was first liquefied by Kamerlingh Onnes of Lieden in 1908. He promptly used helium to discover the phenomenon of superconductivity. Onnes is also credited with coining the term cryogenics.

---

*Additional details on the history of cryogenics may be found in *History and Origins of Cryogenics*, R. G. Scurlock, ed. (Oxford: Oxford University Press, 1991).

During this effort to liquefy gases, the researchers developed various refrigeration, storage, and instrumentation technologies. This work formed the basis of cryogenic knowledge today. As the twentieth century progressed, industrial applications of cryogenics increased, particularly in the area of air liquefaction. The space race of the 1960s greatly increased cryogenic research in the handling of liquid hydrogen and oxygen rocket fuels. Another major trend has been the development of practical superconducting materials in the last 25 years. Today cryogenic research continues, especially in the areas of cryocoolers, He II technology, space cryogenics, and superconductivity (both at liquid helium temperatures and with the more recently discovered high-temperature superconductors that can operate at 70–100 K).

The primary purpose of this handbook is to provide useful information for scientists, engineers, and students involved in the field of cryogenics. It is hoped that readers will find this book useful for looking up a particular equation or data point as well as for getting an overview of a topic in cryogenics.

As seen above, cryogenics is a broad field, and a secondary goal of this work is to bring together surveys of the state of the art of various cryogenic subfields. No single work can completely cover all of cryogenics, and where choices were necessary, emphasis was placed on those areas about which data might not be widely distributed. For example, polymers and composite materials are covered in greater detail than are standard metals.

Chapter 1 discusses the properties of cryogenic fluids. The law of corresponding states is introduced, allowing for the estimate of properties of a wide range of fluids. Tabular and graphical data of the properties of oxygen, helium, nitrogen, argon, and parahydrogen are also included. The properties of various useful materials at cryogenic temperatures are discussed in chapter 2. The materials discussed are composites, polymers, magnetic materials for cryogenic refrigeration, and one of the more technically promising high-temperature superconductors. Data on the phenomena of friction at cryogenic temperatures are also presented. Chapter 3 discusses aspects of heat transfer of particular importance to cryogenics. Covered here are thermal conductivity integrals, thermal contact conductance, correlations for forced-convection heat transfer, boiling limits in liquid helium, and multilayer insulation systems. Cryogenic instrumentation is the subject of chapter 4. The design of measurement systems, determination of uncertainties, and the selection of sensors are all discussed. Detailed data are given on the measurement of temperature, pressure, flow, strain, liquid level, and magnetic field in cryogenic systems. Chapter 5 discusses the proper design of cryostats, including basic design considerations, materials, cold seals, and the proper design of vapor-cooled shields. The design of cryogenic transfer lines is also covered in chapter 5. Chapter 6 addresses refrigerants for normal refrigeration. Small mechanical cryocoolers have become a very important application of cryogenics. Chapter 7 provides data on the various types of cryocoolers (Gifford–McMahon, Joule–Thomson, Stirling, and pulse-tube). The performance and uses of these cryocoolers are compared, and the proper selection of a cryocooler is discussed. Superconducting magnet technology is covered in chapter 8. Data are provided on the technically useful superconductors (NbTi and A-15 compounds). Design of magnets, AC losses, stabilization, quench protection, and insulation are all addressed in detail in this chapter. Equations, tables, and figures of useful information are provided. Chapter 9 covers cryogenic equipment. Extensive data are given on valves, pumps, cold compressors, current leads, and heat exchangers. The calculation of pressure drop in cryogenic transfer systems is also discussed. Chapter 10 addresses He II (superfluid helium). The basic properties of this fluid, including flow and heat transfer, are discussed. Data supporting practical applications of He II are also included. Here, information is given on Kapitza conductance, He II heat exchanger design, pumping methods, and flowmetering techniques. Safety is a vital part of any cryogenic system. In chapter 11, the unique hazards found in cryogenics and ways to reduce them are discussed.

It was clear from the start that this handbook required the contributions of a wide range of experts. I would like to thank all the authors who took time from their busy careers to write a chapter or section for this book. Additional thanks are due to Professor Frederking of UCLA and Professor Van Sciver of Florida State University, who not only wrote chapters but also suggested several contributors. My colleagues at DESY Laboratory were also very supportive of my efforts.

Lisa Ehmer, Carolyn Ormes, and the production staff at Taylor & Francis are to be thanked for their enthusiasm, support, and advice.

Throughout the duration of this work, my wife Shari and daughter Rachel were supportive and understanding. As always, I am indebted to them.

J. G. Weisend II

LIST OF CONTRIBUTORS

V. ARP
Cryodata Inc.
P.O. Box 173
Louisville, CO 80027

J. A. BARCLAY
Cryofuel Systems—University
of Victoria
P.O. Box 3055, Victoria
BC V8W 3P6, Canada

S. S. COURTS
Lake Shore Cryotronics
575 McCorkle Boulevard
Westerville, OH 43802

D. E. DANEY
MS-J580, LANL
Los Alamos, NM 87545

M. DAUGHERTY
24 Oak Grove Drive
Madison, WI 53717

H. DESPORTES
CEA Saclay, DAPIA/SCTM
91191 Gif Sur Yvette Cedex
France

A. DEVRED
CEA Saclay, DAPIA/SCTM
91191 Gif Sur Yvette Cedex
France

J. E. DILLARD
Barber-Nichols Inc.
6325 W 55th Avenue
Arvada, CO 80002

L. DUBAND
Centre d'Etudes Nucleaires
Grenoble, DRFMC/SBT
17 Ave des Martyrs
38054 Grenoble, Cédex 9
France

J. L. DUCHATEAU
CEA Cadarache, DRFC/STID
13108 Saint-Paul-lez-Durance Cedex
France

F. J. EDESKUTY
MS-J576, LANL
Los Alamos, NM 87545

M. D. FORSHA
Barber-Nichols Inc.
6325 W 55th Avenue
Arvada, CO 80002

T. H. K. FREDERKING
UCLA, BH5531 SEAS/Chem E
Los Angeles, CA 90095

R. FLÜKIGER
University of Geneva
DPMC, 24, Quai Ernest Ansermet
Geneva, 1211, Switzerland

J. L. HALL
Jet Propulsion Laboratory
MS 156-316
4800 Oak Grove Drive
Pasadena, CA 91109

G. HARTWIG
Forschungszentrum Karlsruhe
IMF II, Postfach 3640
76021 Karlsruhe, Germany

D. S. HOLMES
Lake Shore Cryotronics
575 McCorkle Boulevard
Westerville, OH 43802

M. KAUSCHKE
Technische Universität Dresden
01062 Dresden, Germany

F. KIRCHER
CEA Saclay, DAPIA/SCTM
91191 Gif Sur Yvette Cedex
France

P. KITTEL
NASA Ames Research Center
MS 234-1, Moffett Field
CA 94035-1000

W. E. KRAUS
Technische Universität Dresden
01062 Dresden, Germany

C. LESMOND
CEA Saclay, DAPIA/SCTM
91191 Gif Sur Yvette Cedex
France

X. Y. LIU
Integrated Manufacturing
Technologies Institute
National Research Council of Canada
800 Collip Circle, London
Ontario, Canada N6G 4X8

G. McINTOSH
Cryogenic Technical Services
164 Primrose Court
Longmont, CO 80501-6036

C. MEURIS
CEA Saclay, DAPIA/SCTM
91191 Gif Sur Yvette Cedex France

V. L. MORRIS
Morris Associates
20952 Mesa Rica Road
Covina, CA 91724

T. NAST
Lockheed Martin Missiles and Space
3251 Hanover Street
Orgn. H121, Building 205
Palo Alto, CA 94304

A. RAVEX
Centre d'Etudes Nucleaires
Grenoble, DRFMC/SBT
17 Ave des Martyrs
38054 Grenoble, Cédex 9, France

J. M. REY
CEA Saclay, DAPIA/SCTM
91191 Gif Sur Yvette Cedex, France

L. J. SALERNO
NASA Ames Research Center
MS 234-1, Moffett Field
CA 94035-1000

M. SHIOTSU
Kyoto University
Department of Energy Science
and Technology
Gokasho, Uji
Kyoto 611, Japan

S. W. VAN SCIVER
NHMFL / FSU
1800 E. Paul Dirac Drive
Tallahassee, FL 32310

J. G. WEISEND II
MKS, DESY Laboratory
Notkestrasse 85
22607 Hamburg
Germany

ONE

PROPERTIES OF CRYOGENIC FLUIDS

V. Arp

Cryodata Inc., P.O. Box 173, Louisville, CO 80027

J. G. Weisend II

MKS, DESY Laboratory, Notkestrasse 85, 22607 Hamburg, Germany

1-1 INTRODUCTION

Cryogenic fluids may loosely be defined as those fluids whose normal boiling temperatures at atmospheric pressure are below 273 K. This definition includes the more common cryogens such as helium, hydrogen, neon, nitrogen, oxygen, argon, krypton, xenon, methane, ethane, and propane. Carbon dioxide should be included even though a pressure of over 5 atmospheres is required to maintain it in liquid form. Other fluids that fit the definition but are rarely used at temperatures below 273 K include carbon monoxide, nitrogen trifluoride, hydrogen sulfide, and some higher hydrocarbons.

The chemical reactivity of cryogenic fluids varies from nil for the noble gases to potentially explosive for hydrogen and the hydrocarbons and very dangerously reactive for liquid oxygen.

A general description of thermophysical fluid properties is given in Section 1-2 of this chapter. Tables of properties for particular fluids (He, Ar, H_2, N_2, O_2) are presented in section 1-3.

1-2 THERMOPHYSICAL PROPERTIES OF FLUIDS

Thermophysical fluid properties may be subdivided into state properties and transport properties. State properties relate to a static fluid element essentially unperturbed by any temperature gradient or fluid motion; they include pressure, volume, and temperature relationships, specific heats, compressibilities, and energies. These are reviewed in section 1-2-1.

Transport properties relate to the transport of energy or momentum through the fluid. They are more difficult to calculate from first principles, but adequate empirical descriptions exist. The thermal conductivity and viscosity of fluids are reviewed in section 1-2-2.

Computer programs are widely used to calculate fluid properties. Some available programs are discussed in section 1-2-3.

1-2-1 Fluid State Properties

The Fluid Phase Diagram. The fluid phase diagram for oxygen, Figure 1-1, is typical of that for all fluids except helium. The pressure, density, and temperature at the critical point are denoted P_c, ρ_c, and T_c, respectively. These critical parameters provide the scaling by which state properties of various fluids may be compared one with another. The melting and saturation lines intersect at the triple point, which is identified with P_t, ρ_t, and T_t. It is important to note that the saturation line exhibits an apparent extension above T_c shown as a dashed line in Fig. 1-1. The dashed line is known as the transposed critical line or the critical isochore and is the locus of peaks in some fluid properties, as is discussed later (e.g., specific heat). The peaks diminish in size as the temperature is raised, becoming ill-defined at several times T_c.

The phase diagram for helium, Fig. 1-2, is unique in that the melting line and the saturation line do not intersect even at the limit of absolute zero temperature but are

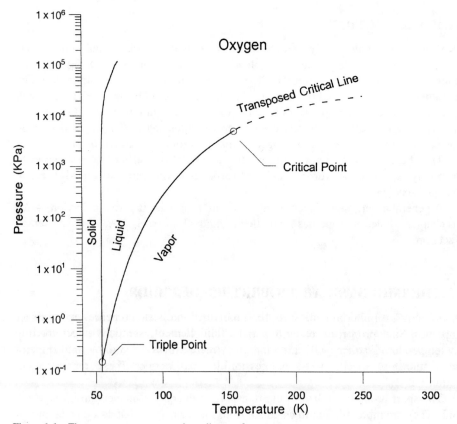

Figure 1-1   The pressure–temperature phase diagram for oxygen.

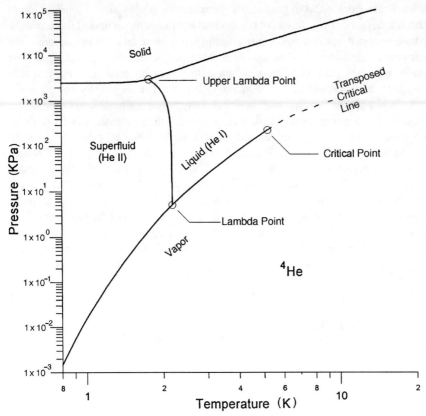

Figure 1-2 The pressure–temperature phase diagram for ^{4}He.

separated by the superfluid range (often denoted He II) and the lambda line. Above the critical temperature, helium exhibits a transposed critical line and properties that are consonant with those of other fluids.

One other special feature of helium should be mentioned. The ordinary helium atom is of mass 4, ^{4}He. In any container of helium, about 10^{-4} % of the helium atoms will be the rare ^{3}He isotope. When ^{3}He is prepared in pure liquid form (generally by radioactive decay of ^{3}Li), its properties are much different from those presented in Fig. 1-2. For example, ^{3}He does not become superfluid until cooled to a few millikelvin, where it then can exist in two alternative superfluid states. Although ^{3}He is fascinating to study, it is so rare that we do not consider it further in this chapter.

Hydrogen also deserves special attention. It can be in either of two molecular states: para-hydrogen, with the two nuclear spins opposing each other, and ortho-hydrogen, with the two nuclear spins parallel to each other. It happens that para-hydrogen has the lower ground-state energy and is the preferred state at low temperature. At room temperature, the thermal energy is enough to keep both quantum states fully occupied, which means that 3/4 of the hydrogen molecules will be in the ortho state, and the remainder will be in the para state. This 3/4–1/4 mixture is termed normal hydrogen. At liquid temperature, all the hydrogen molecules will eventually revert to the para state. However, the transition rate from ortho to para at low temperature is very slow (hours or days) unless catalyzed, and it is possible to obtain normal liquid hydrogen in the laboratory. At intermediate temperatures it is possible in principle to achieve an equilibrium hydrogen with intermediate ortho–para ratios; however, this equilibrium state is rarely achieved in ordinary laboratory practice. The problem with this ortho–para conversion is that it releases heat, causing boil-off of surrounding liquid. This is usually solved using catalysts in the hydrogen liquefier to create nominally pure para-hydrogen liquid.

It turns out that some normal hydrogen properties differ measurably from those of para-hydrogen. The most prominent differences are in specific heats, illustrated in Fig. 1-3, and thermal conductivity, illustrated in Fig. 1-4. The specific heat differences are pronounced roughly in the range of 50 to 400 K and disappear in the liquid range, even at high density. The conductivity differences appear below about 300 K and are most prominent in the compressed liquid. (It is possible that the greater critical point enhancement seen for the normal hydrogen in Fig. 1-4 is an artifact of the fitting process.) It is interesting to note that, by contrast, the differences between the viscosity of para and normal hydrogen are essentially negligible, as seen in Fig. 1-5. Other properties

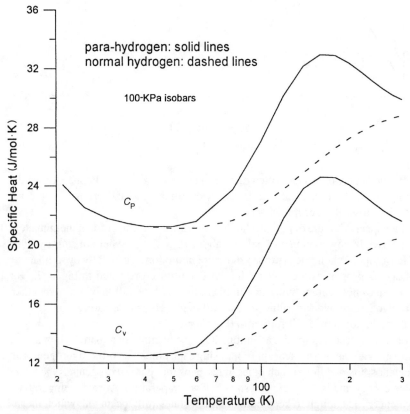

Figure 1-3 Comparison of specific heat for normal and para-hydrogen (solid line = normal hydrogen, dashed line = para-hydrogen).

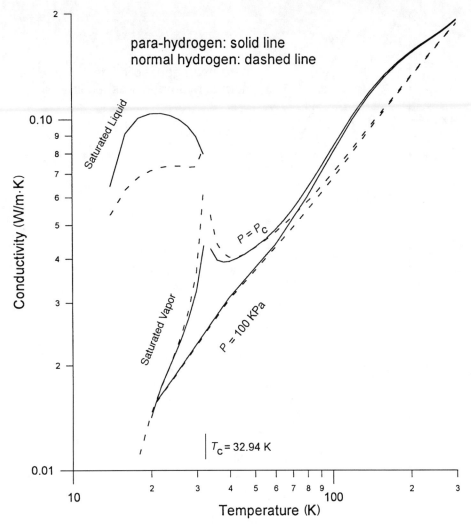

Figure 1-4 Comparison of the thermal conductivity for normal and para-hydrogen (solid line = normal hydrogen, dashed line = para-hydrogen.)

that share this approximate equality are the density, expansivity, compressibility, sound velocity, and triple and critical point parameters.

In the following presentation, many thermodynamic quantities have been normalized to the critical pressure, temperature, or density. Table 1-1 lists triple point and critical point values for many cryogens. Also listed is the normal boiling point, NBP, at standard atmospheric pressure.

Scaling laws. Figure 1-6 shows the pressure as a function of temperature along the saturation line for several fluids. By normalizing the pressure and temperature to their respective critical values for each fluid, one finds that the saturation pressures differ by no

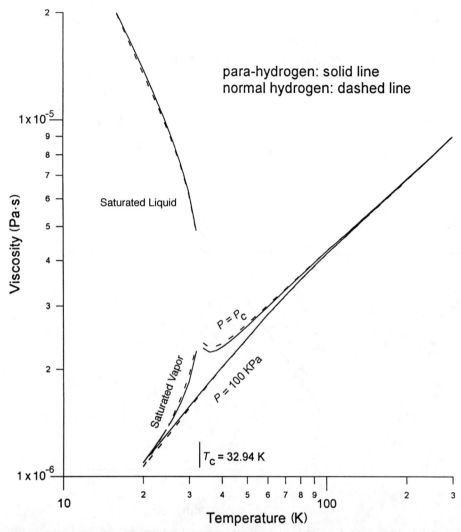

Figure 1-5 Comparison of viscosity for normal and para-hydrogen (solid line = normal hydrogen, dashed line = para-hydrogen).

more than a few percent from each other, except for hydrogen and helium. The location of the triple point along the quasiuniversal saturation line shows no obvious correlation with any other fluid property.

The slope of the saturation lines on the log–log graph of Fig. 1-6 is about 7 for most fluids and about 4 for helium. An easy way to remember the Clausius–Clapeyron equation is to recognize that this (dimensionless) slope is equal to the ratio of latent heat to PdV work in a liquid-to-vapor transition at constant pressure.

Hydrogen and helium properties are influenced by quantum effects at low temperatures and thus do not scale as well to properties of other fluids. For hydrogen, the scaling is further confused by two different forms of hydrogen, para-hydrogen and

Table 1-1 Critical point, triple point and normal boiling point properties for various cryogenic fluids

	Temperatures (K)			Pressure (kPa)		Critical density (kg/m^3)
	Triple point	Normal boiling point	Critical point	Triple point	Critical point	
Helium	2.1768[a]	4.222	5.1953	5.048	227.46	69.64
Hydrogen	13.8	20.28	32.94	7.042	1283.8	31.36
Neon	24.5561	27.09	44.44	43.35	2703	483.23
Nitrogen	63.15	77.36	126.26	12.46	3399	313.11
Oxygen	54.36	90.19	154.58	0.148	5043	436.14
Argon	83.8	87.28	150.86	68.9	4906	535.70
Krypton	115.76	119.77	209.39	73.2	5496	910.75
Xenon	161.36	165.04	289.74	81.6	5821	1100
CO_2	216.58	(−)	304.21	518.16	7384	466.51
Methane	90.69	111.63	190.55	11.7	4599	162.65
Ethane	90.35	184.55	305.33	0.0011	4871	206.73
Propane	85.47	231.07	369.85	0.1×10^{-6}	4248	220.49
Ammonia	195.49	239.81	406.65	0.0662	11627	237.57

[a] Triple point values for helium are those of the lambda point.

ortho-hydrogen, discussed in the preceding paragraphs. The quantum effects in helium properties are evidenced by the superfluid phase seen in Fig. 1-2.

For other cryogens, it is generally true that properties can be scaled from one fluid to another with an accuracy that is adequate for understanding and review of properties, as in this chapter. Evidence for this is seen in Fig. 1-6 and can be developed for other parameters if necessary. This scaleability of fluid properties is known generally as the "law of corresponding states."

As an example, if you wished to use these figures to find the density of xenon at 200 K and 580 kPa, you would divide these values respectively by the critical temperature and pressure for xenon listed in Table 1-1 and find the intersection of these reduced values on Fig. 1-7. The corresponding y coordinate would then be multiplied by the critical density (also found in Table 1-1) to yield the desired density (in this case it is ≈ 44 kg/m^3). More accurate data may be found using the tables in section 1-3 or the computer codes described in section 1-2-3.

Most properties in Figs. 1-7 to 1-13 have been calculated from an accurate state equation for oxygen. The figures would be little changed had they been calculated from an accurate state equation for any of the other cryogens.

Nomenclature and definitions. The use of dimensionless parameters makes it easier to scale properties from one fluid to another. The following scaling factors and definitions are useful:

Gas constant = energy per mole = $R = 8.31441 \pm 0.00026$ J·mol^{-1}·K^{-1}. For a fluid of known molecular weight, M, it is common practice to define an effective gas constant by the quotient R/M with units of energy/mass. This permits easy translation into other units systems.

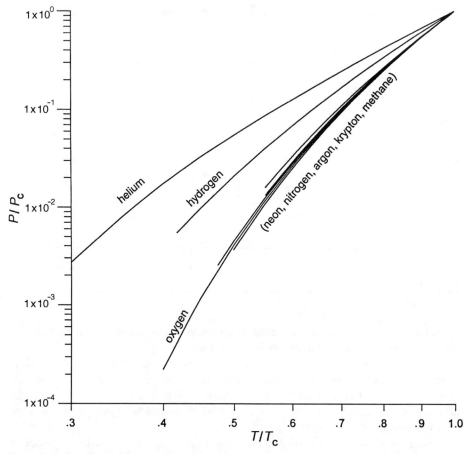

Figure 1-6 The saturation pressure as a function of temperature for several fluids. Numerical values have been normalized to the critical pressure and the critical temperature for each fluid.

Internal energy, enthalpy, Helmholtz energy, Gibbs energy, latent heat = U, H, A, G, and L, respectively, can all be normalized by dividing by RT_c.

Entropy and specific heats = $S, C_P,$ and C_V and can be normalized by dividing by R.

Dimensionless thermodynamic derivatives:

$$\text{Thermal expansivity} = \alpha = (T/V)(\partial V/\partial T)_P \qquad (1\text{-}1)$$

$$\text{Isothermal compressibility} = K_T = (P/\rho)(\partial \rho/\partial P)_T \qquad (1\text{-}2)$$

$$\text{Isentropic compressibility} = K_S = (P/\rho)(\partial \rho/\partial P)_S \qquad (1\text{-}3)$$

$$\text{Isenthalpic compressibility} = K_H = (P/\rho)(\partial \rho/\partial P)_H \qquad (1\text{-}4)$$

$$\text{Joule–Thomson coefficient}: \psi = (P/T)(\partial T/\partial P)_H \qquad (1\text{-}5)$$

$$\text{Grüneisen parameter} = \phi = (1/\rho)(\partial P/\partial U)_V \qquad (1\text{-}6)$$

(sometimes called the energy derivative)

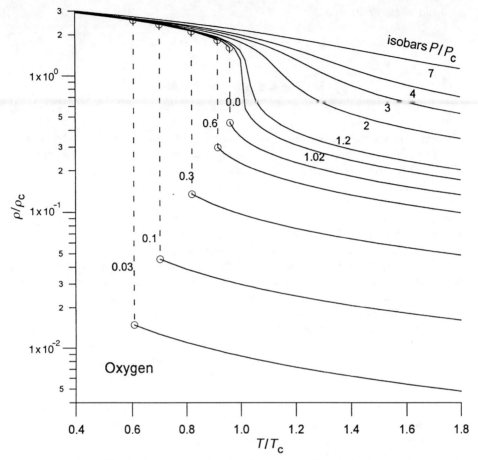

Figure 1-7 Isobars of density for oxygen as a function of temperature. Numerical values have been normalized to the critical pressure, density, and temperature.

Dimensioned properties:

Velocity of sound $= c$ SI units are $\mathrm{m \cdot s^{-1}}$
Viscosity $= \mu$ SI units are $\mathrm{Pa \cdot s}$ or $\mathrm{kg \cdot m^{-1} \cdot s^{-1}}$
Thermal conductivity $= \lambda$ SI units are $\mathrm{W \cdot m^{-1} \cdot K^{-1}}$

The following identities have been found to be very useful when manipulating thermodynamic parameters and equations:

$$\gamma = C_\mathrm{P}/C_\mathrm{V} = K_\mathrm{T}/K_\mathrm{S} = 1 + \alpha\phi \tag{1-7}$$

$$c^2 = P/(K_\mathrm{S}\rho) = \phi C_\mathrm{P} T/\alpha \tag{1-8}$$

$$K_\mathrm{H} = K_\mathrm{S}(1 + \phi) \tag{1-9}$$

$$\psi = \phi K_\mathrm{S}(1 - 1/\alpha) \tag{1-10}$$

In the ideal gas limit,

$$\alpha = K_T = K_H = 1, \tag{1-11}$$
$$\psi = 0 \tag{1-12}$$
$$\gamma = 1 + \phi = 5/3 \text{ for monatomic gases,}$$
$$7/5 \text{ for diatomic gases.} \tag{1-13}$$

Density. The normalized densities (ρ/ρ_c) (for oxygen) are shown in Fig. 1-7 as a function of normalized temperature (T/T_c), along lines of constant normalized pressure (P/P_c). The circles connected by dotted lines are saturated liquid and vapor states on the saturation line.

Specific heats. In Figs. 1-8 and 1-9 the oxygen specific heats C_P/R and C_V/R are plotted as a function of T/T_c along selected isobars from $P/P_c = 0.03$ to $P/P_c = 7$. On both figures, the circles connected by dashed lines are, respectively, saturated liquid and vapor states on the saturation line. It should be noted that the specific heat curves for the monatomic gases would be reduced in magnitude by an amount 1.0 (in C/R units).

Note the dramatic difference between these two figures. The peaks in C_P for $P/P_c > 1$ lie on the transposed critical line; C_P rises to infinity at the critical temperature and to very high values over an appreciable temperature range. On the other hand, C_V exhibits much less temperature variation over the whole range and has a visible rise of only a few percent very close to the critical temperature. In fact, theory says that C_V does go to infinity at the critical point, but the peak is so narrow that our accurate fluid properties equation gives no more than a hint of it. The same dramatic difference is seen in Fig. 1-10, where the specific heats along the saturation line and the transposed critical line are plotted. It should be further noted that isobars for the specific heat ratio $\gamma = C_P/C_V$ also rise to high peaks along the transposed critical line in a way that is qualitatively similar to the C_P data.

Thermal expansivity. The normalized thermal expansivity (for oxygen) is plotted Fig. 1-11 as a function of normalized temperature (T/T_c) along isobars P/P_c. As with the C_P plots, the circles lie on the saturation line, and the peaks lie on the transposed critical line.

Compressibility and sound velocity. Isothermal and isentropic compressibilities, K_T and K_S, are plotted in Figs. 1-12 and 1-13 as functions of reduced temperature (T/T_c) along isobars (P/P_c). It is important to note the qualitative difference between these two figures. The isothermal compressibility is sharply peaked along the transposed critical line, whereas the isentropic compressibility shows no hint of any enhancement in the transposed critical range. Sound velocities, in Fig. 1-14, are calculated from the isothermal compressibility and are plotted as a function of temperature along isobars. For an ideal gas, the sound velocity is

$$c_i = (\gamma R T)^{0.5} \tag{1-14}$$

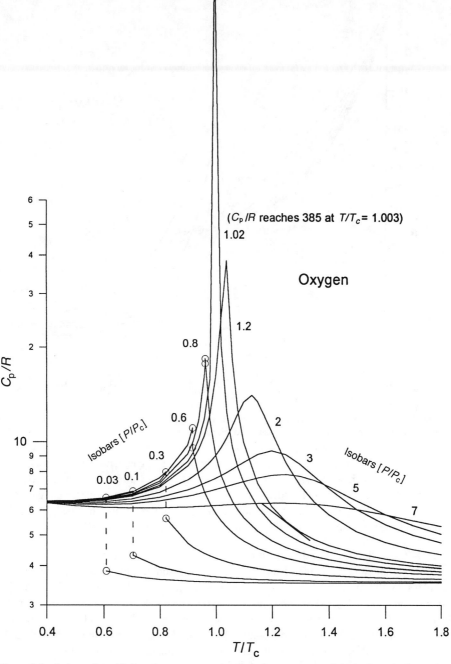

Figure 1-8 Isobars of specific heat for oxygen as a function of temperature. (C_p/R is dimensionless; other normalizing parameters are the critical pressure and temperature).

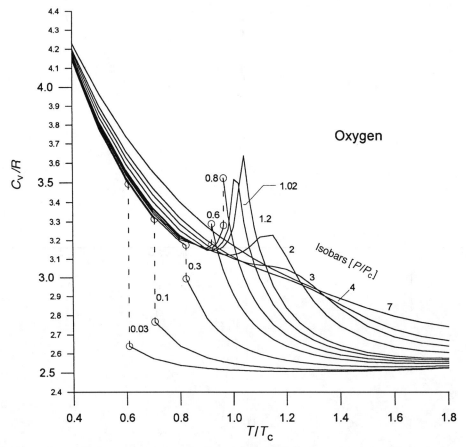

Figure 1-9 Isobars of specific heat for oxygen as a function of temperature. C_V/R is dimensionless; other normalizing parameters are the critical pressure and temperature).

where $\gamma = 5/3$ for an monatomic gas, $7/5$ for diatomic gas. The sound velocities in Fig. 1-14 have been normalized by dividing by the ideal gas value of the sound velocity at that temperature (i.e., using the ideal gas value of γ rather than the γ that would be calculated at that state point). For pressures less than the critical pressure, the ideal gas prediction yields a reasonable estimate for sound velocity at temperatures above about 1.1 T_c.

The J–T coefficient. The Joule–Thomson (ψ) coefficient is a measure of cooling (or warming) that can be obtained from an infinitesimal isenthalpic expansion. The dimensionless coefficient is plotted in Fig. 1-15 as a function of reduced temperature (T/T_c) along isobars (P/P_c). At supercritical pressures, the peaks of the curves lie approximately along the transposed critical line. The value of ψ at the critical point is equal to the value of PV/RT at the critical point, which is 0.288 for oxygen and is typically 0.25 to 0.3 for most fluids. Away from the critical point, values of ψ will always be less.

Theoretical framework. The state equation is a single thermodynamic function from which all static properties of the fluid can be derived. In principle, the state equation

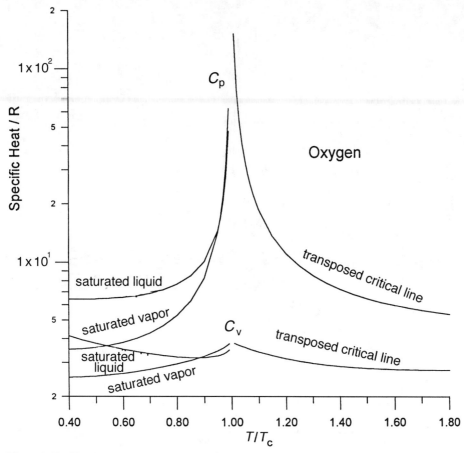

Figure 1-10   The dimensionless specific heats C_p/R and C_v/R for saturated liquid, saturated vapor, and along the transposed critical line as a function of normalized temperature, T/T_c.

of a pure fluid can be developed from a mathematical description of the interaction of a single molecule with all of its neighbors. The natural coordinates used in such theoretical development are the interatomic spacing (i.e., the density) and the temperature. It is very difficult to derive an accurate state equation by just this process; nevertheless, most commonly used (empirical) fluid state equations do utilize density and temperature as the two independent thermodynamic parameters. The ideal gas equation provides the simplest example. It may be written in terms of the Helmholtz potential $A(\rho, T)$ as

$$A(\rho, T) = RT(\log \rho - a \log T + S_0) \qquad (1\text{-}15)$$

where the constant $a = 3/2$ for a monatomic gas, $5/2$ for a diatomic gas, and so forth. The S_0 is an adjustable constant that sets the zero of entropy. All state properties can be obtained from $A(\rho, T)$ using classical thermodynamics relationships.

Virial state equations add an extra term or two to describe dense single- phase fluids with reasonable accuracy, such as

$$P(\rho, T) = \rho RT[1 + B(T)\rho + C(T)\rho^2] \qquad (1\text{-}16)$$

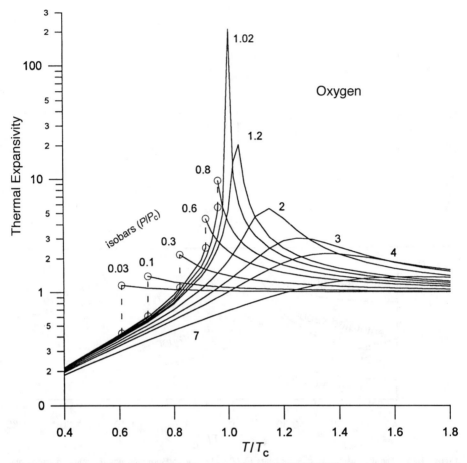

Figure 1-11 Isobars of the dimensionless thermal expansivity $(T/V)(\partial V/\partial T)_P$ for oxygen as a function of temperature. Normalizing parameters are the critical pressure and temperature.

with the caution that there is some theoretical uncertainty whether the second term should be written as shown above or as $C(T)\rho^2 \log(\rho)$. Virial equations can be useful for calculations in a restricted fluid range, but the coefficients B and C are not conveniently tabulated in the literature for most fluids. To calculate specific heats and compressibilities, it is necessary to evaluate the first and second temperature derivatives of B and C.

Virial equations are sometimes generalized by replacing the term $[1 + B(T)\rho + C(T)\rho^2]$ with a single parameter Z, usually called the "compressibility factor." Graphs of Z as a function of P and T are available for many cryogenic fluids, and a few equations for $Z(P, T)$ have been published. However, equations of this form have not been successful in predicting compressed liquid properties.

The van der Waals equation is representative of several fairly simple equations that predict fluid critical points and liquid–vapor separation with semiquantitative accuracy. These equations are used for quantitative calculations only in the absence of more accurate equations, as discussed in the next paragraph.

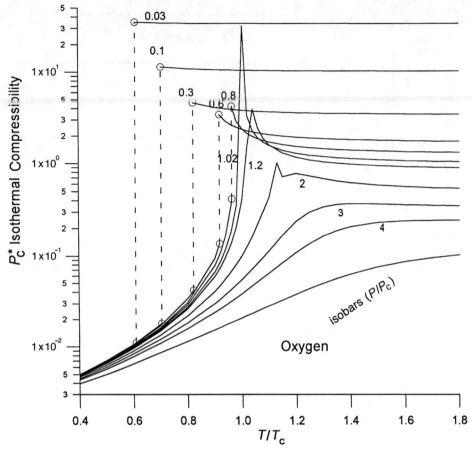

Figure 1-12 Isobars of the dimensionless isothermal compressibility $(P_c/\rho)(\partial\rho/\partial P)_T$ for oxygen as a function of temperature. Normalizing parameters are the critical pressure and temperature. The small glitch in $P/P_c = 2$ for $T/T_c \approx 1$ is most probably due to residual errors in the state equation.

State equations, which are the accepted standard in commerce, typically have 20 to 50 adjustable parameters in the expression for $A(\rho, T)$ carefully fitted by least-squares analysis to a variety of experimental data for any particular fluid. A common equation of this type is the Benedict–Webb–Rubin (BWR) [1] equation with 32 adjustable parameters. Many of the newer state equations (e.g., for halogenated hydrocarbon refrigerants, ammonia, and water) are based on a more generalized potential function sometimes referred to as the Wagner equation [2]. These multiparameter equations are practical for use only in computerized form.

Influence of the critical point. Figures 1-8 to 1-12 show that many derivative properties (specific heats, expansivity, isothermal compressibilities, etc.) diverge to infinity as the critical point is approached. Extensive theoretical and experimental studies of critical-point phenomena have yielded specialized equations that do describe individual

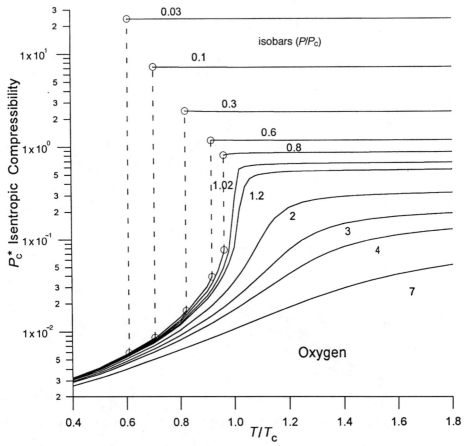

Figure 1-13 Isobars of the dimensionless isentropic compressibility $(P_c/\rho)(\partial\rho/\partial P)_S$ for oxygen as a function of temperature. Normalizing parameters are the critical pressure and temperature.

fluid properties asymptotic to the critical point. However, such equations are always nonanalytic at the critical point, and it has proven mathematically impossible to include these asymptotically correct equations within a thermodynamic potential function (e.g., in a BWR or Wagner-type equation). The important conclusion for this work is that the fluid properties illustrated here are increasingly inaccurate as the critical point is approached. The inaccuracy may be quite significant when the density is within about 20% of the critical density **and** the temperature is within about 2% of the critical temperature.

Strongly and weakly divergent parameters, the critical point, and liquid–vapor mixtures. Strongly divergent parameters are those that become large at appreciable distances from the critical point and along the transposed critical line. From Figs. 1-8 to 1-12, it can be seen that these parameters include α, C_P, K_T, and γ. These strongly divergent parameters are undefined, or may be said to equal infinity, in a liquid–vapor

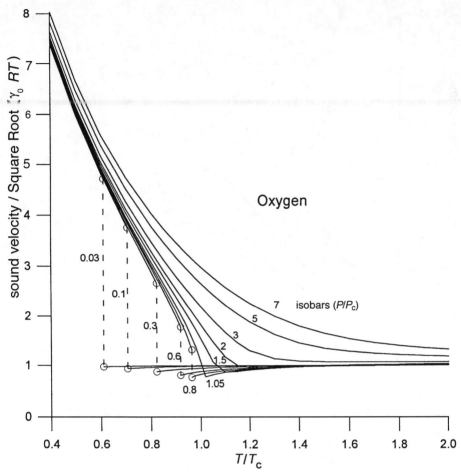

Figure 1-14 Isobars of the sound velocity for oxygen as a function of temperature. The sound velocity has been normalized by dividing by the square root of $(\gamma_0 RT)$, where γ_0 is the specific heat ratio C_p/C_v for the ideal gas. The temperatures and pressures have been normalized by their critical values.

mixture. Weakly divergent parameters are those that appear essentially unperturbed by proximity to the critical point until they are extremely close to the critical point, where they do diverge to infinity. Available state equations or graphs usually do not display the divergence. Weakly divergent parameters include C_V, K_S, K_H, $(1/\phi)$, and $(1/c)$. All of these weakly divergent state parameters can be defined for a constant-volume container of a liquid–vapor mixture in terms of the saturated liquid properties, the saturated vapor properties, and the vapor mass fraction, if one assumes complete thermodynamic equilibrium between liquid and vapor. This is in interesting contrast to the strongly divergent parameters that cannot be defined for such a container. However, such definitions of mixture properties are rarely published or used. In practice, the condition of complete thermodynamic equilibrium for a liquid–vapor mixture may be hard to establish. For example, the predicted sound velocity in a liquid–vapor mixture is extremely low, much

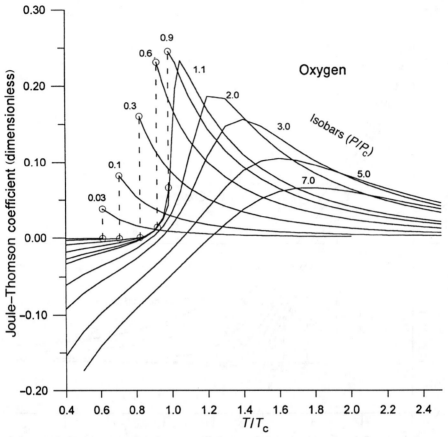

Figure 1-15 Isobars of the dimensionless Joule–Thomson coefficient $(P/T)(\partial T/\partial P)_H$ for oxygen as a function of temperature. Normalizing parameters are the critical pressure and temperature.

lower than the measured sound velocity, simply because the relaxation time for liquid–vapor equilibrium is much longer than the period of the sound wave.

Parameters that remain finite at the critical point include ψ and the product ϕK_S.

1-2-2 Thermal Conductivity and Viscosity

Thermal conductivity and viscosity are properties related to the transfer of energy and momentum through the fluid. These properties are not predictable from the state equation, nor are they easily predictable from models of molecular interactions. However, their qualitative behavior is fairly easy to describe.

Superfluid helium is a special case, because energy and mass transfer mechanisms are closely related to extended state properties (i.e., to second and fourth sound velocities, the superfluid density fraction, and the mutual friction parameter). A discussion of superfluid transfer processes is given in chapter 10 of this handbook.

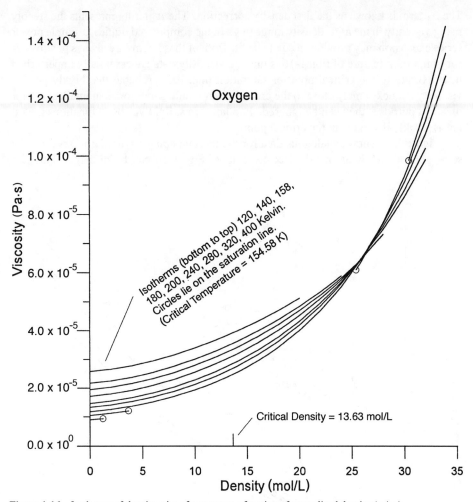

Figure 1-16   Isotherms of the viscosity of oxygen as a function of normalized density (ρ/ρ_c).

Isotherms of the viscosity, μ, of oxygen as a function of density are shown in Fig. 1-16. The equivalent curves for other fluids are qualitatively very similar. The first point to note is that the ideal gas state $\mu_0(T)$ (i.e., the y-intercepts in Fig. 1-16) can be approximated by the equation

$$\mu_0 = \text{const. } T^n, \text{ with } n \approx 0.7 \tag{1-17}$$

The constant will be unique for each fluid.

For nonzero fluid density, the viscosity data are fitted to reasonable accuracy by an equation

$$\mu = \mu_0(T) + \mu_1(T)\rho + \mu_2(\rho, T) \tag{1-18}$$

The μ_1 term is known as the first density correction. The μ_2 term represents the steeply rising viscosity in the high-density range (e.g., in the compressed liquid); a simple power series expansion may provide an adequate fit. Both of these terms are always positive. A very important feature of Fig. 1-16 is that the viscosity data are essentially unperturbed by proximity to the critical point or saturation line. It is probable that highly precise viscosity data extremely close to the critical point would show some anomalies, but for practical purposes they can be ignored. In other terms, fluid viscosity functions are (at most) weakly divergent at the critical point.

Figure 1-17 shows analogous data for the thermal conductivity, λ, of oxygen. The same general trends as in the viscosity data of Fig. 1-16 can be discerned but with

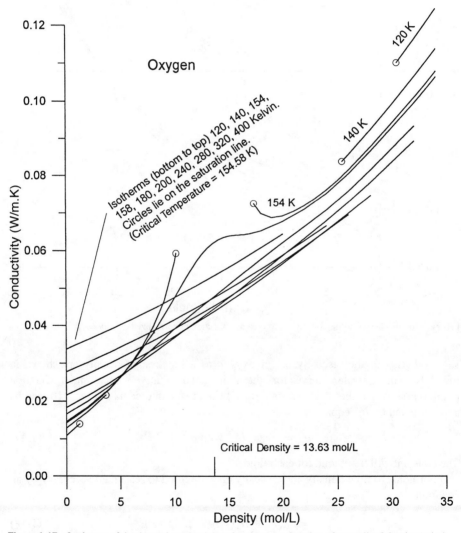

Figure 1-17   Isotherms of the thermal conductivity of oxygen as a function of normalized density (ρ/ρ_c).

added superposition of a significant perturbation when the density and temperature are not too far from their critical values or the saturation line. In other terms, the thermal conductivity function is strongly divergent at the critical point.

It is found that the ideal gas thermal conductivity is fitted approximately by the analog to Eq. (1-17), that is

$$\lambda_0 = \text{const. } T^n, \text{ with } n \approx 0.7 \qquad (1\text{-}19)$$

However, Eq. (1.18) is replaced by

$$\lambda = \lambda_0(T) + \lambda_1(T)\rho + \lambda_2(\rho, T) + \lambda_c(\rho/\rho_c, T/T_c) \qquad (1\text{-}20)$$

where the λ_c term represents the critical anomaly. Fairly complex equations for λ_c have been considered. For accurate work, it is best to use existing computer programs to calculate the thermal conductivity outside of the ideal gas limit.

The Prandtl number, Pr, is a dimensionless parameter that occurs prominently in heat and mass transfer studies. Conceptually it is a ratio of energy transferred by convection to energy transferred by conduction. It is defined as

$$Pr = \mu C_P/\lambda \qquad (1\text{-}21)$$

For most common fluids, the Prandtl number is about 0.7, except close to the critical point where the divergence in all three parameters μ, C_P, and λ is important. Values of Pr close to the critical point have not been widely studied to our knowledge. Predicted values of the Prandtl number for oxygen near its critical point are shown in Fig. 1-18. The Prandtl number is strongly divergent near the critical point.

1-2-3 Computer Programs for Fluid Properties

Fluid properties are available in computer form from several sources. The U.S. Department of Commerce offers the NIST-12 "standard reference" program, formerly distributed under the name MIPROPS [3]. This program contains properties of 17 fluids, including transport properties, where they are available. The Center for Advanced Thermodynamics at the University of Idaho offers ALLPROPS, which contains state properties of 42 fluids but no transport properties [4]. Cryodata, Inc., offers GASPAK, which contains properties of 32 fluids [5], including transport properties, where they are available. The NIST-12 program uses only BWR equations, whereas ALLPROPS and GAS-PAK include BWR equations as a subset of Wagner-type equations. All three of these computer programs are directly referenced to high-quality professional publications of fluid properties data. Special programs for helium properties, including superfluid properties down to 0.8 K and near-lambda-line properties, are available (a) as a subset of NIST-12 and (b) from Cryodata, Inc.

Information on where to order these programs is listed in section 1-4.

1-3 TABULAR DATA FOR PARTICULAR FLUIDS

This section contains property tables (1-3 to 1-27) for the following fluids: helium, nitrogen, argon, oxygen, and para-hydrogen. The tabular data listed here have been generated

Table 1-2 Estimated accuracies for tabulated data

Fluid	ρ (%)	S, H (%)	C_p (%)	μ, k (%)
He	0.5	5	5	5
H_2	0.25	2.5	2.5	5
N_2	0.2	2	5–10	5–10
A_2	0.2	2	5–10	5–10
O_2	0.1	2	2–5	2–5

using the Cryodata HEPAK (for He) and GASPAK (for all other fluids) programs. The accuracy of the programs and thus of these tables is given in Table 1-2. An exception to the listed accuracy occurs in the critical region. This region is defined as being within 20% of the critical density at temperatures within 2% of the critical temperature. The errors in this region are very high, and calculations in this region should be avoided if possible.

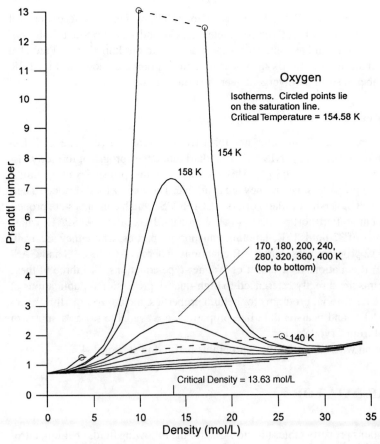

Figure 1-18 Isotherms of the Prandtl number of oxygen as a function of normalized density (ρ/ρ_c).

Table 1-3 Saturation properties of helium (Liquid properties are shown in the first row of each temperature)

P (Pa)	T (K)	ρ (kg/m^3)	C_p (J/kg · K)	S (J/kg · K)	H (J/kg)	μ (Pa · s)	k (W/m · K)
0.2116E+6	5.100	93.88	0.3878E+5	4922.	0.1739E+5	0.2510E−5	0.1986E−1
0.2116E+6	5.100	45.89	0.6087E+5	6752.	0.2673E+5	0.1803E−5	0.1577E−1
0.1960E+6	5.000	100.9	0.2010E+5	4664.	0.1592E+5	0.2636E−5	0.1930E−1
0.1960E+6	5.000	39.33	0.3327E+5	7063.	0.2794E+5	0.1700E−5	0.1386E−1
0.1813E+6	4.900	106.1	0.1359E+5	4463.	0.1478E+5	0.2736E−5	0.1908E−1
0.1813E+6	4.900	34.36	0.2251E+5	7321.	0.2881E+5	0.1617E−5	0.1263E−1
0.1674E+6	4.800	110.2	0.1051E+5	4296.	0.1384E+5	0.2820E−5	0.1897E−1
0.1674E+6	4.800	30.44	0.1732E+5	7539.	0.2945E+5	0.1547E−5	0.1176E−1
0.1543E+6	4.700	113.5	8763.	4151.	0.1304E+5	0.2890E−5	0.1890E−1
0.1543E+6	4.700	27.22	0.1437E+5	7732.	0.2991E+5	0.1484E−5	0.1109E−1
0.1419E+6	4.600	116.3	7590.	4018.	0.1231E+5	0.2954E−5	0.1884E−1
0.1419E+6	4.600	24.49	0.1250E+5	7906.	0.3024E+5	0.1428E−5	0.1054E−1
0.1303E+6	4.500	118.9	6742.	3893.	0.1164E+5	0.3014E−5	0.1880E−1
0.1303E+6	4.500	22.12	0.1122E+5	8067.	0.3047E+5	0.1376E−5	0.1007E−1
0.1193E+6	4.400	121.3	6097.	3774.	0.1102E+5	0.3071E−5	0.1875E−1
0.1193E+6	4.400	20.03	0.1029E+5	8218.	0.3062E+5	0.1327E−5	0.9664E−2
0.1089E+6	4.300	123.4	5587.	3661.	0.1045E+5	0.3126E−5	0.1870E−1
0.1089E+6	4.300	18.17	9582.	8363.	0.3071E+5	0.1280E−5	0.9299E−2
0.9923E+5	4.200	125.4	5170.	3551.	9901.	0.3179E−5	0.1864E−1
0.9923E+5	4.200	16.49	9033.	8504.	0.3074E+5	0.1236E−5	0.8966E−2
0.9014E+5	4.100	127.2	4820.	3444.	9386.	0.3230E−5	0.1857E−1
0.9014E+5	4.100	14.96	8595.	8641.	0.3073E+5	0.1193E−5	0.8656E−2
0.8162E+5	4.000	128.9	4519.	3340.	8899.	0.3280E−5	0.1848E−1
0.8162E+5	4.000	13.56	8238.	8776.	0.3068E+5	0.1152E−5	0.8365E−2
0.7366E+5	3.900	130.5	4254.	3239.	8437.	0.3329E−5	0.1837E−1
0.7366E+5	3.900	12.29	7942.	8911.	0.3060E+5	0.1113E−5	0.8087E−2
0.6625E+5	3.800	132.0	4017.	3140.	7998.	0.3377E−5	0.1825E−1
0.6625E+5	3.800	11.11	7694.	9046.	0.3048E+5	0.1074E−5	0.7820E−2
0.5935E+5	3.700	133.5	3801.	3042.	7580.	0.3409E−5	0.1810E−1
0.5935E+5	3.700	10.03	7484.	9181.	0.3034E+5	0.1038E−5	0.7561E−2
0.5296E+5	3.600	134.8	3601.	2946.	7183.	0.3472E−5	0.1794E−1
0.5296E+5	3.600	9.033	7305.	9318.	0.3017E+5	0.1004E−5	0.7310E−2
0.4704E+5	3.500	136.1	3413.	2852.	6806.	0.3564E−5	0.1775E−1
0.4704E+5	3.500	8.114	7150.	9458.	0.2997E+5	0.9718E−6	0.7065E−2
0.4159E+5	3.400	137.3	3233.	2760.	6448.	0.3619E−5	−
0.4159E+5	3.400	7.267	7015.	9600.	0.2975E+5	0.9377E−6	0.6854E−2
0.3659E+5	3.300	138.4	3061.	2670.	6108.	0.3642E−5	−
0.3659E+5	3.300	6.486	6897.	9747.	0.2952E+5	0.9044E−6	0.6626E−2
0.3201E+5	3.200	139.4	2896.	2581.	5787.	0.3638E−5	−
0.3201E+5	3.200	5.767	6792.	9897.	0.2926E+5	0.8716E−6	0.6401E−2
0.2784E+5	3.100	140.4	2740.	2494.	5483.	0.3612E−5	−
0.2784E+5	3.100	5.106	6700.	0.1005E+5	0.2898E+5	0.8394E−6	0.6178E−2

(Continues)

Table 1-3 (*Continued*)

P (Pa)	T (K)	ρ (kg/m³)	C_p (J/kg · K)	S (J/kg · K)	H (J/kg)	μ (Pa · s)	k (W/m · K)
0.2405E+5	3.000	141.4	2597.	2408.	5195.	0.3569E−5	–
0.2405E+5	3.000	4.499	6616.	0.1022E+5	0.2869E+5	0.8078E−6	0.5959E−2
0.2063E+5	2.900	142.2	2486.	2324.	4923.	0.3513E−5	–
0.2063E+5	2.900	3.942	6540.	0.1039E+5	0.2838E+5	0.7767E−6	0.5741E−2
0.1755E+5	2.800	143.0	2403.	2240.	4662.	0.3448E−5	–
0.1755E+5	2.800	3.433	6470.	0.1057E+5	0.2806E+5	0.7461E−6	0.5526E−2
0.1481E+5	2.700	143.8	2351.	2155.	4408.	0.3372E−5	–
0.1481E+5	2.700	2.970	6406.	0.1076E+5	0.2772E+5	0.7160E−6	0.5312E−2
0.1237E+5	2.600	144.4	2320.	2068.	4161.	0.3284E−5	–
0.1237E+5	2.600	2.549	6344.	0.1096E+5	0.2737E+5	0.6863E−6	0.5101E−2
0.1023E+5	2.500	145.0	2284.	1980.	3922.	0.3178E−5	–
0.1023E+5	2.500	2.170	6285.	0.1117E+5	0.2700E+5	0.6570E−6	0.4892E−2
8354.	2.400	145.5	2375.	1886.	3678.	0.3044E−5	–
8354.	2.400	1.828	6228.	0.1140E+5	0.2663E+5	0.6281E−6	0.4684E−2
6730.	2.300	145.9	2685.	1780.	3418.	0.2865E−5	–
6730.	2.300	1.523	6170.	0.1165E+5	0.2624E+5	0.5996E−6	0.4479E−2
5335.	2.200	146.1	4222.	1638.	3090.	0.2604E−5	–
5335.	2.200	1.251	6111.	0.1192E+5	0.2585E+5	0.5714E−6	0.4274E−2
4141.	2.100	145.9	7244.	1256.	2261.	0.1867E−5	–
4141.	2.100	1.008	6046.	0.1223E+5	0.2545E+5	0.5435E−6	0.4071E−2
3129.	2.000	145.7	5187.	957.8	1642.	0.1488E−5	–
3129.	2.000	0.7936	5975.	0.1258E+5	0.2504E+5	0.5160E−6	0.3870E−2
2299.	1.900	145.5	3893.	727.0	1186.	0.1336E−5	–
2299.	1.900	0.6090	5898.	0.1298E+5	0.2463E+5	0.4887E−6	0.3669E−2
1638.	1.800	145.4	2938.	543.7	842.2	0.1300E−5	–
1638.	1.800	0.4547	5818.	0.1343E+5	0.2420E+5	0.4617E−6	0.3471E−2
1128.	1.700	145.3	2193.	398.1	583.6	0.1316E−5	–
1128.	1.700	0.3292	5736.	0.1393E+5	0.2377E+5	0.4350E−6	0.3273E−2
746.4	1.600	145.3	1603.	283.9	392.3	0.1354E−5	–
746.4	1.600	0.2301	5654.	0.1449E+5	0.2332E+5	0.4086E−6	0.3077E−2
471.5	1.500	145.2	1138.	196.2	254.3	0.1413E−5	–
471.5	1.500	0.1542	5574.	0.1513E+5	0.2287E+5	0.3824E−6	0.2882E−2
282.0	1.400	145.2	779.7	130.8	157.9	0.1522E−5	–
282.0	1.400	0.9836E−1	5496.	0.1586E+5	0.2240E+5	0.3565E−6	0.2688E−2
157.9	1.300	145.2	511.1	83.57	93.15	0.1735E−5	–
157.9	1.300	0.5906E−1	5424.	0.1670E+5	0.2192E+5	0.3307E−6	0.2494E−2
81.48	1.200	145.2	317.6	50.96	51.76	0.2135E−5	–
81.48	1.200	0.3292E−1	5360.	0.1767E+5	0.2144E+5	0.3050E−6	0.2301E−2
38.00	1.100	145.2	185.2	29.56	26.76	–	–
38.00	1.100	0.1671E−1	5305.	0.1882E+5	0.2095E+5	–	–
15.57	1.000	145.2	100.2	16.34	12.68	–	–
15.57	1.000	0.7516E−2	5262.	0.2019E+5	0.2044E+5	–	–

Table 1-4 Helium properties along the 10^5 pascal (1 bar) isobar

T (K)	ρ (kg/m^3)	C_p (J/kg · K)	S (J/kg · K)	H (J/kg)	μ (Pa · s)	k (W/m · K)
300.0	0.1604	5193.	0.3161E+5	0.1574E+7	0.1993E−4	0.1560
290.0	0.1659	5193.	0.3144E+5	0.1522E+7	0.1947E−4	0.1524
280.0	0.1718	5193.	0.3125E+5	0.1470E+7	0.1901E−4	0.1487
270.0	0.1782	5193.	0.3106E+5	0.1418E+7	0.1855E−4	0.1450
260.0	0.1851	5193.	0.3087E+5	0.1366E+7	0.1808E−4	0.1413
250.0	0.1925	5193.	0.3066E+5	0.1314E+7	0.1760E−4	0.1375
240.0	0.2005	5193.	0.3045E+5	0.1262E+7	0.1712E−4	0.1337
230.0	0.2092	5193.	0.3023E+5	0.1210E+7	0.1664E−4	0.1299
220.0	0.2187	5193.	0.3000E+5	0.1158E+7	0.1614E−4	0.1260
210.0	0.2291	5193.	0.2976E+5	0.1106E+7	0.1565E−4	0.1220
200.0	0.2405	5193.	0.2951E+5	0.1054E+7	0.1514E−4	0.1180
190.0	0.2532	5193.	0.2924E+5	0.1002E+7	0.1463E−4	0.1139
180.0	0.2672	5193.	0.2896E+5	0.9503E+6	0.1411E−4	0.1098
170.0	0.2829	5193.	0.2866E+5	0.8984E+6	0.1358E−4	0.1056
160.0	0.3006	5193.	0.2835E+5	0.8465E+6	0.1305E−4	0.1013
150.0	0.3206	5193.	0.2801E+5	0.7946E+6	0.1250E−4	0.9694E−1
140.0	0.3435	5193.	0.2765E+5	0.7426E+6	0.1194E−4	0.9250E−1
130.0	0.3699	5194.	0.2727E+5	0.6907E+6	0.1138E−4	0.8797E−1
120.0	0.4007	5194.	0.2685E+5	0.6387E+6	0.1079E−4	0.8333E−1
110.0	0.4371	5194.	0.2640E+5	0.5868E+6	0.1020E−4	0.7859E−1
100.0	0.4807	5194.	0.2591E+5	0.5349E+6	0.9778E−5	0.7371E−1
95.00	0.5060	5195.	0.2564E+5	0.5089E+6	0.9467E−5	0.7122E−1
90.00	0.5340	5195.	0.2536E+5	0.4829E+6	0.9152E−5	0.6870E−1
85.00	0.5654	5195.	0.2506E+5	0.4569E+6	0.8831E−5	0.6613E−1
80.00	0.6007	5195.	0.2475E+5	0.4310E+6	0.8503E−5	0.6352E−1
75.00	0.6407	5196.	0.2441E+5	0.4050E+6	0.8169E−5	0.6086E−1
70.00	0.6864	5196.	0.2405E+5	0.3790E+6	0.7827E−5	0.5815E−1
65.00	0.7391	5197.	0.2367E+5	0.3530E+6	0.7477E−5	0.5538E−1
60.00	0.8006	5198.	0.2325E+5	0.3270E+6	0.7116E−5	0.5255E−1
55.00	0.8733	5199.	0.2280E+5	0.3010E+6	0.6745E−5	0.4965E−1
50.00	0.9605	5201.	0.2230E+5	0.2750E+6	0.6360E−5	0.4668E−1
45.00	1.067	5203.	0.2176E+5	0.2490E+6	0.5960E−5	0.4361E−1
40.00	1.200	5206.	0.2114E+5	0.2230E+6	0.5542E−5	0.4044E−1
35.00	1.372	5211.	0.2045E+5	0.1970E+6	0.5101E−5	0.3715E−1
30.00	1.601	5218.	0.1964E+5	0.1709E+6	0.4634E−5	0.3372E−1
25.00	1.923	5229.	0.1869E+5	0.1448E+6	0.4131E−5	0.3009E−1
22.00	2.187	5240.	0.1802E+5	0.1291E+6	0.3808E−5	0.2779E−1
20.00	2.408	5250.	0.1752E+5	0.1186E+6	0.3582E−5	0.2620E−1
18.00	2.680	5264.	0.1697E+5	0.1081E+6	0.3345E−5	0.2454E−1
16.00	3.023	5282.	0.1635E+5	0.9754E+5	0.3097E−5	0.2281E−1
14.00	3.468	5310.	0.1564E+5	0.8695E+5	0.2835E−5	0.2098E−1
12.00	4.074	5353.	0.1482E+5	0.7629E+5	0.2557E−5	0.1903E−1
10.00	4.949	5426.	0.1384E+5	0.6552E+5	0.2258E−5	0.1689E−1
9.000	5.555	5485.	0.1326E+5	0.6006E+5	0.2100E−5	0.1573E−1

(Continues)

Table 1-4 (*Continued*)

T (K)	ρ (kg/m^3)	C_p (J/kg · K)	S (J/kg · K)	H (J/kg)	μ (Pa · s)	k (W/m · K)
8.000	6.344	5575.	0.1261E+5	0.5454E+5	0.1935E−5	0.1449E−1
7.000	7.426	5724.	0.1186E+5	0.4889E+5	0.1761E−5	0.1316E−1
6.000	9.028	6011.	0.1096E+5	0.4305E+5	0.1579E−5	0.1174E−1
5.000	11.78	6735.	9803.	0.3674E+5	0.1389E−5	0.1022E−1
4.900	12.18	6870.	9666.	0.3606E+5	0.1369E−5	0.1006E−1
4.800	12.62	7027.	9523.	0.3536E+5	0.1350E−5	0.9901E−2
4.700	13.11	7213.	9373.	0.3465E+5	0.1331E−5	0.9743E−2
4.600	13.64	7436.	9215.	0.3392E+5	0.1312E−5	0.9586E−2
4.500	14.25	7710.	9049.	0.3316E+5	0.1293E−5	0.9429E−2
4.400	14.94	8056.	8872.	0.3237E+5	0.1274E−5	0.9275E−2
4.300	15.75	8508.	8682.	0.3155E+5	0.1256E−5	0.9125E−2
4.200	125.4	5161	3550.	9902.	0.3181E−5	0.1865E−1
4.100	127.8	4734.	3431.	9408.	0.3256E−5	0.1865E−1
4.000	129.9	4396.	3318.	8952.	0.3327E−5	0.1862E−1
3.900	131.7	4116.	3210.	8527.	0.3393E−5	0.1856E−1
3.800	133.5	3874.	3107.	8128.	0.3456E−5	0.1847E−1
3.700	135.1	3659.	3006.	7751.	0.3508E−5	0.1835E−1
3.600	136.5	3463.	2909.	7395.	0.3585E−5	0.1820E−1
3.500	137.9	3281.	2814.	7058.	0.3674E−5	0.1803E−1
3.400	139.1	3108.	2721.	6739.	0.3718E−5	−
3.300	140.3	2943.	2631.	6436.	0.3730E−5	−
3.200	141.4	2784.	2543.	6150.	0.3715E−5	−
3.100	142.4	2634.	2457.	5879.	0.3681E−5	−
3.000	143.3	2496.	2373.	5623.	0.3634E−5	−
2.900	144.2	2387.	2291.	5380.	0.3578E−5	−
2.800	145.0	2308.	2209.	5147.	0.3515E−5	−
2.700	145.7	2259.	2126.	4919.	0.3445E−5	−
2.600	146.3	2233.	2042.	4696.	0.3364E−5	−
2.500	146.9	2204.	1957.	4479.	0.3266E−5	−
2.400	147.4	2282.	1866.	4257.	0.3140E−5	−
2.300	147.8	2562.	1764.	4017.	0.2968E−5	−
2.200	148.0	3777.	1631.	3719.	0.2715E−5	−
2.100	147.7	7400.	1268.	2940.	0.1971E−5	−
2.000	147.5	5249.	965.7	2319.	0.1555E−5	−
1.900	147.3	3927.	732.7	1864.	0.1389E−5	−
1.800	147.2	2959.	548.0	1522.	0.1347E−5	−
1.700	147.1	2207.	401.4	1265.	0.1359E−5	−
1.600	147.0	1614.	286.5	1075.	0.1392E−5	−
1.500	147.0	1147.	198.2	938.4	0.1447E−5	−
1.400	146.9	787.1	132.1	842.5	0.1557E−5	−
1.300	146.9	517.0	84.45	777.9	0.1784E−5	−
1.200	146.9	322.3	51.42	736.6	0.2221E−5	−
1.100	146.9	188.6	29.66	711.5	−	−
1.000	146.9	102.3	16.19	697.2	−	−

Table 1-5 Helium properties along the 2×10^5 pascal (2 bar) isobar

T (K)	ρ (kg/m³)	C_p (J/kg · K)	S (J/kg · K)	H (J/kg)	μ (Pa · s)	k (W/m · K)
300.0	0.3206	5193.	0.3017E+5	0.1574E+7	0.1993E−4	0.1561
290.0	0.3317	5193.	0.3000E+5	0.1522E+7	0.1948E−4	0.1524
280.0	0.3435	5193.	0.2981E+5	0.1470E+7	0.1902E−4	0.1488
270.0	0.3562	5193.	0.2962E+5	0.1418E+7	0.1855E−4	0.1451
260.0	0.3699	5193.	0.2943E+5	0.1366E+7	0.1808E−4	0.1414
250.0	0.3847	5193.	0.2923E+5	0.1314E+7	0.1761E−4	0.1376
240.0	0.4007	5193.	0.2901E+5	0.1262E+7	0.1713E−4	0.1338
230.0	0.4181	5193.	0.2879E+5	0.1210E+7	0.1664E−4	0.1299
220.0	0.4371	5193.	0.2856E+5	0.1158E+7	0.1615E−4	0.1260
210.0	0.4579	5193.	0.2832E+5	0.1106E+7	0.1565E−4	0.1221
200.0	0.4807	5193.	0.2807E+5	0.1055E+7	0.1515E−4	0.1181
190.0	0.5060	5193.	0.2780E+5	0.1003E+7	0.1464E−4	0.1140
180.0	0.5340	5193.	0.2752E+5	0.9507E+6	0.1412E−4	0.1099
170.0	0.5654	5193.	0.2722E+5	0.8987E+6	0.1359E−4	0.1056
160.0	0.6007	5194.	0.2691E+5	0.8468E+6	0.1306E−4	0.1014
150.0	0.6406	5194.	0.2657E+5	0.7949E+6	0.1251E−4	0.9702E−1
140.0	0.6863	5194.	0.2621E+5	0.7429E+6	0.1195E−4	0.9258E−1
130.0	0.7390	5194.	0.2583E+5	0.6910E+6	0.1139E−4	0.8805E−1
120.0	0.8004	5195.	0.2541E+5	0.6390E+6	0.1081E−4	0.8342E−1
110.0	0.8730	5195.	0.2496E+5	0.5871E+6	0.1021E−4	0.7867E−1
100.0	0.9600	5196.	0.2447E+5	0.5351E+6	0.9791E−5	0.7380E−1
95.00	1.010	5196.	0.2420E+5	0.5092E+6	0.9480E−5	0.7131E−1
90.00	1.066	5197.	0.2392E+5	0.4832E+6	0.9165E−5	0.6878E−1
85.00	1.129	5197.	0.2362E+5	0.4572E+6	0.8845E−5	0.6622E−1
80.00	1.199	5198.	0.2331E+5	0.4312E+6	0.8518E−5	0.6361E−1
75.00	1.279	5199.	0.2297E+5	0.4052E+6	0.8184E−5	0.6095E−1
70.00	1.370	5200.	0.2261E+5	0.3792E+6	0.7843E−5	0.5824E−1
65.00	1.475	5201.	0.2223E+5	0.3532E+6	0.7493E−5	0.5548E−1
60.00	1.598	5203.	0.2181E+5	0.3272E+6	0.7134E−5	0.5265E−1
55.00	1.742	5205.	0.2136E+5	0.3012E+6	0.6763E−5	0.4976E−1
50.00	1.916	5209.	0.2086E+5	0.2752E+6	0.6379E−5	0.4678E−1
45.00	2.129	5213.	0.2031E+5	0.2491E+6	0.5981E−5	0.4372E−1
40.00	2.395	5219.	0.1970E+5	0.2230E+6	0.5564E−5	0.4056E−1
35.00	2.737	5228.	0.1900E+5	0.1969E+6	0.5126E−5	0.3728E−1
30.00	3.194	5242.	0.1819E+5	0.1707E+6	0.4661E−5	0.3386E−1
25.00	3.839	5264.	0.1724E+5	0.1445E+6	0.4163E−5	0.3025E−1
22.00	4.371	5286.	0.1656E+5	0.1287E+6	0.3844E−5	0.2798E−1
20.00	4.818	5306.	0.1606E+5	0.1181E+6	0.3621E−5	0.2640E−1
18.00	5.370	5334.	0.1550E+5	0.1074E+6	0.3389E−5	0.2477E−1
16.00	6.071	5372.	0.1487E+5	0.9672E+5	0.3146E−5	0.2307E−1
14.00	6.994	5429.	0.1415E+5	0.8593E+5	0.2891E−5	0.2127E−1
12.00	8.271	5520.	0.1330E+5	0.7499E+5	0.2622E−5	0.1937E−1
10.00	10.18	5685.	0.1228E+5	0.6380E+5	0.2337E−5	0.1731E−1
9.000	11.56	5828.	0.1168E+5	0.5805E+5	0.2188E−5	0.1620E−1
8.000	13.45	6064.	0.1098E+5	0.5211E+5	0.2036E−5	0.1504E−1
7.000	16.26	6519.	0.1014E+5	0.4585E+5	0.1882E−5	0.1383E−1
6.000	21.26	7737.	9057.	0.3884E+5	0.1734E−5	0.1277E−1

(Continues)

Table 1-5 (*Continued*)

T (K)	ρ (kg/m³)	C_p (J/kg · K)	S (J/kg · K)	H (J/kg)	μ (Pa · s)	k (W/m · K)
5.000	102.8	0.1658E+5	4608.	0.1568E+5	0.2683E−5	0.1929E−1
4.900	110.1	0.1016E+5	4354.	0.1442E+5	0.2847E−5	0.1929E−1
4.800	114.8	7942.	4170.	0.1353E+5	0.2964E−5	0.1935E−1
4.700	118.5	6752.	4016.	0.1280E+5	0.3061E−5	0.1942E−1
4.600	121.6	5984.	3880.	0.1216E+5	0.3147E−5	0.1947E−1
4.500	124.3	5434.	3755.	0.1159E+5	0.3225E−5	0.1950E−1
4.400	126.6	5014.	3638.	0.1107E+5	0.3298E−5	0.1951E−1
4.300	128.8	4676.	3526.	0.1059E+5	0.3366E−5	0.1950E−1
4.200	130.7	4395.	3420.	0.1014E+5	0.3432E−5	0.1946E−1
4.100	132.5	4153.	3317.	9709.	0.3496E−5	0.1939E−1
4.000	134.1	3940.	3217.	9305.	0.3557E−5	0.1930E−1
3.900	135.6	3747.	3120.	8920.	0.3617E−5	0.1919E−1
3.800	137.1	3570.	3025.	8555.	0.3675E−5	0.1905E−1
3.700	138.4	3404.	2932.	8206.	0.3734E−5	0.1889E−1
3.600	139.7	3246.	2841.	7874.	0.3809E−5	0.1871E−1
3.500	140.8	3093.	2751.	7557.	0.3869E−5	0.1851E−1
3.400	141.9	2943.	2664.	7255.	0.3881E−5	−
3.300	143.0	2797.	2578.	6968.	0.3867E−5	−
3.200	143.9	2653.	2494.	6695.	0.3834E−5	−
3.100	144.8	2515.	2412.	6437.	0.3787E−5	−
3.000	145.7	2387.	2332.	6192.	0.3733E−5	−
2.900	146.4	2281.	2253.	5960.	0.3674E−5	−
2.800	147.1	2209.	2175.	5738.	0.3613E−5	−
2.700	147.8	2169.	2096.	5520.	0.3547E−5	−
2.600	148.3	2153.	2016.	5306.	0.3471E−5	−
2.500	148.8	2133.	1934.	5098.	0.3379E−5	−
2.400	149.3	2195.	1847.	4885.	0.3260E−5	−
2.300	149.6	2445.	1749.	4655.	0.3095E−5	−
2.200	149.9	3419.	1625.	4375.	0.2846E−5	−
2.100	149.6	7586.	1285.	3647.	0.2100E−5	−
2.000	149.3	5323.	976.6	3015.	0.1633E−5	−
1.900	149.0	3972.	740.7	2554.	0.1446E−5	−
1.800	148.9	2990.	554.0	2208.	0.1395E−5	−
1.700	148.7	2230.	405.9	1949.	0.1401E−5	−
1.600	148.6	1631.	289.7	1757.	0.1429E−5	−
1.500	148.6	1160.	200.5	1619.	0.1480E−5	−
1.400	148.5	796.9	133.7	1522.	0.1591E−5	−
1.300	148.5	524.4	85.34	1456.	0.1830E−5	−
1.200	148.5	327.6	51.81	1414.	0.2301E−5	−
1.100	148.5	192.1	29.68	1389.	−	−
1.000	148.5	104.2	15.95	1374.	−	−

Table 1-6 Helium properties along the 5×10^5 pascal (5 bar) isobar

T (K)	ρ (kg/m^3)	C_p (J/kg · K)	S (J/kg · K)	H (J/kg)	μ (Pa · s)	k (W/m · K)
300.0	0.8005	5193.	0.2827E+5	0.1575E+7	0.1994E−4	0.1563
290.0	0.8281	5193.	0.2809E+5	0.1523E+7	0.1949E−4	0.1527
280.0	0.8575	5193.	0.2791E+5	0.1471E+7	0.1903E−4	0.1490
270.0	0.8892	5193.	0.2772E+5	0.1419E+7	0.1857E−4	0.1453
260.0	0.9233	5193.	0.2753E+5	0.1367E+7	0.1810E−4	0.1416
250.0	0.9601	5193.	0.2732E+5	0.1315E+7	0.1762E−4	0.1378
240.0	1.000	5193.	0.2711E+5	0.1263E+7	0.1715E−4	0.1340
230.0	1.043	5193.	0.2689E+5	0.1211E+7	0.1666E−4	0.1302
220.0	1.091	5193.	0.2666E+5	0.1159E+7	0.1617E−4	0.1263
210.0	1.142	5193.	0.2642E+5	0.1107E+7	0.1567E−4	0.1223
200.0	1.199	5193.	0.2616E+5	0.1056E+7	0.1517E−4	0.1183
190.0	1.262	5193.	0.2590E+5	0.1004E+7	0.1466E−4	0.1142
180.0	1.332	5194.	0.2562E+5	0.9516E+6	0.1414E−4	0.1101
170.0	1.410	5194.	0.2532E+5	0.8997E+6	0.1362E−4	0.1059
160.0	1.498	5194.	0.2500E+5	0.8478E+6	0.1308E−4	0.1016
150.0	1.597	5195.	0.2467E+5	0.7958E+6	0.1254E−4	0.9727E−1
140.0	1.710	5195.	0.2431E+5	0.7439E+6	0.1199E−4	0.9284E−1
130.0	1.841	5196.	0.2393E+5	0.6919E+6	0.1142E−4	0.8831E−1
120.0	1.994	5197.	0.2351E+5	0.6400E+6	0.1084E−4	0.8368E−1
110.0	2.174	5198.	0.2306E+5	0.5880E+6	0.1024E−4	0.7894E−1
100.0	2.390	5199.	0.2256E+5	0.5360E+6	0.9829E−5	0.7408E−1
95.00	2.514	5200.	0.2230E+5	0.5100E+6	0.9520E−5	0.7160E−1
90.00	2.653	5202.	0.2201E+5	0.4840E+6	0.9206E−5	0.6908E−1
85.00	2.808	5203.	0.2172E+5	0.4580E+6	0.8887E−5	0.6652E−1
80.00	2.982	5205.	0.2140E+5	0.4320E+6	0.8561E−5	0.6391E−1
75.00	3.179	5207.	0.2107E+5	0.4059E+6	0.8229E−5	0.6127E−1
70.00	3.405	5210.	0.2071E+5	0.3799E+6	0.7890E−5	0.5857E−1
65.00	3.665	5213.	0.2032E+5	0.3538E+6	0.7542E−5	0.5582E−1
60.00	3.968	5218.	0.1990E+5	0.3278E+6	0.7185E−5	0.5300E−1
55.00	4.326	5224.	0.1945E+5	0.3017E+6	0.6817E−5	0.5013E−1
50.00	4.756	5231.	0.1895E+5	0.2755E+6	0.6437E−5	0.4718E−1
45.00	5.281	5242.	0.1840E+5	0.2493E+6	0.6042E−5	0.4415E−1
40.00	5.940	5257.	0.1778E+5	0.2231E+6	0.5631E−5	0.4103E−1
35.00	6.789	5278.	0.1708E+5	0.1968E+6	0.5199E−5	0.3780E−1
30.00	7.929	5312.	0.1626E+5	0.1703E+6	0.4744E−5	0.3445E−1
25.00	9.547	5368.	0.1529E+5	0.1436E+6	0.4260E−5	0.3095E−1
22.00	10.90	5422.	0.1460E+5	0.1274E+6	0.3952E−5	0.2876E−1
20.00	12.05	5472.	0.1408E+5	0.1165E+6	0.3740E−5	0.2726E−1
18.00	13.49	5541.	0.1350E+5	0.1055E+6	0.3520E−5	0.2572E−1
16.00	15.35	5641.	0.1284E+5	0.9434E+5	0.3294E−5	0.2413E−1
14.00	17.89	5796.	0.1208E+5	0.8292E+5	0.3061E−5	0.2249E−1
12.00	21.60	6065.	0.1116E+5	0.7108E+5	0.2824E−5	0.2081E−1
10.00	27.76	6635.	0.1001E+5	0.5847E+5	0.2592E−5	0.1911E−1
9.000	32.87	7241.	9285.	0.5156E+5	0.2488E−5	0.1831E−1
8.000	41.34	8505.	8366.	0.4378E+5	0.2412E−5	0.1767E−1

(Continues)

Table 1-6 (*Continued*)

T (K)	ρ (kg/m^3)	C_p (J/kg·K)	S (J/kg·K)	H (J/kg)	μ (Pa·s)	k (W/m·K)
7.000	59.44	0.1165E+5	7047.	0.3393E+5	0.2443E−5	0.1787E−1
6.000	102.1	0.1004E+5	5121.	0.2142E+5	0.2942E−5	0.2118E−1
5.000	129.0	4846.	3901.	0.1466E+5	0.3573E−5	0.2186E−1
4.900	130.7	4632.	3806.	0.1418E+5	0.3629E−5	0.2183E−1
4.800	132.4	4440.	3712.	0.1373E+5	0.3685E−5	0.2179E−1
4.700	133.9	4265.	3620.	0.1329E+5	0.3741E−5	0.2173E−1
4.600	135.4	4104.	3531.	0.1288E+5	0.3797E−5	0.2166E−1
4.500	136.8	3955.	3442.	0.1247E+5	0.3853E−5	0.2156E−1
4.400	138.1	3815.	3355.	0.1209E+5	0.3909E−5	0.2145E−1
4.300	139.4	3684.	3269.	0.1171E+5	0.3964E−5	0.2133E−1
4.200	140.6	3558.	3183.	0.1135E+5	0.4020E−5	0.2118E−1
4.100	141.8	3438.	3099.	0.1100E+5	0.4076E−5	0.2102E−1
4.000	142.9	3321.	3016.	0.1066E+5	0.4133E−5	0.2084E−1
3.900	143.9	3206.	2933.	0.1033E+5	0.4188E−5	0.2064E−1
3.800	145.0	3093.	2851.	0.1002E+5	0.4244E−5	0.2042E−1
3.700	145.9	2979.	2770.	9716.	0.4320E−5	0.2019E−1
3.600	146.8	2864.	2690.	9424.	0.4387E−5	0.1994E−1
3.500	147.7	2748.	2611.	9143.	0.4384E−5	0.1967E−1
3.400	148.5	2629.	2533.	8874.	0.4338E−5	−
3.300	149.3	2508.	2457.	8617.	0.4277E−5	−
3.200	150.1	2385.	2381.	8373.	0.4209E−5	−
3.100	150.8	2265.	2307.	8140.	0.4140E−5	−
3.000	151.4	2151.	2235.	7920.	0.4075E−5	−
2.900	152.0	2053.	2164.	7710.	0.4017E−5	−
2.800	152.5	1993.	2095.	7513.	0.3962E−5	−
2.700	153.0	1973.	2024.	7318.	0.3909E−5	−
2.600	153.5	1976.	1951.	7125.	0.3852E−5	−
2.500	153.8	1973.	1876.	6933.	0.3782E−5	−
2.400	154.2	1985.	1798.	6743.	0.3685E−5	−
2.300	154.5	2153.	1710.	6537.	0.3539E−5	−
2.200	154.8	2696.	1605.	6301.	0.3308E−5	−
2.100	154.5	8523.	1352.	5761.	0.2629E−5	−
2.000	154.0	5604.	1021.	5081.	0.1922E−5	−
1.900	153.7	4146.	773.9	4599.	0.1634E−5	−
1.800	153.4	3117.	579.2	4238.	0.1537E−5	−
1.700	153.2	2327.	424.8	3968.	0.1520E−5	−
1.600	153.1	1705.	303.5	3767.	0.1533E−5	−
1.500	153.0	1216.	210.0	3622.	0.1575E−5	−
1.400	152.9	838.0	139.9	3520.	0.1687E−5	−
1.300	152.8	553.1	88.99	3451.	0.1954E−5	−
1.200	152.8	346.4	53.57	3407.	0.2500E−5	−
1.100	152.8	203.1	30.17	3380.	−	−
1.000	152.8	109.3	15.70	3365.	−	−

Table 1-7 Helium properties along the 20×10^5 pascal (20 bar) isobar

T (k)	ρ (kg/m³)	C_p (J/kg · K)	S (J/kg · K)	H (J/kg)	μ (Pa · s)	k (W/m · K)
300.0	3.180	5192.	0.2539E+5	0.1580E+7	0.2000E−4	0.1574
290.0	3.289	5192.	0.2522E+5	0.1528E+7	0.1955E−4	0.1538
280.0	3.405	5192.	0.2503E+5	0.1476E+7	0.1909E−4	0.1501
270.0	3.530	5192.	0.2484E+5	0.1424E+7	0.1863E−4	0.1464
260.0	3.664	5192.	0.2465E+5	0.1372E+7	0.1817E−4	0.1427
250.0	3.809	5192.	0.2444E+5	0.1320E+7	0.1770E−4	0.1390
240.0	3.965	5193.	0.2423E+5	0.1268E+7	0.1723E−4	0.1352
230.0	4.135	5193.	0.2401E+5	0.1216E+7	0.1675E−4	0.1313
220.0	4.321	5193.	0.2378E+5	0.1164E+7	0.1627E−4	0.1274
210.0	4.523	5194.	0.2354E+5	0.1112E+7	0.1578E−4	0.1235
200.0	4.746	5194.	0.2329E+5	0.1060E+7	0.1528E−4	0.1195
190.0	4.992	5195.	0.2302E+5	0.1008E+7	0.1478E−4	0.1155
180.0	5.264	5196.	0.2274E+5	0.9565E+6	0.1427E−4	0.1113
170.0	5.568	5197.	0.2244E+5	0.9045E+6	0.1375E−4	0.1072
160.0	5.910	5198.	0.2213E+5	0.8526E+6	0.1322E−4	0.1029
150.0	6.296	5199.	0.2179E+5	0.8006E+6	0.1268E−4	0.9862E−1
140.0	6.736	5201.	0.2143E+5	0.7486E+6	0.1214E−4	0.9423E−1
130.0	7.242	5204.	0.2105E+5	0.6966E+6	0.1158E−4	0.8975E−1
120.0	7.832	5208.	0.2063E+5	0.6445E+6	0.1101E−4	0.8518E−1
110.0	8.526	5212.	0.2018E+5	0.5924E+6	0.1042E−4	0.8052E−1
100.0	9.355	5218.	0.1968E+5	0.5403E+6	0.1002E−4	0.7575E−1
95.00	9.834	5222.	0.1941E+5	0.5142E+6	0.9713E−5	0.7332E−1
90.00	10.36	5227.	0.1913E+5	0.4880E+6	0.9405E−5	0.7086E−1
85.00	10.96	5233.	0.1883E+5	0.4619E+6	0.9092E−5	0.6837E−1
80.00	11.62	5239.	0.1851E+5	0.4357E+6	0.8774E−5	0.6584E−1
75.00	12.37	5248.	0.1817E+5	0.4095E+6	0.8449E−5	0.6328E−1
70.00	13.23	5258.	0.1781E+5	0.3832E+6	0.8119E−5	0.6069E−1
65.00	14.22	5271.	0.1742E+5	0.3569E+6	0.7781E−5	0.5805E−1
60.00	15.37	5287.	0.1700E+5	0.3305E+6	0.7435E−5	0.5538E−1
55.00	16.72	5308.	0.1654E+5	0.3040E+6	0.7080E−5	0.5266E−1
50.00	18.35	5335.	0.1603E+5	0.2774E+6	0.6715E−5	0.4991E−1
45.00	20.34	5373.	0.1547E+5	0.2506E+6	0.6340E−5	0.4711E−1
40.00	22.84	5424.	0.1483E+5	0.2237E+6	0.5953E−5	0.4426E−1
35.00	26.08	5498.	0.1410E+5	0.1964E+6	0.5554E−5	0.4139E−1
30.00	30.47	5609.	0.1325E+5	0.1686E+6	0.5142E−5	0.3848E−1
25.00	36.84	5789.	0.1221E+5	0.1402E+6	0.4722E−5	0.3557E−1
22.00	42.29	5954.	0.1146E+5	0.1226E+6	0.4471E−5	0.3384E−1
20.00	47.04	6101.	0.1088E+5	0.1105E+6	0.4307E−5	0.3272E−1
18.00	53.13	6288.	0.1023E+5	0.9814E+5	0.4150E−5	0.3164E−1
16.00	61.22	6517.	9478.	0.8534E+5	0.4010E−5	0.3065E−1
14.00	72.39	6766.	8590.	0.7205E+5	0.3902E−5	0.2985E−1
12.00	88.17	6892.	7534.	0.5835E+5	0.3866E−5	0.2946E−1
10.00	109.3	6420.	6307.	0.4488E+5	0.3985E−5	0.2988E−1
9.000	120.9	5814.	5662.	0.3874E+5	0.4137E−5	0.3034E−1
8.000	132.1	5074.	5021.	0.3329E+5	0.4367E−5	0.3074E−1

(Continues)

Table 1-7 (*Continued*)

T (k)	ρ (kg/m^3)	C_p (J/kg · K)	S (J/kg · K)	H (J/kg)	μ (Pa · s)	k (W/m · K)
7.000	142.3	4333.	4394.	0.2859E+5	0.4690E−5	0.3075E−1
6.000	151.3	3652.	3781.	0.2461E+5	0.5131E−5	0.3008E−1
5.000	158.9	3047.	3173.	0.2126E+5	0.5730E−5	0.2841E−1
4.900	159.6	2990.	3112.	0.2096E+5	0.5801E−5	0.2818E−1
4.800	160.2	2933.	3051.	0.2067E+5	0.5874E−5	0.2793E−1
4.700	160.9	2876.	2990.	0.2038E+5	0.5948E−5	0.2767E−1
4.600	161.5	2819.	2929.	0.2009E+5	0.6025E−5	0.2740E−1
4.500	162.1	2762.	2867.	0.1981E+5	0.6105E−5	0.2712E−1
4.400	162.7	2704.	2806.	0.1954E+5	0.6186E−5	0.2682E−1
4.300	163.3	2645.	2744.	0.1927E+5	0.6270E−5	0.2650E−1
4.200	163.9	2585.	2683.	0.1901E+5	0.6355E−5	0.2618E−1
4.100	164.4	2523.	2621.	0.1875E+5	0.6443E−5	0.2583E−1
4.000	164.9	2459.	2560.	0.1851E+5	0.6534E−5	0.2548E−1
3.900	165.5	2392.	2498.	0.1826E+5	0.6626E−5	0.2511E−1
3.800	166.0	2321.	2437.	0.1803E+5	0.6720E−5	0.2472E−1
3.700	166.4	2247.	2376.	0.1780E+5	0.6810E−5	0.2432E−1
3.600	166.9	2167.	2316.	0.1758E+5	0.6774E−5	0.2391E−1
3.500	167.3	2083.	2256.	0.1737E+5	0.6533E−5	0.2348E−1
3.400	167.8	1993.	2197.	0.1716E+5	0.6364E−5	−
3.300	168.2	1898.	2139.	0.1697E+5	0.6192E−5	−
3.200	168.5	1799.	2082.	0.1678E+5	0.6035E−5	−
3.100	168.9	1699.	2026.	0.1661E+5	0.5906E−5	−
3.000	169.3	1602.	1972.	0.1644E+5	0.5817E−5	−
2.900	169.6	1517.	1919.	0.1629E+5	0.5773E−5	−
2.800	169.9	1463.	1867.	0.1614E+5	0.5776E−5	−
2.700	170.2	1480.	1811.	0.1599E+5	0.5822E−5	−
2.600	170.4	1525.	1751.	0.1583E+5	0.5904E−5	−
2.500	170.7	1562.	1688.	0.1567E+5	0.6008E−5	−
2.400	171.0	1511.	1624.	0.1552E+5	0.6111E−5	−
2.300	171.3	1413.	1565.	0.1538E+5	0.6181E−5	−
2.200	171.5	1429.	1502.	0.1524E+5	0.6172E−5	−
2.100	171.7	1529.	1433.	0.1509E+5	0.6029E−5	−
2.000	171.8	1926.	1351.	0.1492E+5	0.5664E−5	−
1.900	171.2	7070.	1121.	0.1448E+5	0.4183E−5	−
1.800	170.2	4570.	816.8	0.1391E+5	0.2826E−5	−
1.700	169.6	3215.	597.5	0.1353E+5	0.2274E−5	−
1.600	169.2	2290.	432.5	0.1325E+5	0.2045E−5	−
1.500	168.9	1620.	307.7	0.1306E+5	0.1968E−5	−
1.400	168.7	1126.	214.0	0.1292E+5	0.2016E−5	−
1.300	168.6	764.2	144.8	0.1283E+5	0.2260E−5	−
1.200	168.5	503.2	94.83	0.1277E+5	0.2856E−5	−
1.100	168.4	320.7	59.60	0.1273E+5	−	−
1.000	168.4	197.9	35.38	0.1270E+5	−	−

Table 1-8 Saturation properties of nitrogen (Liquid properties are shown in the first row of each temperature)

P (Pa)	T (K)	ρ (kg/m^3)	C_p (J/kg · K)	S (J/kg · K)	H (J/kg)	μ (Pa · s)	k (W/m · K)
0.3367E+7	126.0	377.0	0.7409E+5	4118.	0.1724E+5	0.2177E−4	0.6504E−1
0.3367E+7	126.0	253.5	0.1220E+6	4330.	0.4388E+5	0.1493E−4	0.6494E−1
0.3071E+7	124.0	457.1	8718.	3985.	−78.92	0.2854E−4	0.5908E−1
0.3071E+7	124.0	179.2	0.1191E+5	4487.	0.6211E+5	0.1213E−4	0.3438E−1
0.2799E+7	122.0	495.5	5663.	3912.	−9681.	0.3271E−4	0.6145E−1
0.2799E+7	122.0	148.4	6780.	4559.	0.6927E+5	0.1111E−4	0.2711E−1
0.2534E+7	120.0	523.7	4515.	3852.	−0.1748E+5	0.3629E−4	0.6427E−1
0.2534E+7	120.0	126.5	4850.	4615.	0.7411E+5	0.1042E−4	0.2301E−1
0.2287E+7	118.0	547.8	3849.	3797.	−0.2448E+5	0.3974E−4	0.6741E−1
0.2287E+7	118.0	109.4	3845.	4662.	0.7766E+5	0.9883E−5	0.2031E−1
0.2061E+7	116.0	569.0	3414.	3745.	−0.3094E+5	0.4316E−4	0.7082E−1
0.2061E+7	116.0	95.12	3217.	4704.	0.8045E+5	0.9438E−5	0.1835E−1
0.1851E+7	114.0	588.0	3116.	3696.	−0.3697E+5	0.4656E−4	0.7433E−1
0.1851E+7	114.0	82.88	2786.	4744.	0.8271E+5	0.9052E−5	0.1686E−1
0.1657E+7	112.0	605.3	2902.	3648.	−0.4267E+5	0.4997E−4	0.7785E−1
0.1657E+7	112.0	72.44	2485.	4782.	0.8443E+5	0.8714E−5	0.1570E−1
0.1478E+7	110.0	621.2	2743.	3602.	−0.4811E+5	0.5343E−4	0.8136E−1
0.1478E+7	110.0	63.42	2264.	4817.	0.8572E+5	0.8412E−5	0.1475E−1
0.1313E+7	108.0	636.2	2619.	3556.	−0.5335E+5	0.5698E−4	0.8481E−1
0.1313E+7	108.0	55.54	2095.	4851.	0.8665E+5	0.8137E−5	0.1394E−1
0.1162E+7	106.0	650.2	2522.	3511.	−0.5842E+5	0.6065E−4	0.8821E−1
0.1162E+7	106.0	48.61	1964.	4884.	0.8728E+5	0.7884E−5	0.1324E−1
0.1023E+7	104.0	663.6	2442.	3466.	−0.6334E+5	0.6447E−4	0.9156E−1
0.1023E+7	104.0	42.49	1859.	4917.	0.8765E+5	0.7648E−5	0.1263E−1
0.8975E+6	102.0	676.4	2377.	3421.	−0.6815E+5	0.6846E−4	0.9486E−1
0.8975E+6	102.0	37.07	1774.	4949.	0.8779E+5	0.7426E−5	0.1207E−1
0.7830E+6	100.0	688.7	2323.	3376.	−0.7285E+5	0.7266E−4	0.9813E−1
0.7830E+6	100.0	32.26	1704.	4981.	0.8771E+5	0.7216E−5	0.1156E−1
0.6795E+6	98.00	700.6	2277.	3331.	−0.7747E+5	0.7710E−4	0.1014
0.6795E+6	98.00	27.98	1646.	5013.	0.8745E+5	0.7016E−5	0.1109E−1
0.5862E+6	96.00	712.1	2238.	3286.	−0.8201E+5	0.8181E−4	0.1046
0.5862E+6	96.00	24.18	1597.	5046.	0.8703E+5	0.6824E−5	0.1065E−1
0.5027E+6	94.00	723.2	2204.	3240.	−0.8647E+5	0.8685E−4	0.1077
0.5027E+6	94.00	20.81	1556.	5079.	0.8644E+5	0.6640E−5	0.1024E−1
0.4282E+6	92.00	734.1	2174.	3194.	−0.9088E+5	0.9225E−4	0.1109
0.4282E+6	92.00	17.83	1520.	5112.	0.8572E+5	0.6462E−5	0.9856E−2
0.3621E+6	90.00	744.6	2148.	3147.	−0.9523E+5	0.9806E−4	0.1140
0.3621E+6	90.00	15.19	1489.	5147.	0.8486E+5	0.6289E−5	0.9495E−2
0.3038E+6	88.00	755.0	2125.	3100.	−0.9953E+5	0.1044E−3	0.1171
0.3038E+6	88.00	12.86	1462.	5183.	0.8388E+5	0.6121E−5	0.9152E−2
0.2528E+6	86.00	765.1	2105.	3051.	−0.1038E+6	0.1112E−3	0.1201
0.2528E+6	86.00	10.81	1437.	5220.	0.8280E+5	0.5957E−5	0.8827E−2
0.2085E+6	84.00	775.0	2087.	3002.	−0.1080E+6	0.1187E−3	0.1232
0.2085E+6	84.00	9.028	1414.	5259.	0.8161E+5	0.5796E−5	0.8517E−2
0.1702E+6	82.00	784.7	2072.	2953.	−0.1122E+6	0.1270E−3	0.1261
0.1702E+6	82.00	7.475	1393.	5299.	0.8033E+5	0.5639E−5	0.8220E−2
0.1375E+6	80.00	794.2	2058.	2902.	−0.1163E+6	0.1361E−3	0.1291

(*Continues*)

Table 1-8 (Continued)

P (Pa)	T (K)	ρ (kg/m³)	C_p (J/kg·K)	S (J/kg·K)	H (J/kg)	μ (Pa·s)	k (W/m·K)
0.1375E+6	80.00	6.132	1372.	5342.	0.7896E+5	0.5484E−5	0.7935E−2
0.1098E+6	78.00	803.6	2046.	2850.	−0.1205E+6	0.1463E−3	0.1320
0.1098E+6	78.00	4.979	1351.	5387.	0.7751E+5	0.5331E−5	0.7658E−2
0.8655E+5	76.00	812.8	2035.	2797.	−0.1246E+6	0.1578E−3	0.1349
0.8655E+5	76.00	3.998	1330.	5435.	0.7598E+5	0.5179E−5	0.7389E−2
0.6727E+5	74.00	822.0	2027.	2743.	−0.1286E+6	0.1707E−3	0.1377
0.6727E+5	74.00	3.171	1309.	5486.	0.7440E+5	0.5029E−5	0.7126E−2
0.5149E+5	72.00	830.9	2020.	2688.	−0.1327E+6	0.1855E−3	0.1404
0.5149E+5	72.00	2.480	1287.	5540.	0.7275E+5	0.4880E−5	0.6865E−2
0.3875E+5	70.00	839.8	2015.	2631.	−0.1367E+6	0.2025E−3	0.1431
0.3875E+5	70.00	1.909	1265.	5598.	0.7104E+5	0.4731E−5	0.6605E−2
0.2862E+5	68.00	848.6	2013.	2573.	−0.1408E+6	0.2223E−3	0.1457
0.2862E+5	68.00	1.445	1242.	5661.	0.6928E+5	0.4583E−5	0.6343E−2
0.2070E+5	66.00	857.4	2013.	2513.	−0.1448E+6	0.2456E−3	0.1482
0.2070E+5	66.00	1.073	1219.	5728.	0.6748E+5	0.4433E−5	0.6076E−2
0.1463E+5	64.00	866.0	2016.	2451.	−0.1488E+6	0.2733E−3	0.1506
0.1463E+5	64.00	0.7791	1197.	5802.	0.6563E+5	0.4282E−5	0.5800E−2

Table 1-9 Nitrogen properties along the 1×10^5 pascal (1 bar) isobar

T (K)	ρ (kg/m³)	C_p (J/kg·K)	S (J/kg·K)	H (J/kg)	μ (Pa·s)	k (W/m·K)
300.0	1.123	1041.	6846.	0.3114E+6	0.1795E−4	0.2578E−1
295.0	1.142	1041.	6828.	0.3062E+6	0.1772E−4	0.2544E−1
290.0	1.162	1041.	6810.	0.3010E+6	0.1749E−4	0.2509E−1
285.0	1.183	1041.	6792.	0.2958E+6	0.1725E−4	0.2475E−1
280.0	1.204	1041.	6774.	0.2906E+6	0.1702E−4	0.2440E−1
275.0	1.226	1041.	6755.	0.2854E+6	0.1678E−4	0.2405E−1
270.0	1.249	1041.	6736.	0.2802E+6	0.1654E−4	0.2369E−1
265.0	1.272	1041.	6717.	0.2750E+6	0.1630E−4	0.2334E−1
260.0	1.297	1041.	6697.	0.2698E+6	0.1605E−4	0.2298E−1
255.0	1.322	1041.	6677.	0.2646E+6	0.1580E−4	0.2261E−1
250.0	1.349	1041.	6656.	0.2594E+6	0.1555E−4	0.2225E−1
245.0	1.376	1041.	6635.	0.2542E+6	0.1530E−4	0.2188E−1
240.0	1.405	1041.	6613.	0.2490E+6	0.1505E−4	0.2151E−1
235.0	1.435	1042.	6592.	0.2438E+6	0.1479E−4	0.2113E−1
230.0	1.467	1042.	6569.	0.2385E+6	0.1453E−4	0.2075E−1
225.0	1.499	1042.	6546.	0.2333E+6	0.1427E−4	0.2037E−1
220.0	1.534	1042.	6523.	0.2281E+6	0.1401E−4	0.1999E−1
215.0	1.570	1042.	6499.	0.2229E+6	0.1374E−4	0.1960E−1
210.0	1.607	1042.	6474.	0.2177E+6	0.1347E−4	0.1920E−1
205.0	1.647	1043.	6449.	0.2125E+6	0.1320E−4	0.1881E−1
200.0	1.688	1043.	6423.	0.2073E+6	0.1292E−4	0.1840E−1
195.0	1.732	1043.	6397.	0.2021E+6	0.1265E−4	0.1800E−1
190.0	1.778	1044.	6370.	0.1968E+6	0.1237E−4	0.1759E−1
185.0	1.827	1044.	6342.	0.1916E+6	0.1208E−4	0.1718E−1
180.0	1.878	1044.	6314.	0.1864E+6	0.1180E−4	0.1676E−1
175.0	1.932	1045.	6284.	0.1812E+6	0.1151E−4	0.1634E−1
170.0	1.990	1045.	6254.	0.1760E+6	0.1121E−4	0.1591E−1

(Continues)

Table 1-9 (*Continued*)

T (K)	ρ (kg/m³)	C_p (J/kg · K)	S (J/kg · K)	H (J/kg)	μ (Pa · s)	k (W/m · K)
165.0	2.051	1046.	6223.	0.1707E+6	0.1092E−4	0.1548E−1
160.0	2.116	1046.	6190.	0.1655E+6	0.1062E−4	0.1504E−1
155.0	2.185	1047.	6157.	0.1603E+6	0.1032E−4	0.1461E−1
150.0	2.259	1048.	6123.	0.1550E+6	0.1001E−4	0.1417E−1
145.0	2.339	1049.	6087.	0.1498E+6	0.9703E−5	0.1372E−1
140.0	2.424	1050.	6050.	0.1445E+6	0.9392E−5	0.1327E−1
135.0	2.516	1051.	6012.	0.1393E+6	0.9077E−5	0.1282E−1
130.0	2.615	1052.	5973.	0.1340E+6	0.8760E−5	0.1237E−1
125.0	2.723	1054.	5931.	0.1288E+6	0.8440E−5	0.1192E−1
120.0	2.840	1056.	5888.	0.1235E+6	0.8117E−5	0.1146E−1
115.0	2.968	1058.	5843.	0.1182E+6	0.7792E−5	0.1100E−1
110.0	3.109	1060.	5796.	0.1129E+6	0.7464E−5	0.1055E−1
105.0	3.264	1063.	5747.	0.1076E+6	0.7134E−5	0.1009E−1
100.0	3.436	1066.	5695.	0.1023E+6	0.6803E−5	0.9637E−2
99.00	3.473	1067.	5684.	0.1012E+6	0.6736E−5	0.9546E−2
98.00	3.510	1068.	5673.	0.1001E+6	0.6670E−5	0.9455E−2
97.00	3.549	1069.	5662.	0.9908E+5	0.6603E−5	0.9365E−2
96.00	3.588	1070.	5651.	0.9801E+5	0.6536E−5	0.9274E−2
95.00	3.628	1072.	5640.	0.9694E+5	0.6469E−5	0.9183E−2
94.00	3.670	1073.	5629.	0.9587E+5	0.6403E−5	0.9093E−2
93.00	3.712	1074.	5617.	0.9479E+5	0.6336E−5	0.9002E−2
92.00	3.755	1076.	5606.	0.9372E+5	0.6269E−5	0.8911E−2
91.00	3.799	1078.	5594.	0.9264E+5	0.6202E−5	0.8821E−2
90.00	3.845	1081.	5582.	0.9156E+5	0.6135E−5	0.8730E−2
89.00	3.892	1084.	5570.	0.9048E+5	0.6068E−5	0.8639E−2
88.00	3.940	1087.	5558.	0.8939E+5	0.6000E−5	0.8548E−2
87.00	3.989	1092.	5545.	0.8830E+5	0.5933E−5	0.8457E−2
86.00	4.040	1097.	5532.	0.8721E+5	0.5866E−5	0.8366E−2
85.00	4.092	1104.	5520.	0.8611E+5	0.5798E−5	0.8274E−2
84.00	4.146	1113.	5506.	0.8500E+5	0.5731E−5	0.8183E−2
83.00	4.201	1125.	5493.	0.8388E+5	0.5663E−5	0.8091E−2
82.00	4.258	1141.	5479.	0.8275E+5	0.5596E−5	0.7999E−2
81.00	4.318	1163.	5465.	0.8160E+5	0.5528E−5	0.7906E−2
80.00	4.380	1191.	5451.	0.8042E+5	0.5460E−5	0.7813E−2
79.00	4.444	1230.	5435.	0.7921E+5	0.5392E−5	0.7720E−2
78.00	4.512	1284.	5419.	0.7796E+5	0.5324E−5	0.7626E−2
77.00	808.2	2040.	2824.	−0.1225E+6	0.1519E−3	0.1334
76.00	812.9	2035.	2797.	−0.1245E+6	0.1578E−3	0.1349
75.00	817.5	2031.	2770.	−0.1266E+6	0.1641E−3	0.1363
74.00	822.0	2027.	2743.	−0.1286E+6	0.1708E−3	0.1377
73.00	826.6	2023.	2716.	−0.1306E+6	0.1779E−3	0.1391
72.00	831.1	2020.	2688.	−0.1327E+6	0.1856E−3	0.1404
71.00	835.5	2017.	2659.	−0.1347E+6	0.1938E−3	0.1418
70.00	840.0	2015.	2631.	−0.1367E+6	0.2027E−3	0.1431
69.00	844.4	2013.	2602.	−0.1387E+6	0.2122E−3	0.1444
68.00	848.8	2012.	2573.	−0.1407E+6	0.2225E−3	0.1457
67.00	853.1	2012.	2543.	−0.1427E+6	0.2337E−3	0.1470
66.00	857.5	2013.	2512.	−0.1447E+6	0.2458E−3	0.1483
65.00	861.8	2014.	2482.	−0.1468E+6	0.2591E−3	0.1495
64.00	866.2	2016.	2450.	−0.1488E+6	0.2736E−3	0.1507

Table 1-10 Nitrogen properties along the 2×10^5 pascal (2 bar) isobar

T (K)	ρ (kg/m^3)	C_p (J/kg · K)	S (J/kg · K)	H (J/kg)	μ (Pa · s)	k (W/m · K)
300.0	2.247	1042.	6639.	0.3112E+6	0.1797E−4	0.2584E−1
295.0	2.285	1042.	6622.	0.3060E+6	0.1774E−4	0.2550E−1
290.0	2.325	1042.	6604.	0.3008E+6	0.1751E−4	0.2516E−1
285.0	2.366	1042.	6586.	0.2956E+6	0.1727E−4	0.2481E−1
280.0	2.408	1043 .	6567.	0.2903E+6	0.1704E−4	0.2446E−1
275.0	2.453	1043.	6549.	0.2851E+6	0.1680E−4	0.2411E−1
270.0	2.498	1043.	6529.	0.2799E+6	0.1656E−4	0.2376E−1
265.0	2.546	1043.	6510.	0.2747E+6	0.1631E−4	0.2341E−1
260.0	2.595	1043.	6490.	0.2695E+6	0.1607E−4	0.2305E−1
255.0	2.646	1043.	6470.	0.2643E+6	0.1582E−4	0.2269E−1
250.0	2.700	1044.	6449.	0.2590E+6	0.1557E−4	0.2232E−1
245.0	2.755	1044.	6428.	0.2538E+6	0.1532E−4	0.2196E−1
240.0	2.813	1044.	6407.	0.2486E+6	0.1507E−4	0.2159E−1
235.0	2.874	1044.	6385.	0.2434E+6	0.1481E−4	0.2121E−1
230.0	2.937	1045.	6362.	0.2382E+6	0.1455E−4	0.2084E−1
225.0	3.003	1045.	6339.	0.2329E+6	0.1429E−4	0.2046E−1
220.0	3.072	1046.	6316.	0.2277E+6	0.1403E−4	0.2007E−1
215.0	3.144	1046.	6292.	0.2225E+6	0.1376E−4	0.1969E−1
210.0	3.220	1046.	6267.	0.2173E+6	0.1349E−4	0.1929E−1
205.0	3.300	1047.	6242.	0.2120E+6	0.1322E−4	0.1890E−1
200.0	3.384	1047.	6216.	0.2068E+6	0.1295E−4	0.1850E−1
195.0	3.472	1048.	6189.	0.2015E+6	0.1267E−4	0.1810E−1
190.0	3.565	1049.	6162.	0.1963E+6	0.1239E−4	0.1769E−1
185.0	3.664	1049.	6134.	0.1911E+6	0.1211E−4	0.1728E−1
180.0	3.768	1050.	6105.	0.1858E+6	0.1182E−4	0.1687E−1
175.0	3.878	1051.	6076.	0.1806E+6	0.1153E−4	0.1645E−1
170.0	3.995	1052.	6045.	0.1753E+6	0.1124E−4	0.1603E−1
165.0	4.119	1053.	6014.	0.1700E+6	0.1095E−4	0.1560E−1
160.0	4.252	1055.	5982.	0.1648E+6	0.1065E−4	0.1517E−1
155.0	4.394	1056.	5948.	0.1595E+6	0.1035E−4	0.1474E−1
150.0	4.545	1058.	5913.	0.1542E+6	0.1005E−4	0.1430E−1
145.0	4.708	1059.	5877.	0.1489E+6	0.9738E−5	0.1386E−1
140.0	4.884	1061.	5840.	0.1436E+6	0.9428E−5	0.1342E−1
135.0	5.074	1064.	5802.	0.1383E+6	0.9115E−5	0.1298E−1
130.0	5.279	1067.	5761.	0.1330E+6	0.8799E−5	0.1254E−1
125.0	5.503	1070.	5720.	0.1276E+6	0.8480E−5	0.1209E−1
120.0	5.748	1074.	5676.	0.1223E+6	0.8159E−5	0.1164E−1
115.0	6.017	1078.	5630.	0.1169E+6	0.7836E−5	0.1120E−1
110.0	6.315	1084.	5582.	0.1115E+6	0.7510E−5	0.1075E−1
105.0	6.646	1090.	5531.	0.1061E+6	0.7182E−5	0.1031E−1
100.0	7.017	1100.	5478.	0.1006E+6	0.6853E−5	0.9872E−2
99.00	7.096	1103.	5467.	0.9948E+5	0.6787E−5	0.9785E−2
98.00	7.178	1106.	5456.	0.9838E+5	0.6721E−5	0.9697E−2
97.00	7.262	1109.	5444.	0.9727E+5	0.6655E−5	0.9610E−2
96.00	7.348	1113.	5433.	0.9616E+5	0.6589E−5	0.9523E−2
95.00	7.437	1118.	5421.	0.9504E+5	0.6523E−5	0.9436E−2
94.00	7.528	1123.	5409.	0.9392E+5	0.6456E−5	0.9350E−2
93.00	7.621	1130.	5397.	0.9279E+5	0.6390E−5	0.9263E−2
92.00	7.718	1138.	5385.	0.9166E+5	0.6323E−5	0.9177E−2
91.00	7.817	1148.	5372.	0.9052E+5	0.6257E−5	0.9090E−2

(Continues)

Table 1-10 (*Continued*)

T (K)	ρ (kg/m^3)	C_p (J/kg · K)	S (J/kg · K)	H (J/kg)	μ (Pa · s)	k (W/m · K)
90.00	7.920	1161.	5360.	0.8936E+5	0.6191E−5	0.9004E−2
89.00	8.027	1177.	5347.	0.8820E+5	0.6124E−5	0.8918E−2
88.00	8.137	1198.	5333.	0.8701E+5	0.6058E−5	0.8832E−2
87.00	8.251	1225.	5319.	0.8580E+5	0.5991E−5	0.8746E−2
86.00	8.371	1262.	5305.	0.8455E+5	0.5924E−5	0.8661E−2
85.00	8.496	1310.	5290.	0.8327E+5	0.5858E−5	0.8575E−2
84.00	8.628	1376.	5274.	0.8193E+5	0.5791E−5	0.8490E−2
83.00	779.9	2079.	2978.	−0.1101E+6	0.1228E−3	0.1247
82.00	784.8	2071.	2952.	−0.1122E+6	0.1270E−3	0.1262
81.00	789.6	2064.	2927.	−0.1142E+6	0.1315E−3	0.1277
80.00	794.4	2057.	2901.	−0.1163E+6	0.1363E−3	0.1292
79.00	799.1	2051.	2876.	−0.1184E+6	0.1412E−3	0.1306
78.00	803.8	2045.	2850.	−0.1204E+6	0.1465E−3	0.1321
77.00	808.5	2039.	2823.	−0.1224E+6	0.1521E−3	0.1335
76.00	813.1	2034.	2797.	−0.1245E+6	0.1580E−3	0.1350
75.00	817.7	2030.	2770.	−0.1265E+6	0.1643E−3	0.1364
74.00	822.3	2026.	2742.	−0.1285E+6	0.1710E−3	0.1378
73.00	826.8	2022.	2715.	−0.1306E+6	0.1782E−3	0.1392
72.00	831.3	2019.	2687.	−0.1326E+6	0.1859E−3	0.1405
71.00	835.7	2016.	2659.	−0.1346E+6	0.1941E−3	0.1419
70.00	840.2	2014.	2630.	−0.1366E+6	0.2029E−3	0.1432
69.00	844.6	2013.	2601.	−0.1386E+6	0.2125E−3	0.1445
68.00	849.0	2012.	2572.	−0.1406E+6	0.2228E−3	0.1458
67.00	853.3	2012.	2542.	−0.1427E+6	0.2340E−3	0.1471
66.00	857.7	2012.	2512.	−0.1447E+6	0.2461E−3	0.1483
65.00	862.0	2013.	2481.	−0.1467E+6	0.2594E−3	0.1496
64.00	866.4	2016.	2450.	−0.1487E+6	0.2739E−3	0.1508

Table 1-11 Nitrogen properties along the 5×10^5 pascal (5 bar) isobar

T (k)	ρ (kg/m^3)	C_p (J/kg · K)	S (J/kg · K)	H (J/kg)	μ (Pa · s)	k (W/m · K)
300.0	5.620	1047.	6365.	0.3105E+6	0.1802E−4	0.2603E−1
295.0	5.717	1047.	6348.	0.3053E+6	0.1779E−4	0.2569E−1
290.0	5.817	1048.	6330.	0.3001E+6	0.1756E−4	0.2535E−1
285.0	5.920	1048.	6312.	0.2948E+6	0.1732E−4	0.2501E−1
280.0	6.028	1048.	6293.	0.2896E+6	0.1709E−4	0.2466E−1
275.0	6.139	1049.	6274.	0.2843E+6	0.1685E−4	0.2432E−1
270.0	6.255	1049.	6255.	0.2791E+6	0.1661E−4	0.2397E−1
265.0	6.375	1050.	6235.	0.2738E+6	0.1637E−4	0.2362E−1
260.0	6.500	1050.	6215.	0.2686E+6	0.1612E−4	0.2326E−1
255.0	6.630	1051.	6195.	0.2633E+6	0.1588E−4	0.2291E−1
250.0	6.765	1051.	6174.	0.2581E+6	0.1563E−4	0.2255E−1
245.0	6.906	1052.	6153.	0.2528E+6	0.1538E−4	0.2219E−1
240.0	7.054	1053.	6131.	0.2476E+6	0.1513E−4	0.2182E−1
235.0	7.208	1053.	6109.	0.2423E+6	0.1487E−4	0.2145E−1
230.0	7.369	1054.	6086.	0.2370E+6	0.1462E−4	0.2108E−1
225.0	7.537	1055.	6063.	0.2318E+6	0.1436E−4	0.2071E−1

(*Continues*)

Table 1-11 (*Continued*)

T (k)	ρ (kg/m³)	C_p (J/kg · K)	S (J/kg · K)	H (J/kg)	μ (Pa · s)	k (W/m · K)
220.0	7.714	1056.	6039.	0.2265E+6	0.1410E−4	0.2033E−1
215.0	7.899	1057.	6015.	0.2212E+6	0.1383E−4	0.1995E−1
210.0	8.094	1058.	5990.	0.2159E+6	0.1357E−4	0.1957E−1
205.0	8.299	1060.	5965.	0.2106E+6	0.1330E−4	0.1918E−1
200.0	8.515	1061.	5939.	0.2053E+6	0.1302E−4	0.1879E−1
195.0	8.743	1063.	5912.	0.2000E+6	0.1275E−4	0.1840E−1
190.0	8.984	1064.	5884.	0.1947E+6	0.1247E−4	0.1800E−1
185.0	9.239	1066.	5856.	0.1894E+6	0.1219E−4	0.1760E−1
180.0	9.510	1068.	5826.	0.1840E+6	0.1191E−4	0.1720E−1
175.0	9.798	1071.	5796.	0.1787E+6	0.1162E−4	0.1679E−1
170.0	10.11	1073.	5765.	0.1733E+6	0.1133E−4	0.1638E−1
165.0	10.43	1076.	5733.	0.1679E+6	0.1104E−4	0.1597E−1
160.0	10.79	1080.	5700.	0.1625E+6	0.1075E−4	0.1556E−1
155.0	11.16	1084.	5666.	0.1571E+6	0.1045E−4	0.1514E−1
150.0	11.57	1088.	5630.	0.1517E+6	0.1015E−4	0.1473E−1
145.0	12.01	1093.	5593.	0.1463E+6	0.9845E−5	0.1431E−1
140.0	12.49	1099.	5554.	0.1408E+6	0.9539E−5	0.1389E−1
135.0	13.01	1106.	5514.	0.1353E+6	0.9231E−5	0.1347E−1
130.0	13.59	1114.	5473.	0.1297E+6	0.8920E−5	0.1306E−1
125.0	14.22	1124.	5429.	0.1241E+6	0.8607E−5	0.1264E−1
120.0	14.92	1136.	5382.	0.1185E+6	0.8292E−5	0.1223E−1
115.0	15.71	1152.	5334.	0.1127E+6	0.7975E−5	0.1182E−1
110.0	16.61	1173.	5282.	0.1069E+6	0.7657E−5	0.1142E−1
105.0	17.64	1207.	5227.	0.1010E+6	0.7339E−5	0.1103E−1
100.0	18.85	1276.	5166.	0.9480E+5	0.7019E−5	0.1065E−1
99.00	19.12	1300.	5154.	0.9352E+5	0.6956E−5	0.1058E−1
98.00	19.40	1328.	5140.	0.9220E+5	0.6892E−5	0.1051E−1
97.00	19.69	1364.	5126.	0.9086E+5	0.6828E−5	0.1044E−1
96.00	20.00	1411.	5112.	0.8947E+5	0.6765E−5	0.1037E−1
95.00	20.33	1470.	5097.	0.8803E+5	0.6701E−5	0.1030E−1
94.00	20.68	1548.	5081.	0.8652E+5	0.6638E−5	0.1023E−1
93.00	728.8	2187.	3217.	−0.8867E+5	0.8957E−4	0.1094
92.00	734.4	2172.	3193.	−0.9085E+5	0.9240E−4	0.1110
91.00	739.8	2158.	3170.	−0.9301E+5	0.9532E−4	0.1126
90.00	745.2	2145.	3146.	−0.9516E+5	0.9835E−4	0.1142
89.00	750.5	2132.	3122.	−0.9730E+5	0.1015E−3	0.1158
88.00	755.7	2121.	3098.	−0.9943E+5	0.1048E−3	0.1173
87.00	760.9	2111.	3074.	−0.1015E+6	0.1082E−3	0.1189
86.00	765.9	2101.	3049.	−0.1037E+6	0.1117E−3	0.1204
85.00	771.0	2091.	3025.	−0.1057E+6	0.1155E−3	0.1220
84.00	775.9	2083.	3000.	−0.1078E+6	0.1193E−3	0.1235
83.00	780.8	2074.	2975.	−0.1099E+6	0.1234E−3	0.1250
82.00	785.7	2067.	2950.	−0.1120E+6	0.1277E−3	0.1265
81.00	790.5	2060.	2925.	−0.1140E+6	0.1322E−3	0.1280
80.00	795.3	2053.	2899.	−0.1161E+6	0.1369E−3	0.1295
79.00	800.0	2047.	2873.	−0.1182E+6	0.1419E−3	0.1310
78.00	804.7	2041.	2847.	−0.1202E+6	0.1472E−3	0.1324
77.00	809.3	2036.	2821.	−0.1222E+6	0.1528E−3	0.1338
76.00	813.9	2031.	2795.	−0.1243E+6	0.1587E−3	0.1353

(*Continues*)

Table 1-11 (*Continued*)

T (k)	ρ (kg/m^3)	C_p (J/kg·K)	S (J/kg·K)	H (J/kg)	μ (Pa·s)	k (W/m·K)
75.00	818.4	2027.	2768.	−0.1263E+6	0.1651E−3	0.1367
74.00	823.0	2023.	2740.	−0.1283E+6	0.1718E−3	0.1381
73.00	827.5	2020.	2713.	−0.1303E+6	0.1790E−3	0.1394
72.00	831.9	2017.	2685.	−0.1324E+6	0.1867E−3	0.1408
71.00	836.4	2014.	2657.	−0.1344E+6	0.1949E−3	0.1421
70.00	840.8	2012.	2628.	−0.1364E+6	0.2038E−3	0.1435
69.00	845.2	2011.	2599.	−0.1384E+6	0.2133E−3	0.1448
68.00	849.6	2010.	2570.	−0.1404E+6	0.2237E−3	0.1461
67.00	853.9	2010.	2540.	−0.1424E+6	0.2349E−3	0.1473
66.00	858.3	2011.	2510.	−0.1444E+6	0.2471E−3	0.1486
65.00	862.6	2012.	2479.	−0.1464E+6	0.2604E−3	0.1498
64.00	866.9	2014.	2448.	−0.1485E+6	0.2750E−3	0.1510

Table 1-12 Nitrogen properties along the 20×10^5 pascal (20 bar) isobar

T k	ρ (kg/m^3)	C_p (J/kg·K)	S (J/kg·K)	H (J/kg)	μ (Pa·s)	k (W/m·K)
300.0	22.52	1071.	5944.	0.3073E+6	0.1827E−4	0.2695E−1
295.0	22.93	1073.	5926.	0.3019E+6	0.1805E−4	0.2663E−1
290.0	23.34	1074.	5907.	0.2966E+6	0.1782E−4	0.2630E−1
285.0	23.77	1076.	5889.	0.2912E+6	0.1759E−4	0.2598E−1
280.0	24.22	1077.	5870.	0.2858E+6	0.1736E−4	0.2566E−1
275.0	24.69	1079.	5850.	0.2804E+6	0.1713E−4	0.2533E−1
270.0	25.18	1081.	5830.	0.2750E+6	0.1690E−4	0.2501E−1
265.0	25.69	1083.	5810.	0.2696E+6	0.1666E−4	0.2468E−1
260.0	26.22	1085.	5790.	0.2642E+6	0.1643E−4	0.2435E−1
255.0	26.77	1088.	5768.	0.2587E+6	0.1619E−4	0.2402E−1
250.0	27.35	1090.	5747.	0.2533E+6	0.1595E−4	0.2368E−1
245.0	27.96	1093.	5725.	0.2478E+6	0.1571E−4	0.2335E−1
240.0	28.60	1096.	5702.	0.2424E+6	0.1546E−4	0.2302E−1
235.0	29.27	1100.	5679.	0.2369E+6	0.1522E−4	0.2268E−1
230.0	29.98	1103.	5655.	0.2314E+6	0.1497E−4	0.2234E−1
225.0	30.72	1107.	5631.	0.2258E+6	0.1472E−4	0.2201E−1
220.0	31.51	1112.	5606.	0.2203E+6	0.1447E−4	0.2167E−1
215.0	32.34	1117.	5581.	0.2147E+6	0.1422E−4	0.2133E−1
210.0	33.23	1122.	5554.	0.2091E+6	0.1396E−4	0.2099E−1
205.0	34.17	1128.	5527.	0.2035E+6	0.1371E−4	0.2065E−1
200.0	35.17	1135.	5499.	0.1978E+6	0.1345E−4	0.2031E−1
195.0	36.24	1143.	5470.	0.1921E+6	0.1319E−4	0.1997E−1
190.0	37.38	1151.	5441.	0.1864E+6	0.1293E−4	0.1963E−1
185.0	38.62	1161.	5410.	0.1806E+6	0.1266E−4	0.1929E−1
180.0	39.95	1172.	5378.	0.1748E+6	0.1240E−4	0.1896E−1
175.0	41.40	1185.	5345.	0.1689E+6	0.1213E−4	0.1863E−1
170.0	42.98	1200.	5310.	0.1629E+6	0.1187E−4	0.1831E−1
165.0	44.72	1218.	5274.	0.1569E+6	0.1160E−4	0.1801E−1

(Continues)

Table 1-12 (*Continued*)

T k	ρ (kg/m^3)	C_p (J/kg · K)	S (J/kg · K)	H (J/kg)	μ (Pa · s)	k (W/m · K)
160.0	46.63	1239.	5236.	0.1508E+6	0.1133E−4	0.1771E−1
155.0	48.77	1264.	5196.	0.1445E+6	0.1107E−4	0.1744E−1
150.0	51.18	1296.	5154.	0.1381E+6	0.1080E−4	0.1719E−1
145.0	53.92	1335.	5110.	0.1315E+6	0.1054E−4	0.1697E−1
140.0	57.09	1388.	5062.	0.1247E+6	0.1028E−4	0.1679E−1
135.0	60.85	1459.	5010.	0.1176E+6	0.1003E−4	0.1667E−1
130.0	65.43	1564.	4954.	0.1101E+6	0.9792E−5	0.1661E−1
125.0	71.28	1737.	4889.	0.1019E+6	0.9574E−5	0.1668E−1
120.0	79.38	2090.	4812.	0.9244E+5	0.9395E−5	0.1698E−1
115.0	579.7	3226.	3719.	−0.3411E+5	0.4503E−4	0.7275E−1
110.0	627.4	2644.	3591.	−0.4852E+5	0.5488E−4	0.8285E−1
105.0	664.4	2397.	3474.	−0.6106E+5	0.6468E−4	0.9190E−1
100.0	696.2	2259.	3361.	−0.7266E+5	0.7528E−4	0.1003
99.00	702.1	2238.	3338.	−0.7491E+5	0.7755E−4	0.1020
98.00	707.9	2219.	3316.	−0.7714E+5	0.7988E−4	0.1036
97.00	713.6	2202.	3293.	−0.7935E+5	0.8228E−4	0.1052
96.00	719.2	2186.	3270.	−0.8154E+5	0.8475E−4	0.1068
95.00	724.7	2171.	3247.	−0.8372E+5	0.8730E−4	0.1084
94.00	730.2	2157.	3224.	−0.8589E+5	0.8993E−4	0.1100
93.00	735.5	2144.	3201.	−0.8804E+5	0.9265E−4	0.1115
92.00	740.8	2132.	3178.	−0.9017E+5	0.9547E−4	0.1131
91.00	746.0	2121.	3155.	−0.9230E+5	0.9839E−4	0.1147
90.00	751.1	2110.	3132.	−0.9442E+5	0.1014E−3	0.1162
89.00	756.2	2100.	3108.	−0.9652E+5	0.1046E−3	0.1177
88.00	761.2	2091.	3085.	−0.9862E+5	0.1079E−3	0.1192
87.00	766.2	2082.	3061.	−0.1007E+6	0.1113E−3	0.1208
86.00	771.1	2074.	3037.	−0.1028E+6	0.1149E−3	0.1223
85.00	775.9	2067.	3012.	−0.1049E+6	0.1186E−3	0.1238
84.00	780.7	2060.	2988.	−0.1069E+6	0.1225E−3	0.1252
83.00	785.4	2053.	2963.	−0.1090E+6	0.1266E−3	0.1267
82.00	790.2	2046.	2939.	−0.1110E+6	0.1309E−3	0.1282
81.00	794.8	2041.	2914.	−0.1131E+6	0.1355E−3	0.1296
80.00	799.4	2035.	2888.	−0.1151E+6	0.1403E−3	0.1311
79.00	804.0	2030.	2863.	−0.1171E+6	0.1453E−3	0.1325
78.00	808.6	2025.	2837.	−0.1192E+6	0.1507E−3	0.1339
77.00	813.1	2021.	2811.	−0.1212E+6	0.1563E−3	0.1353
76.00	817.6	2017.	2784.	−0.1232E+6	0.1623E−3	0.1367
75.00	822.0	2013.	2758.	−0.1252E+6	0.1687E−3	0.1381
74.00	826.5	2010.	2731.	−0.1272E+6	0.1755E−3	0.1394
73.00	830.8	2008.	2703.	−0.1292E+6	0.1828E−3	0.1408
72.00	835.2	2005.	2676.	−0.1312E+6	0.1906E−3	0.1421
71.00	839.6	2004.	2648.	−0.1333E+6	0.1989E−3	0.1434
70.00	843.9	2002.	2619.	−0.1353E+6	0.2079E−3	0.1447
69.00	848.2	2002.	2590.	−0.1373E+6	0.2176E−3	0.1460
68.00	852.5	2001.	2561.	−0.1393E+6	0.2281E−3	0.1472
67.00	856.7	2002.	2531.	−0.1413E+6	0.2395E−3	0.1485
66.00	861.0	2003.	2501.	−0.1433E+6	0.2518E−3	0.1497
65.00	865.2	2005.	2471.	−0.1453E+6	0.2653E−3	0.1509
64.00	869.5	2008.	2440.	−0.1473E+6	0.2801E−3	0.1521

Table 1-13 Saturation properties of oxygen (Liquid properties are shown in the first row of each temperature)

P (Pa)	T (K)	ρ (kg/m)^3	C_p (J/kg · K)	S (J/kg · K)	H (J/kg)	μ (Pa · s)	k (W/m · K)
0.4226E+7	150.0	677.0	5356.	3953.	−6606.	0.4310E−4	0.7168E−1
0.4226E+7	150.0	214.0	6491.	4484.	0.7308E+5	0.1516E−4	0.3419E−1
0.3901E+7	148.0	712.0	4223.	3908.	−0.1369E+5	0.4697E−4	0.7384E−1
0.3901E+7	148.0	186.3	4678.	4528.	0.7790E+5	0.1427E−4	0.2998E−1
0.3595E+7	146.0	741.7	3590.	3868.	−0.2001E+5	0.5059E−4	0.7614E−1
0.3595E+7	146.0	164.3	3701.	4564.	0.8158E+5	0.1358E−4	0.2703E−1
0.3308E+7	144.0	767.9	3183.	3831.	−0.2584E+5	0.5408E−4	0.7856E−1
0.3308E+7	144.0	146.0	3089.	4597.	0.8448E+5	0.1301E−4	0.2481E−1
0.3039E+7	142.0	791.6	2899.	3795.	−0.3129E+5	0.5751E−4	0.8109E−1
0.3039E+7	142.0	130.4	2671.	4627.	0.8683E+5	0.1253E−4	0.2305E−1
0.2788E+7	140.0	813.2	2691.	3761.	−0.3645E+5	0.6091E−4	0.8367E−1
0.2788E+7	140.0	116.7	2369.	4655.	0.8873E+5	0.1211E−4	0.2162E−1
0.2551E+7	138.0	833.3	2532.	3727.	−0.4137E+5	0.6432E−4	0.8629E−1
0.2551E+7	138.0	104.7	2140.	4681.	0.9026E+5	0.1173E−4	0.2043E−1
0.2330E+7	136.0	852.0	2407.	3695.	−0.4610E+5	0.6775E−4	0.8893E−1
0.2330E+7	136.0	94.11	1961.	4706.	0.9149E+5	0.1139E−4	0.1939E−1
0.2123E+7	134.0	869.7	2306.	3663.	−0.5067E+5	0.7123E−4	0.9156E−1
0.2123E+7	134.0	84.61	1817.	4731.	0.9245E+5	0.1108E−4	0.1848E−1
0.1929E+7	132.0	886.5	2223.	3631.	−0.5510E+5	0.7478E−4	0.9419E−1
0.1929E+7	132.0	76.06	1699.	4754.	0.9319E+5	0.1079E−4	0.1767E−1
0.1749E+7	130.0	902.5	2153.	3600.	−0.5941E+5	0.7842E−4	0.9682E−1
0.1749E+7	130.0	68.35	1600.	4778.	0.9372E+5	0.1052E−4	0.1693E−1
0.1581E+7	128.0	917.8	2094.	3568.	−0.6363E+5	0.8215E−4	0.9944E−1
0.1581E+7	128.0	61.37	1516.	4801.	0.9408E+5	0.1027E−4	0.1626E−1
0.1425E+7	126.0	932.5	2043.	3537.	−0.6775E+5	0.8601E−4	0.1021
0.1425E+7	126.0	55.04	1443.	4823.	0.9427E+5	0.1003E−4	0.1563E−1
0.1280E+7	124.0	946.8	1999.	3506.	−0.7179E+5	0.9000E−4	0.1047
0.1280E+7	124.0	49.29	1380.	4846.	0.9431E+5	0.9799E−5	0.1504E−1
0.1146E+7	122.0	960.5	1961.	3475.	−0.7575E+5	0.9414E−4	0.1073
0.1146E+7	122.0	44.06	1325.	4868.	0.9422E+5	0.9579E−5	0.1449E−1
0.1022E+7	120.0	973.9	1927.	3444.	−0.7966E+5	0.9844E−4	0.1100
0.1022E+7	120.0	39.30	1276.	4891.	0.9400E+5	0.9367E−5	0.1397E−1
0.9085E+6	118.0	986.8	1897.	3413.	−0.8350E+5	0.1029E−3	0.1127
0.9085E+6	118.0	34.97	1233.	4914.	0.9367E+5	0.9163E−5	0.1348E−1
0.8043E+6	116.0	999.4	1871.	3381.	−0.8729E+5	0.1076E−3	0.1154
0.8043E+6	116.0	31.04	1194.	4937.	0.9323E+5	0.8964E−5	0.1301E−1
0.7090E+6	114.0	1012.	1847.	3349.	−0.9103E+5	0.1125E−3	0.1181
0.7090E+6	114.0	27.46	1160.	4961.	0.9268E+5	0.8770E−5	0.1256E−1
0.6222E+6	112.0	1024.	1826.	3317.	−0.9473E+5	0.1176E−3	0.1208
0.6222E+6	112.0	24.22	1129.	4985.	0.9204E+5	0.8581E−5	0.1213E−1
0.5434E+6	110.0	1035.	1807.	3285.	−0.9839E+5	0.1230E−3	0.1236
0.5434E+6	110.0	21.28	1101.	5010.	0.9130E+5	0.8397E−5	0.1172E−1
0.4722E+6	108.0	1047.	1790.	3253.	−0.1020E+6	0.1286E−3	0.1263
0.4722E+6	108.0	18.62	1077.	5035.	0.9048E+5	0.8215E−5	0.1133E−1
0.4081E+6	106.0	1058.	1774.	3220.	−0.1056E+6	0.1345E−3	0.1291
0.4081E+6	106.0	16.23	1055.	5061.	0.8958E+5	0.8037E−5	0.1096E−1
0.3506E+6	104.0	1069.	1761.	3186.	−0.1092E+6	0.1408E−3	0.1320
0.3506E+6	104.0	14.08	1036.	5088.	0.8859E+5	0.7861E−5	0.1060E−1

(Continues)

Table 1-13 (*Continued*)

P (Pa)	T (K)	ρ (kg/m)^3	C_p (J/kg · K)	S (J/kg · K)	H (J/kg)	μ (Pa · s)	k (W/m · K)
0.2994E+6	102.0	1080.	1748.	3152.	−0.1127E+6	0.1474E−3	0.1348
0.2994E+6	102.0	12.15	1020.	5115.	0.8754E+5	0.7688E−5	0.1025E−1
0.2540E+6	100.0	1091.	1737.	3118.	−0.1162E+6	0.1543E−3	0.1377
0.2540E+6	100.0	10.42	1006.	5144.	0.8641E+5	0.7516E−5	0.9919E−2
0.2139E+6	98.00	1101.	1728.	3083.	−0.1197E+6	0.1617E−3	0.1405
0.2139E+6	98.00	8.892	994.8	5174.	0.8521E+5	0.7347E−5	0.9599E−2
0.1789E+6	96.00	1112.	1719.	3048.	−0.1231E+6	0.1695E−3	0.1434
0.1789E+6	96.00	7.535	985.6	5205.	0.8395E+5	0.7179E−5	0.9291E−2
0.1483E+6	94.00	1122.	1711.	3012.	−0.1266E+6	0.1777E−3	0.1463
0.1483E+6	94.00	6.341	978.5	5238.	0.8262E+5	0.7012E−5	0.8994E−2
0.1219E+6	92.00	1132.	1705.	2975.	−0.1300E+6	0.1865E−3	0.1492
0.1219E+6	92.00	5.295	973.5	5272.	0.8124E+5	0.6846E−5	0.8708E−2
0.9931E+5	90.00	1142.	1699.	2938.	−0.1334E+6	0.1957E−3	0.1521
0.9931E+5	90.00	4.385	970.3	5307.	0.7980E+5	0.6682E−5	0.8433E−2
0.8007E+5	88.00	1152.	1694.	2900.	−0.1368E+6	0.2056E−3	0.1550
0.8007E+5	88.00	3.599	968.8	5345.	0.7832E+5	0.6518E−5	0.8167E−2
0.6387E+5	86.00	1162.	1690.	2861.	−0.1402E+6	0.2161E−3	0.1578
0.6387E+5	86.00	2.925	968.7	5385.	0.7678E+5	0.6354E−5	0.7911E−2
0.5035E+5	84.00	1171.	1686.	2821.	−0.1436E+6	0.2272E−3	0.1606
0.5035E+5	84.00	2.352	969.8	5427.	0.7521E+5	0.6191E−5	0.7663E−2
0.3919E+5	82.00	1181.	1684.	2781.	−0.1470E+6	0.2391E−3	0.1634
0.3919E+5	82.00	1.869	971.7	5471.	0.7360E+5	0.6028E−5	0.7423E−2
0.3009E+5	80.00	1190.	1681.	2739.	−0.1504E+6	0.2517E−3	0.1661
0.3009E+5	80.00	1.467	974.0	5518.	0.7195E+5	0.5866E−5	0.7191E−2
0.2276E+5	78.00	1200.	1680.	2697.	−0.1537E+6	0.2651E−3	0.1688
0.2276E+5	78.00	1.135	976.4	5569.	0.7027E+5	0.5703E−5	0.6964E−2
0.1695E+5	76.00	1209.	1679.	2653.	−0.1571E+6	0.2794E−3	0.1714
0.1695E+5	76.00	0.8655	978.3	5623.	0.6857E+5	0.5540E−5	0.6744E−2
0.1240E+5	74.00	1219.	1678.	2608.	−0.1604E+6	0.2946E−3	0.1739
0.1240E+5	74.00	0.6491	979.4	5680.	0.6684E+5	0.5376E−5	0.6527E−2
8895.	72.00	1228.	1678.	2562.	−0.1638E+6	0.3107E−3	0.1763
8895.	72.00	0.4780	979.2	5742.	0.6510E+5	0.5211E−5	0.6314E−2
6251.	70.00	1237.	1678.	2515.	−0.1672E+6	0.3278E−3	0.1786
6251.	70.00	0.3451	977.6	5809.	0.6335E+5	0.5045E−5	0.6101E−2
4295.	68.00	1246.	1678.	2467.	−0.1705E+6	0.3459E−3	0.1808
4295.	68.00	0.2438	974.4	5880.	0.6158E+5	0.4878E−5	0.5888E−2
2878.	66.00	1255.	1677.	2416.	−0.1739E+6	0.3649E−3	0.1829
2878.	66.00	0.1682	969.5	5958.	0.5980E+5	0.4708E−5	0.5672E−2
1876.	64.00	1264.	1677.	2365.	−0.1772E+6	0.3848E−3	0.1848
1876.	64.00	0.1130	963.2	6041.	0.5802E+5	0.4535E−5	0.5448E−2
1187.	62.00	1273.	1675.	2312.	−0.1806E+6	0.4054E−3	0.1866
1187.	62.00	0.7378E−1	955.7	6131.	0.5623E+5	0.4359E−5	0.5213E−2
726.8	60.00	1282.	1673.	2257.	−0.1839E+6	0.4266E−3	0.1883
726.8	60.00	0.4666E−1	947.6	6229.	0.5444E+5	0.4179E−5	0.4962E−2
429.1	58.00	1291.	1671.	2200.	−0.1873E+6	0.4479E−3	0.1898
429.1	58.00	0.2849E−1	939.5	6336.	0.5264E+5	0.3993E−5	0.4688E−2
243.4	56.00	1299.	1671.	2141.	−0.1906E+6	0.4687E−3	0.1913
243.4	56.00	0.1674E−1	931.9	6451.	0.5084E+5	0.3800E−5	0.4382E−2

Table 1-14 Oxygen properties along the 1×10^5 pascal (1 bar) isobar

T (k)	ρ (kg/m^3)	C_p (J/kg·K)	S (J/kg·K)	H (J/kg)	μ (Pa·s)	k (W/m·K)
300.0	1.284	919.9	6416.	0.2730E+6	0.2063E−4	0.2629E−1
295.0	1.305	919.2	6400.	0.2684E+6	0.2035E−4	0.2591E−1
290.0	1.328	918.6	6385.	0.2638E+6	0.2007E−4	0.2553E−1
285.0	1.351	918.0	6369.	0.2592E+6	0.1979E−4	0.2515E−1
280.0	1.376	917.4	6353.	0.2546E+6	0.1951E−4	0.2477E−1
275.0	1.401	916.9	6336.	0.2500E+6	0.1923E−4	0.2439E−1
270.0	1.427	916.4	6319.	0.2454E+6	0.1894E−4	0.2401E−1
265.0	1.454	916.0	6302.	0.2409E+6	0.1865E−4	0.2362E−1
260.0	1.482	915.7	6285.	0.2363E+6	0.1836E−4	0.2324E−1
255.0	1.511	915.3	6267.	0.2317E+6	0.1806E−4	0.2285E−1
250.0	1.542	915.1	6249.	0.2271E+6	0.1777E−4	0.2246E−1
245.0	1.573	914.8	6230.	0.2225E+6	0.1747E−4	0.2207E−1
240.0	1.606	914.6	6211.	0.2180E+6	0.1716E−4	0.2167E−1
235.0	1.641	914.5	6192.	0.2134E+6	0.1686E−4	0.2128E−1
230.0	1.676	914.4	6172.	0.2088E+6	0.1655E−4	0.2088E−1
225.0	1.714	914.3	6152.	0.2043E+6	0.1624E−4	0.2048E−1
220.0	1.753	914.3	6132.	0.1997E+6	0.1593E−4	0.2008E−1
215.0	1.794	914.3	6111.	0.1951E+6	0.1561E−4	0.1967E−1
210.0	1.837	914.4	6089.	0.1905E+6	0.1529E−4	0.1926E−1
205.0	1.883	914.5	6067.	0.1860E+6	0.1497E−4	0.1885E−1
200.0	1.930	914.7	6045.	0.1814E+6	0.1464E−4	0.1843E−1
195.0	1.980	914.9	6022.	0.1768E+6	0.1431E−4	0.1801E−1
190.0	2.033	915.1	5998.	0.1722E+6	0.1398E−4	0.1759E−1
185.0	2.088	915.5	5973.	0.1677E+6	0.1365E−4	0.1716E−1
180.0	2.147	915.8	5948.	0.1631E+6	0.1331E−4	0.1673E−1
175.0	2.209	916.3	5922.	0.1585E+6	0.1297E−4	0.1629E−1
170.0	2.275	916.8	5896.	0.1539E+6	0.1262E−4	0.1585E−1
165.0	2.345	917.4	5869.	0.1493E+6	0.1227E−4	0.1541E−1
160.0	2.420	918.0	5840.	0.1448E+6	0.1192E−4	0.1495E−1
155.0	2.499	918.8	5811.	0.1402E+6	0.1156E−4	0.1450E−1
150.0	2.584	919.7	5781.	0.1356E+6	0.1121E−4	0.1404E−1
145.0	2.676	920.7	5750.	0.1310E+6	0.1084E−4	0.1357E−1
140.0	2.774	921.8	5717.	0.1264E+6	0.1048E−4	0.1310E−1
135.0	2.879	923.1	5684.	0.1217E+6	0.1011E−4	0.1263E−1
130.0	2.993	924.6	5649.	0.1171E+6	0.9739E−5	0.1215E−1
125.0	3.117	926.2	5613.	0.1125E+6	0.9365E−5	0.1168E−1
120.0	3.252	927.9	5575.	0.1079E+6	0.8989E−5	0.1120E−1
115.0	3.400	929.7	5535.	0.1032E+6	0.8610E−5	0.1072E−1
110.0	3.562	931.5	5494.	0.9857E+5	0.8228E−5	0.1024E−1
105.0	3.742	933.1	5451.	0.9391E+5	0.7845E−5	0.9775E−2
100.0	3.941	935.1	5405.	0.8924E+5	0.7459E−5	0.9315E−2
99.00	3.984	935.7	5396.	0.8830E+5	0.7382E−5	0.9224E−2
98.00	4.027	936.6	5386.	0.8736E+5	0.7304E−5	0.9134E−2
97.00	4.072	937.6	5377.	0.8643E+5	0.7227E−5	0.9044E−2

(Continues)

Table 1-14 (*Continued*)

T (k)	ρ (kg/m³)	C_p (J/kg · K)	S (J/kg · K)	H (J/kg)	μ (Pa · s)	k (W/m · K)
96.00	4.117	939.1	5367.	0.8549E+5	0.7149E−5	0.8955E−2
95.00	4.164	941.2	5357.	0.8455E+5	0.7071E−5	0.8867E−2
94.00	4.212	944.0	5347.	0.8361E+5	0.6994E−5	0.8779E−2
93.00	4.261	947.8	5337.	0.8266E+5	0.6916E−5	0.8693E−2
92.00	4.312	953.2	5327.	0.8171E+5	0.6838E−5	0.8606E−2
91.00	4.363	960.7	5316.	0.8075E+5	0.6760E−5	0.8521E−2
90.00	1142.	1699.	2938.	−0.1334E+6	0.1957E−3	0.1521
89.00	1147.	1696.	2919.	−0.1351E+6	0.2006E−3	0.1535
88.00	1152.	1694.	2900.	−0.1368E+6	0.2056E−3	0.1550
87.00	1157.	1691.	2880.	−0.1385E+6	0.2108E−3	0.1564
86.00	1162.	1689.	2861.	−0.1402E+6	0.2162E−3	0.1578
85.00	1167.	1688.	2841.	−0.1419E+6	0.2217E−3	0.1592
84.00	1171.	1686.	2821.	−0.1436E+6	0.2273E−3	0.1606
83.00	1176.	1685.	2801.	−0.1453E+6	0.2332E−3	0.1620
82.00	1181.	1683.	2781.	−0.1470E+6	0.2392E−3	0.1634
81.00	1186.	1682.	2760.	−0.1486E+6	0.2454E−3	0.1648
80.00	1191.	1681.	2739.	−0.1503E+6	0.2519E−3	0.1662
79.00	1195.	1680.	2718.	−0.1520E+6	0.2585E−3	0.1675
78.00	1200.	1680.	2697.	−0.1537E+6	0.2653E−3	0.1688
77.00	1205.	1679.	2675.	−0.1554E+6	0.2724E−3	0.1701
76.00	1209.	1679.	2653.	−0.1570E+6	0.2796E−3	0.1714
75.00	1214.	1678.	2631.	−0.1587E+6	0.2871E−3	0.1727
74.00	1219.	1678.	2608.	−0.1604E+6	0.2948E−3	0.1739
73.00	1223.	1678.	2585.	−0.1621E+6	0.3028E−3	0.1752
72.00	1228.	1678.	2562.	−0.1638E+6	0.3110E−3	0.1764
71.00	1233.	1678.	2539.	−0.1654E+6	0.3194E−3	0.1775
70.00	1237.	1678.	2515.	−0.1671E+6	0.3281E−3	0.1787
69.00	1242.	1678.	2491.	−0.1688E+6	0.3370E−3	0.1798
68.00	1246.	1678.	2466.	−0.1705E+6	0.3462E−3	0.1809
67.00	1251.	1678.	2441.	−0.1721E+6	0.3556E−3	0.1819
66.00	1255.	1677.	2416.	−0.1738E+6	0.3652E−3	0.1829
65.00	1260.	1677.	2391.	−0.1755E+6	0.3750E−3	0.1839
64.00	1264.	1676.	2365.	−0.1772E+6	0.3851E−3	0.1848
63.00	1269.	1676.	2338.	−0.1788E+6	0.3953E−3	0.1858
62.00	1273.	1675.	2311.	−0.1805E+6	0.4058E−3	0.1866
61.00	1278.	1674.	2284.	−0.1822E+6	0.4163E−3	0.1875
60.00	1282.	1673.	2257.	−0.1839E+6	0.4269E−3	0.1883
59.00	1287.	1672.	2228.	−0.1855E+6	0.4376E−3	0.1891
58.00	1291.	1671.	2200.	−0.1872E+6	0.4483E−3	0.1898
57.00	1295.	1670.	2171.	−0.1889E+6	0.4588E−3	0.1906
56.00	1299.	1670.	2141.	−0.1906E+6	0.4691E−3	0.1913

Table 1-15 Oxygen properties along the 2×10^5 pascal (2 bar) isobar

T (k)	ρ (kg/m³)	C_p (J/kg·K)	S (J/kg·K)	H (J/kg)	μ (Pa·s)	k (W/m·K)
300.0	2.569	921.5	6235.	0.2727E+6	0.2064E−4	0.2633E−1
295.0	2.613	920.8	6220.	0.2681E+6	0.2036E−4	0.2596E−1
290.0	2.658	920.3	6204.	0.2635E+6	0.2008E−4	0.2558E−1
285.0	2.705	919.7	6188.	0.2589E+6	0.1980E−4	0.2520E−1
280.0	2.754	919.3	6172.	0.2543E+6	0.1952E−4	0.2482E−1
275.0	2.804	918.8	6155.	0.2497E+6	0.1924E−4	0.2444E−1
270.0	2.857	918.5	6138.	0.2451E+6	0.1895E−4	0.2406E−1
265.0	2.911	918.1	6121.	0.2405E+6	0.1866E−4	0.2368E−1
260.0	2.967	917.9	6104.	0.2360E+6	0.1837E−4	0.2329E−1
255.0	3.026	917.7	6086.	0.2314E+6	0.1808E−4	0.2291E−1
250.0	3.087	917.5	6068.	0.2268E+6	0.1778E−4	0.2252E−1
245.0	3.151	917.4	6049.	0.2222E+6	0.1748E−4	0.2213E−1
240.0	3.217	917.3	6030.	0.2176E+6	0.1718E−4	0.2174E−1
235.0	3.287	917.3	6011.	0.2130E+6	0.1687E−4	0.2135E−1
230.0	3.359	917.4	5991.	0.2084E+6	0.1657E−4	0.2095E−1
225.0	3.435	917.5	5971.	0.2038E+6	0.1626E−4	0.2055E−1
220.0	3.514	917.7	5950.	0.1993E+6	0.1594E−4	0.2015E−1
215.0	3.597	917.9	5929.	0.1947E+6	0.1563E−4	0.1975E−1
210.0	3.684	918.3	5908.	0.1901E+6	0.1531E−4	0.1934E−1
205.0	3.776	918.6	5886.	0.1855E+6	0.1499E−4	0.1893E−1
200.0	3.872	919.1	5863.	0.1809E+6	0.1466E−4	0.1852E−1
195.0	3.973	919.6	5840.	0.1763E+6	0.1433E−4	0.1811E−1
190.0	4.080	920.2	5816.	0.1717E+6	0.1400E−4	0.1769E−1
185.0	4.193	921.0	5791.	0.1671E+6	0.1367E−4	0.1726E−1
180.0	4.312	921.8	5766.	0.1625E+6	0.1333E−4	0.1684E−1
175.0	4.439	922.7	5740.	0.1579E+6	0.1299E−4	0.1641E−1
170.0	4.573	923.8	5713.	0.1533E+6	0.1264E−4	0.1597E−1
165.0	4.716	925.0	5686.	0.1486E+6	0.1229E−4	0.1553E−1
160.0	4.869	926.5	5657.	0.1440E+6	0.1194E−4	0.1509E−1
155.0	5.032	928.1	5628.	0.1394E+6	0.1159E−4	0.1464E−1
150.0	5.207	929.9	5597.	0.1347E+6	0.1123E−4	0.1419E−1
145.0	5.395	932.1	5566.	0.1301E+6	0.1087E−4	0.1374E−1
140.0	5.598	934.5	5533.	0.1254E+6	0.1051E−4	0.1328E−1
135.0	5.817	937.3	5499.	0.1207E+6	0.1014E−4	0.1283E−1
130.0	6.056	940.4	5463.	0.1160E+6	0.9768E−5	0.1237E−1
125.0	6.316	943.9	5426.	0.1113E+6	0.9396E−5	0.1191E−1
120.0	6.600	947.7	5388.	0.1066E+6	0.9020E−5	0.1145E−1
115.0	6.914	951.9	5347.	0.1018E+6	0.8643E−5	0.1100E−1
110.0	7.262	956.2	5305.	0.9707E+5	0.8262E−5	0.1055E−1
105.0	7.650	961.6	5260.	0.9228E+5	0.7880E−5	0.1012E−1
100.0	8.087	973.5	5213.	0.8744E+5	0.7496E−5	0.9702E−2
99.00	8.181	978.3	5203.	0.8647E+5	0.7419E−5	0.9621E−2
98.00	8.278	984.6	5193.	0.8549E+5	0.7341E−5	0.9541E−2
97.00	1107.	1723.	3066.	−0.1214E+6	0.1655E−3	0.1420

(*Continues*)

Table 1-15 (*Continued*)

T (k)	ρ (kg/m^3)	C_p (J/kg · K)	S (J/kg · K)	H (J/kg)	μ (Pa · s)	k (W/m · K)
96.00	1112.	1719.	3048.	−0.1231E+6	0.1695E−3	0.1434
95.00	1117.	1715.	3030.	−0.1249E+6	0.1736E−3	0.1449
94.00	1122.	1711.	3012.	−0.1266E+6	0.1778E−3	0.1463
93.00	1127.	1707.	2993.	−0.1283E+6	0.1821E−3	0.1478
92.00	1132.	1704.	2975.	−0.1300E+6	0.1866E−3	0.1492
91.00	1137.	1701.	2956.	−0.1317E+6	0.1912E−3	0.1507
90.00	1142.	1698.	2938.	−0.1334E+6	0.1959E−3	0.1521
89.00	1147.	1696.	2919.	−0.1351E+6	0.2008E−3	0.1536
88.00	1152.	1693.	2899.	−0.1368E+6	0.2058E−3	0.1550
87.00	1157.	1691.	2880.	−0.1385E+6	0.2110E−3	0.1564
86.00	1162.	1689.	2861.	−0.1402E+6	0.2164E−3	0.1578
85.00	1167.	1687.	2841.	−0.1418E+6	0.2219E−3	0.1593
84.00	1172.	1686.	2821.	−0.1435E+6	0.2275E−3	0.1607
83.00	1176.	1684.	2801.	−0.1452E+6	0.2334E−3	0.1621
82.00	1181.	1683.	2780.	−0.1469E+6	0.2394E−3	0.1634
81.00	1186.	1682.	2760.	−0.1486E+6	0.2457E−3	0.1648
80.00	1191.	1681.	2739.	−0.1503E+6	0.2521E−3	0.1662
79.00	1195.	1680.	2718.	−0.1519E+6	0.2587E−3	0.1675
78.00	1200.	1679.	2696.	−0.1536E+6	0.2656E−3	0.1689
77.00	1205.	1679.	2675.	−0.1553E+6	0.2726E−3	0.1702
76.00	1210.	1679.	2653.	−0.1570E+6	0.2799E−3	0.1715
75.00	1214.	1678.	2630.	−0.1587E+6	0.2874E−3	0.1727
74.00	1219.	1678.	2608.	−0.1603E+6	0.2951E−3	0.1740
73.00	1223.	1678.	2585.	−0.1620E+6	0.3031E−3	0.1752
72.00	1228.	1678.	2562.	−0.1637E+6	0.3112E−3	0.1764
71.00	1233.	1678.	2538.	−0.1654E+6	0.3197E−3	0.1776
70.00	1237.	1678.	2515.	−0.1670E+6	0.3284E−3	0.1787
69.00	1242.	1678.	2490.	−0.1687E+6	0.3373E−3	0.1798
68.00	1246.	1677.	2466.	−0.1704E+6	0.3465E−3	0.1809
67.00	1251.	1677.	2441.	−0.1721E+6	0.3559E−3	0.1819
66.00	1255.	1677.	2416.	−0.1738E+6	0.3655E−3	0.1829
65.00	1260.	1677.	2390.	−0.1754E+6	0.3754E−3	0.1839
64.00	1264.	1676.	2364.	−0.1771E+6	0.3854E−3	0.1849
63.00	1269.	1676.	2338.	−0.1788E+6	0.3957E−3	0.1858
62.00	1273.	1675.	2311.	−0.1805E+6	0.4061E−3	0.1867
61.00	1278.	1674.	2284.	−0.1821E+6	0.4167E−3	0.1875
60.00	1282.	1673.	2256.	−0.1838E+6	0.4273E−3	0.1883
59.00	1287.	1672.	2228.	−0.1855E+6	0.4380E−3	0.1891
58.00	1291.	1671.	2200.	−0.1872E+6	0.4486E−3	0.1899
57.00	1295.	1670.	2171.	−0.1888E+6	0.4592E−3	0.1906
56.00	1300.	1670.	2141.	−0.1905E+6	0.4695E−3	0.1913

Table 1-16 Oxygen properties along the 5×10^5 pascal (5 bar) isobar

T (k)	ρ (kg/m^3)	C_p (J/kg·K)	S (J/kg·K)	H (J/kg)	μ (Pa·s)	k (W/m·K)
300.0	6.434	926.1	5995.	0.2720E+6	0.2067E−4	0.2647E−1
295.0	6.545	925.7	5980.	0.2674E+6	0.2040E−4	0.2610E−1
290.0	6.660	925.4	5964.	0.2627E+6	0.2012E−4	0.2573E−1
285.0	6.779	925.1	5948.	0.2581E+6	0.1984E−4	0.2535E−1
280.0	6.902	924.8	5931.	0.2535E+6	0.1956E−4	0.2498E−1
275.0	7.030	924.7	5915.	0.2489E+6	0.1927E−4	0.2460E−1
270.0	7.163	924.6	5898.	0.2442E+6	0.1899E−4	0.2422E−1
265.0	7.301	924.5	5880.	0.2396E+6	0.1870E−4	0.2384E−1
260.0	7.445	924.6	5863.	0.2350E+6	0.1841E−4	0.2346E−1
255.0	7.594	924.7	5845.	0.2304E+6	0.1812E−4	0.2308E−1
250.0	7.750	924.9	5827.	0.2258E+6	0.1782E−4	0.2270E−1
245.0	7.913	925.2	5808.	0.2211E+6	0.1752E−4	0.2232E−1
240.0	8.082	925.6	5789.	0.2165E+6	0.1722E−4	0.2193E−1
235.0	8.259	926.1	5769.	0.2119E+6	0.1692E−4	0.2155E−1
230.0	8.445	926.6	5749.	0.2072E+6	0.1661E−4	0.2116E−1
225.0	8.639	927.3	5729.	0.2026E+6	0.1630E−4	0.2077E−1
220.0	8.843	928.1	5708.	0.1980E+6	0.1599E−4	0.2038E−1
215.0	9.057	929.1	5687.	0.1933E+6	0.1568E−4	0.1998E−1
210.0	9.282	930.1	5665.	0.1887E+6	0.1536E−4	0.1959E−1
205.0	9.518	931.3	5642.	0.1840E+6	0.1504E−4	0.1919E−1
200.0	9.768	932.7	5619.	0.1794E+6	0.1472E−4	0.1879E−1
195.0	10.03	934.3	5596.	0.1747E+6	0.1439E−4	0.1839E−1
190.0	10.31	936.1	5572.	0.1700E+6	0.1406E−4	0.1798E−1
185.0	10.61	938.1	5547.	0.1653E+6	0.1373E−4	0.1758E−1
180.0	10.92	940.4	5521.	0.1606E+6	0.1339E−4	0.1717E−1
175.0	11.25	943.0	5494.	0.1559E+6	0.1305E−4	0.1676E−1
170.0	11.61	946.0	5467.	0.1512E+6	0.1271E−4	0.1634E−1
165.0	11.99	949.5	5439.	0.1465E+6	0.1237E−4	0.1593E−1
160.0	12.40	953.5	5409.	0.1417E+6	0.1202E−4	0.1551E−1
155.0	12.84	958.0	5379.	0.1369E+6	0.1167E−4	0.1510E−1
150.0	13.32	963.4	5347.	0.1321E+6	0.1131E−4	0.1468E−1
145.0	13.84	969.5	5315.	0.1273E+6	0.1095E−4	0.1427E−1
140.0	14.40	976.7	5281.	0.1224E+6	0.1059E−4	0.1385E−1
135.0	15.02	985.1	5245.	0.1175E+6	0.1023E−4	0.1344E−1
130.0	15.70	994.8	5208.	0.1126E+6	0.9865E−5	0.1304E−1
125.0	16.46	1006.	5168.	0.1076E+6	0.9497E−5	0.1264E−1
120.0	17.31	1020.	5127.	0.1025E+6	0.9126E−5	0.1226E−1
115.0	18.27	1038.	5083.	0.9737E+5	0.8753E−5	0.1190E−1
110.0	19.37	1072.	5036.	0.9211E+5	0.8378E−5	0.1156E−1
105.0	1064.	1766.	3202.	−0.1073E+6	0.1378E−3	0.1306
100.0	1092.	1735.	3117.	−0.1161E+6	0.1548E−3	0.1378
99.00	1097.	1730.	3100.	−0.1178E+6	0.1584E−3	0.1392
98.00	1102.	1725.	3082.	−0.1195E+6	0.1622E−3	0.1406
97.00	1107.	1721.	3064.	−0.1213E+6	0.1661E−3	0.1421

(Continues)

Table 1-16 (*Continued*)

T (k)	ρ (kg/m³)	C_p (J/kg · K)	S (J/kg · K)	H (J/kg)	μ (Pa · s)	k (W/m · K)
96.00	1113.	1717.	3047.	−0.1230E+6	0.1701E−3	0.1435
95.00	1118.	1713.	3029.	−0.1247E+6	0.1742E−3	0.1450
94.00	1123.	1709.	3010.	−0.1264E+6	0.1784E−3	0.1464
93.00	1128.	1706.	2992.	−0.1281E+6	0.1827E−3	0.1479
92.00	1133.	1702.	2974.	−0.1298E+6	0.1872E−3	0.1493
91.00	1138.	1699.	2955.	−0.1315E+6	0.1918E−3	0.1508
90.00	1143.	1697.	2936.	−0.1332E+6	0.1965E−3	0.1522
89.00	1148.	1694.	2917.	−0.1349E+6	0.2014E−3	0.1536
88.00	1153.	1692.	2898.	−0.1366E+6	0.2064E−3	0.1551
87.00	1158.	1690.	2879.	−0.1383E+6	0.2116E−3	0.1565
86.00	1163.	1688.	2859.	−0.1400E+6	0.2170E−3	0.1579
85.00	1167.	1686.	2840.	−0.1417E+6	0.2225E−3	0.1593
84.00	1172.	1684.	2820.	−0.1434E+6	0.2282E−3	0.1608
83.00	1177.	1683.	2800.	−0.1450E+6	0.2341E−3	0.1621
82.00	1182.	1682.	2779.	−0.1467E+6	0.2401E−3	0.1635
81.00	1187.	1681.	2759.	−0.1484E+6	0.2463E−3	0.1649
80.00	1191.	1680.	2738.	−0.1501E+6	0.2528E−3	0.1663
79.00	1196.	1679.	2717.	−0.1518E+6	0.2594E−3	0.1676
78.00	1201.	1679.	2695.	−0.1534E+6	0.2663E−3	0.1689
77.00	1205.	1678.	2674.	−0.1551E+6	0.2733E−3	0.1702
76.00	1210.	1678.	2652.	−0.1568E+6	0.2806E−3	0.1715
75.00	1215.	1677.	2629.	−0.1585E+6	0.2881E−3	0.1728
74.00	1219.	1677.	2607.	−0.1602E+6	0.2959E−3	0.1740
73.00	1224.	1677.	2584.	−0.1618E+6	0.3038E−3	0.1753
72.00	1229.	1677.	2561.	−0.1635E+6	0.3121E−3	0.1764
71.00	1233.	1677.	2538.	−0.1652E+6	0.3205E−3	0.1776
70.00	1238.	1677.	2514.	−0.1669E+6	0.3292E−3	0.1788
69.00	1242.	1677.	2490.	−0.1685E+6	0.3382E−3	0.1799
68.00	1247.	1677.	2465.	−0.1702E+6	0.3473E−3	0.1809
67.00	1251.	1677.	2440.	−0.1719E+6	0.3568E−3	0.1820
66.00	1256.	1677.	2415.	−0.1736E+6	0.3664E−3	0.1830
65.00	1260.	1676.	2389.	−0.1753E+6	0.3763E−3	0.1840
64.00	1265.	1676.	2363.	−0.1769E+6	0.3864E−3	0.1849
63.00	1269.	1675.	2337.	−0.1786E+6	0.3967E−3	0.1858
62.00	1274.	1674.	2310.	−0.1803E+6	0.4071E−3	0.1867
61.00	1278.	1673.	2283.	−0.1820E+6	0.4177E−3	0.1876
60.00	1283.	1672.	2255.	−0.1836E+6	0.4284E−3	0.1884
59.00	1287.	1671.	2227.	−0.1853E+6	0.4391E−3	0.1891
58.00	1291.	1670.	2199.	−0.1870E+6	0.4498E−3	0.1899
57.00	1296.	1669.	2170.	−0.1886E+6	0.4604E−3	0.1906
56.00	1300.	1669.	2140.	−0.1903E+6	0.4707E−3	0.1913

Table 1-17 Oxygen properties along the 20×10^5 pascal (20 bar) isobar

T (k)	ρ (kg/m^3)	C_p (J/kg·K)	S (J/kg·K)	H (J/kg)	μ (Pa·s)	k (W/m·K)
300.0	25.97	950.1	5625.	0.2683E+6	0.2088E−4	0.2720E−1
295.0	26.44	950.8	5609.	0.2636E+6	0.2061E−4	0.2685E−1
290.0	26.92	951.5	5593.	0.2588E+6	0.2034E−4	0.2649E−1
285.0	27.43	952.5	5576.	0.2541E+6	0.2006E−4	0.2613E−1
280.0	27.96	953.5	5559.	0.2493E+6	0.1979E−4	0.2578E−1
275.0	28.51	954.8	5542.	0.2445E+6	0.1951E−4	0.2542E−1
270.0	29.08	956.2	5525.	0.2398E+6	0.1923E−4	0.2507E−1
265.0	29.68	957.9	5507.	0.2350E+6	0.1895E−4	0.2471E−1
260.0	30.30	959.7	5489.	0.2302E+6	0.1867E−4	0.2436E−1
255.0	30.96	961.8	5470.	0.2254E+6	0.1838E−4	0.2401E−1
250.0	31.64	964.1	5451.	0.2206E+6	0.1809E−4	0.2366E−1
245.0	32.36	966.8	5431.	0.2157E+6	0.1780E−4	0.2331E−1
240.0	33.12	969.7	5411.	0.2109E+6	0.1751E−4	0.2296E−1
235.0	33.92	973.0	5391.	0.2060E+6	0.1722E−4	0.2261E−1
230.0	34.76	976.7	5370.	0.2012E+6	0.1692E−4	0.2227E−1
225.0	35.64	980.8	5348.	0.1963E+6	0.1662E−4	0.2192E−1
220.0	36.58	985.5	5326.	0.1914E+6	0.1632E−4	0.2158E−1
215.0	37.58	990.8	5304.	0.1864E+6	0.1602E−4	0.2125E−1
210.0	38.64	996.7	5280.	0.1815E+6	0.1572E−4	0.2091E−1
205.0	39.77	1003.	5256.	0.1765E+6	0.1541E−4	0.2058E−1
200.0	40.99	1011.	5231.	0.1714E+6	0.1510E−4	0.2026E−1
195.0	42.29	1020.	5206.	0.1663E+6	0.1479E−4	0.1994E−1
190.0	43.69	1030.	5179.	0.1612E+6	0.1448E−4	0.1964E−1
185.0	45.21	1042.	5151.	0.1560E+6	0.1416E−4	0.1934E−1
180.0	46.86	1056.	5123.	0.1508E+6	0.1384E−4	0.1905E−1
175.0	48.66	1072.	5093.	0.1455E+6	0.1353E−4	0.1878E−1
170.0	50.65	1092.	5061.	0.1401E+6	0.1321E−4	0.1852E−1
165.0	52.86	1116.	5028.	0.1346E+6	0.1289E−4	0.1829E−1
160.0	55.34	1145.	4994.	0.1289E+6	0.1257E−4	0.1808E−1
155.0	58.16	1182.	4957.	0.1231E+6	0.1225E−4	0.1790E−1
150.0	61.40	1230.	4917.	0.1171E+6	0.1193E−4	0.1777E−1
145.0	65.22	1296.	4874.	0.1108E+6	0.1162E−4	0.1769E−1
140.0	69.86	1396.	4827.	0.1041E+6	0.1131E−4	0.1769E−1
135.0	75.79	1582.	4774.	0.9667E+5	0.1102E−4	0.1783E−1
130.0	904.7	2136.	3597.	−0.5948E+5	0.7895E−4	0.9707E−1
125.0	944.1	1993.	3516.	−0.6977E+5	0.8923E−4	0.1039
120.0	979.1	1900.	3437.	−0.7949E+5	0.1002E−3	0.1107
115.0	1011.	1834.	3358.	−0.8882E+5	0.1122E−3	0.1174
110.0	1041.	1786.	3277.	−0.9786E+5	0.1255E−3	0.1243
105.0	1069.	1750.	3195.	−0.1067E+6	0.1404E−3	0.1313
100.0	1096.	1723.	3110.	−0.1154E+6	0.1574E−3	0.1384
99.00	1101.	1719.	3093.	−0.1171E+6	0.1611E−3	0.1398
98.00	1106.	1715.	3076.	−0.1188E+6	0.1649E−3	0.1412

(Continues)

Table 1-17 (*Continued*)

T (k)	ρ (kg/m³)	C_p (J/kg · K)	S (J/kg · K)	H (J/kg)	μ (Pa · s)	k (W/m · K)
97.00	1111.	1711.	3058.	−0.1205E+6	0.1688E−3	0.1426
96.00	1116.	1707.	3040.	−0.1222E+6	0.1728E−3	0.1441
95.00	1121.	1703.	3022.	−0.1239E+6	0.1769E−3	0.1455
94.00	1126.	1700.	3004.	−0.1256E+6	0.1812E−3	0.1469
93.00	1131.	1697.	2986.	−0.1273E+6	0.1856E−3	0.1484
92.00	1136.	1694.	2968.	−0.1290E+6	0.1901E−3	0.1498
91.00	1141.	1692.	2949.	−0.1307E+6	0.1947E−3	0.1513
90.00	1146.	1689.	2931.	−0.1324E+6	0.1995E−3	0.1527
89.00	1151.	1687.	2912.	−0.1341E+6	0.2044E−3	0.1541
88.00	1156.	1685.	2893.	−0.1358E+6	0.2095E−3	0.1555
87.00	1161.	1683.	2874.	−0.1375E+6	0.2147E−3	0.1570
86.00	1166.	1682.	2854.	−0.1392E+6	0.2201E−3	0.1584
85.00	1170.	1680.	2835.	−0.1408E+6	0.2257E−3	0.1598
84.00	1175.	1679.	2815.	−0.1425E+6	0.2314E−3	0.1612
83.00	1180.	1678.	2795.	−0.1442E+6	0.2373E−3	0.1626
82.00	1185.	1677.	2774.	−0.1459E+6	0.2434E−3	0.1639
81.00	1189.	1676.	2754.	−0.1476E+6	0.2497E−3	0.1653
80.00	1194.	1675.	2733.	−0.1492E+6	0.2562E−3	0.1667
79.00	1199.	1675.	2712.	−0.1509E+6	0.2629E−3	0.1680
78.00	1203.	1674.	2690.	−0.1526E+6	0.2698E−3	0.1693
77.00	1208.	1674.	2669.	−0.1543E+6	0.2770E−3	0.1706
76.00	1212.	1674.	2647.	−0.1559E+6	0.2843E−3	0.1719
75.00	1217.	1674.	2625.	−0.1576E+6	0.2919E−3	0.1731
74.00	1222.	1674.	2602.	−0.1593E+6	0.2997E−3	0.1744
73.00	1226.	1674.	2580.	−0.1609E+6	0.3078E−3	0.1756
72.00	1231.	1674.	2556.	−0.1626E+6	0.3161E−3	0.1768
71.00	1235.	1674.	2533.	−0.1643E+6	0.3246E−3	0.1779
70.00	1240.	1674.	2509.	−0.1660E+6	0.3334E−3	0.1791
69.00	1244.	1674.	2485.	−0.1676E+6	0.3425E−3	0.1802
68.00	1249.	1674.	2461.	−0.1693E+6	0.3518E−3	0.1812
67.00	1253.	1674.	2436.	−0.1710E+6	0.3613E−3	0.1823
66.00	1258.	1674.	2411.	−0.1727E+6	0.3711E−3	0.1833
65.00	1262.	1673.	2385.	−0.1743E+6	0.3811E−3	0.1843
64.00	1267.	1673.	2359.	−0.1760E+6	0.3913E−3	0.1852
63.00	1271.	1672.	2333.	−0.1777E+6	0.4017E−3	0.1861
62.00	1276.	1671.	2306.	−0.1794E+6	0.4123E−3	0.1870
61.00	1280.	1670.	2279.	−0.1810E+6	0.4230E−3	0.1878
60.00	1284.	1669.	2251.	−0.1827E+6	0.4338E−3	0.1886
59.00	1289.	1668.	2223.	−0.1844E+6	0.4446E−3	0.1894
58.00	1293.	1666.	2195.	−0.1860E+6	0.4555E−3	0.1902
57.00	1297.	1665.	2166.	−0.1877E+6	0.4662E−3	0.1909
56.00	1302.	1664.	2136.	−0.1894E+6	0.4767E−3	0.1916

Table 1-18 Saturation properties of argon (Liquid properties are shown in the first row of each temperature)

P (PA)	T (K)	ρ (kg/m³)	C_p (J/kg·K)	S (J/kg·K)	H (J/kg)	μ (Pa·s)	k (W/m·K)
0.4744E+7	150.0	694.6	0.1667E+5	2155.	−0.1832E+5	0.3763E−4	0.5475E−1
0.4744E+7	150.0	390.9	0.2109E+5	2363.	0.1300E+5	0.2093E−4	0.4324E−1
0.4380E+7	148.0	774.5	6257.	2101.	−0.2684E+5	0.4443E−4	0.5262E−1
0.4380E+7	148.0	317.6	8130.	2426.	0.2138E+5	0.1831E−4	0.3099E−1
0.4044E+7	146.0	830.6	3927.	2061.	−0.3312E+5	0.5010E−4	0.5379E−1
0.4044E+7	146.0	266.7	4471.	2476.	0.2754E+5	0.1669E−4	0.2452E−1
0.3733E+7	144.0	874.3	3008.	2028.	−0.3827E+5	0.5513E−4	0.5561E−1
0.3733E+7	144.0	230.3	3103.	2515.	0.3192E+5	0.1561E−4	0.2081E−1
0.3442E+7	142.0	910.9	2518.	1999.	−0.4276E+5	0.5983E−4	0.5769E−1
0.3442E+7	142.0	202.0	2401.	2548.	0.3529E+5	0.1478E−4	0.1835E−1
0.3170E+7	140.0	942.9	2213.	1972.	−0.4684E+5	0.6436E−4	0.5993E−1
0.3170E+7	140.0	178.8	1980.	2578.	0.3796E+5	0.1412E−4	0.1660E−1
0.2911E+7	138.0	971.4	2006.	1947.	−0.5061E+5	0.6878E−4	0.6226E−1
0.2911E+7	138.0	159.5	1703.	2604.	0.4010E+5	0.1357E−4	0.1529E−1
0.2668E+7	136.0	997.5	1854.	1923.	−0.5416E+5	0.7318E−4	0.6465E−1
0.2668E+7	136.0	142.9	1504.	2629.	0.4186E+5	0.1309E−4	0.1426E−1
0.2441E+7	134.0	1022.	1737.	1899.	−0.5753E+5	0.7762E−4	0.6707E−1
0.2441E+7	134.0	128.2	1353.	2652.	0.4335E+5	0.1266E−4	0.1341E−1
0.2227E+7	132.0	1045.	1644.	1877.	−0.6076E+5	0.8213E−4	0.6950E−1
0.2227E+7	132.0	115.2	1235.	2675.	0.4460E+5	0.1228E−4	0.1270E−1
0.2027E+7	130.0	1066.	1569.	1854.	−0.6387E+5	0.8672E−4	0.7192E−1
0.2027E+7	130.0	103.6	1140.	2697.	0.4565E+5	0.1192E−4	0.1208E−1
0.1841E+7	128.0	1087.	1507.	1832.	−0.6688E+5	0.9143E−4	0.7433E−1
0.1841E+7	128.0	93.11	1062.	2718.	0.4653E+5	0.1159E−4	0.1154E−1
0.1667E+7	126.0	1106.	1455.	1811.	−0.6980E+5	0.9627E−4	0.7671E−1
0.1667E+7	126.0	83.66	997.2	2739.	0.4725E+5	0.1129E−4	0.1105E−1
0.1505E+7	124.0	1125.	1411.	1789.	−0.7264E+5	0.1013E−3	0.7909E−1
0.1505E+7	124.0	75.10	942.2	2760.	0.4784E+5	0.1100E−4	0.1061E−1
0.1355E+7	122.0	1143.	1373.	1768.	−0.7542E+5	0.1065E−3	0.8146E−1
0.1355E+7	122.0	67.33	895.1	2781.	0.4830E+5	0.1073E−4	0.1020E−1
0.1216E+7	120.0	1160.	1340.	1746.	−0.7813E+5	0.1118E−3	0.8382E−1
0.1216E+7	120.0	60.26	854.4	2802.	0.4865E+5	0.1047E−4	0.9827E−2
0.1087E+7	118.0	1177.	1312.	1725.	−0.8080E+5	0.1174E−3	0.8619E−1
0.1087E+7	118.0	53.84	818.8	2823.	0.4889E+5	0.1023E−4	0.9476E−2
0.9683E+6	116.0	1194.	1287.	1703.	−0.8341E+5	0.1233E−3	0.8856E−1

(Continues)

Table 1-18 (*Continued*)

P (PA)	T (K)	ρ (kg/m³)	C_p (J/kg · K)	S (J/kg · K)	H (J/kg)	μ (Pa · s)	k (W/m · K)
0.9683E+6	116.0	47.99	787.5	2845.	0.4905E+5	0.9991E−5	0.9147E−2
0.8592E+6	114.0	1210.	1265.	1682.	−0.8598E+5	0.1295E−3	0.9096E−1
0.8592E+6	114.0	42.66	759.8	2866.	0.4911E+5	0.9765E−5	0.8836E−2
0.7591E+6	112.0	1225.	1246.	1660.	−0.8851E+5	0.1359E−3	0.9337E−1
0.7591E+6	112.0	37.82	735.2	2888.	0.4909E+5	0.9546E−5	0.8543E−2
0.6678E+6	110.0	1240.	1229.	1638.	−0.9101E+5	0.1427E−3	0.9582E−1
0.6678E+6	110.0	33.42	713.1	2910.	0.4900E+5	0.9335E−5	0.8264E−2
0.5846E+6	108.0	1255.	1213.	1616.	−0.9347E+5	0.1499E−3	0.9830E−1
0.5846E+6	108.0	29.42	693.2	2933.	0.4883E+5	0.9129E−5	0.7999E−2
0.5092E+6	106.0	1270.	1199.	1594.	−0.9591E+5	0.1575E−3	0.1008
0.5092E+6	106.0	25.80	675.3	2957.	0.4860E+5	0.8930E−5	0.7747E−2
0.4411E+6	104.0	1284.	1186.	1572.	−0.9831E+5	0.1656E−3	0.1034
0.4411E+6	104.0	22.53	659.1	2981.	0.4830E+5	0.8735E−5	0.7506E−2
0.3799E+6	102.0	1298.	1174.	1549.	−0.1007E+6	0.1742E−3	0.1060
0.3799E+6	102.0	19.59	644.4	3005.	0.4794E+5	0.8545E−5	0.7276E−2
0.3252E+6	100.0	1312.	1163.	1526.	−0.1030E+6	0.1834E−3	0.1087
0.3252E+6	100.0	16.94	631.0	3031.	0.4752E+5	0.8359E−5	0.7057E−2
0.2765E+6	98.00	1325.	1153.	1503.	−0.1054E+6	0.1932E−3	0.1115
0.2765E+6	98.00	14.57	618.8	3057.	0.4705E+5	0.8177E−5	0.6846E−2
0.2335E+6	96.00	1339.	1144.	1479.	−0.1077E+6	0.2038E−3	0.1144
0.2335E+6	96.00	12.45	607.7	3085.	0.4653E+5	0.7998E−5	0.6645E−2
0.1956E+6	94.00	1352.	1136.	1455.	−0.1100E+6	0.2151E−3	0.1174
0.1956E+6	94.00	10.57	597.6	3114.	0.4597E+5	0.7822E−5	0.6452E−2
0.1626E+6	92.00	1365.	1130.	1431.	−0.1123E+6	0.2273E−3	0.1205
0.1626E+6	92.00	8.917	588.3	3144.	0.4535E+5	0.7650E−5	0.6266E−2
0.1339E+6	90.00	1377.	1124.	1407.	−0.1145E+6	0.2405E−3	0.1237
0.1339E+6	90.00	7.461	579.9	3175.	0.4470E+5	0.7479E−5	0.6088E−2
0.1093E+6	88.00	1390.	1121.	1381.	−0.1168E+6	0.2548E−3	0.1270
0.1093E+6	88.00	6.191	572.3	3208.	0.4400E+5	0.7311E−5	0.5917E−2
0.8826E+5	86.00	1402.	1119.	1356.	−0.1190E+6	0.2704E−3	0.1306
0.8826E+5	86.00	5.090	565.4	3242.	0.4327E+5	0.7145E−5	0.5752E−2
0.7052E+5	84.00	1414.	1122.	1329.	−0.1213E+6	0.2874E−3	0.1343
0.7052E+5	84.00	4.144	559.1	3279.	0.4250E+5	0.6981E−5	0.5593E−2

Table 1-19 Argon properties along the 1×10^5 pascal (1 bar) isobar

T (K)	ρ (kg/m^3)	C_p (J/kg·K)	S (J/kg·K)	H (J/kg)	μ (Pa·s)	k (W/m·K)
300.0	1.602	521.5	3879.	0.1561E+6	0.2290E−4	0.1791E−1
295.0	1.630	521.6	3870.	0.1535E+6	0.2258E−4	0.1766E−1
290.0	1.658	521.6	3861.	0.1509E+6	0.2225E−4	0.1741E−1
285.0	1.687	521.7	3852.	0.1483E+6	0.2193E−4	0.1715E−1
280.0	1.717	521.8	3843.	0.1457E+6	0.2160E−4	0.1689E−1
275.0	1.749	521.8	3833.	0.1430E+6	0.2127E−4	0.1664E−1
270.0	1.781	521.9	3824.	0.1404E+6	0.2093E−4	0.1637E−1
265.0	1.815	521.9	3814.	0.1378E+6	0.2060E−4	0.1611E−1
260.0	1.850	522.0	3804.	0.1352E+6	0.2026E−4	0.1585E−1
255.0	1.886	522.1	3794.	0.1326E+6	0.1992E−4	0.1558E−1
250.0	1.924	522.2	3784.	0.1300E+6	0.1957E−4	0.1531E−1
245.0	1.964	522.3	3773.	0.1274E+6	0.1923E−4	0.1504E−1
240.0	2.005	522.4	3762.	0.1248E+6	0.1888E−4	0.1477E−1
235.0	2.048	522.5	3751.	0.1222E+6	0.1852E−4	0.1450E−1
230.0	2.093	522.6	3740.	0.1195E+6	0.1817E−4	0.1422E−1
225.0	2.140	522.7	3729.	0.1169E+6	0.1781E−4	0.1394E−1
220.0	2.189	522.9	3717.	0.1143E+6	0.1746E−4	0.1366E−1
215.0	2.240	523.0	3705.	0.1117E+6	0.1709E−4	0.1338E−1
210.0	2.294	523.2	3693.	0.1091E+6	0.1673E−4	0.1310E−1
205.0	2.350	523.4	3680.	0.1065E+6	0.1636E−4	0.1282E−1
200.0	2.409	523.6	3667.	0.1039E+6	0.1599E−4	0.1253E−1
195.0	2.472	523.8	3654.	0.1012E+6	0.1562E−4	0.1224E−1
190.0	2.537	524.0	3640.	0.9862E+5	0.1525E−4	0.1195E−1
185.0	2.607	524.3	3626.	0.9600E+5	0.1487E−4	0.1166E−1
180.0	2.680	524.6	3612.	0.9338E+5	0.1449E−4	0.1137E−1
175.0	2.758	524.9	3597.	0.9075E+5	0.1411E−4	0.1107E−1
170.0	2.840	525.3	3582.	0.8813E+5	0.1373E−4	0.1078E−1
165.0	2.927	525.8	3566.	0.8550E+5	0.1334E−4	0.1048E−1
160.0	3.020	526.3	3550.	0.8287E+5	0.1296E−4	0.1018E−1
155.0	3.119	526.9	3533.	0.8023E+5	0.1257E−4	0.9880E−2
150.0	3.226	527.5	3516.	0.7760E+5	0.1218E−4	0.9579E−2
149.0	3.248	527.7	3512.	0.7707E+5	0.1210E−4	0.9519E−2
148.0	3.270	527.8	3509.	0.7654E+5	0.1202E−4	0.9458E−2
147.0	3.293	528.0	3505.	0.7602E+5	0.1194E−4	0.9398E−2
146.0	3.316	528.2	3502.	0.7549E+5	0.1186E−4	0.9338E−2
145.0	3.339	528.3	3498.	0.7496E+5	0.1178E−4	0.9277E−2
144.0	3.363	528.5	3494.	0.7443E+5	0.1171E−4	0.9217E−2
143.0	3.387	528.7	3491.	0.7390E+5	0.1163E−4	0.9157E−2
142.0	3.411	528.9	3487.	0.7337E+5	0.1155E−4	0.9096E−2
141.0	3.436	529.1	3483.	0.7284E+5	0.1147E−4	0.9036E−2
140.0	3.461	529.3	3480.	0.7232E+5	0.1139E−4	0.8975E−2
139.0	3.487	529.5	3476.	0.7179E+5	0.1131E−4	0.8915E−2
138.0	3.513	529.7	3472.	0.7126E+5	0.1123E−4	0.8854E−2
137.0	3.539	529.9	3468.	0.7073E+5	0.1115E−4	0.8794E−2
136.0	3.566	530.1	3464.	0.7020E+5	0.1108E−4	0.8733E−2
135.0	3.593	530.4	3460.	0.6967E+5	0.1100E−4	0.8673E−2
134.0	3.620	530.6	3456.	0.6914E+5	0.1092E−4	0.8612E−2
133.0	3.648	530.8	3452.	0.6861E+5	0.1084E−4	0.8552E−2
132.0	3.677	531.1	3448.	0.6807E+5	0.1076E−4	0.8492E−2

(Continues)

Table 1-19 (*Continued*)

T (K)	ρ (kg/m^3)	C_p (J/kg · K)	S (J/kg · K)	H (J/kg)	μ (Pa · s)	k (W/m · K)
131.0	3.706	531.4	3444.	0.6754E+5	0.1068E−4	0.8431E−2
130.0	3.735	531.7	3440.	0.6701E+5	0.1060E−4	0.8371E−2
129.0	3.765	532.0	3436.	0.6648E+5	0.1052E−4	0.8310E−2
128.0	3.795	532.3	3432.	0.6595E+5	0.1044E−4	0.8250E−2
127.0	3.826	532.6	3428.	0.6542E+5	0.1037E−4	0.8189E−2
126.0	3.858	532.9	3424.	0.6488E+5	0.1029E−4	0.8129E−2
125.0	3.889	533.2	3419.	0.6435E+5	0.1021E−4	0.8069E−2
124.0	3.922	533.6	3415.	0.6382E+5	0.1013E−4	0.8008E−2
123.0	3.955	534.0	3411.	0.6328E+5	0.1005E−4	0.7948E−2
122.0	3.989	534.3	3406.	0.6275E+5	0.9970E−5	0.7888E−2
121.0	4.023	534.7	3402.	0.6221E+5	0.9891E−5	0.7828E−2
120.0	4.058	535.2	3398.	0.6168E+5	0.9812E−5	0.7767E−2
119.0	4.093	535.6	3393.	0.6114E+5	0.9733E−5	0.7707E−2
118.0	4.129	536.0	3389.	0.6061E+5	0.9654E−5	0.7647E−2
117.0	4.166	536.5	3384.	0.6007E+5	0.9575E−5	0.7587E−2
116.0	4.203	537.0	3379.	0.5953E+5	0.9496E−5	0.7527E−2
115.0	4.241	537.5	3375.	0.5900E+5	0.9417E−5	0.7468E−2
114.0	4.280	538.0	3370.	0.5846E+5	0.9338E−5	0.7408E−2
113.0	4.320	538.6	3365.	0.5792E+5	0.9259E−5	0.7348E−2
112.0	4.360	539.2	3360.	0.5738E+5	0.9180E−5	0.7288E−2
111.0	4.401	539.8	3356.	0.5684E+5	0.9101E−5	0.7229E−2
110.0	4.443	540.4	3351.	0.5630E+5	0.9023E−5	0.7169E−2
109.0	4.486	541.1	3346.	0.5576E+5	0.8944E−5	0.7110E−2
108.0	4.530	541.8	3341.	0.5522E+5	0.8865E−5	0.7051E−2
107.0	4.575	542.6	3336.	0.5468E+5	0.8787E−5	0.6992E−2
106.0	4.620	543.3	3331.	0.5414E+5	0.8708E−5	0.6933E−2
105.0	4.667	544.2	3326.	0.5359E+5	0.8630E−5	0.6874E−2
104.0	4.714	545.0	3320.	0.5305E+5	0.8551E−5	0.6815E−2
103.0	4.763	545.9	3315.	0.5250E+5	0.8473E−5	0.6756E−2
102.0	4.813	546.9	3310.	0.5195E+5	0.8394E−5	0.6697E−2
101.0	4.863	547.9	3304.	0.5141E+5	0.8316E−5	0.6639E−2
100.0	4.915	548.9	3299.	0.5086E+5	0.8238E−5	0.6581E−2
99.00	4.968	550.0	3293.	0.5031E+5	0.8160E−5	0.6523E−2
98.00	5.023	551.2	3288.	0.4976E+5	0.8082E−5	0.6464E−2
97.00	5.078	552.4	3282.	0.4921E+5	0.8004E−5	0.6407E−2
96.00	5.135	553.7	3276.	0.4865E+5	0.7926E−5	0.6349E−2
95.00	5.194	555.1	3271.	0.4810E+5	0.7848E−5	0.6291E−2
94.00	5.254	556.6	3265.	0.4754E+5	0.7770E−5	0.6234E−2
93.00	5.315	558.1	3259.	0.4699E+5	0.7693E−5	0.6177E−2
92.00	5.378	559.8	3253.	0.4643E+5	0.7615E−5	0.6120E−2
91.00	5.442	561.5	3247.	0.4587E+5	0.7538E−5	0.6063E−2
90.00	5.509	563.4	3240.	0.4530E+5	0.7460E−5	0.6006E−2
89.00	5.577	565.3	3234.	0.4474E+5	0.7383E−5	0.5950E−2
88.00	5.647	567.4	3228.	0.4417E+5	0.7306E−5	0.5894E−2
87.00	1396.	1120.	1369.	−0.1179E+6	0.2625E−3	0.1288
86.00	1402.	1119.	1356.	−0.1190E+6	0.2705E−3	0.1306
85.00	1408.	1120.	1343.	−0.1202E+6	0.2788E−3	0.1324
84.00	1414.	1121.	1329.	−0.1213E+6	0.2875E−3	0.1343

Table 1-20 Argon properties along the 2×10^5 pascal (2 bar) isobar

T (K)	ρ (kg/m^3)	C_p (J/kg · K)	S (J/kg · K)	H (J/kg)	μ (Pa · s)	k (W/m · K)
300.0	3.207	522.8	3734.	0.1559E+6	0.2292E−4	0.1795E−1
295.0	3.262	522.9	3725.	0.1533E+6	0.2260E−4	0.1770E−1
290.0	3.318	523.0	3716.	0.1507E+6	0.2227E−4	0.1745E−1
285.0	3.377	523.1	3707.	0.1481E+6	0.2195E−4	0.1719E−1
280.0	3.438	523.2	3698.	0.1454E+6	0.2162E−4	0.1694E−1
275.0	3.501	523.3	3689.	0.1428E+6	0.2129E−4	0.1668E−1
270.0	3.566	523.4	3679.	0.1402E+6	0.2095E−4	0.1642E−1
265.0	3.634	523.6	3669.	0.1376E+6	0.2062E−4	0.1616E−1
260.0	3.704	523.7	3659.	0.1350E+6	0.2028E−4	0.1590E−1
255.0	3.778	523.9	3649.	0.1323E+6	0.1994E−4	0.1563E−1
250.0	3.854	524.0	3639.	0.1297E+6	0.1959E−4	0.1536E−1
245.0	3.933	524.2	3628.	0.1271E+6	0.1925E−4	0.1509E−1
240.0	4.016	524.4	3617.	0.1245E+6	0.1890E−4	0.1482E−1
235.0	4.103	524.6	3606.	0.1219E+6	0.1855E−4	0.1455E−1
230.0	4.193	524.9	3595.	0.1192E+6	0.1819E−4	0.1428E−1
225.0	4.288	525.1	3583.	0.1166E+6	0.1784E−4	0.1400E−1
220.0	4.386	525.4	3572.	0.1140E+6	0.1748E−4	0.1372E−1
215.0	4.490	525.7	3560.	0.1114E+6	0.1712E−4	0.1345E−1
210.0	4.599	526.1	3547.	0.1087E+6	0.1675E−4	0.1316E−1
205.0	4.713	526.4	3534.	0.1061E+6	0.1639E−4	0.1288E−1
200.0	4.833	526.8	3521.	0.1035E+6	0.1602E−4	0.1260E−1
195.0	4.959	527.3	3508.	0.1008E+6	0.1565E−4	0.1231E−1
190.0	5.092	527.8	3494.	0.9819E+5	0.1528E−4	0.1202E−1
185.0	5.233	528.3	3480.	0.9555E+5	0.1490E−4	0.1174E−1
180.0	5.382	529.0	3466.	0.9291E+5	0.1452E−4	0.1145E−1
175.0	5.540	529.7	3451.	0.9026E+5	0.1414E−4	0.1116E−1
170.0	5.707	530.5	3436.	0.8761E+5	0.1376E−4	0.1086E−1
165.0	5.886	531.4	3420.	0.8496E+5	0.1338E−4	0.1057E−1
160.0	6.076	532.4	3403.	0.8230E+5	0.1299E−4	0.1028E−1
155.0	6.279	533.6	3386.	0.7963E+5	0.1260E−4	0.9981E−2
150.0	6.497	535.0	3369.	0.7696E+5	0.1221E−4	0.9686E−2
149.0	6.542	535.4	3365.	0.7643E+5	0.1213E−4	0.9626E−2
148.0	6.589	535.7	3362.	0.7589E+5	0.1206E−4	0.9567E−2
147.0	6.635	536.0	3358.	0.7536E+5	0.1198E−4	0.9508E−2
146.0	6.683	536.3	3354.	0.7482E+5	0.1190E−4	0.9449E−2
145.0	6.731	536.7	3351.	0.7428E+5	0.1182E−4	0.9390E−2
144.0	6.780	537.1	3347.	0.7375E+5	0.1174E−4	0.9331E−2
143.0	6.830	537.4	3343.	0.7321E+5	0.1166E−4	0.9271E−2
142.0	6.880	537.8	3340.	0.7267E+5	0.1159E−4	0.9212E−2
141.0	6.931	538.2	3336.	0.7213E+5	0.1151E−4	0.9153E−2
140.0	6.983	538.6	3332.	0.7159E+5	0.1143E−4	0.9094E−2
139.0	7.036	539.1	3328.	0.7106E+5	0.1135E−4	0.9035E−2
138.0	7.090	539.5	3324.	0.7052E+5	0.1127E−4	0.8975E−2
137.0	7.144	540.0	3320.	0.6998E+5	0.1119E−4	0.8916E−2
136.0	7.200	540.4	3316.	0.6944E+5	0.1111E−4	0.8857E−2
135.0	7.256	540.9	3312.	0.6890E+5	0.1104E−4	0.8798E−2
134.0	7.313	541.4	3308.	0.6835E+5	0.1096E−4	0.8739E−2
133.0	7.371	542.0	3304.	0.6781E+5	0.1088E−4	0.8680E−2
132.0	7.431	542.5	3300.	0.6727E+5	0.1080E−4	0.8621E−2

(Continues)

Table 1-20 (*Continued*)

T (K)	ρ (kg/m^3)	C_p (J/kg · K)	S (J/kg · K)	H (J/kg)	μ (Pa · s)	k (W/m · K)
131.0	7.491	543.1	3296.	0.6673E+5	0.1072E−4	0.8562E−2
130.0	7.552	543.7	3292.	0.6618E+5	0.1064E−4	0.8503E−2
129.0	7.614	544.3	3288.	0.6564E+5	0.1056E−4	0.8444E−2
128.0	7.678	545.0	3283.	0.6510E+5	0.1049E−4	0.8386E−2
127.0	7.742	545.6	3279.	0.6455E+5	0.1041E−4	0.8327E−2
126.0	7.808	546.3	3275.	0.6400E+5	0.1033E−4	0.8268E−2
125.0	7.875	547.1	3270.	0.6346E+5	0.1025E−4	0.8210E−2
124.0	7.943	547.8	3266.	0.6291E+5	0.1017E−4	0.8151E−2
123.0	8.012	548.6	3262.	0.6236E+5	0.1009E−4	0.8093E−2
122.0	8.083	549.4	3257.	0.6181E+5	0.1001E−4	0.8034E−2
121.0	8.155	550.3	3253.	0.6126E+5	0.9934E−5	0.7976E−2
120.0	8.228	551.2	3248.	0.6071E+5	0.9855E−5	0.7918E−2
119.0	8.303	552.1	3243.	0.6016E+5	0.9777E−5	0.7860E−2
118.0	8.379	553.1	3239.	0.5961E+5	0.9698E−5	0.7802E−2
117.0	8.457	554.1	3234.	0.5905E+5	0.9619E−5	0.7744E−2
116.0	8.537	555.2	3229.	0.5850E+5	0.9541E−5	0.7686E−2
115.0	8.618	556.3	3224.	0.5794E+5	0.9462E−5	0.7629E−2
114.0	8.700	557.5	3220.	0.5739E+5	0.9384E−5	0.7571E−2
113.0	8.785	558.7	3215.	0.5683E+5	0.9305E−5	0.7514E−2
112.0	8.871	560.0	3210.	0.5627E+5	0.9227E−5	0.7457E−2
111.0	8.959	561.3	3205.	0.5571E+5	0.9148E−5	0.7400E−2
110.0	9.049	562.8	3200.	0.5515E+5	0.9070E−5	0.7343E−2
109.0	9.141	564.3	3194.	0.5458E+5	0.8991E−5	0.7286E−2
108.0	9.235	565.8	3189.	0.5402E+5	0.8913E−5	0.7230E−2
107.0	9.332	567.5	3184.	0.5345E+5	0.8835E−5	0.7173E−2
106.0	9.430	569.2	3179.	0.5288E+5	0.8757E−5	0.7117E−2
105.0	9.531	571.0	3173.	0.5231E+5	0.8679E−5	0.7061E−2
104.0	9.634	573.0	3168.	0.5174E+5	0.8601E−5	0.7005E−2
103.0	9.740	575.0	3162.	0.5117E+5	0.8523E−5	0.6950E−2
102.0	9.849	577.1	3157.	0.5059E+5	0.8445E−5	0.6895E−2
101.0	9.960	579.4	3151.	0.5001E+5	0.8367E−5	0.6840E−2
100.0	10.07	581.8	3145.	0.4943E+5	0.8289E−5	0.6785E−2
99.00	10.19	584.4	3139.	0.4885E+5	0.8212E−5	0.6730E−2
98.00	10.31	587.1	3133.	0.4826E+5	0.8134E−5	0.6676E−2
97.00	10.44	589.9	3127.	0.4768E+5	0.8057E−5	0.6622E−2
96.00	10.56	593.0	3121.	0.4708E+5	0.7979E−5	0.6568E−2
95.00	10.69	596.2	3115.	0.4649E+5	0.7902E−5	0.6515E−2
94.00	1352.	1136.	1455.	−0.1100E+6	0.2151E−3	0.1174
93.00	1358.	1133.	1443.	−0.1111E+6	0.2211E−3	0.1189
92.00	1365.	1129.	1431.	−0.1123E+6	0.2274E−3	0.1205
91.00	1371.	1126.	1419.	−0.1134E+6	0.2339E−3	0.1221
90.00	1377.	1124.	1406.	−0.1145E+6	0.2407E−3	0.1237
89.00	1384.	1122.	1394.	−0.1156E+6	0.2477E−3	0.1254
88.00	1390.	1120.	1381.	−0.1168E+6	0.2551E−3	0.1271
87.00	1396.	1119.	1368.	−0.1179E+6	0.2627E−3	0.1288
86.00	1402.	1119.	1355.	−0.1190E+6	0.2707E−3	0.1306
85.00	1408.	1119.	1342.	−0.1201E+6	0.2791E−3	0.1325
84.00	1414.	1121.	1329.	−0.1212E+6	0.2878E−3	0.1344

Table 1-21 Argon properties along the 5×10^5 pascal (5 bar) isobar

T (K)	ρ (kg/m^3)	C_p (J/kg · K)	S (J/kg · K)	H (J/kg)	μ (Pa · s)	k (W/m · K)
300.0	8.032	526.4	3542.	0.1553E+6	0.2297E-4	0.1807E-1
295.0	8.170	526.7	3533.	0.1527E+6	0.2265E-4	0.1783E-1
290.0	8.313	526.9	3524.	0.1501E+6	0.2233E-4	0.1757E-1
285.0	8.462	527.2	3515.	0.1474E+6	0.2200E-4	0.1732E-1
280.0	8.615	527.5	3505.	0.1448E+6	0.2167E-4	0.1707E-1
275.0	8.775	527.8	3496.	0.1421E+6	0.2134E-4	0.1681E-1
270.0	8.941	528.1	3486.	0.1395E+6	0.2101E-4	0.1656E-1
265.0	9.113	528.5	3476.	0.1369E+6	0.2068E-4	0.1630E-1
260.0	9.292	528.9	3466.	0.1342E+6	0.2034E-4	0.1604E-1
255.0	9.479	529.3	3456.	0.1316E+6	0.2000E-4	0.1578E-1
250.0	9.673	529.7	3446.	0.1289E+6	0.1966E-4	0.1552E-1
245.0	9.876	530.2	3435.	0.1263E+6	0.1931E-4	0.1525E-1
240.0	10.09	530.7	3424.	0.1236E+6	0.1897E-4	0.1498E-1
235.0	10.31	531.2	3413.	0.1210E+6	0.1862E-4	0.1472E-1
230.0	10.54	531.9	3401.	0.1183E+6	0.1826E-4	0.1445E-1
225.0	10.78	532.5	3390.	0.1157E+6	0.1791E-4	0.1418E-1
220.0	11.04	533.2	3378.	0.1130E+6	0.1755E-4	0.1391E-1
215.0	11.30	534.0	3365.	0.1103E+6	0.1719E-4	0.1363E-1
210.0	11.58	534.9	3353.	0.1076E+6	0.1683E-4	0.1336E-1
205.0	11.88	535.9	3340.	0.1050E+6	0.1647E-4	0.1308E-1
200.0	12.19	536.9	3327.	0.1023E+6	0.1610E-4	0.1281E-1
195.0	12.52	538.1	3313.	0.9960E+5	0.1573E-4	0.1253E-1
190.0	12.86	539.4	3299.	0.9691E+5	0.1536E-4	0.1225E-1
185.0	13.23	540.9	3285.	0.9421E+5	0.1499E-4	0.1197E-1
180.0	13.62	542.6	3270.	0.9150E+5	0.1461E-4	0.1169E-1
175.0	14.04	544.5	3255.	0.8878E+5	0.1424E-4	0.1141E-1
170.0	14.48	546.7	3239.	0.8605E+5	0.1386E-4	0.1113E-1
165.0	14.96	549.2	3222.	0.8331E+5	0.1348E-4	0.1085E-1
160.0	15.47	552.1	3205.	0.8056E+5	0.1309E-4	0.1057E-1
155.0	16.01	555.5	3188.	0.7779E+5	0.1271E-4	0.1029E-1
150.0	16.60	559.4	3170.	0.7500E+5	0.1232E-4	0.1002E-1
149.0	16.73	560.3	3166.	0.7444E+5	0.1225E-4	0.9960E-2
148.0	16.85	561.2	3162.	0.7388E+5	0.1217E-4	0.9905E-2
147.0	16.98	562.2	3158.	0.7332E+5	0.1209E-4	0.9849E-2
146.0	17.11	563.1	3154.	0.7276E+5	0.1201E-4	0.9794E-2
145.0	17.25	564.1	3150.	0.7219E+5	0.1194E-4	0.9739E-2
144.0	17.38	565.2	3147.	0.7163E+5	0.1186E-4	0.9683E-2
143.0	17.52	566.3	3143.	0.7106E+5	0.1178E-4	0.9628E-2
142.0	17.66	567.4	3139.	0.7050E+5	0.1170E-4	0.9573E-2
141.0	17.80	568.6	3135.	0.6993E+5	0.1163E-4	0.9518E-2
140.0	17.94	569.8	3131.	0.6936E+5	0.1155E-4	0.9463E-2
139.0	18.09	571.0	3127.	0.6879E+5	0.1147E-4	0.9408E-2
138.0	18.24	572.3	3122.	0.6822E+5	0.1139E-4	0.9354E-2
137.0	18.39	573.7	3118.	0.6764E+5	0.1132E-4	0.9299E-2
136.0	18.55	575.1	3114.	0.6707E+5	0.1124E-4	0.9245E-2
135.0	18.71	576.6	3110.	0.6649E+5	0.1116E-4	0.9190E-2
134.0	18.87	578.1	3105.	0.6592E+5	0.1108E-4	0.9136E-2
133.0	19.03	579.7	3101.	0.6534E+5	0.1101E-4	0.9082E-2
132.0	19.20	581.4	3097.	0.6476E+5	0.1093E-4	0.9028E-2

(*Continues*)

Table 1-21 (*Continued*)

T (K)	ρ (kg/m^3)	C_p (J/kg · K)	S (J/kg · K)	H (J/kg)	μ (Pa · s)	k (W/m · K)
131.0	19.37	583.1	3092.	0.6418E+5	0.1085E−4	0.8975E−2
130.0	19.55	584.9	3088.	0.6359E+5	0.1077E−4	0.8921E−2
129.0	19.72	586.8	3083.	0.6301E+5	0.1070E−4	0.8868E−2
128.0	19.91	588.8	3079.	0.6242E+5	0.1062E−4	0.8815E−2
127.0	20.09	590.9	3074.	0.6183E+5	0.1054E−4	0.8762E−2
126.0	20.28	593.1	3069.	0.6124E+5	0.1046E−4	0.8709E−2
125.0	20.48	595.3	3065.	0.6064E+5	0.1039E−4	0.8657E−2
124.0	20.68	597.7	3060.	0.6004E+5	0.1031E−4	0.8605E−2
123.0	20.88	600.2	3055.	0.5945E+5	0.1023E−4	0.8553E−2
122.0	21.09	602.8	3050.	0.5884E+5	0.1015E−4	0.8501E−2
121.0	21.30	605.6	3045.	0.5824E+5	0.1008E−4	0.8450E−2
120.0	21.52	608.5	3040.	0.5763E+5	0.9999E−5	0.8399E−2
119.0	21.74	611.5	3035.	0.5702E+5	0.9921E−5	0.8348E−2
118.0	21.97	614.7	3030.	0.5641E+5	0.9844E−5	0.8297E−2
117.0	22.21	618.1	3025.	0.5579E+5	0.9767E−5	0.8247E−2
116.0	22.45	621.7	3019.	0.5517E+5	0.9690E−5	0.8198E−2
115.0	22.70	625.4	3014.	0.5455E+5	0.9613E−5	0.8148E−2
114.0	22.95	629.4	3008.	0.5392E+5	0.9536E−5	0.8100E−2
113.0	23.21	633.6	3003.	0.5329E+5	0.9459E−5	0.8051E−2
112.0	23.48	638.1	2997.	0.5266E+5	0.9382E−5	0.8003E−2
111.0	23.76	642.8	2991.	0.5202E+5	0.9306E−5	0.7956E−2
110.0	24.04	647.8	2986.	0.5137E+5	0.9229E−5	0.7909E−2
109.0	24.34	653.2	2980.	0.5072E+5	0.9153E−5	0.7862E−2
108.0	24.64	658.8	2974.	0.5006E+5	0.9076E−5	0.7816E−2
107.0	24.96	664.9	2967.	0.4940E+5	0.9000E−5	0.7771E−2
106.0	25.28	671.4	2961.	0.4873E+5	0.8924E−5	0.7727E−2
105.0	1277.	1192.	1583.	−0.9710E+5	0.1616E−3	0.1021
104.0	1284.	1185.	1571.	−0.9829E+5	0.1658E−3	0.1034
103.0	1292.	1179.	1560.	−0.9947E+5	0.1701E−3	0.1048
102.0	1299.	1173.	1548.	−0.1007E+6	0.1745E−3	0.1061
101.0	1306.	1167.	1537.	−0.1018E+6	0.1791E−3	0.1075
100.0	1313.	1162.	1525.	−0.1030E+6	0.1838E−3	0.1089
99.00	1319.	1157.	1514.	−0.1041E+6	0.1887E−3	0.1103
98.00	1326.	1152.	1502.	−0.1053E+6	0.1938E−3	0.1117
97.00	1333.	1147.	1490.	−0.1064E+6	0.1990E−3	0.1131
96.00	1340.	1143.	1478.	−0.1076E+6	0.2044E−3	0.1146
95.00	1346.	1138.	1466.	−0.1087E+6	0.2100E−3	0.1161
94.00	1353.	1134.	1454.	−0.1099E+6	0.2158E−3	0.1176
93.00	1359.	1131.	1442.	−0.1110E+6	0.2219E−3	0.1191
92.00	1366.	1128.	1430.	−0.1121E+6	0.2281E−3	0.1207
91.00	1372.	1125.	1418.	−0.1133E+6	0.2347E−3	0.1223
90.00	1378.	1122.	1405.	−0.1144E+6	0.2415E−3	0.1239
89.00	1385.	1120.	1393.	−0.1155E+6	0.2485E−3	0.1256
88.00	1391.	1119.	1380.	−0.1166E+6	0.2559E−3	0.1273
87.00	1397.	1118.	1367.	−0.1177E+6	0.2635E−3	0.1290
86.00	1403.	1118.	1354.	−0.1189E+6	0.2715E−3	0.1308
85.00	1409.	1118.	1341.	−0.1200E+6	0.2799E−3	0.1327
84.00	1415.	1120.	1328.	−0.1211E+6	0.2887E−3	0.1345

Table 1-22 Argon properties along the 20×10^5 pascal (20 bar) isobar

T (K)	ρ (kg/m^3)	C_p (J/kg $\cdot$ K)	S (J/kg $\cdot$ K)	H (J/kg)	μ (Pa $\cdot$ s)	k (W/m $\cdot$ K)
300.0	32.40	545.0	3246.	0.1525E+6	0.2327E−4	0.1869E−1
295.0	32.99	546.0	3236.	0.1497E+6	0.2296E−4	0.1845E−1
290.0	33.60	547.1	3227.	0.1470E+6	0.2264E−4	0.1821E−1
285.0	34.23	548.3	3218.	0.1443E+6	0.2232E−4	0.1798E−1
280.0	34.88	549.6	3208.	0.1415E+6	0.2200E−4	0.1774E−1
275.0	35.57	550.9	3198.	0.1388E+6	0.2168E−4	0.1750E−1
270.0	36.28	552.4	3188.	0.1360E+6	0.2135E−4	0.1726E−1
265.0	37.03	553.9	3177.	0.1332E+6	0.2103E−4	0.1702E−1
260.0	37.80	555.6	3167.	0.1305E+6	0.2070E−4	0.1678E−1
255.0	38.62	557.4	3156.	0.1277E+6	0.2037E−4	0.1654E−1
250.0	39.47	559.4	3145.	0.1249E+6	0.2003E−4	0.1630E−1
245.0	40.37	561.6	3134.	0.1221E+6	0.1970E−4	0.1606E−1
240.0	41.31	564.0	3122.	0.1193E+6	0.1936E−4	0.1582E−1
235.0	42.30	566.5	3110.	0.1165E+6	0.1902E−4	0.1557E−1
230.0	43.34	569.4	3098.	0.1136E+6	0.1868E−4	0.1533E−1
225.0	44.44	572.5	3085.	0.1108E+6	0.1834E−4	0.1509E−1
220.0	45.61	576.0	3073.	0.1079E+6	0.1800E−4	0.1485E−1
215.0	46.84	579.9	3059.	0.1050E+6	0.1765E−4	0.1462E−1
210.0	48.16	584.3	3046.	0.1021E+6	0.1730E−4	0.1438E−1
205.0	49.56	589.2	3031.	0.9915E+5	0.1695E−4	0.1415E−1
200.0	51.05	594.7	3017.	0.9619E+5	0.1660E−4	0.1392E−1
195.0	52.66	601.1	3002.	0.9320E+5	0.1625E−4	0.1369E−1
190.0	54.39	608.4	2986.	0.9018E+5	0.1590E−4	0.1347E−1
185.0	56.25	616.8	2970.	0.8712E+5	0.1555E−4	0.1326E−1
180.0	58.28	626.7	2953.	0.8401E+5	0.1520E−4	0.1305E−1
175.0	60.49	638.3	2935.	0.8085E+5	0.1484E−4	0.1285E−1
170.0	62.92	652.3	2916.	0.7762E+5	0.1449E−4	0.1267E−1
165.0	65.61	669.2	2896.	0.7432E+5	0.1414E−4	0.1249E−1
160.0	68.61	690.1	2875.	0.7092E+5	0.1380E−4	0.1233E−1
155.0	72.00	716.4	2853.	0.6741E+5	0.1345E−4	0.1218E−1
150.0	75.88	750.3	2829.	0.6375E+5	0.1311E−4	0.1206E−1
149.0	76.73	758.4	2824.	0.6299E+5	0.1304E−4	0.1203E−1
148.0	77.61	766.9	2819.	0.6223E+5	0.1298E−4	0.1201E−1
147.0	78.51	775.9	2814.	0.6146E+5	0.1291E−4	0.1199E−1
146.0	79.44	785.5	2808.	0.6068E+5	0.1285E−4	0.1197E−1
145.0	80.41	795.8	2803.	0.5989E+5	0.1278E−4	0.1196E−1
144.0	81.41	806.7	2797.	0.5909E+5	0.1272E−4	0.1194E−1
143.0	82.45	818.5	2792.	0.5827E+5	0.1265E−4	0.1193E−1
142.0	83.53	831.1	2786.	0.5745E+5	0.1259E−4	0.1191E−1
141.0	84.66	844.7	2780.	0.5661E+5	0.1252E−4	0.1190E−1
140.0	85.83	859.4	2774.	0.5576E+5	0.1246E−4	0.1190E−1
139.0	87.05	875.3	2768.	0.5489E+5	0.1240E−4	0.1189E−1
138.0	88.33	892.6	2761.	0.5401E+5	0.1234E−4	0.1189E−1
137.0	89.67	911.4	2755.	0.5311E+5	0.1228E−4	0.1189E−1
136.0	91.08	932.1	2748.	0.5219E+5	0.1222E−4	0.1189E−1
135.0	92.56	954.8	2741.	0.5124E+5	0.1216E−4	0.1189E−1
134.0	94.12	980.0	2734.	0.5028E+5	0.1210E−4	0.1190E−1
133.0	95.77	1008.	2726.	0.4928E+5	0.1205E−4	0.1192E−1

(Continues)

Table 1-22 (*Continued*)

T (K)	ρ (kg/m^3)	C_p (J/kg · K)	S (J/kg · K)	H (J/kg)	μ (Pa · s)	k (W/m · K)
132.0	97.53	1039.	2719.	0.4826E+5	0.1199E−4	0.1193E−1
131.0	99.40	1075.	2711.	0.4720E+5	0.1194E−4	0.1196E−1
130.0	101.4	1115.	2702.	0.4611E+5	0.1189E−4	0.1199E−1
129.0	1077.	1531.	1843.	−0.6541E+5	0.8926E−4	0.7323E−1
128.0	1089.	1496.	1831.	−0.6693E+5	0.9190E−4	0.7456E−1
127.0	1099.	1465.	1819.	−0.6841E+5	0.9454E−4	0.7588E−1
126.0	1110.	1437.	1808.	−0.6986E+5	0.9720E−4	0.7717E−1
125.0	1120.	1412.	1796.	−0.7128E+5	0.9988E−4	0.7845E−1
124.0	1130.	1389.	1785.	−0.7268E+5	0.1026E−3	0.7972E−1
123.0	1139.	1369.	1774.	−0.7406E+5	0.1053E−3	0.8097E−1
122.0	1149.	1350.	1763.	−0.7542E+5	0.1081E−3	0.8222E−1
121.0	1158.	1333.	1752.	−0.7676E+5	0.1109E−3	0.8345E−1
120.0	1167.	1317.	1741.	−0.7809E+5	0.1138E−3	0.8468E−1
119.0	1176.	1303.	1730.	−0.7940E+5	0.1167E−3	0.8591E−1
118.0	1184.	1289.	1719.	−0.8069E+5	0.1197E−3	0.8713E−1
117.0	1193.	1277.	1708.	−0.8197E+5	0.1227E−3	0.8835E−1
116.0	1201.	1265.	1697.	−0.8324E+5	0.1258E−3	0.8957E−1
115.0	1209.	1254.	1686.	−0.8450E+5	0.1289E−3	0.9079E−1
114.0	1217.	1244.	1675.	−0.8575E+5	0.1321E−3	0.9202E−1
113.0	1225.	1235.	1664.	−0.8699E+5	0.1354E−3	0.9324E−1
112.0	1233.	1226.	1654.	−0.8822E+5	0.1388E−3	0.9447E−1
111.0	1240.	1218.	1643.	−0.8945E+5	0.1422E−3	0.9570E−1
110.0	1248.	1210.	1632.	−0.9066E+5	0.1458E−3	0.9694E−1
109.0	1255.	1202.	1621.	−0.9187E+5	0.1494E−3	0.9819E−1
108.0	1263.	1195.	1610.	−0.9306E+5	0.1531E−3	0.9945E−1
107.0	1270.	1189.	1598.	−0.9426E+5	0.1570E−3	0.1007
106.0	1277.	1182.	1587.	−0.9544E+5	0.1609E−3	0.1020
105.0	1284.	1176.	1576.	−0.9662E+5	0.1650E−3	0.1033
104.0	1291.	1171.	1565.	−0.9779E+5	0.1692E−3	0.1046
103.0	1298.	1165.	1554.	−0.9896E+5	0.1735E−3	0.1059
102.0	1305.	1160.	1542.	−0.1001E+6	0.1780E−3	0.1072
101.0	1312.	1155.	1531.	−0.1013E+6	0.1825E−3	0.1086
100.0	1319.	1150.	1519.	−0.1024E+6	0.1873E−3	0.1099
99.00	1325.	1145.	1508.	−0.1036E+6	0.1922E−3	0.1113
98.00	1332.	1141.	1496.	−0.1047E+6	0.1973E−3	0.1127
97.00	1339.	1137.	1485.	−0.1059E+6	0.2025E−3	0.1141
96.00	1345.	1133.	1473.	−0.1070E+6	0.2080E−3	0.1156
95.00	1352.	1129.	1461.	−0.1081E+6	0.2136E−3	0.1170
94.00	1358.	1125.	1449.	−0.1093E+6	0.2195E−3	0.1185
93.00	1364.	1122.	1437.	−0.1104E+6	0.2256E−3	0.1201
92.00	1371.	1119.	1425.	−0.1115E+6	0.2319E−3	0.1216
91.00	1377.	1117.	1413.	−0.1126E+6	0.2384E−3	0.1232
90.00	1383.	1114.	1400.	−0.1137E+6	0.2453E−3	0.1248
89.00	1389.	1113.	1388.	−0.1148E+6	0.2524E−3	0.1265
88.00	1395.	1111.	1375.	−0.1160E+6	0.2598E−3	0.1282
87.00	1401.	1111.	1363.	−0.1171E+6	0.2676E−3	0.1299
86.00	1407.	1111.	1350.	−0.1182E+6	0.2756E−3	0.1317
85.00	1413.	1112.	1337.	−0.1193E+6	0.2841E−3	0.1335

Table 1-23 Saturation properties of para hydrogen (Liquid properties are shown in the first row of each temperature)

P (Pa)	T (K)	ρ (kg/m^3)	C_p (J/kg·K)	S (J/kg·K)	H (J/kg)	μ (Pa·s)	k (W/m·K)
0.1119E+7	32.00	45.73	0.6880E+5	0.1504E+5	−0.2357E+5	0.4886E−5	0.8000E−1
0.1119E+7	32.00	17.65	0.9627E+5	0.2088E+5	0.1635E+6	0.2248E−5	0.4358E−1
0.1038E+7	31.50	48.37	0.4716E+5	0.1451E+5	−0.4201E+5	0.5286E−5	0.8292E−1
0.1038E+7	31.50	15.31	0.6270E+5	0.2155E+5	0.1799E+6	0.2107E−5	0.3953E−1
0.9616E+6	31.00	50.47	0.3695E+5	0.1407E+5	−0.5736E+5	0.5637E−5	0.8536E−1
0.9616E+6	31.00	13.54	0.4720E+5	0.2211E+5	0.1919E+6	0.2002E−5	0.3663E−1
0.8895E+6	30.50	52.26	0.3088E+5	0.1367E+5	−0.7093E+5	0.5966E−5	0.8751E−1
0.8895E+6	30.50	12.09	0.3831E+5	0.2259E+5	0.2011E+6	0.1916E−5	0.3436E−1
0.8214E+6	30.00	53.85	0.2684E+5	0.1331E+5	−0.8322E+5	0.6282E−5	0.8945E−1
0.8214E+6	30.00	10.86	0.3256E+5	0.2303E+5	0.2085E+6	0.1844E−5	0.3248E−1
0.7573E+6	29.50	55.28	0.2395E+5	0.1297E+5	−0.9453E+5	0.6590E−5	0.9120E−1
0.7573E+6	29.50	9.797	0.2855E+5	0.2344E+5	0.2144E+6	0.1780E−5	0.3088E−1
0.6967E+6	29.00	56.59	0.2177E+5	0.1265E+5	−0.1051E+6	0.6894E−5	0.9281E−1
0.6967E+6	29.00	8.861	0.2559E+5	0.2382E+5	0.2192E+6	0.1723E−5	0.2949E−1
0.6397E+6	28.50	57.80	0.2005E+5	0.1234E+5	−0.1149E+6	0.7199E−5	0.9427E−1
0.6397E+6	28.50	8.026	0.2331E+5	0.2419E+5	0.2230E+6	0.1672E−5	0.2824E−1
0.5861E+6	28.00	58.92	0.1865E+5	0.1204E+5	−0.1243E+6	0.7505E−5	0.9561E−1
0.5861E+6	28.00	7.276	0.2152E+5	0.2455E+5	0.2261E+6	0.1624E−5	0.2711E−1
0.5357E+6	27.50	59.97	0.1749E+5	0.1175E+5	−0.1331E+6	0.7816E−5	0.9683E−1
0.5357E+6	27.50	6.598	0.2006E+5	0.2490E+5	0.2285E+6	0.1579E−5	0.2608E−1
0.4885E+6	27.00	60.97	0.1650E+5	0.1147E+5	−0.1416E+6	0.8132E−5	0.9794E−1
0.4885E+6	27.00	5.982	0.1886E+5	0.2524E+5	0.2304E+6	0.1538E−5	0.2512E−1
0.4443E+6	26.50	61.91	0.1564E+5	0.1120E+5	−0.1496E+6	0.8456E−5	0.9895E−1
0.4443E+6	26.50	5.421	0.1786E+5	0.2558E+5	0.2316E+6	0.1498E−5	0.2423E−1
0.4029E+6	26.00	62.80	0.1489E+5	0.1093E+5	−0.1574E+6	0.8789E−5	0.9986E−1
0.4029E+6	26.00	4.907	0.1700E+5	0.2592E+5	0.2325E+6	0.1461E−5	0.2338E−1
0.3643E+6	25.50	63.65	0.1422E+5	0.1066E+5	−0.1648E+6	0.9132E−5	0.1007
0.3643E+6	25.50	4.437	0.1626E+5	0.2625E+5	0.2329E+6	0.1425E−5	0.2259E−1
0.3284E+6	25.00	64.47	0.1362E+5	0.1040E+5	−0.1719E+6	0.9487E−5	0.1014
0.3284E+6	25.00	4.006	0.1563E+5	0.2659E+5	0.2328E+6	0.1390E−5	0.2182E−1
0.2951E+6	24.50	65.25	0.1308E+5	0.1015E+5	−0.1787E+6	0.9855E−5	0.1021
0.2951E+6	24.50	3.610	0.1507E+5	0.2693E+5	0.2325E+6	0.1357E−5	0.2109E−1
0.2642E+6	24.00	66.00	0.1257E+5	9895.	−0.1853E+6	0.1024E−4	0.1027
0.2642E+6	24.00	3.246	0.1458E+5	0.2727E+5	0.2318E+6	0.1325E−5	0.2037E−1
0.2357E+6	23.50	66.72	0.1211E+5	9645.	−0.1917E+6	0.1064E−4	0.1032
0.2357E+6	23.50	2.912	0.1414E+5	0.2762E+5	0.2307E+6	0.1294E−5	0.1967E−1
0.2094E+6	23.00	67.41	0.1168E+5	9398.	−0.1978E+6	0.1105E−4	0.1036

(*Continues*)

Table 1-23 (*Continued*)

P (Pa)	T (K)	ρ (kg/m³)	C_p (J/kg·K)	S (J/kg·K)	H (J/kg)	μ (Pa·s)	k (W/m·K)
0.2094E+6	23.00	2.606	0.1375E+5	0.2797E+5	0.2294E+6	0.1263E−5	0.1898E−1
0.1853E+6	22.50	68.08	0.1127E+5	9154.	−0.2037E+6	0.1149E−4	0.1039
0.1853E+6	22.50	2.325	0.1341E+5	0.2833E+5	0.2278E+6	0.1234E−5	0.1827E−1
0.1632E+6	22.00	68.73	0.1088E+5	8911.	−0.2095E+6	0.1195E−4	0.1042
0.1632E+6	22.00	2.067	0.1310E+5	0.2870E+5	0.2260E+6	0.1205E−5	0.1755E−1
0.1431E+6	21.50	69.35	0.1051E+5	8671.	−0.2150E+6	0.1243E−4	0.1043
0.1431E+6	21.50	1.832	0.1282E+5	0.2908E+5	0.2239E+6	0.1176E−5	0.1680E−1
0.1247E+6	21.00	69.96	0.1016E+5	8433.	−0.2203E+6	0.1294E−4	0.1043
0.1247E+6	21.00	1.617	0.1257E+5	0.2947E+5	0.2215E+6	0.1148E−5	0.1599E−1
0.1082E+6	20.50	70.54	9816.	8196.	−0.2255E+6	0.1347E−4	0.1043
0.1082E+6	20.50	1.421	0.1234E+5	0.2987E+5	0.2190E+6	0.1121E−5	0.1511E−1
0.9326E+5	20.00	71.11	9485.	7961.	−0.2304E+6	0.1404E−4	0.1040
0.9326E+5	20.00	1.243	0.1213E+5	0.3029E+5	0.2162E+6	0.1094E−5	0.1412E−1
0.7989E+5	19.50	71.66	9163.	7728.	−0.2352E+6	0.1463E−4	0.1036
0.7989E+5	19.50	1.082	0.1194E+5	0.3072E+5	0.2132E+6	0.1067E−5	0.1300E−1
0.6796E+5	19.00	72.20	8851.	7497.	−0.2398E+6	0.1526E−4	0.1030
0.6796E+5	19.00	0.9362	0.1177E+5	0.3118E+5	0.2101E+6	0.1040E−5	0.1168E−1
0.5739E+5	18.50	72.71	8547.	7267.	−0.2443E+6	0.1593E−4	0.1021
0.5739E+5	18.50	0.8052	0.1161E+5	0.3165E+5	0.2067E+6	0.1013E−5	0.1013E−1
0.4807E+5	18.00	73.22	8255.	7039.	−0.2486E+6	0.1664E−4	0.1010
0.4807E+5	18.00	0.6879	0.1147E+5	0.3214E+5	0.2032E+6	0.9863E−6	0.8262E−2
0.3992E+5	17.50	73.71	7976.	6812.	−0.2527E+6	0.1740E−4	0.9938E−1
0.3992E+5	17.50	0.5834	0.1134E+5	0.3266E+5	0.1996E+6	0.9593E−6	0.5991E−2
0.3284E+5	17.00	74.19	7717.	6586.	−0.2567E+6	0.1820E−4	0.9730E−1
0.3284E+5	17.00	0.4907	0.1122E+5	0.3320E+5	0.1958E+6	0.9321E−6	0.3204E−2
0.2674E+5	16.50	74.66	7486.	6360.	−0.2606E+6	0.1905E−4	0.9461E−1
0.2674E+5	16.50	0.4092	0.1111E+5	0.3378E+5	0.1918E+6	0.9044E−6	−0.2401E−3
0.2153E+5	16.00	75.12	7296.	6133.	−0.2643E+6	0.1995E−4	0.9114E−1
0.2153E+5	16.00	0.3378	0.1101E+5	0.3439E+5	0.1877E+6	0.8759E−6	−0.4521E−2
0.1712E+5	15.50	75.56	7168.	5905.	−0.2680E+6	0.2092E−4	0.8670E−1
0.1712E+5	15.50	0.2759	0.1092E+5	0.3504E+5	0.1835E+6	0.8465E−6	−0.9866E−2
0.1343E+5	15.00	76.00	7130.	5671.	−0.2716E+6	0.2194E−4	0.8102E−1
0.1343E+5	15.00	0.2227	0.1084E+5	0.3573E+5	0.1792E+6	0.8157E−6	−0.1656E−1
0.1038E+5	14.50	76.44	7227.	5429.	−0.2752E+6	0.2304E−4	0.7378E−1
0.1038E+5	14.50	0.1773	0.1076E+5	0.3646E+5	0.1748E+6	0.7831E−6	−0.2497E−1
7896.	14.00	76.87	7524.	5171.	−0.2789E+6	0.2420E−4	0.6457E−1
7896.	14.00	0.1392	0.1070E+5	0.3725E+5	0.1702E+6	0.7481E−6	−0.3556E−1

Table 1-24 Para hydrogen properties along the 1×10^5 pascal (1 bar) isobar

T (K)	ρ (kg/m^3)	C_p (J/kg · K)	S (J/kg · K)	H (J/kg)	μ (Pa · s)	k (W/m · K)
300.0	0.8077E−1	0.1485E+5	0.6493E+5	0.4228E+7	0.8952E−5	0.1916
295.0	0.8214E−1	0.1488E+5	0.6468E+5	0.4154E+7	0.8851E−5	0.1896
290.0	0.8356E−1	0.1492E+5	0.6443E+5	0.4079E+7	0.8749E−5	0.1876
285.0	0.8502E−1	0.1496E+5	0.6417E+5	0.4004E+7	0.8647E−5	0.1857
280.0	0.8654E−1	0.1500E+5	0.6390E+5	0.3930E+7	0.8544E−5	0.1838
275.0	0.8811E−1	0.1504E+5	0.6363E+5	0.3854E+7	0.8440E−5	0.1820
270.0	0.8974E−1	0.1509E+5	0.6336E+5	0.3779E+7	0.8336E−5	0.1802
265.0	0.9144E−1	0.1514E+5	0.6307E+5	0.3704E+7	0.8230E−5	0.1784
260.0	0.9319E−1	0.1520E+5	0.6278E+5	0.3628E+7	0.8124E−5	0.1766
255.0	0.9502E−1	0.1526E+5	0.6249E+5	0.3551E+7	0.8017E−5	0.1749
250.0	0.9692E−1	0.1532E+5	0.6219E+5	0.3475E+7	0.7910E−5	0.1732
245.0	0.9890E−1	0.1539E+5	0.6188E+5	0.3398E+7	0.7801E−5	0.1714
240.0	0.1010	0.1546E+5	0.6156E+5	0.3321E+7	0.7692E−5	0.1697
235.0	0.1031	0.1553E+5	0.6123E+5	0.3244E+7	0.7582E−5	0.1680
230.0	0.1053	0.1560E+5	0.6090E+5	0.3166E+7	0.7471E−5	0.1662
225.0	0.1077	0.1568E+5	0.6055E+5	0.3088E+7	0.7359E−5	0.1644
220.0	0.1101	0.1576E+5	0.6020E+5	0.3009E+7	0.7246E−5	0.1626
215.0	0.1127	0.1584E+5	0.5984E+5	0.2930E+7	0.7132E−5	0.1607
210.0	0.1154	0.1592E+5	0.5946E+5	0.2851E+7	0.7018E−5	0.1587
205.0	0.1182	0.1600E+5	0.5908E+5	0.2771E+7	0.6902E−5	0.1567
200.0	0.1211	0.1607E+5	0.5868E+5	0.2691E+7	0.6785E−5	0.1546
195.0	0.1243	0.1615E+5	0.5827E+5	0.2610E+7	0.6668E−5	0.1524
190.0	0.1275	0.1621E+5	0.5785E+5	0.2529E+7	0.6549E−5	0.1500
185.0	0.1310	0.1627E+5	0.5742E+5	0.2448E+7	0.6429E−5	0.1476
180.0	0.1346	0.1632E+5	0.5697E+5	0.2367E+7	0.6308E−5	0.1450
175.0	0.1385	0.1635E+5	0.5651E+5	0.2285E+7	0.6186E−5	0.1422
170.0	0.1425	0.1637E+5	0.5604E+5	0.2203E+7	0.6062E−5	0.1393
165.0	0.1468	0.1637E+5	0.5555E+5	0.2121E+7	0.5938E−5	0.1362
160.0	0.1514	0.1635E+5	0.5505E+5	0.2039E+7	0.5812E−5	0.1329
155.0	0.1563	0.1630E+5	0.5453E+5	0.1958E+7	0.5685E−5	0.1294
150.0	0.1615	0.1622E+5	0.5400E+5	0.1876E+7	0.5556E−5	0.1258
145.0	0.1671	0.1610E+5	0.5345E+5	0.1796E+7	0.5426E−5	0.1219
140.0	0.1731	0.1596E+5	0.5289E+5	0.1715E+7	0.5294E−5	0.1179
135.0	0.1795	0.1577E+5	0.5231E+5	0.1636E+7	0.5160E−5	0.1136
130.0	0.1864	0.1554E+5	0.5172E+5	0.1558E+7	0.5025E−5	0.1092
125.0	0.1939	0.1528E+5	0.5111E+5	0.1481E+7	0.4888E−5	0.1046
120.0	0.2020	0.1498E+5	0.5050E+5	0.1405E+7	0.4749E−5	0.9987E−1
115.0	0.2108	0.1463E+5	0.4987E+5	0.1331E+7	0.4608E−5	0.9498E−1
110.0	0.2204	0.1425E+5	0.4922E+5	0.1259E+7	0.4464E−5	0.8998E−1
105.0	0.2309	0.1385E+5	0.4857E+5	0.1189E+7	0.4318E−5	0.8492E−1
100.0	0.2425	0.1343E+5	0.4790E+5	0.1120E+7	0.4170E−5	0.7982E−1
98.00	0.2475	0.1325E+5	0.4763E+5	0.1094E+7	0.4110E−5	0.7778E−1
96.00	0.2527	0.1308E+5	0.4736E+5	0.1067E+7	0.4049E−5	0.7574E−1
94.00	0.2581	0.1291E+5	0.4709E+5	0.1041E+7	0.3988E−5	0.7372E−1
92.00	0.2637	0.1274E+5	0.4681E+5	0.1016E+7	0.3926E−5	0.7170E−1
90.00	0.2696	0.1257E+5	0.4654E+5	0.9904E+6	0.3863E−5	0.6970E−1
88.00	0.2757	0.1240E+5	0.4626E+5	0.9654E+6	0.3800E−5	0.6773E−1
86.00	0.2822	0.1224E+5	0.4597E+5	0.9408E+6	0.3737E−5	0.6577E−1

(Continues)

Table 1-24 (*Continued*)

T (K)	ρ (kg/m³)	C_p (J/kg · K)	S (J/kg · K)	H (J/kg)	μ (Pa · s)	k (W/m · K)
84.00	0.2890	0.1208E+5	0.4569E+5	0.9165E+6	0.3673E−5	0.6384E−1
82.00	0.2961	0.1193E+5	0.4540E+5	0.8925E+6	0.3608E−5	0.6194E−1
80.00	0.3035	0.1178E+5	0.4510E+5	0.8688E+6	0.3542E−5	0.6007E−1
78.00	0.3114	0.1163E+5	0.4481E+5	0.8453E+6	0.3476E−5	0.5824E−1
76.00	0.3196	0.1149E+5	0.4451E+5	0.8222E+6	0.3409E−5	0.5645E−1
74.00	0.3283	0.1136E+5	0.4420E+5	0.7994E+6	0.3342E−5	0.5471E−1
72.00	0.3375	0.1124E+5	0.4389E+5	0.7768E+6	0.3273E−5	0.5301E−1
70.00	0.3473	0.1113E+5	0.4358E+5	0.7544E+6	0.3204E−5	0.5135E−1
68.00	0.3576	0.1103E+5	0.4326E+5	0.7322E+6	0.3133E−5	0.4975E−1
66.00	0.3686	0.1093E+5	0.4293E+5	0.7103E+6	0.3062E−5	0.4820E−1
64.00	0.3802	0.1085E+5	0.4259E+5	0.6885E+6	0.2990E−5	0.4670E−1
62.00	0.3927	0.1077E+5	0.4225E+5	0.6669E+6	0.2917E−5	0.4524E−1
60.00	0.4060	0.1071E+5	0.4190E+5	0.6454E+6	0.2842E−5	0.4384E−1
58.00	0.4202	0.1065E+5	0.4154E+5	0.6240E+6	0.2767E−5	0.4248E−1
56.00	0.4355	0.1061E+5	0.4116E+5	0.6028E+6	0.2690E−5	0.4116E−1
54.00	0.4520	0.1058E+5	0.4078E+5	0.5816E+6	0.2612E−5	0.3988E−1
52.00	0.4697	0.1055E+5	0.4038E+5	0.5605E+6	0.2533E−5	0.3862E−1
50.00	0.4890	0.1054E+5	0.3997E+5	0.5394E+6	0.2452E−5	0.3738E−1
48.00	0.5099	0.1053E+5	0.3954E+5	0.5183E+6	0.2370E−5	0.3615E−1
46.00	0.5327	0.1053E+5	0.3909E+5	0.4973E+6	0.2287E−5	0.3492E−1
44.00	0.5577	0.1053E+5	0.3862E+5	0.4762E+6	0.2202E−5	0.3367E−1
42.00	0.5853	0.1054E+5	0.3813E+5	0.4551E+6	0.2116E−5	0.3239E−1
40.00	0.6158	0.1055E+5	0.3762E+5	0.4340E+6	0.2028E−5	0.3107E−1
38.00	0.6497	0.1058E+5	0.3707E+5	0.4129E+6	0.1939E−5	0.2970E−1
36.00	0.6877	0.1062E+5	0.3650E+5	0.3917E+6	0.1849E−5	0.2827E−1
34.00	0.7307	0.1066E+5	0.3589E+5	0.3704E+6	0.1757E−5	0.2678E−1
33.00	0.7543	0.1069E+5	0.3557E+5	0.3598E+6	0.1710E−5	0.2601E−1
32.00	0.7797	0.1072E+5	0.3524E+5	0.3491E+6	0.1664E−5	0.2524E−1
31.00	0.8068	0.1076E+5	0.3490E+5	0.3383E+6	0.1617E−5	0.2445E−1
30.00	0.8360	0.1080E+5	0.3455E+5	0.3275E+6	0.1570E−5	0.2366E−1
29.00	0.8676	0.1085E+5	0.3418E+5	0.3167E+6	0.1522E−5	0.2287E−1
28.00	0.9018	0.1091E+5	0.3380E+5	0.3058E+6	0.1475E−5	0.2207E−1
27.00	0.9391	0.1098E+5	0.3340E+5	0.2949E+6	0.1428E−5	0.2128E−1
26.00	0.9798	0.1107E+5	0.3299E+5	0.2839E+6	0.1380E−5	0.2048E−1
25.00	1.025	0.1117E+5	0.3255E+5	0.2727E+6	0.1333E−5	0.1968E−1
24.00	1.074	0.1130E+5	0.3209E+5	0.2615E+6	0.1285E−5	0.1885E−1
23.00	1.129	0.1146E+5	0.3161E+5	0.2501E+6	0.1238E−5	0.1796E−1
22.00	1.191	0.1167E+5	0.3109E+5	0.2386E+6	0.1190E−5	0.1696E−1
21.00	1.262	0.1195E+5	0.3055E+5	0.2268E+6	0.1143E−5	0.1576E−1
20.00	71.12	9482.	7960.	−0.2304E+6	0.1404E−4	0.1041
19.00	72.23	8838.	7490.	−0.2395E+6	0.1530E−4	0.1031
18.00	73.28	8239.	7029.	−0.2480E+6	0.1670E−4	0.1011
17.00	74.26	7701.	6574.	−0.2560E+6	0.1828E−4	0.9744E−1
16.00	75.19	7282.	6121.	−0.2635E+6	0.2005E−4	0.9129E−1
15.00	76.08	7119.	5658.	−0.2707E+6	0.2206E−4	0.8117E−1
14.00	76.94	7517.	5158.	−0.2779E+6	0.2433E−4	0.6471E−1

Table 1-25 Para hydrogen properties along the 2×10^5 pascal (2 bar) isobar

T (K)	ρ (kg/m^3)	C_p (J/kg·K)	S (J/kg·K)	H (J/kg)	μ (Pa·s)	k (W/m·K)
300.0	0.1614	0.1485E+5	0.6207E+5	0.4228E+7	0.8953E−5	0.1917
295.0	0.1642	0.1488E+5	0.6182E+5	0.4154E+7	0.8852E−5	0.1897
290.0	0.1670	0.1492E+5	0.6157E+5	0.4080E+7	0.8751E−5	0.1877
285.0	0.1699	0.1496E+5	0.6131E+5	0.4005E+7	0.8648E−5	0.1858
280.0	0.1730	0.1500E+5	0.6104E+5	0.3930E+7	0.8545E−5	0.1839
275.0	0.1761	0.1505E+5	0.6077E+5	0.3855E+7	0.8442E−5	0.1821
270.0	0.1794	0.1510E+5	0.6050E+5	0.3779E+7	0.8337E−5	0.1803
265.0	0.1828	0.1515E+5	0.6021E+5	0.3704E+7	0.8232E−5	0.1785
260.0	0.1863	0.1520E+5	0.5992E+5	0.3628E+7	0.8126E−5	0.1767
255.0	0.1899	0.1526E+5	0.5963E+5	0.3552E+7	0.8019E−5	0.1750
250.0	0.1937	0.1533E+5	0.5933E+5	0.3475E+7	0.7912E−5	0.1733
245.0	0.1977	0.1539E+5	0.5902E+5	0.3399E+7	0.7803E−5	0.1716
240.0	0.2018	0.1546E+5	0.5870E+5	0.3321E+7	0.7694E−5	0.1698
235.0	0.2061	0.1553E+5	0.5837E+5	0.3244E+7	0.7584E−5	0.1681
230.0	0.2105	0.1561E+5	0.5804E+5	0.3166E+7	0.7473E−5	0.1663
225.0	0.2152	0.1569E+5	0.5769E+5	0.3088E+7	0.7361E−5	0.1645
220.0	0.2201	0.1577E+5	0.5734E+5	0.3009E+7	0.7248E−5	0.1627
215.0	0.2252	0.1585E+5	0.5698E+5	0.2930E+7	0.7134E−5	0.1608
210.0	0.2306	0.1593E+5	0.5660E+5	0.2851E+7	0.7020E−5	0.1589
205.0	0.2362	0.1601E+5	0.5622E+5	0.2771E+7	0.6904E−5	0.1568
200.0	0.2421	0.1608E+5	0.5582E+5	0.2691E+7	0.6788E−5	0.1547
195.0	0.2483	0.1615E+5	0.5541E+5	0.2610E+7	0.6670E−5	0.1525
190.0	0.2549	0.1622E+5	0.5499E+5	0.2529E+7	0.6551E−5	0.1502
185.0	0.2618	0.1628E+5	0.5456E+5	0.2448E+7	0.6431E−5	0.1477
180.0	0.2690	0.1633E+5	0.5411E+5	0.2366E+7	0.6310E−5	0.1451
175.0	0.2767	0.1636E+5	0.5365E+5	0.2285E+7	0.6188E−5	0.1423
170.0	0.2849	0.1638E+5	0.5318E+5	0.2203E+7	0.6065E−5	0.1394
165.0	0.2935	0.1638E+5	0.5269E+5	0.2121E+7	0.5940E−5	0.1363
160.0	0.3027	0.1636E+5	0.5218E+5	0.2039E+7	0.5815E−5	0.1331
155.0	0.3125	0.1631E+5	0.5167E+5	0.1957E+7	0.5687E−5	0.1296
150.0	0.3229	0.1623E+5	0.5113E+5	0.1876E+7	0.5559E−5	0.1260
145.0	0.3340	0.1612E+5	0.5058E+5	0.1795E+7	0.5429E−5	0.1221
140.0	0.3460	0.1597E+5	0.5002E+5	0.1715E+7	0.5297E−5	0.1181
135.0	0.3588	0.1578E+5	0.4944E+5	0.1635E+7	0.5164E−5	0.1138
130.0	0.3727	0.1556E+5	0.4885E+5	0.1557E+7	0.5029E−5	0.1094
125.0	0.3876	0.1530E+5	0.4825E+5	0.1480E+7	0.4892E−5	0.1048
120.0	0.4038	0.1500E+5	0.4763E+5	0.1404E+7	0.4753E−5	0.1001
115.0	0.4215	0.1466E+5	0.4700E+5	0.1330E+7	0.4612E−5	0.9519E−1
110.0	0.4407	0.1428E+5	0.4635E+5	0.1258E+7	0.4469E−5	0.9020E−1
105.0	0.4619	0.1388E+5	0.4570E+5	0.1187E+7	0.4323E−5	0.8514E−1
100.0	0.4851	0.1346E+5	0.4503E+5	0.1119E+7	0.4174E−5	0.8005E−1
98.00	0.4951	0.1329E+5	0.4476E+5	0.1092E+7	0.4114E−5	0.7802E−1
96.00	0.5055	0.1312E+5	0.4449E+5	0.1066E+7	0.4054E−5	0.7599E−1
94.00	0.5164	0.1295E+5	0.4421E+5	0.1040E+7	0.3992E−5	0.7396E−1
92.00	0.5277	0.1278E+5	0.4394E+5	0.1014E+7	0.3931E−5	0.7195E−1
90.00	0.5395	0.1261E+5	0.4366E+5	0.9884E+6	0.3869E−5	0.6996E−1
88.00	0.5519	0.1245E+5	0.4338E+5	0.9634E+6	0.3806E−5	0.6799E−1
86.00	0.5649	0.1229E+5	0.4309E+5	0.9386E+6	0.3742E−5	0.6603E−1

(*Continues*)

Table 1-25 (*Continued*)

T (K)	ρ (kg/m^3)	C_p (J/kg · K)	S (J/kg · K)	H (J/kg)	μ (Pa · s)	k (W/m · K)
84.00	0.5785	0.1213E+5	0.4280E+5	0.9142E+6	0.3678E−5	0.6411E−1
82.00	0.5928	0.1198E+5	0.4251E+5	0.8901E+6	0.3614E−5	0.6221E−1
80.00	0.6079	0.1183E+5	0.4222E+5	0.8663E+6	0.3548E−5	0.6035E−1
78.00	0.6237	0.1169E+5	0.4192E+5	0.8428E+6	0.3482E−5	0.5853E−1
76.00	0.6404	0.1155E+5	0.4162E+5	0.8196E+6	0.3416E−5	0.5675E−1
74.00	0.6580	0.1143E+5	0.4131E+5	0.7966E+6	0.3348E−5	0.5501E−1
72.00	0.6766	0.1131E+5	0.4100E+5	0.7738E+6	0.3280E−5	0.5331E−1
70.00	0.6964	0.1120E+5	0.4069E+5	0.7513E+6	0.3211E−5	0.5167E−1
68.00	0.7173	0.1110E+5	0.4036E+5	0.7290E+6	0.3140E−5	0.5007E−1
66.00	0.7396	0.1101E+5	0.4003E+5	0.7069E+6	0.3069E−5	0.4852E−1
64.00	0.7633	0.1093E+5	0.3970E+5	0.6850E+6	0.2997E−5	0.4703E−1
62.00	0.7886	0.1086E+5	0.3935E+5	0.6632E+6	0.2924E−5	0.4559E−1
60.00	0.8157	0.1081E+5	0.3899E+5	0.6415E+6	0.2850E−5	0.4419E−1
58.00	0.8448	0.1076E+5	0.3863E+5	0.6199E+6	0.2775E−5	0.4284E−1
56.00	0.8761	0.1073E+5	0.3825E+5	0.5985E+6	0.2699E−5	0.4153E−1
54.00	0.9098	0.1070E+5	0.3786E+5	0.5770E+6	0.2621E−5	0.4026E−1
52.00	0.9464	0.1069E+5	0.3746E+5	0.5556E+6	0.2543E−5	0.3902E−1
50.00	0.9861	0.1069E+5	0.3704E+5	0.5343E+6	0.2462E−5	0.3779E−1
48.00	1.029	0.1069E+5	0.3660E+5	0.5129E+6	0.2381E−5	0.3657E−1
46.00	1.077	0.1071E+5	0.3615E+5	0.4915E+6	0.2298E−5	0.3536E−1
44.00	1.129	0.1073E+5	0.3567E+5	0.4700E+6	0.2214E−5	0.3412E−1
42.00	1.187	0.1077E+5	0.3517E+5	0.4485E+6	0.2128E−5	0.3286E−1
40.00	1.252	0.1081E+5	0.3464E+5	0.4270E+6	0.2041E−5	0.3156E−1
38.00	1.324	0.1087E+5	0.3409E+5	0.4053E+6	0.1953E−5	0.3022E−1
36.00	1.406	0.1096E+5	0.3350E+5	0.3835E+6	0.1863E−5	0.2881E−1
34.00	1.499	0.1107E+5	0.3287E+5	0.3614E+6	0.1772E−5	0.2736E−1
33.00	1.551	0.1114E+5	0.3254E+5	0.3503E+6	0.1726E−5	0.2661E−1
32.00	1.608	0.1122E+5	0.3219E+5	0.3391E+6	0.1680E−5	0.2585E−1
31.00	1.669	0.1131E+5	0.3184E+5	0.3279E+6	0.1633E−5	0.2509E−1
30.00	1.735	0.1142E+5	0.3146E+5	0.3165E+6	0.1587E−5	0.2432E−1
29.00	1.808	0.1155E+5	0.3107E+5	0.3050E+6	0.1540E−5	0.2355E−1
28.00	1.887	0.1171E+5	0.3067E+5	0.2934E+6	0.1494E−5	0.2278E−1
27.00	1.976	0.1191E+5	0.3024E+5	0.2816E+6	0.1447E−5	0.2202E−1
26.00	2.075	0.1215E+5	0.2978E+5	0.2696E+6	0.1400E−5	0.2125E−1
25.00	2.187	0.1247E+5	0.2930E+5	0.2573E+6	0.1354E−5	0.2049E−1
24.00	2.315	0.1290E+5	0.2878E+5	0.2446E+6	0.1307E−5	0.1971E−1
23.00	2.465	0.1348E+5	0.2822E+5	0.2314E+6	0.1261E−5	0.1888E−1
22.00	68.79	0.1085E+5	8901.	−0.2092E+6	0.1199E−4	0.1043
21.00	70.07	0.1011E+5	8414.	−0.2196E+6	0.1301E−4	0.1046
20.00	71.25	9434.	7937.	−0.2294E+6	0.1415E−4	0.1043
19.00	72.36	8801.	7470.	−0.2385E+6	0.1541E−4	0.1034
18.00	73.39	8209.	7010.	−0.2470E+6	0.1682E−4	0.1013
17.00	74.36	7678.	6557.	−0.2550E+6	0.1840E−4	0.9765E−1
16.00	75.28	7264.	6105.	−0.2624E+6	0.2018E−4	0.9148E−1
15.00	76.16	7107.	5643.	−0.2696E+6	0.2220E−4	0.8135E−1
14.00	77.01	7510.	5143.	−0.2768E+6	0.2448E−4	0.6487E−1

Table 1-26 Para hydrogen properties along the 5×10^5 pascal (5 bar) isobar

T (K)	ρ (kg/m^3)	C_p (J/kg · K)	S (J/kg · K)	H (J/kg)	μ (Pa · s)	k (W/m · K)
300.0	0.4029	0.1486E+5	0.5829E+5	0.4230E+7	0.8957E−5	0.1919
295.0	0.4097	0.1489E+5	0.5804E+5	0.4156E+7	0.8857E−5	0.1899
290.0	0.4168	0.1493E+5	0.5779E+5	0.4081E+7	0.8755E−5	0.1880
285.0	0.4241	0.1497E+5	0.5753E+5	0.4006E+7	0.8653E−5	0.1861
280.0	0.4316	0.1501E+5	0.5726E+5	0.3931E+7	0.8550E−5	0.1842
275.0	0.4394	0.1506E+5	0.5699E+5	0.3856E+7	0.8446E−5	0.1824
270.0	0.4476	0.1511E+5	0.5671E+5	0.3781E+7	0.8342E−5	0.1806
265.0	0.4560	0.1516E+5	0.5643E+5	0.3705E+7	0.8237E−5	0.1788
260.0	0.4647	0.1522E+5	0.5614E+5	0.3629E+7	0.8131E−5	0.1770
255.0	0.4738	0.1528E+5	0.5585E+5	0.3553E+7	0.8024E−5	0.1753
250.0	0.4833	0.1534E+5	0.5554E+5	0.3476E+7	0.7917E−5	0.1736
245.0	0.4932	0.1541E+5	0.5523E+5	0.3399E+7	0.7808E−5	0.1719
240.0	0.5034	0.1548E+5	0.5491E+5	0.3322E+7	0.7699E−5	0.1702
235.0	0.5141	0.1555E+5	0.5459E+5	0.3245E+7	0.7589E−5	0.1684
230.0	0.5253	0.1563E+5	0.5425E+5	0.3167E+7	0.7478E−5	0.1667
225.0	0.5369	0.1570E+5	0.5391E+5	0.3088E+7	0.7367E−5	0.1649
220.0	0.5491	0.1578E+5	0.5355E+5	0.3010E+7	0.7254E−5	0.1631
215.0	0.5619	0.1586E+5	0.5319E+5	0.2931E+7	0.7141E−5	0.1612
210.0	0.5752	0.1595E+5	0.5282E+5	0.2851E+7	0.7026E−5	0.1593
205.0	0.5893	0.1603E+5	0.5243E+5	0.2771E+7	0.6911E−5	0.1572
200.0	0.6040	0.1610E+5	0.5203E+5	0.2691E+7	0.6794E−5	0.1551
195.0	0.6195	0.1618E+5	0.5162E+5	0.2610E+7	0.6677E−5	0.1529
190.0	0.6358	0.1625E+5	0.5120E+5	0.2529E+7	0.6558E−5	0.1506
185.0	0.6530	0.1631E+5	0.5077E+5	0.2448E+7	0.6439E−5	0.1481
180.0	0.6711	0.1636E+5	0.5032E+5	0.2366E+7	0.6318E−5	0.1455
175.0	0.6903	0.1639E+5	0.4986E+5	0.2284E+7	0.6196E−5	0.1428
170.0	0.7107	0.1641E+5	0.4939E+5	0.2202E+7	0.6073E−5	0.1399
165.0	0.7322	0.1642E+5	0.4889E+5	0.2120E+7	0.5949E−5	0.1368
160.0	0.7552	0.1640E+5	0.4839E+5	0.2038E+7	0.5823E−5	0.1335
155.0	0.7796	0.1635E+5	0.4787E+5	0.1956E+7	0.5696E−5	0.1301
150.0	0.8057	0.1627E+5	0.4734E+5	0.1875E+7	0.5568E−5	0.1265
145.0	0.8336	0.1616E+5	0.4679E+5	0.1793E+7	0.5438E−5	0.1226
140.0	0.8635	0.1602E+5	0.4622E+5	0.1713E+7	0.5307E−5	0.1186
135.0	0.8956	0.1584E+5	0.4564E+5	0.1633E+7	0.5174E−5	0.1144
130.0	0.9303	0.1562E+5	0.4505E+5	0.1555E+7	0.5040E−5	0.1100
125.0	0.9678	0.1536E+5	0.4444E+5	0.1477E+7	0.4903E−5	0.1054
120.0	1.009	0.1507E+5	0.4382E+5	0.1401E+7	0.4765E−5	0.1007
115.0	1.053	0.1473E+5	0.4318E+5	0.1327E+7	0.4625E−5	0.9581E−1
110.0	1.101	0.1436E+5	0.4254E+5	0.1254E+7	0.4482E−5	0.9085E−1
105.0	1.155	0.1397E+5	0.4188E+5	0.1183E+7	0.4337E−5	0.8581E−1
100.0	1.213	0.1356E+5	0.4121E+5	0.1114E+7	0.4190E−5	0.8075E−1
98.00	1.239	0.1339E+5	0.4093E+5	0.1087E+7	0.4130E−5	0.7872E−1
96.00	1.265	0.1323E+5	0.4066E+5	0.1061E+7	0.4070E−5	0.7671E−1
94.00	1.292	0.1306E+5	0.4038E+5	0.1034E+7	0.4009E−5	0.7470E−1
92.00	1.321	0.1290E+5	0.4010E+5	0.1008E+7	0.3948E−5	0.7270E−1
90.00	1.351	0.1274E+5	0.3982E+5	0.9826E+6	0.3886E−5	0.7072E−1
88.00	1.383	0.1258E+5	0.3954E+5	0.9573E+6	0.3824E−5	0.6876E−1
86.00	1.416	0.1243E+5	0.3925E+5	0.9323E+6	0.3761E−5	0.6683E−1

(Continues)

Table 1-26 (*Continued*)

T (K)	ρ (kg/m³)	C_p (J/kg·K)	S (J/kg·K)	H (J/kg)	μ (Pa·s)	k (W/m·K)
84.00	1.451	0.1228E+5	0.3896E+5	0.9076E+6	0.3697E−5	0.6492E−1
82.00	1.487	0.1213E+5	0.3867E+5	0.8832E+6	0.3633E−5	0.6304E−1
80.00	1.526	0.1199E+5	0.3837E+5	0.8591E+6	0.3569E−5	0.6120E−1
78.00	1.566	0.1186E+5	0.3807E+5	0.8352E+6	0.3503E−5	0.5939E−1
76.00	1.609	0.1174E+5	0.3776E+5	0.8116E+6	0.3437E−5	0.5763E−1
74.00	1.655	0.1162E+5	0.3745E+5	0.7883E+6	0.3370E−5	0.5591E−1
72.00	1.703	0.1152E+5	0.3713E+5	0.7651E+6	0.3303E−5	0.5423E−1
70.00	1.754	0.1142E+5	0.3681E+5	0.7422E+6	0.3234E−5	0.5261E−1
68.00	1.809	0.1133E+5	0.3648E+5	0.7195E+6	0.3165E−5	0.5104E−1
66.00	1.867	0.1126E+5	0.3614E+5	0.6969E+6	0.3095E−5	0.4952E−1
64.00	1.929	0.1120E+5	0.3580E+5	0.6744E+6	0.3024E−5	0.4805E−1
62.00	1.996	0.1115E+5	0.3544E+5	0.6521E+6	0.2952E−5	0.4664E−1
60.00	2.067	0.1112E+5	0.3508E+5	0.6298E+6	0.2879E−5	0.4528E−1
58.00	2.145	0.1110E+5	0.3470E+5	0.6076E+6	0.2805E−5	0.4396E−1
56.00	2.229	0.1109E+5	0.3431E+5	0.5854E+6	0.2730E−5	0.4269E−1
54.00	2.320	0.1110E+5	0.3391E+5	0.5632E+6	0.2654E−5	0.4146E−1
52.00	2.419	0.1113E+5	0.3349E+5	0.5410E+6	0.2577E−5	0.4026E−1
50.00	2.529	0.1117E+5	0.3305E+5	0.5187E+6	0.2499E−5	0.3908E−1
48.00	2.649	0.1123E+5	0.3259E+5	0.4963E+6	0.2419E−5	0.3792E−1
46.00	2.783	0.1131E+5	0.3211E+5	0.4737E+6	0.2338E−5	0.3676E−1
44.00	2.933	0.1142E+5	0.3161E+5	0.4510E+6	0.2256E−5	0.3560E−1
42.00	3.102	0.1156E+5	0.3107E+5	0.4280E+6	0.2173E−5	0.3442E−1
40.00	3.294	0.1173E+5	0.3051E+5	0.4048E+6	0.2089E−5	0.3321E−1
38.00	3.517	0.1198E+5	0.2990E+5	0.3811E+6	0.2004E−5	0.3198E−1
36.00	3.778	0.1232E+5	0.2924E+5	0.3568E+6	0.1918E−5	0.3071E−1
34.00	4.092	0.1279E+5	0.2852E+5	0.3317E+6	0.1832E−5	0.2942E−1
33.00	4.275	0.1312E+5	0.2814E+5	0.3188E+6	0.1789E−5	0.2877E−1
32.00	4.480	0.1352E+5	0.2773E+5	0.3054E+6	0.1746E−5	0.2812E−1
31.00	4.714	0.1404E+5	0.2729E+5	0.2917E+6	0.1704E−5	0.2748E−1
30.00	4.985	0.1473E+5	0.2682E+5	0.2773E+6	0.1662E−5	0.2687E−1
29.00	5.306	0.1570E+5	0.2631E+5	0.2621E+6	0.1621E−5	0.2628E−1
28.00	5.697	0.1714E+5	0.2573E+5	0.2458E+6	0.1581E−5	0.2575E−1
27.00	61.01	0.1645E+5	0.1146E+5	−0.1416E+6	0.8146E−5	0.9803E−1
26.00	63.09	0.1463E+5	0.1088E+5	−0.1571E+6	0.8895E−5	0.1005
25.00	64.90	0.1331E+5	0.1033E+5	−0.1710E+6	0.9663E−5	0.1023
24.00	66.50	0.1227E+5	9811.	−0.1838E+6	0.1047E−4	0.1037
23.00	67.95	0.1140E+5	9308.	−0.1956E+6	0.1134E−4	0.1047
22.00	69.28	0.1064E+5	8819.	−0.2066E+6	0.1228E−4	0.1053
21.00	70.51	9944.	8340.	−0.2169E+6	0.1331E−4	0.1055
20.00	71.65	9302.	7871.	−0.2265E+6	0.1446E−4	0.1051
19.00	72.72	8695.	7410.	−0.2355E+6	0.1573E−4	0.1041
18.00	73.72	8124.	6956.	−0.2439E+6	0.1715E−4	0.1020
17.00	74.66	7610.	6506.	−0.2518E+6	0.1876E−4	0.9827E−1
16.00	75.56	7212.	6058.	−0.2592E+6	0.2056E−4	0.9205E−1
15.00	76.41	7070.	5599.	−0.2663E+6	0.2261E−4	0.8187E−1
14.00	77.24	7489.	5101.	−0.2735E+6	0.2491E−4	0.6535E−1

Table 1-27 Para hydrogen properties along the 20×10^5 pascal (20 bar) isobar

T (K)	ρ (kg/m^3)	C_p (J/kg·K)	S (J/kg·K)	H (J/kg)	μ (Pa·s)	k (W/m·K)
300.0	1.597	0.1490E+5	0.5256E+5	0.4237E+7	0.8982E−5	0.1933
295.0	1.624	0.1493E+5	0.5231E+5	0.4163E+7	0.8882E−5	0.1913
290.0	1.652	0.1497E+5	0.5206E+5	0.4088E+7	0.8781E−5	0.1894
285.0	1.680	0.1501E+5	0.5179E+5	0.4013E+7	0.8679E−5	0.1875
280.0	1.710	0.1506E+5	0.5153E+5	0.3938E+7	0.8577E−5	0.1856
275.0	1.741	0.1511E+5	0.5126E+5	0.3863E+7	0.8474E−5	0.1838
270.0	1.773	0.1516E+5	0.5098E+5	0.3787E+7	0.8370E−5	0.1820
265.0	1.806	0.1521E+5	0.5069E+5	0.3711E+7	0.8266E−5	0.1803
260.0	1.841	0.1527E+5	0.5040E+5	0.3635E+7	0.8161E−5	0.1786
255.0	1.877	0.1534E+5	0.5011E+5	0.3558E+7	0.8055E−5	0.1769
250.0	1.914	0.1540E+5	0.4980E+5	0.3481E+7	0.7948E−5	0.1752
245.0	1.953	0.1547E+5	0.4949E+5	0.3404E+7	0.7840E−5	0.1735
240.0	1.993	0.1555E+5	0.4917E+5	0.3327E+7	0.7732E−5	0.1718
235.0	2.035	0.1562E+5	0.4884E+5	0.3249E+7	0.7623E−5	0.1701
230.0	2.079	0.1570E+5	0.4851E+5	0.3170E+7	0.7513E−5	0.1684
225.0	2.125	0.1579E+5	0.4816E+5	0.3092E+7	0.7403E−5	0.1666
220.0	2.173	0.1587E+5	0.4780E+5	0.3012E+7	0.7291E−5	0.1648
215.0	2.224	0.1596E+5	0.4744E+5	0.2933E+7	0.7179E−5	0.1630
210.0	2.277	0.1604E+5	0.4706E+5	0.2853E+7	0.7065E−5	0.1611
205.0	2.332	0.1613E+5	0.4667E+5	0.2773E+7	0.6951E−5	0.1591
200.0	2.390	0.1621E+5	0.4628E+5	0.2692E+7	0.6836E−5	0.1570
195.0	2.451	0.1629E+5	0.4586E+5	0.2610E+7	0.6720E−5	0.1549
190.0	2.516	0.1636E+5	0.4544E+5	0.2529E+7	0.6603E−5	0.1526
185.0	2.584	0.1643E+5	0.4500E+5	0.2447E+7	0.6485E−5	0.1502
180.0	2.656	0.1649E+5	0.4455E+5	0.2364E+7	0.6366E−5	0.1476
175.0	2.732	0.1654E+5	0.4409E+5	0.2282E+7	0.6246E−5	0.1450
170.0	2.812	0.1657E+5	0.4361E+5	0.2199E+7	0.6125E−5	0.1421
165.0	2.898	0.1658E+5	0.4311E+5	0.2116E+7	0.6003E−5	0.1391
160.0	2.989	0.1657E+5	0.4260E+5	0.2033E+7	0.5880E−5	0.1359
155.0	3.087	0.1654E+5	0.4208E+5	0.1951E+7	0.5755E−5	0.1325
150.0	3.191	0.1647E+5	0.4153E+5	0.1868E+7	0.5630E−5	0.1289
145.0	3.303	0.1638E+5	0.4098E+5	0.1786E+7	0.5503E−5	0.1252
140.0	3.423	0.1626E+5	0.4040E+5	0.1704E+7	0.5375E−5	0.1212
135.0	3.552	0.1609E+5	0.3982E+5	0.1623E+7	0.5245E−5	0.1171
130.0	3.692	0.1590E+5	0.3921E+5	0.1543E+7	0.5115E−5	0.1128
125.0	3.844	0.1566E+5	0.3859E+5	0.1465E+7	0.4982E−5	0.1083
120.0	4.009	0.1540E+5	0.3796E+5	0.1387E+7	0.4849E−5	0.1037
115.0	4.191	0.1509E+5	0.3731E+5	0.1311E+7	0.4713E−5	0.9899E−1
110.0	4.390	0.1476E+5	0.3665E+5	0.1236E+7	0.4577E−5	0.9417E−1
105.0	4.611	0.1441E+5	0.3597E+5	0.1163E+7	0.4438E−5	0.8928E−1
100.0	4.856	0.1405E+5	0.3528E+5	0.1092E+7	0.4298E−5	0.8439E−1
98.00	4.962	0.1391E+5	0.3499E+5	0.1064E+7	0.4241E−5	0.8244E−1
96.00	5.074	0.1376E+5	0.3471E+5	0.1036E+7	0.4184E−5	0.8050E−1
94.00	5.190	0.1362E+5	0.3442E+5	0.1009E+7	0.4127E−5	0.7857E−1
92.00	5.313	0.1349E+5	0.3413E+5	0.9818E+6	0.4069E−5	0.7666E−1
90.00	5.442	0.1336E+5	0.3383E+5	0.9549E+6	0.4011E−5	0.7477E−1
88.00	5.579	0.1323E+5	0.3353E+5	0.9284E+6	0.3953E−5	0.7290E−1

(Continues)

Table 1-27 (*Continued*)

T (K)	ρ (kg/m^3)	C_p (J/kg · K)	S (J/kg · K)	H (J/kg)	μ (Pa · s)	k (W/m · K)
86.00	5.722	0.1311E+5	0.3323E+5	0.9020E+6	0.3894E−5	0.7106E−1
84.00	5.874	0.1300E+5	0.3292E+5	0.8759E+6	0.3835E−5	0.6926E−1
82.00	6.036	0.1290E+5	0.3261E+5	0.8500E+6	0.3776E−5	0.6749E−1
80.00	6.207	0.1281E+5	0.3229E+5	0.8243E+6	0.3717E−5	0.6577E−1
78.00	6.389	0.1273E+5	0.3197E+5	0.7988E+6	0.3657E−5	0.6409E−1
76.00	6.584	0.1266E+5	0.3164E+5	0.7734E+6	0.3597E−5	0.6246E−1
74.00	6.793	0.1261E+5	0.3130E+5	0.7481E+6	0.3537E−5	0.6089E−1
72.00	7.016	0.1257E+5	0.3096E+5	0.7229E+6	0.3476E−5	0.5937E−1
70.00	7.257	0.1255E+5	0.3061E+5	0.6978E+6	0.3416E−5	0.5792E−1
68.00	7.518	0.1256E+5	0.3024E+5	0.6727E+6	0.3355E−5	0.5653E−1
66.00	7.802	0.1259E+5	0.2987E+5	0.6476E+6	0.3294E−5	0.5522E−1
64.00	8.111	0.1265E+5	0.2948E+5	0.6223E+6	0.3233E−5	0.5397E−1
62.00	8.450	0.1274E+5	0.2908E+5	0.5970E+6	0.3172E−5	0.5281E−1
60.00	8.824	0.1287E+5	0.2866E+5	0.5713E+6	0.3112E−5	0.5172E−1
58.00	9.241	0.1305E+5	0.2822E+5	0.5454E+6	0.3052E−5	0.5071E−1
56.00	9.708	0.1330E+5	0.2775E+5	0.5191E+6	0.2993E−5	0.4979E−1
54.00	10.24	0.1361E+5	0.2727E+5	0.4922E+6	0.2936E−5	0.4896E−1
52.00	10.85	0.1403E+5	0.2674E+5	0.4646E+6	0.2881E−5	0.4824E−1
50.00	11.56	0.1460E+5	0.2618E+5	0.4360E+6	0.2829E−5	0.4763E−1
48.00	12.40	0.1537E+5	0.2557E+5	0.4060E+6	0.2781E−5	0.4717E−1
46.00	13.43	0.1649E+5	0.2490E+5	0.3742E+6	0.2742E−5	0.4692E−1
44.00	14.75	0.1819E+5	0.2413E+5	0.3397E+6	0.2716E−5	0.4701E−1
42.00	16.54	0.2106E+5	0.2322E+5	0.3007E+6	0.2714E−5	0.4769E−1
40.00	19.24	0.2670E+5	0.2207E+5	0.2537E+6	0.2767E−5	0.4963E−1
38.00	24.21	0.4078E+5	0.2040E+5	0.1885E+6	0.2980E−5	0.5480E−1
36.00	36.23	0.6039E+5	0.1751E+5	0.8177E+5	0.3906E−5	0.7016E−1
34.00	48.68	0.3043E+5	0.1500E+5	−6254.	0.5457E−5	0.8656E−1
33.00	52.39	0.2423E+5	0.1419E+5	−0.3327E+5	0.6081E−5	0.9136E−1
32.00	55.32	0.2062E+5	0.1351E+5	−0.5555E+5	0.6657E−5	0.9515E−1
31.00	57.78	0.1822E+5	0.1289E+5	−0.7490E+5	0.7216E−5	0.9830E−1
30.00	59.92	0.1648E+5	0.1233E+5	−0.9221E+5	0.7776E−5	0.1009
29.00	61.81	0.1514E+5	0.1179E+5	−0.1080E+6	0.8350E−5	0.1031
28.00	63.52	0.1405E+5	0.1128E+5	−0.1226E+6	0.8949E−5	0.1050
27.00	65.09	0.1314E+5	0.1079E+5	−0.1362E+6	0.9583E−5	0.1064
26.00	66.53	0.1235E+5	0.1030E+5	−0.1489E+6	0.1026E−4	0.1076
25.00	67.87	0.1165E+5	9834.	−0.1609E+6	0.1099E−4	0.1086
24.00	69.12	0.1101E+5	9372.	−0.1722E+6	0.1179E−4	0.1092
23.00	70.29	0.1042E+5	8916.	−0.1829E+6	0.1267E−4	0.1096
22.00	71.39	9853.	8466.	−0.1931E+6	0.1364E−4	0.1098
21.00	72.43	9310.	8020.	−0.2026E+6	0.1472E−4	0.1095
20.00	73.42	8781.	7579.	−0.2117E+6	0.1593E−4	0.1089
19.00	74.35	8264.	7142.	−0.2202E+6	0.1729E−4	0.1075
18.00	75.23	7766.	6709.	−0.2282E+6	0.1882E−4	0.1051
17.00	76.07	7315.	6278.	−0.2358E+6	0.2054E−4	0.1012
16.00	76.86	6976.	5846.	−0.2429E+6	0.2248E−4	0.9475E−1
15.00	77.62	6893.	5401.	−0.2498E+6	0.2467E−4	0.8437E−1

Notice that for the fluids other than helium, there are cases where the listed entropy and enthalpy values are negative. Although this may seem counterintuitive, recall that entropy and enthalpy are not absolute and must be compared with a reference value. The third law of thermodynamics defines a fluid's entropy as zero at zero temperature and defined pressure. From this definition, a standard reference value (usually at 1 atmosphere and 298 K) may be calculated. In general, the reference values for entropy and enthalpy used in GASPAK and HEPAK agree with those recommended by the CODATA and organization. In some cases, the absolute values of entropy and enthalpy in these tables may differ from those in other sources, but the differences between any two states (which are the only physically meaningful values) will be the same.

1-4 SOURCES FOR FLUID PROPERTY COMPUTER PROGRAMS

1. ALL PROPS
Center for Applied Thermodynamic Studies
College of Engineering
University of Idaho
Moscow, ID 83843

2. NIST-12
Office of Standard Reference Data
National Institute of Standards and Technology
Gaithersburg, MD 20899

3. GASPAK AND HEPAK
Cryodata, Inc.
P.O. Box 173
Louisville, CO 80027

REFERENCES

1. Benedict, M., Webb, G. B., and Rubin, L. C., "An Empirical Equation for Thermodynamic Properties of Light Hydrocarbons and their Mixtures I: Methane, Ethane, Propane, and *n*-Butane," *J. Chem. Phys.* 8 (1940):334–345.
2. Schmidt, R., and Wagner, W., "A New Form of the Equation of State for Pure Substances and Its Application to Oxygen," *Fluid Phase Equilibria* 19 (1985):175–200.
3. Haynes, W. M., and Friend, D. G., "Reference Data for Thermophysical Properties of Cryogenic Fluids," *Adv. Cryog. Eng.* 39 (1994):1865–1874.
4. Lemmon, E. W., Jacobsen, R. T., Penoncello, S. G., and Beyerlein, S. W., "Computer Programs for the Calculation of Thermodynamic Properties of Cryogens and Other Fluids," *Adv. Cryog. Eng.* 39 (1994): 1891–1897.
5. Cryodata, Inc., P.O. Box 173, Louisville, CO 80027.

TWO

PROPERTIES OF CRYOGENIC MATERIALS

T. H. K. Frederking

UCLA, BH5531 SEAS/Chem E,
Los Angeles, CA 90095

J. A. Barclay

Cryofuel Systems—University of Victoria,
P.O. Box 3055, Victoria, BC V8W 3P6, Canada

R. Flükiger

University of Geneva, DPMC, 24, Quai Ernest
Ansermet, Geneva, 1211, Switzerland

X. Y. Liu

Integrated Manufacturing Technologies Institute,
National Research Council of Canada, 800 Collip
Circle, London, Ontario, Canada N6G 4X8

J. L. Hall

Jet Propulsion Laboratory, MS 156-316, 4800 Oak
Grove Drive, Pasadena, CA 91109

G. Hartwig

Forschungszentrum Karlsruhe, IMF II
Postfach 3640, 76021 Karlsruhe, Germany

V. L. Morris

Morris Associates, 20952 Mesa Rica Road,
Covina, CA 91724

2-1 FRICTION COEFFICIENTS AND RELATED PHENOMENA

T. H. K. Frederking

UCLA, BH5531 SEAS/Chem E, Los Angeles, CA 90095

2-1-1 Introduction

This section addresses tribology at low temperatures (T). Tribology, the study of friction, considers, among other phenomena, friction forces that act at the external boundary common to two materials. The real interface usually has a nonplanar (i.e., imperfect) domain structure with departures from a mathematical plane. Therefore, considerable complexity involving numerous material combinations is encountered. Data at low T are scarce; consequently, various tribology subdisciplines outside the cryotemperature range are mentioned. Often, room temperature data are the only results that provide order of magnitude (OOM) hints.

Examples of tribology phenomena are Earth tectonics [1], traction on tires for road vehicles, dissipation of energy reduction in oil-lubricated bearings, drag reduction in dilute polymer–water solutions [2], and polymer-coated windings in magnets and electrical systems.

Static friction is required at the tires of road vehicles for force transmission. The order of the friction coefficient is unity on dry roads but 0.1 or less on wet or icy roads. Similarly, gear trains with polymer belts require sufficient friction.

Dynamic conditions are encountered in bearings. A lowering of friction by oil films aims at reducing losses associated with energy dissipation. Huge economic benefits derive from an improved bearing tribology.

Polymers* play an important role as construction materials (e.g., Kevlar [3]) and as insulators (e.g., Kapton) in magnets and other electrical systems. Sliding motion is characterized by a friction coefficient on the order of magnitude of 0.4 up to $10\,\text{N/mm}^2$.

Solid lubricants may replace liquids. Examples are molybdenum disulfide (MoS_2), graphite, and carbides. An early literature compilation of NASA is Ref. [4] (compare also Clauss 1972 [20]).

Nanotribology [5,6] is a recent subdiscipline aiming at optimization of lubrication in advanced small-scale systems. Examples of related physics investigations are found in Refs. [7] and [8].

At low temperatures (T), naturally the question of T-effects on friction arises. Early data indicate that in some cases the friction coefficient decreases as T is lowered [9]. Other results show a constant coefficient [10]. Recent work indicates the additional possibility of a friction coefficient increase as T is decreased.

In the following subsections, static [11] and dynamic friction coefficients are addressed. Next, experimental methods simulating complex tribology scenarios are outlined. Subsequently, applied superconductivity magnet phenomena are outlined. They constitute a significant part (partially unexplored) of the cryotechnology spectrum. The magnets pose challenges of quantification of friction. Related magnet tribology in static and dynamic scenarios will be discussed.

Because of considerable tribology complexity, it is emphasized that data may be interpreted from more than only one point of view.

2-1-2 Phenomena of Static and Dynamic Friction

Static phenomena are characterized by the ability to avoid slippage in a restricted range of parameters. An example is the ladder placed at standard gravity at a vertical wall. At a particular angle, a static limit is reached. Dynamic phenomena are initiated. This point of view has been extended to some magnet winding systems. At a certain limiting parameter set, static phenomena are replaced by dynamic events. They include stick-slip known from other areas of tribology. Thus, static tribology is replaced by dynamic tribology at a particular set of parameters. At present, magnet experience indicates a predominance of sliding motion in large-scale systems. This implies a great significance of dynamic tribology in experiments.

---

*Additional information on the use of polymers in cryogenics can be found in section 2-5 of this chapter.

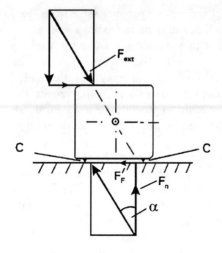

Figure 2-1 Schematic of a static friction model system. Two model asperities (cones C) indicate symbolically real conditions of a rough surface (F_{ext} denotes externally applied force, F_n is the normal reaction force component, and F_F signifies the tangential reaction force component, which is equal to the friction force).

Dynamic phenomena are characterized by relative motion of the two materials once forces have been switched on. An example is the start-up of magnet operation. The individual winding "sees" a magnet-field-related resulting force. The hoop-stress-related normal force component and the tangential component are superposed vectorially. As the electrical current and the associated magnetic field are increased, the forces increase. During this energization process, there exists a finite chance that static conditions will be changed to dynamic phenomena. Relative motion of a winding takes place with respect to an adjacent winding or substrate material. Upon initiation of relative motion, dynamic friction is established. We turn next to a quantification of simplified tribology.

Static friction (zero relative motion). Figure 2-1 presents an ideal static system schematically and symbolically. The force F is applied externally to the body located above a plane symbolizing a substrate material. Two cone-shaped asperities are protruding from the upper body. The cones constitute "macroroughness" replacing symbolically numerous microasperities of the real surface. For an applied normal force F_n there is a relatively large tangential component in the contact plane.

As a result of external force application, first elastic deformation takes place in the low force range. Included in Fig. 2-1 are reactive force components. The normal force component F_n counteracts the applied force in the vertical direction. The tangential component F_F represents the static friction and is in the range $0 < \alpha < \alpha_0$; $F_F = F_n \tan \alpha$. For the tribostatics up to the limiting angle there exists a limiting envelope of the static range. The limiting topology is an α_0-cone for an ideal sphere geometry. There is a limiting wedge for the ideal cylinder. Thus, static friction conditions are realized ideally when the following inequality is satisfied:

$$F_F < F_n \tan \alpha_0 \qquad (2\text{-}1)$$

The ideal topology limit is characterized by the following static friction coefficient:

$$\mu_0 = F_{F_0}/F_n = \tan \alpha_0 \qquad (2\text{-}2)$$

This friction coefficient μ_0 depends on material and surface parameters. Because real surfaces are not ideal, there are departures from the ideal limiting topology.

In this context, we note elastic deformation by normal force alone for a sphere pair or sphere-plane, sphere-cylinder geometry, and others. For the simple systems, the Hertz theory is available for the quantification of elastic deformations (e.g., Ref. [12]). A pair of identical materials, for instance, is characterized by the following results: the ratio of the deformed domain radius to the sphere radius is proportional to the third root of the applied (normal) force and proportional to the reciprocal third root of Young's modulus.

The general dependence of deformation on the specific normal force "pressure" is more complicated than the Hertz theory. Further complexity arises from coatings. There is the additional tangential component. Thus, the static friction coefficient depends on a multitude of parameters. Among them are the surface domain compositions, structure, and concentration of chemical and physical "impurities." Further, the presence of fluid films and solid coatings is important as well as the related temperature and pressure-dependent thermophysical properties. As the external force is increased, shear causes plastic deformation or fracture of the cone-like asperities indicated in Fig. 2-1.

Dynamic friction—Coulomb's law. Dynamic friction involves sliding at a relative velocity $v > 0$. As the applied force is increased beyond the static limit, there is a transition into the dynamic range characterized by relative motion of the two materials. In experiments simulating the friction of complex systems, usually one material is kept stationary, and the second one is moving with the speed v. For the dynamic range, Coulomb's law describes the phenomena using a dynamic friction coefficient (μ_d) (Fig. 2-2).

$$\mu = F_F/F_n = \tan \beta \tag{2-3}$$

In Fig. 2-2, F_{ext} is the externally applied force. Further, the components of the reactive force are shown with friction F_F and normal force F_n. Friction acts in the tangential plane.

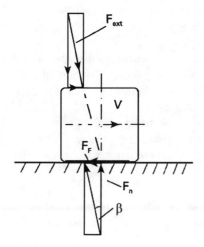

Figure 2-2 Schematic of a dynamic friction model (v is the relative velocity between the upper body and the lower substrate, R_{ext} is the externally applied force, F_n denotes the normal reaction force component, and F_F is the tangential [friction] force component).

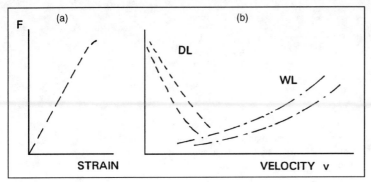

Figure 2-3 Schematic representation of force conditions for various groups of phenomena for (a) force (F) versus strain and (b) force versus velocity (v). (DL denotes the dry lubircation regime, and WL signifies the wet lubricant such as the organic lubricant film in the hydrodynamic region.)

Comparing Figs. 2-1 and 2-2 for the same normal force, we have a decreased dynamic tangential force compared with the static range. For polymer-coated metals, the dynamic friction coefficient (μ) is below unity. Thus, the angle β is less than 45°. The dynamic μ-values depend on the parameters for static friction discussed above. In addition, the lubrication technique applied to the bodies is important (e.g., "dry friction," special coatings, presence of fluid lubricant). Thus, there is no constant friction coefficient in Coulomb's law in general (see Fig. 2-3).

Complicated conditions are created in superconducting magnets. In some winding geometries using the composite NbTi–Cu, the domain structure involves the material sequence copper–Formvar–cryoliquid residue/solid condensate–Formvar–copper. Each subdomain in general has individual Young modulus values and shear modulus values. They do not necessarily match each other. In cryoliquid-free magnets, there is no fluid matter within the contact domains.

It has been remarked that very small dynamic friction coefficients ($\mu_d = 0.05$) have been observed with ice–ice systems. The sliding velocity has been on the order of magnitude of 1 cm/s [13].

Stick–slip phenomena. In a friction simulation test with two material pairs (one stationary, one moving), well-defined conditions are aimed at. First, small, finite velocities ($v > 0$) are imposed. The external load is increased and with it the tangential reactive force component F_F. Eventually, the static limit is exceeded. A possible consequence is local yielding of surface asperity material and local slippage. The force is reduced to a low level. Upon continued application of shear, pressure builds up again, and a second slip event takes place. Aside from steady sliding, oscillations are possible as well. For magnets, these scenarios have been studied at low temperatures (e.g., Refs. [14] and [15]).

Stick–slip phenomena are not restricted to magnet scenarios. They have been observed in several tribology areas. Common features are observed for both metals and nonmetals.

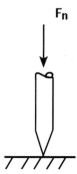

Figure 2-4 Schematic representation of pin-on-disk/plate geometry. The force F_n is applied in the vertical direction.

2-1-3 Experimental Methods

Examples of experimental systems are shown schematically in Figs. 2-4 to 2-8 (e.g., Refs. [15–17] and others. Figure 2-4 displays the pin-on-plate system. The pin is moved across the surface of the disk, permitting plowing action in some materials. The results are relatively high friction coefficients on the order of magnitude of unity for metal–metal systems, (e.g., Refs. [9] and [10]).

Figure 2-5 schematically depicts the arrangement of Artoos et al. [17]. A flat slab of one material is placed into a clamping system whose fingers consist of the second material. The normal force is applied to the clamps in a horizontal direction. Reciprocating motion permits repetitive load cycles.

Figure 2-6 schematically displays the disk–disk geometry of Kensley and Iwasa [15, 16]. The upper rotating disk is in contact with a lower stationary disk. Several variations of this geometry have been developed [15].

Figure 2-7 shows a schematic drawing of the tribology simulation system for superconducting composite samples of Ref. [18]. There is a helical Cu-wire clamping scheme around the central, vertical conductor. The lacquer-coated Cu-helix, in turn, is located inside a clamping system applying a normal force. The assembly is surrounded by a magnet coil providing a longitudinal field with respect to the vertical conductor (transverse to the Cu-helix). Upon external force (F_{ext}) application, significant

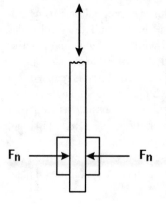

Figure 2-5 Schematic representation of a slab sample with a second material arranged as a clamping finger pair geometry (from Ref. [17]). The normal force F_n is applied in the horizontal direction.

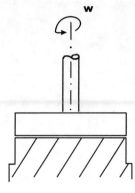

Figure 2-6 Schematic of a tribology system with stationary disk-moving disk geometry (form Ref. [15]). The upper disk is rotating with angular velocity (ω); the lower disk is stationary.

friction arises during relative motion of the sample with respect to stationary surroundings. The sample is pulled with a speed of 0.02 to 0.2 mm/min. Aside from friction force information, quench zone formation-related flux motion is detected by a pickup coil (not shown in Fig. 2-7). Thus, the quench kinetics are monitored in the system.

Figure 2-8 presents another tribology system for a composite, Formvar-insulated NbTi–Cu conductor, (Ref. [19]). A calorimetric technique is used in He II in conjunction

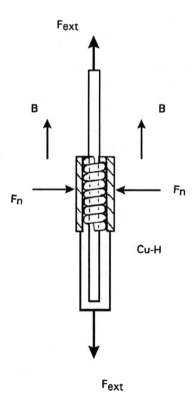

Figure 2-7 Schematic of a tribology simulation system for composite superconductor samples with an externally applied longitudinal field for the vertical sample (B denotes the externally applied magnetic field, Cu–H is the copper conductor helix, F_{ext} is the externally applied pulling force, and F_n signifies normal force).

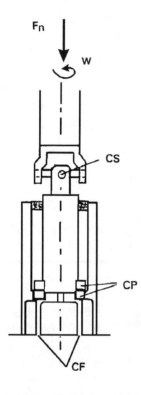

Figure 2-8 Schematic of a tribology simulation system for superconductor–superconductor friction measurements using a calorimetric technique (CS denotes cardanic suspension, CF signifies the superfluid He II counterflow ducts for calorimetry, and F_n is the applied normal force).

with the dissipation of friction energy. The latter is removed via counterflow channels. The normal force F_n is applied from the top via a cardanic suspension.

Concerning other diagnostic tools, the technique of acoustic emission (AE) is mentioned (e.g., Ref. [21]). The AE is capable of registering internal friction events (e.g., prequench and quench activities inside a superconducting material). Results suggest that tribology surface-domain events are potentially accessible to AE methods.

2-1-4 Friction Data

Figure 2-9 is a plot of high friction coefficients of investigators (Refs. [9,10]), as compiled by Kim in 1978 [22]. The data show a weak temperature dependence of the friction factor for Cu–Cu and a noticeable T-dependence for Ni–Ni. Plowing action of the pin-slab system (Fig. 2-4) causes relatively high friction coefficients.

Figure 2-10 shows recent pin-on-slab data reported by Yokoi and Okada [23] for an applied force of 3 kgf (approximately 30 N). A hard pin of 18-8 stainless steel has been used on soft plates of PTFE and Al–4% Cu at 300 and 16 K. The friction force versus load function observed is slightly nonlinear. There are oscillations at relatively low load.

Figure 2-11 shows selected friction data of the Francis Bitter National Magnet Laboratory (FBNML) (Ref. [15]). Included are "peak" friction coefficient ($\mu = \mu_d$) results deduced from the maximum values of a series of dynamic friction experiments

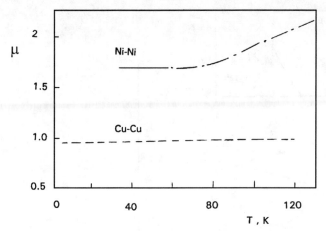

Figure 2-9 Friction coefficients near and above unity caused in part by the plowing action of the pin-on-slab geometry (Ni–Ni from Ref. [9]; Cu–Cu from Ref. [10]).

of Kensley and Iwasa [15]. In the dynamic runs, the velocity v is increased. Associated with the v-rise is an increase of the friction up to a particular point, the "peak." At this high-load condition, a sudden drop in the friction coefficient occurs. The peak value is designated as μ_p. The stick–slip sequence is interpreted as local surface stress release. The inset of Fig. 2-11 displays the stick–slip event schematically. There are several types of post-peak phenomena, including oscillations (e.g., Ref. [15]).

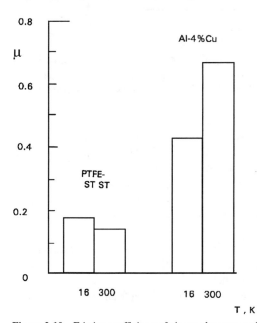

Figure 2-10 Friction coefficients of pin-on-plate tests at 16 and 300 K (from Ref. [23]).

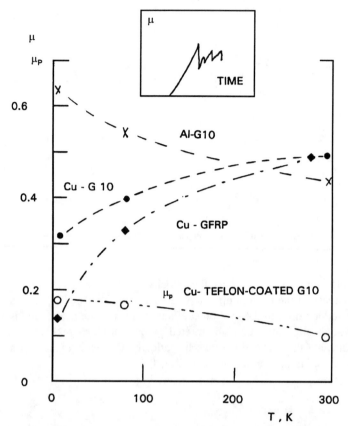

Figure 2-11 Friction coefficients versus temperature (from Refs. [15] and [24]). The μ values were derived from Ref. [15]. ●= Cu–G10; x-Al-G10. The μ_p values constitute "peak" results of the stick–slip sequences for (○) Cu-teflon-coated G10 [15] and (◊) Cu-GFRP plate [24]. The inset schematically shows μ versus time stick–slip record on the basis of Ref. [15].

The friction data of Fig. 2-11 are representative examples for specific conditions [15]. For instance, the dynamic coefficient (μ) for the pair Cu–G10 shows a monotonic increase with temperature. In contrast, the pair Al–G10 displays a decrease of μ as T is increased. The peak data μ_p (T) show a weak decrease as T is raised. An additional set of data of Ref. [24] is included in Fig. 2-11 for copper in contact with GFRP. These latter results are quite consistent with the Cu–G10 results [15] as far as $d\mu/dT$ and the magnitude are concerned.

Figure 2-12 shows dynamic friction coefficients for various pairs investigated at CERN [17]. The data are in part very close to the FBNML results [15]. The low value of an MoS_2 varnish layer near 0.05 has been achieved at room temperature. At low T, this attractive feature got lost: relatively high μ-values have been found instead with the coatings used in Ref. [17].

The comparison of various results suggests that a large set of variables affects low-temperature tribology. Improvements are possible in various directions. For instance,

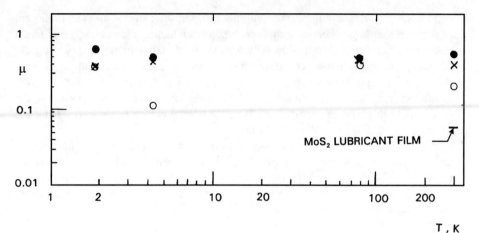

T , K

Figure 2-12 The dynamic friction coefficient versus temperature [17] for (●) stainless steel/mild steel, (x) Al–Vetronite [G10], and (○) stainless steel–Vetronite.

for magnets, extreme cases of construction approaches are "perfect clamping" and low-friction sliding across relatively small distances. Particular magnet aspects are outlined in section 2-1-5.

2-1-5 Magnet Tribology and Related Parameters*

After introduction of a classification scheme, magnet tribology is considered. Friction modeling approaches and related quench parameters are addressed. Consequences for magnet construction are outlined.

Classification scheme. In a simplified classification scheme of magnet-related friction scenarios, three different categories are distinguished: (1) magnetic flux motion at small externally applied mechanical stresses (e.g., fast flux jumps); (2) zero magnetic field tribology, including non-elastic and stick–slip events; and (3) magnet tribology with combinations of magnet-induced flux motion, mechanical-stress-induced plastic flow, and related jumps and stick–slip phenomena in finite fields.

1. Magnetic flux motion phenomena have been studied at small mechanical forces. At very small fields in the Meissner state, a superconductor with partially adiabatic walls undergoes magneto-caloric cooling. At enhanced fields, flux jump patterns are established with associated magneto-thermal heating. During increasing field ramping and decreasing ramping, nonlinear oscillations are possible.
2. In a zero externally applied magnetic field, the effect of the Earth's field is negligible for large structures. Deformations at large forces are encountered in (local) plastic regimes at large strains. The deformation characteristics in general are nonlinear. Suitable stress

---

*Additional information on superconducting magnet systems may be found in chapter 8 of this handbook.

conditions may trigger nonlinear oscillations. Further, stick-slip events are reminiscent of serrated yielding observed with Type II superconducting filaments–normal metal composite conductors. Plastic flow is favored in "soft" stabilizer material of low yield point (e.g., copper). In most composite conductors, there are stabilizer materials (Cu, Al) aside from type II filaments (e.g., NbTi), AC barriers, (e.g., Cu–Ni), and electrical insulation (e.g., Kapton). As a result of the plastic flow of copper, one portion of the system is highly mobile, whereas the Type II material is locally stressed. This leads to serrated yielding (e.g., Refs. [18],[25],[44].)

3. In magnet tribology, the general stress situation involves superpositions of field effects and friction forces. There is a finite probability of magnetic hoop stress effects, plastic deformation, and field-related property changes. Reference [18] provides an example of quench domain phenomena. Cyclic loading–unloading sequences ("training") may raise the quench limits of a magnet.

Small-scale versus large-scale magnets. In small laboratory magnets and in low-field, moderate size windings (e.g., MRI type systems), epoxy-potted coils and similar techniques have been employed for mechanical stability of windings. Epoxy cracking may be encountered upon excessive stress accumulation. Suitable filler–epoxy combinations have been developed to avoid quenches. Examples of epoxy phenomena are given in Refs. [30–32].

In large magnets with large forces, winding displacement is accompanied by dynamic friction events. Therefore, simple tribology models have aimed at parameters delineating characteristic "critical" quantities associated with a quench. Examples of parameters related to quenches and magnet tribology are the minimum quench energy (MQE) and energy density, respectively, the minimum propagating zone (MPZ), and the maximum adiabatic zone (MAZ).

The models considered are based on investigators of the UCLA Cryolab (e.g., Refs. [19],[22],[26], and [27]). The characteristic parameter MPZ and quench consequences have been discussed in detail by Wilson [29]; compare also [40],[41]. The minimum propagating zone is written as

$$\text{MPZ} = [A/I][2k(T_c - T_\infty)/\rho_{el}]^{1/2} \qquad (2\text{-}4)$$

where k is thermal conductivity, ρ_{el} is normal state electrical resistivity, I is electrical current, A is cross section for the current, and I/A is current density. As the thermal conductivity (k) is a function of temperature, the MPZ is temperature dependent. For a composite low-T_c superconductor, MPZ may reach the order of magnitude of 1 cm.

Maximum adiabatic zone [MAZ]. The MAZ represents the dynamic friction-related distance at which the tribology-caused dissipation leads to a temperature rise to the superconducting phase boundary. The MAZ may be significantly shorter than the MPZ of a composite conductor. This indicates the sensitivity of low-T_c superconductors to tribology disturbances. The characteristic length MAZ is large when the T-span from the magnet operation temperature to the superconducting transition temperature is large. The associated enthalpy change of the adiabatic composite conductor has been considered for low-T_c superconductors (i.e., a composite of NbTi–Cu [19], [27]). The enthalpy differential increment per unit volume is $(\rho\, c_p)dT$ (specific heat per unit volume = product of the density ρ and the specific heat c_p at constant pressure). For the composite conductor, various contributions to the thermal energy are summed up, noting dominant Debye T^3-law contributions for low-T_c systems.

The friction model [26,27] in a winding system has presumed an external force with a normal and tangential field-induced force component. This is expressed parametrically by a load factor based on the magnetic pressure $\Delta P_m = B^2/(2\mu_0)$; B induction; $\mu_0 = 1.256 \times 10^{-6}$ H/m. For MAZ evaluation, the enthalpy difference ΔH, up to the transition temperature T_c, is equal to the frictional energy dissipation. For a conductor of square cross section (a^2), the MAZ condition has been expressed per volume (V). The simplified form of this equation is written parametrically in terms of a load factor (LF) [19] as follows:

$$\Delta H/V = (LF)\,\Delta P_m\,\mu\, MAZ/a \qquad (2\text{-}5)$$

In a related model, a body sliding on an inclined plate has been considered an analog case of the single magnet section "seeing" the external field [27].

In general, the friction coefficient varies with temperature. In fast events, the sliding details of dynamic friction during adiabatic dissipation depend on the temperature variation of the friction coefficient. In this area, detailed tribology calculations have been presented by Maksimov [28]. There are two classes of slide responses, depending on a positive $(d\mu/dT)$ or a negative value $(d\mu/dT)$. In addition, a relaxation of the adiabatic condition alters the results of the tribology modeling. Heat removal increases the tolerated displacements beyond the MAZ values of the adiabatic case.

For illustration, Fig. 2-13 displays some MAZ functions based on the tribology model versions of Refs. [19] and [22]. It is seen that the "conventional" friction coefficients of the preceding figures lead to rather small MAZ values tolerated prior to a quench. They are on the order of magnitude of 0.1 mm. A substantial reduction to $\mu = 0.05$ improves the displacement (MAZ) margin, provided T is not too close to T_c.

Minimum quench energy [MQE]. Once a minimum quench domain of minimum length (MPZ) has been created, there is a minimum quench energy associated with the MPZ. The order of magnitude of the MQE is assessed: the zone is in the normal state acting as "critical nucleus domain." The related excess temperature of this normal zone extends beyond T_c. A simple zone model is based on a Gaussian bell function:

$$\Delta T = \Delta T_{max} \exp(-\xi^2) \qquad (2\text{-}6)$$

The dimensionless distance is $\xi = x/MPZ$, where x is the axial position coordinate of a composite conductor with adiabatic outer boundary and with fluid contact at $T = T_\infty$ at large x far from the MPZ. The maximum excess temperature ΔT_{max} is on the order of magnitude (OOM) of T_c, noting the superconductor operating rule of thumb of $(T_c/2)$. Thus, we have $\Delta T_{max} = OOM\, T_c$. The definite integral of Eq. (2-4) (i.e., of f(x)dx from very large negative to very large positive values) has the value $\pi^{1/2}(MPZ) = OOM(MPZ)$. Using this result, the order of magnitude of the minimum quench energy is determined by

$$MQE = OOM[(MPZ)A](\rho c_p)T_c \qquad (2\text{-}7)$$

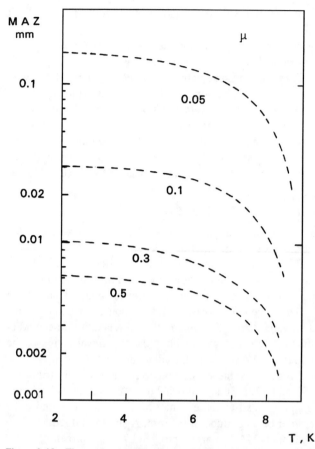

Figure 2-13 The maximum adiabatic zone [MAZ] length versus temperature for various friction coefficients (load factor-0.1, $B = 5$ T; from Refs. [19] and [22]).

The related energy density is MQE/V, where the volume is $V = A$ (MPZ). For low-T_c materials without significant magnetic moment contributions, we note the low-T molar specific heat (Debye function)

$$c_m = 233.8R(T/\Theta_D)^3 \qquad (2\text{-}8)$$

($233.8R = 1944$ kJ/(kmol · K) and kJ/(kg-atom · K), respectively; R is the universal gas constant. For example, if Debye temperature $\Theta_D = 350$ K and $T = 7$ K, $c_m = 0.015$ SI units. For a molar–atomic volume of OOM 10, the volumetric specific heat has the OOM of 1.5 mJ/(cc K).

At room temperature, the results are as follows: Dulong–Petit value of the lattice specific heat of $3R$ equals approximately 25 J/mol · K, and for the same molar volume, $(\rho c_p) = $ OOM 2.5 J/(cc K). This is three orders above the low-T_c MQE density value.

For high-T_c superconductors, operated at relatively low T, the rare-earth magnetic moment contribution raises the volumetric specific heat in comparison with low T_c. As T is raised, the enhanced lattice specific heat increases the volumetric specific heat to the order of magnitude of 0.01 J/(cc K). Thus, there is a possibility of magnetic contributions to the specific heat when T is not too high. For elevated temperatures (e.g., $1/10$ of the Debye temperature) the lattice contributions rise rapidly. This removes the low-T_c sensitivity of the example above (Fig. 2-13).

For $T_c = $ OOM10 K, the MQE per volume is in the OOM range of 0.015 J/cc. At $T_c = 100$ K, the volumetric MQE rises to the OOM of 0.1 to 1 J/cc. The MQE values are compared with the tribology-related energy density.

The tribology-induced volumetric energy dissipation is assessed on the basis of (local) deformation beyond the 0.2% limit. As cyclic loading and unloading are conducted, a hysteresis loop is covered (see Ref. [18]). The order of magnitude of the plastic deformation is 0.005 or 0.5% strain. The related stress level is presumed to be on the order of magnitude of 500 N/mm^2. The resulting energy per volume has the order of magnitude of 2.5 J/cc. This value of the dissipated energy density is quite high in comparison with MPZ-related magnet tolerances. Thus, absolute dissipation levels have to be kept small by appropriate magnet construction.

Further, the order of magnitude comparison suggests that there is an advantage to using means available of moving away from the liquid helium boiling point. The two alternate routes are low-T_c with relatively high T_c (Nb$_3$Sn) or high-T_c, or hybrid low-T_c/high-T_c. Technological improvements in this direction increase the robustness with respect to friction events.

Consequences for magnet construction. The small magnet and low-field magnet with epoxy potting have been replaced in laboratory experiments by other media. For instance, small pancake windings have been clamped by wax [33]. Upon warm-up, a modification is possible just by remelting the wax.

Large magnets require detailed attention to tribology of sliding conditions because static friction cannot be maintained in general. In view of the large forces, nearly all friction investigators have addressed dynamic friction coefficient measurements.

Thus, a dual approach of constraining windings and using low-friction materials is an option. In this regard, Fig. 2-14 presents clamping approaches schematically.

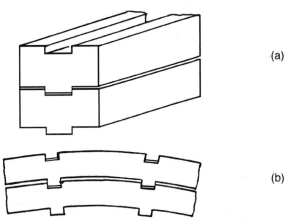

(a)

(b)

Figure 2-14 Schematic examples of geometry constraints for windings. (a) Clamping against lateral (axial) displacements; (b) clamping against tangential displacements.

Figure 2-14(a) depicts prevention of winding motion in axial direction via geometry constraints. Figure 2-14(b) is another possibility using pin-like constraints imposed on the windings. Approaches to problems of this nature are noted in several areas. Examples are high-pressure vessels wrapped as metal or polymer-fiber-reinforced vessels in chemical processing industries and in aerospace. Further, we have closely related winding-system applied technology in the large-scale generator and motor systems of the electrical power industry.

Summarizing remarks, including polymer aspects. It has been found that undesired sudden conductor movement in a winding system is detrimental to stability. In fact, there is an enormously high probability of quench occurrence (e.g., Refs. [34,35]). Aside from the special geometry-enforced stabilization, the option of preload room temperature treatment has been proposed [36]. Despite careful, very tight clamping in support structures, coils have suffered premature quenches [37]. These and other phenomena underline the importance of tribology as one contributing factor out of a set of several others. Jelly-roll windings have been popular, but they turned out to be disturbance-sensitive initially in research and development work. This point has been retested [38], after work approximately 20 years ago, using modern SSC-composite conductors. The test data are interpreted as evidence for conductor motion leading to premature quenches.

Thus, in comparison with early low-T_c "hard" superconductor magneto-mechanics [44], the tribology progress and high-T_c developments encourage continued improvements in the direction of robust magnets. For additional information, Refs. [40] and [41] present numerous details of superconducting magnet issues.

Various polymer results from low temperature to room temperature are summarized in Tables 2-1 and 2-2. Table 2-1 presents a brief overview of low-T results. Table 2-2 focuses on room temperature data.

Table 2-1 Polymers used in low-temperature research

Polymer material	Reference	Remarks
Teflon/polytetra fluoroethylene and polyethylene/high-density Pennlon	[15] Kensley et al. FBNML	Ref. [15] $0.1 < \mu < 0.6$ for the test samples
Nylon 6–Zytel 101 (Dupont)	[15] Kensley et al.	Moisture absorption
G10 glass-fiber-reinforced epoxy	[15],[24]	
G10 vetronite	[17] Artoos et al. CERN	$0.1 < \mu < 0.6$
Formvar [Cu–NbTi]– Formvar [Cu–NbTi]	[19] Kim et al.	He II range $0.6 < \mu < 0.8$

Note: The polymer friction data are supplemented by room temperature results. Note that favorable low-friction coefficients at 300 K have not been reproduced at low T. Instead, at 77 K and lower the friction coefficients have increased. Examples are MoS_2–varnish coating results near 0.06 at room temperature [17] and similar lubrication film data [15]. Ice versus ice has low μ values of 0.05 at 300 K [14].

Table 2-2 Polymer friction results at room temperature

Polymer	Reference	μ (300 K)	Remarks
958-301-coated G10	[15]		Boys Coatings
MLR106-coated G10	[15]	0.05	Research Comp with MoS$_2$
Kevlar (DuPont)	[3]	0.18	
Rulon A	[13]	0.1	
Polyoxymethylen [POM]	[41]	0.4	
(Ultramid-BASF)	[42]	(dry)	up to 10 N/mm^2

Note: Entries are consistent with data of Table 2-1. A low friction coefficient of 0.18 for Kevlar [45] is for a 50-g load, 170 degree wrap angle, and a velocity of 30 cm/s. The rubbing surface is characterized as matte chrome. For other conditions higher μ values are reported. The POM μ data [42] vary from 0.3 to 0.4 at a speed of 0.5 m/s and a load of 1 N/mm^2. The friction coefficient magnitude depends on the roughness (in the range of 0.5 to 3 μm).

In general, magnet friction events involve a set of metallic and nonmetallic materials. In addition, several tribology mechanisms may act simultaneously. In this context acoustic emission (AE) diagnostics have been used extensively [46] to search for details.

ACKNOWLEDGMENTS

I wish to thank my wife Dorothea for a quarter of a century of continuous significant support. The authors of various materials-related sections of this handbook responded generously, and this is appreciated very much. Further inputs came from G. K. White (for permission to use his invited reviews), D. N. Lyon, University of California, Berkeley; T. Collings, Ohio State University, Columbus; F. Fickett, NIST, A. F. Clark, NIST; and V. Arp, NIST-Cryodata; these are acknowledged with thanks. It has been significant that J. L. Olsen, ETH Zurich, and the "Villa Vesta" team of the early low-temperature research, along with collaborators, including the Grassmann Institute, had a substantial part in stimulating solid-state interest. In particular, Peter Wyder, Grenoble, and Klaus Andres, Meissner Institute, Garching, have provided stimulating support and encouragement.

G. Klipping and I. Klipping have given great assistance. Further, quite a few others, too numerous to mention here, gave inputs, and all of these generous synergy efforts are appreciated with special thanks to all.

In the friction area, including superconducting magnet friction, special thanks for input and research results are due G. Bogner, Siemens Research Laboratory; Roger W. Boom; S. Van Sciver, NHMFL; Shlomo Caspi, LBL; R. Scanlan, LBL; Robert Fagaly, Conductus; R. Taylor and Lucky Zoltan, UCLA tokamak; J. A. Burkhart and R. C. Hendricks, NASA Lewis; F. Edeskuty, LANL; Takehiro Ito, Kyushu University; J. Yamamoto, NIFS; T. Mito, NIFS; S. Satoh, NIFS; R. Scurlock, Institute of Cryogenic, University of Southampton, UK; and J. G. Weisend II (DESY).

In addition, other superconductor dissipation work of former and present students and collaborators has been very supportive and is acknowledged with particular appreciation to Yu-Wen Chang [42], T. C. Chuang, C. Linnet, V. Purdy, Y. I. Kim, J. Lee, K. V. Ravikumar, Y. Kamioka, S. Yoshida, the late L. Li-He, W. F. Feng, M. M. Kamegawa, T. Jelmeland, L. Krajewski, and numerous enthusiastic SRP students.

NOMENCLATURE

c_p	Constant pressure specific heat (J/kg · K)
F	Force (N)
T	Temperature (K)
v	Velocity (m/s)
Θ_D	Debye temperature (K)
ρ	density (kg/m^3)
μ_0	Static friction coefficient
μ_D	Dynamic friction coefficient

Subscripts

N	Normal component
F	Friction
Ext	External

REFERENCES

1. Paterson, M. S.,"Experimental Rock Deformation—The Brittle Field," in *Minerals and Rocks*, P. J. Wyle, W. Van Engelhardt, and T. Hahn, eds. (New York: Springer–Verlag, 1978).
2. Rodriguez, F., *Principles of Polymer Systems*, 4th ed. (Washington, D.C.: Taylor & Francis, 1996).
3. Young, H. H., *Kevlar Aramid Fiber* (New York: John Wiley & Sons, 1995).
4. *Bibliography on Solid Lubricants*, National Aeronautics and Space Administration, NASA SP-5037 (U.S. Government Printing Office: Washington, D.C., 1966).
5. Bhushan, B., Israelachvili, J. N., and Landman, U., "Nanotribology: Friction, Wear and Lubrication at the Atomic Scale," *Nature* 374 (1995):607–616.
6. Krim, J., "Friction at the Atomic Scale," *Sci. American* 275 (1996):74–80.
7. Sokoloff, J. B.,"Microscopic Mechanisms for Kinetic Friction: Nearly Frictionless Sliding for Small Solids," *Phys. Rev. B* 52 (1995):7205.
8. Baumberger, T., Caroli, C., Perrin, B., and Ronsin, C., "Nonlinear Analysis of the Stick-Slip Bifurcation in the Creep-Controlled Regime of Dry Friction," *Phys. Rev.* B52 (1995):4005–4010.
9. Bowden, F. P., and Childs, T. H. C., "The Friction and Deformation of Clean Metals at Very Low Temperatures," *Proc. Roy. Soc.* A312 (1969):465–467.
10. Dukhowskii, E. A. et al., "Friction of Analogous Metal Pairs in Liquid and Gaseous Helium at Temperatures of 4.2 K to 80 K," *Dokl. Acad. Nauk SSR Techn. Phys.* 235 (1977):331–334.
11. Michael, P. C. et al., "Mechanical Properties and Static Friction Behaviour of Epoxy Mixes at Room Temperature and at 77 K," *Cryog.* 30 (1990):775–786.
12. Johnson, H. L., *Contact Mechanics* (Cambridge: Cambridge University Press, 1985).
13. Kennedy, F. E., Jr., "Friction," in *Encyclopedia of Physics* (New York: VCh Publishers, 1991), 418.
14. Michael, P. C., Rabinowitz, E., and Iwasa, Y. "Friction and Wear of Polymeric Materials at 293, 77, and 4.2 K," *Cryog.* 31 (1991):695–704.
15. Kensley, R. S., and Iwasa, Y., "Frictional Properties of Metal Insulator Surfaces at Cryogenic Temperatures," *Cryog.* 20 (1980):25–36.
16. Kensley, R. S., M. S. thesis, MIT, 1979.

17. Artoos, K., Clair, D., Poncet, A., and Savary, F., "The Measurements of Friction Coefficient Down to 1.8 K for LHC Magnets," *Cryog.* 34, ICEC Supplement (1994):689–692.
18. Dotsenko, V. I., Kislyak, I. F., and Chaykovskaya, N. M., "Stability of Superconducting Composites During External Friction," *Cryog.* 30 (1990):894–897.
19. Kim, Y. I., Caspi, S., Ravikumar, K. V., and Frederking, T. H. K., "Friction Phenomena in Low-T_c and High-T_c Superconducting Winding Systems," *Cryog.* 32 (1992):498–501. Addendum/Correction 32 (1992):918.
20. Clauss, F. J., *Solid Lubricants and Self-Lubricating Solids* (New York: Academic Press, 1972), 128–193.
21. Ono, K., "Acoustic Emission," in *Fatigue Crack Measurements: Techniques and Applications*, K. Marsh, R. Ritchie, and R. Smith, eds. (West. Midlands, U.K.: Warley, 1991), 173–205.
22. Kim, Y. I., M. S. thesis, UCLA, 1978.
23. Yokoi, K., and Okada, K., "Friction Properties of PTFE, h-BN and Al-4% Cu Alloy in a Vacuum at Super-Low Temperatures," *Cryog.* 34/ICEC15 Supplement (1994):493–496.
24. Takao, T., Tsukamoto, O., and Nishimura, A., "Friction Coefficients Between Conductor and Spacer at 10 Cycles, in *Annual Report National Institute Fusion Science (NIFS)*, Nagoya, Pt. III, C. Namba et al., eds. (Nagoya: NIFS, 1995), 35.
25. Easton, D. S., and Koch, C. C., "Mechanical Properties of Nb–Ti Composites," *Adv. Cryog. Eng.* 22 (1977):453–462.
26. Lee, J. Y., Caspi, S., Kim, Y. I., and Frederking, T. H. K., "Quench Onset Conditions Associated with Friction During Relative Motion of a Composite Conductor Section in a Large Superconducting Magnet," in *Proc. 3rd ANS Topical Meeting on Technology of Controlled Nuclear Fusion* (Santa Fe: NM 1978).
27. Lee, J. Y., Kim, Y. I., Caspi, S., Frederking, T. H. K., "Magnet Safety Properties of Cryo-Energy Systems" *Am. Inst. Ch. Engrs.*, (Paper delivered at the second Intersociety Cryogenic Symposium [AIChE, ASME, IIR], Miami, Florida, New York: 12–16 November 1970).
28. Maksimov, I. L, "Thermal Effects and Low-Temperature Frictional Pair Characteristics," *Adv. Cryog. Mat.* 34 (1988):267–274.
29. Wilson, M. N., *Superconducting Magnets* (New York: Oxford University Press, 1983).
30. Nishijima, S., Okada, T., and Honda, Y., "Evaluation of Epoxy Resin By Positron Annihilation for Cryogenic Use," *Adv. Cryog. Eng. Mat.* 40 (1994):1137–1144.
31. Walsh, R. P., and Reed, R. P., "Thermal Expansion Measurements of Resins (4K–300 K)," *Adv. Cryog. Eng. Mat.* 40 (1994):1145–1151.
32. Michael, P. C., Aized, D., Rabinowicz, E., and Iwasa, Y., "Mechanical Properties and Static Friction Behavior of Epoxy Mixes at Room Temperature and at 77 K," *Cryog.* 30 (1990):775–786.
33. Matsubara, Y., Nihon University, Chiba, Japan, personal communication.
34. Takao, T., Iawasaki, K., and Tsukamoto, O., "Statistical Estimation of Disturbance Energy Due to Conductor Motion in Rotor Windings of Superconducting Generator," *IEEE Trans. Appl. Superconductivity* 5 (1995):361–364.
35. Tsukamoto, O., "Disturbance Due to Conductor Motion and Stability of Large-Scale Superconductors," *Fusion Eng. Design* 20 (1993):361–364.
36. Schmidt, C., and Turck, B., "A Cure Against 'Training' of Superconducting Magnets," *Cryog.* 17 (1977):695–696.
37. Vermilyae, M. E., "Transient Thermal Behavior of Superconducting Coils," in *Proc. 1st. Joint Seminar US–Japan on Magnet Stability-Related Heat Transfer* (1988):191–198; Fukuoka, Japan: Kyushu University, NSF-Japan Soc. Promotion Science, Tokyo.
38. Yoshida, S., Biggins, S. W., Ravikumar, K. V., and Frederking, T. H. K., "Characteristics of an 'Overload' Component for Low-T_c Superconducting Magnet Systems," *IEEE Trans. Appl. Superconductivity* 5 (1995):933–936.
39. Sekiguchi, T., "Symposium on Superconductor Stability," *Cryog.* 31 (1991):488.
40. Dresner, L., *Stability of Superconductors* (New York: Plenum Press, 1995).
41. Iwasa, Y., *Case Studies in Superconducting Magnets—Design and Operational Issues* (New York: Plenum Press, 1994).
42. Klingenspor, H., personal communication; *VDI News* 23 (1977):13.
43. Chang, Yu-Wen, Ph.D. thesis, UCLA, 1971.
44. Kamegawa, M. M., M.S. thesis, UCLA, 1971.

45. Koch, C. C., and Easton, D. S., "A Review of Mechanical Behavior and Stress Effects in Hard Supercon-ductors," *Cryog.* 17 (1977):391–413.
46. DuPont data sheet; courtesy of D. Powell, November, 1996.
47. Yoshimura, H., Ueda, A., Morita, M., Maeda, S., Nagao, M., Shimohata, K., Matsuo, Y., Nagata, Y., Nakamura, S., Yamada, T., and Nakabayashi, Y., "Acoustic Emission Monitoring on a Model Field Winding for the 70 MW Class Superconducting Generator," *Cryog.* 32 (1992):502–507.

2-2 COMPOSITE MATERIALS

V. L. Morris

Morris Associates, 20952 Mesa Rica Road, Covina, CA 91724

2-2-1 Introduction

Composite advantages. Engineered composite structures have an important role to play in the rapidly expanding cryogenics world. For some low-temperature applications, composite materials can meet stringent requirements that metallic materials cannot. For other cryogenic applications, composite technology offers improved performance and lower life-cycle costs.

Advantages of composites include low thermal conductivity, high strength and stiffness, light weight, temperature capability to 1.8 K, tailored structural efficiency, dimensional stability, close tolerances, improved insulation, corrosion resistance, minimum flaw propagation, and low vibration. Perceived disadvantages are lack of a standard composite material database, cost of some materials, complex design parameters, and manufacturing processes that must be carefully controlled.

Scope of discussion. Structural composites currently being used for cryogenic applications are discussed. Background information is available elsewhere. Kasen [1] most admirably covers cryogenic composites through the mid-1980s. Valuable additional data are provided by Clark, Reed, Hartwig, and Evans [2,3,4]. Schwartzberg et al. [5] put together the first available cryogenic composites database. Serafini and Koenig [6] developed cryogenic polymers in the 1960s. Tsai [7] offers composite design expertise. ASM International [8] publishes a reference for composite design, materials, manufacturing processes, quality control, and testing.

Terminology. Composite terms as utilized in this discussion are briefly defined in the nomenclature list.

2-2-2 Composite Materials

Fibers. In composite materials, the fibers provide the primary load-carrying characteristics. Their strength and stiffness are very important. As detailed in Table 2-3, several excellent fibers are available. Quantitative fiber data at cryogenic temperatures are

Table 2-3 Typical properties of fibers at 295 K

Fiber	Tensile strength (MPa)	Tensile modulus (GPa)	Density (g/cc)
E-Glass [8]	3450	72	2.6
S-Glass [8]	4600	85	2.5
Kevlar-49 [9]	3790	124	1.4
Alumina [8]	1450	193	3.2
MS/LM Carbon [10]	4138	228	1.8
MS/MM Carbon [10]	4483	276	1.8
HS/MM Carbon [10]	7007	297	1.8
LS/HM Carbon [10]	2966	359	1.8
MS/VHM Carbon [10]	3938	552	1.9
MS/EHM Carbon [10]	4007	855	2.2

Note: LS, MS, HS = Low, medium, high strength; LM, MM, HM, VHM, EHM = Low, medium, high, very high, extremely high modulus

not available. It is known that the tensile strength of fiberglass at 83 K increases to 5310 MPa (54%) for E-Glass and 8275 MPa (80%) for S-Glass [8].

E-Glass is the lowest-cost fiber followed by S-Glass and then medium strength–low modulus carbon and Kevlar-49. The medium strength and extremely high modulus carbon and alumina fibers are the most expensive. The other carbon fibers are intermediate in price.

Resins. The resin matrix binds the fibers in their proper position, distributes the load between the fibers, protects them from abrasion and environment, provides the interlaminar shear strength, and controls the chemical resistance properties. Even though the elongation to failure of most cured epoxies is relatively low, they provide an unbeatable combination of cryogenic performance, structural excellence, processability, and cost [11]. In addition, epoxies are generally superior to polyesters in resisting moisture and other environmental influences [8]. Typical properties of thermoset resins are presented in Table 2-4. Tensile strength and most other mechanical properties increase at low temperatures [15].

Laminates. Cryogenic composites are typically fabricated by wet winding continuous fibers embedded in resin, winding prepreg tape or tow, laying up or forming woven fabric or other prepregs, or injection molding thermoplastic resins containing discontinuous fibers. The fiber placement is followed by some type of temperature or pressure cure process, or both. Resulting mechanical properties for representative materials are listed in Tables 2-5 and 2-6.

Cooling generally improves mechanical performance, but detailed data are limited. The strength of G-10CR increases ≈100% and the modulus increases ≈30% from 76 to 4 K [1]. From 295 to 20 K compressive strength is reported to increase 55% for S-Glass composite, 27% for Kevlar-49 composite, and 33% for carbon composite whereas modulus increases 16% for S-Glass composite and 32% for Kevlar-49 composite [20]. In general, filament-wound composite material strength increases at least 30%, and modulus increases at least 10% from 295 to 76 K [19].

Table 2-4 Typical properties of thermoset resins at 295 K

	Amine-cured epoxy[a]	Anhydride-cured epoxy[b]	Vinyl ester [8,13]
Tensile strength (MPa)	66	77	83
Tensile modulus (GPa)	3.4	3.4	3.6
Tensile failure strain (%)	32–83	21–41	28–41
Flexural strength (MPa)	110	145	138
Flexural modulus (GPa)	2.8	4.1	3.7
Shear strength (MPa)	59	52	
Shear modulus (GPa)	1.3	1.1	
Compressive strength (MPa)	88	138	
Compressive modulus (GPa)	3.2	3.3	
Compressive strain (%)	4	10	
Density (g/cc)	1.2	1.3	1.2
CTE (cm/cm °C)	47×10^{-6}	80×10^{-6}	65×10^{-6}
Outgassing			
Total mass loss (%)	0.17	0.18	
Collected material (%)	0.01	0.00	
Water vapor (%)	0.07	0.04	

[a] Such as 100 pbw Dow DER 332 or Shell EPON 826 with 45 pbw Huntsman T-403 or Shell EPON Agent Y [9,12,13,14].
[b] Such as Shell 58-68R or US Polymeric E-787 [50 pbw Epon 828/50 pbw Epon 1031/90 pbw NMA/0.55 pbw BDMA] [1,9,14]

Composites reinforced with discontinuous fibers, like Ultem 2100, have lower mechanical properties than those with continuous fibers but also lower thermal conductivity, as shown in Fig. 2-15. Of the continuous fiber–epoxy materials, glass and alumina offer the lowest thermal conductivity above 76 K and so are often the materials of choice for

Table 2-5 Typical properties of composite materials at 295 K

Composite properties	GR-10CR 65-wt% E-Glass Fabric* [1,16]	Ultem 2100 with 10% Chopped Glass Fiber [17]	Ultem 2300 with 30% Chopped Glass Fiber [17]	Quasi-isotropic 60-vol% Continuous MS/LM Carbon* [18]	Quasi-isotropic 60-vol% Continuous LS/HM Carbon* [18]
Strength (MPa)					
Longitudinal (tension)	309 minimum	114	169	552	434
Transverse (tension)	266 minimum	114	169	552	434
Longitudinal (compression)	357 minimum	152	214		
Transverse (compression)	288 minimum	152	214		
Longitudinal (flexural)	412 minimum	193	228		
Transverse (flexural)	330 minimum	193	228		
Shear	45	90	97		
Modulus (GPa)					
Longitudinal	30	4	6	55	131
Transverse	26	4	6	55	131
Shear	10	4	9	19	48
Density (g/cc)	1.8	1.3	1.5	1.5	1.6
CTE (cm/cm °C)		32×10^{-6}	20×10^{-6}	2.9×10^{-6}	0.09×10^{-6}

* In epoxy resin.

Table 2-6 Typical properties of unidirectional composites at 295 K [60-vol% continuous fibers in epoxy resin]

Composite properties	E-Glass [8,9,18]	S-Glass [9,19]	Kevlar-49 [8,19]	MS/LM Carbon [8,18]	MS/MM Carbon [9,19]	HS/MM Carbon [19]	LS/HM Carbon [9,18]
Strength, MPa							
Longitudinal (tension)	1034	1586	1379	1241	2876	3724	1103
Transverse (tension)	48	62	28	45	48	48	31
Longitudinal (comp.)	552	966	276	828	1897	2414	
Transverse (comp.)	138	138	138	138	207	207	
Shear	41	83	55	62	97	97	
Modulus, GPa							
Longitudinal	45	56	76	132	182	189	331
Transverse	12	9	6	10	9	9	6
Shear	4	6	2	7	5	5	4
Density, g/cc	2.1	2.0	1.4	1.5	1.5	1.5	1.6
CTE, cm/cm °C	10^{-6}	10^{-6}	10^{-6}	10^{-6}	10^{-6}	10^{-6}	10^{-6}
Longitudinal	6.7	6.3	−1.9	0.1	−0.3	0.1	0.3
Transverse	31	32	68	16	32	35	18

applications involving ambient to cryogenic temperatures. However, below 76 K, carbon and alumina offer low thermal conductance.

There are four basic fatigue failure mechanisms of composites: layer cracking, delamination, fiber breakage, and fiber–matrix debonding. Fatigue strength involves many variables, including the basic materials, fiber orientation, composite quality, testing parameters, and test specimen configuration. Thus, Fig. 2-16 shows relative fatigue performance of unidirectional reinforced composites assuming all other variables are the same. In general, higher modulus fibers provide the best fatigue strength. The fatigue endurance limits of Kevlar-49 and carbon composites approach 60% of their ultimate tensile strengths [8]. Fatigue performance improves at cryogenic temperatures as indicated by the S-Glass–epoxy data in Fig. 2-16.

Composite structures have low vibration susceptibility because of their high structural dampening properties. They generally do not exhibit creeping tendencies [14], and they have good radiation resistance at ambient and cryogenic temperatures [2].

Comparison with metals. Considerations in selecting a cryogenic material include tension, compression, flexural, shear, and torsion loads; fatigue, deflection, and vibration requirements; creep; temperature gradient; weight allowance; installation geometry; and, of course, cost trade-offs. Composites can often be the material of choice.

One approach to comparing composites and metals is to ratio critical values. For example, a low ratio of thermal conductivity to modulus or strength can improve system performance and reduce costs when structural components are subjected to temperature gradients. Composite materials have the advantage. For another example,

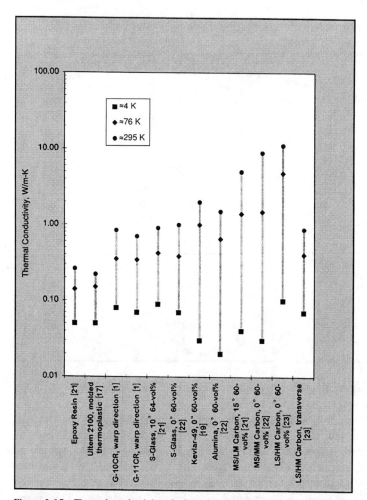

Figure 2-15 Thermal conductivity of selected composite materials.

high ratios of modulus or strength to density reduce weight and thus loads on equipment. Lowest-cost unidirectional E-Glass composites have an equivalent modulus/density ratio to steel or aluminum, but for strength/density the ratio is twice that of steel and five times that of aluminum. Unidirectional carbon composites provide specific tensile strengths that are three to eight times greater and specific moduli that are four to eight times greater than for steel or aluminum. Even quasiisotropic continuous carbon fiber composites have specific strengths and moduli higher than steel or aluminum.

2-2-3 Structural Design

Design approach. The design of composite structures is essentially the same as for metals except that the material must be designed along with the structure. The material consists of hundreds of thousands of continuous fibers that are precisely oriented in patterns to provide strength, stiffness, and other properties in exactly the amount and

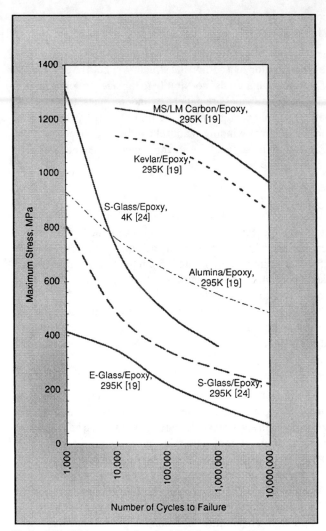

Figure 2-16   Fatigue properties of unidirectional composites.

direction needed. Material design parameters include fiber and matrix selection, fiber direction, fiber content, and fabrication process. Structure design consists of determining thickness, detailing exact configuration, and meeting performance requirements.

One of the composite designer's most difficult tasks is getting someone to accurately define the directions and magnitudes of all system structural and thermal loading requirements on the composite structure. Composites are anisotropic, exhibiting different properties along different axes. Strength, stiffness, thermal expansion, and other properties can vary by more than ten times in different directions. This allows highly efficient structures but also possibly failed structures if requirements are not adequately defined.

Minimum possible cost is almost always a very important design consideration. In addition to material and process costs, this involves designing for least complex structure, minimum part count, integral fittings, loosest possible tolerances, greatest reproducibility, and lowest life-cycle costs.

Design configuration. The configuration of a composite structure should be designed to maximize the advantages of composite materials, not simply to replace the configuration of a metal structure. Typical composite shapes are panels, cylinders, ducts, tubes, struts, cones, straps, rings, and shells. Possible configurations are limited only by the mandrel or mold used for fabrication. A filament winding mandrel can be any shape that does not have a reentrant curve. Injection molding cavities cannot have undercuts that keep the finished structure from being removed.

2-2-4 Composite Structure Uses

Fuel tanks. For a 33% weight savings, McDonnell Douglas is using medium strength–medium modulus carbon–epoxy instead of aluminum for the liquid hydrogen tanks on reusable launch vehicles [25]. The cylindrical tanks are 0.5-cm thick, 2.4 m in diameter, and 4.9 m high with elliptical end domes. They each hold 2700 kg of fuel. The tanks have no liners and no integral reinforcing elements.

Back on Earth, GR-10-type composites are used to support and insulate liquefied natural gas (LNG) tanks, both on ships and in storage facilities [1]. Other composite materials are being utilized for support of vacuum-jacketed LNG fuel tanks on trucks, buses, and trains.

Support straps. Filament-wound straps are utilized to provide structural support and thermal isolation for cryostats and superconducting magnets [26]. They are fabricated with glass, alumina, and carbon fibers in epoxy resin to reduce the parasitic heat flow into the cryogen. Composite straps are found in magnetic resonance imaging and magnetic energy storage systems as well as in space on the Space Shuttle, Hubble Spacecraft, Infrared Astronomical Satellite, and Cosmic Background Explorer. The straps currently range in size from 25 to 965 mm long, 1 to 25 mm wide, 0.31 to 4.39 mm thick, and 3.6 to 38 mm in pin diameter. The small glass–epoxy straps pictured in Fig. 2-17 support the cryogenic bus for the Navy's high-temperature superconductor experiments.

Nested tubes. Nested tubes allow the use of glass composite between ambient and 76 K and carbon composite below 76 K to optimize thermal performance. The first reentrant posts developed by the Fermi National Accelerator Laboratory for superconducting dipole magnets had G-10CR nested support tubes. Switching to carbon–epoxy for the inner tube, as depicted in Fig. 2-18, reduced the overall thermal conductivity [27]. To simplify manufacture, Fermilab then devised two composite tubes connected in series along the thermal path of the assembly: glass–epoxy for 20 to 295 K and carbon–epoxy for 4.5 to 30 K. The overlapped composite tubes are captured and held together through a shrink-fit joint configuration [28].

For the lower load requirements of superconducting quadrupole magnets, Babcock & Wilcox developed thermal isolation supports consisting of three Ultem 2300 molded post segments connected in series [29].

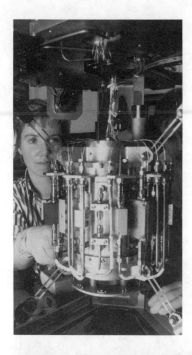

Figure 2-17   Composite support straps. (Courtesy Naval Research Laboratory.)

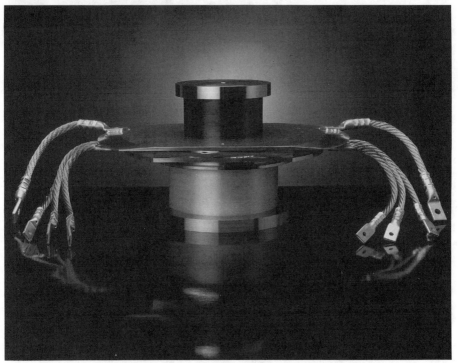

Figure 2-18   Nested composite tubes with heat intercepts. (Courtesy of Fermilab.)

Anchor tie bars. Fermilab also developed composite anchor tie bars for superconducting magnets. Because metals decrease in length at low temperatures, carbon fiber was selected and designed for dimensional stability. When cooled from 295 to 4.5 K, the 305 cm-long-carbon–epoxy structure grows 0.09 cm, whereas its two 15 cm-long-stainless steel ends shrink 0.045 cm for no net dimensional change [27].

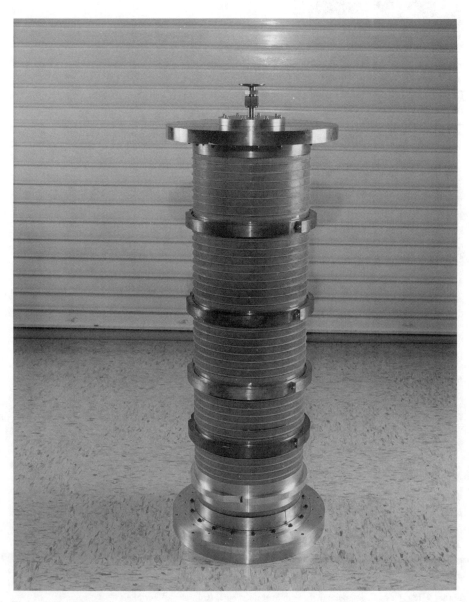

Figure 2-19 Composite necktube with stiffening ribs and metal fittings. (Courtesy Lockheed Martin.)

Dewar necktubes and struts. Lockheed Martin has built a large spacecraft dewar that is 2.2 m in diameter, 3.0-m high, and weighs 842 kg dry. The main aluminum tank contains 2328 L of He II weighing 338 kg at 1.8 K. The aluminum guard tank contains a maximum of 99 L of He I at 4.2 K, which is reduced to 30 L prior to launch using heaters [30]. The main tank is supported by twelve alumina fiber–epoxy struts off the vacuum shell. The guard tank is supported by the 0.51-mm-thick, 328-mm-diameter, 762-mm-long alumina fiber–epoxy necktube shown in Fig. 2-19. It has a 0.03-mm-thick titanium foil liner to provide a low-heat-leak, vacuum-tight cylinder connnecting the main tank to the vacuum shell. The necktube is reinforced on the outside with 33 alumina–epoxy stiffening ribs. The alumina fiber is as stiff as low modulus carbon fiber yet has half the thermal conductivity of glass below 35 K.

Commercial dewars, which are used mainly for medical and biological specimens, utilize low-cost GR-10CR necktubes.

Other applications. Other uses for composite structures include components for airborne magnetohydrodynamic power generators and magnetic fusion energy systems [1]. There are new imaging and spectroscopy applications for magnetic resonance that require composite materials. Compact, rugged, low-cost magnets with optimized suspension systems are needed to make broader applications in medicine possible, as well as industrial applications in process monitoring and nondestructive evaluation [14]. Low-thermal-conductivity, high-mechanical-performance, lightweight structures are also required for numerous applications in the energy, electronics, and transportation areas.

NOMENCLATURE

Alumina A reinforcement fiber of γ-form 85% Al_2O_3–15% SiO_2.

Anisotropic Not isotropic; exhibiting different properties when tested along axes in different directions.

Carbon A reinforcement fiber that is produced by the pyrolysis of organic precursor fibers, such as polyacrylonitrile and pitch, in an inert environment.

Composite material A material created from a fiber reinforcement and a resin matrix material; the constituents retain their identities but act in concert.

Composite structure A filament-wound, tape-wrapped, laid-up, molded, or shaped structure consisting of resin to which reinforcing fibers have been added before the forming operation.

E-Glass A calcium aluminoborosilicate reinforcement fiber.

Epoxy resin A broad range of epichlorohydrin-based resins, catalysts, curing agents, and sometimes other additives.

Fiber A general term used to refer to filamentary materials.

Fiber content The amount of fiber, expressed as volume or weight percent, in a composite.

G-10CR A cryogenic grade material consisting of 7628 fabric woven with continuous E-glass fiber in an amine-cure epoxy resin binder.

Kevlar-49 An organic polymer, in fiber form, composed of aromatic poly-amides having a para-type orientation; a trademark for aramid fiber.

Prepreg A ready-to-use fiber–resin material in either fabric or roving form.

Quasi isotropic Approximating isotrophy by orientation of fibers in several directions.

Resin The thermoset or thermoplastic matrix of a composite material.

S-Glass A magnesium aluminosilicate specially designed to provide high-tensile-strength glass fibers.

Thermoplastic A resin material capable of being repeatedly softened by heating and repeatedly hardened by cooling.

Thermoset A polymer resin that is cured by heat or catalyst into an infusible and insoluble material.

Ultem An amorphous thermoplastic polyetherimide resin.

Unidirectional Orientation of reinforcement fibers in one direction.

Vinyl ester The common name for an unsaturated resin prepared by the reaction of a monofunctional unsaturated acid with a bisphenol diepoxide, which results in better mechanical and chemical characteristics than polyester resin.

REFERENCES

1. Kasen, M. B., "Composites," in *Materials at Low Temperatures*, R. P. Reed and A. F. Clark, eds. (Metals Park, Ohio: American Society for Metals, 1983), 413–463.
2. Clark, A. F., Reed, R. P., and Hartwig, G., *Nonmetallic Materials and Composites at Low Temperatures* (New York: Plenum Press, 1979).
3. Clark, A. F., Reed, R. P., and Hartwig, G., *Nonmetallic Materials and Composites at Low Temperatures 2* (New York: Plenum Press, 1982).
4. Hartwig, G., and Evans, D., *Nonmetallic Materials and Composites at Low Temperatures 3* (New York: Plenum Press, 1986).
5. Schwartzberg, F. H. *Cryogenic Materials Data Handbook* (Revised) Vol. II, AFML-TDR-64-280 (Wright-Patterson Air Force Base, Ohio: Air Force Materials Laboratory, 1970).
6. Serafini, T. T., and Koenig, J. L., *Cryogenic Properties of Polymers* (New York: Marcel Dekker, 1968).
7. Tsai, S. W., *Composites Design*, 4th Ed. (Dayton, Ohio: Think Composites, 1988) and *Introduction to Composite Materials* (Lancaster, Pennsylvania: Technomic Publishing Company, 1980).
8. ASM International Handbook Committee, T. J. Reinhart, Technical Chairman, *Engineered Materials Handbook*, Vol. 1, *Composites* (Metals Park, Ohio: ASM International 1987).
9. Peters, S. T., Humphrey, W. D., and Foral, R. F., *Filament Winding Composite Structure Fabrication* (Covina, California: SAMPE Press, 1991).
10. Product data sheets from Amoco, BASF, Hercules, Hysol-Grafil, Mitsubishi, Toho, and Toray (1995).
11. Will, E. T., "Screening Programme to Select a Resin for Gravity Probe-B Composites," *Cryog.* 32, no. 2, (1992):179–184.
12. Chiao, T. T., and Moore, R. L., "An Epoxy for Advanced Fiber Composites," in *Proc. 29th Ann. Tech. Conf.*, (Washington, D.C.: Reinforced Plastics/Composites Institute, 1974), 7.
13. Product data sheets from Dow, Huntsman, and Shell (1995).
14. Morris, V. L., "Advanced Composite Structures for Superconducting Supercollider," *Supercollider 1*, Michael McAshan, ed. (New York: Plenum Press, 1989):525–535.
15. Reed, R. P., and Walsh, R. P., "Tensile Properties of Resins at Low Temperatures," Paper BZ-9 (Boulder, Colorado: Cryogenic Materials, Inc., 1993).
16. General Dynamics Space Systems Division Specification No. M6A-100102 (1992).
17. GE plastics product data sheets (1996).
18. "Design Guide for Advanced Composites Applications," *Advanced Composites Magazine* (1993):56–57.
19. Morris, V. L., "Advanced Composite Structures for Cryogenic Applications," in *34th International SAMPE Proceedings* (Covina, California; SAMPE Press, 1989), 1867–1876.

20. Abdel Mohsen, H. H., and Abdelsalam, M. K., "Optimal Design of Cryogenic Bucking Cylinder for Space Borne Toroidal Magnets," *Adv. Cryog. Eng.* 35 (1990): 813–814.
21. Parmley, R. T., "Passive Orbital Disconnect Strut Structural Test Program," NASA Contractor Report 177325 (1990).
22. National Institute of Standards and Technology (NIST) Data (1983–1990)
23. Stampfl, E., Personal communication, Aerospace Corporation, Los Angeles, California (1991).
24. Morris, E. E., "Filament Wound Composite Thermal Isolator Structures for Cryogenic Dewars and Instruments," in *Composites for Extreme Environments*, N. R. Adsit, ed. (Philadelphia: American Society for Testing and Materials, 1982), 95–117.
25. McConnell, V. P., "DC-XA Spacecraft to Fly First Composite Liquid Hydrogen Fuel Tank," *High-Performance Composites* 4, no. 2 (1996):80–82.
26. Morris, V. L., "Engineered Composite Structures for Cryogenic Systems," *Adv. Cryog. Eng.* 39 (1994): 2021–2039.
27. Nicol, T. H., Niemann, R. C., and Gonczy, J. D., "Design and Analysis of the SSC Dipole Magnet Suspension System," in *Supercollider 1*, Michael McAshan, ed. (New York: Plenum Press, 1989), 637–649.
28. Boroski, W. N., Nichol, T. H., Ruschman, M. K., and Schoo, C. J., "Thermal and Structural Performance of a Single Tube Support Post for the SSC Dipole Magnet Cryostat," *Adv. Cryog. Eng.* 39 (1994):1699–1705.
29. Hiller, M. W., and Waynert, J. A., "A Cryogenic Support Post for the SSC Quadrupole Magnets," in *Supercollider 4*, Michael McAshan, ed. (New York: Plenum Press, 1992).
30. Parmley, R., *Progress Report on the Relativity Mission Superfluid Helium Flight Dewar*, Lockheed Martin (Palo Alto California: Palo Alto Research Laboratory, 1995).

2-3 CRITICAL CURRENT-DENSITY IN Bi,Pb(2223) TAPES

R. Flükiger

University of Geneva, DPMC, 24, Quai Ernest Ansermet, Geneva, 1211, Switzerland

2-3-1 Introduction

The development of superconducting tapes for industrial applications started immediately after the discovery of the high T_c compounds $Bi_2Sr_2Ca_2Cu_3O_{10}$ (or Bi-2223), with $T_c = 110$ K, and $Bi_2Sr_2Ca_1Cu_2O_8$ (or Bi-2212), with $T_c = 92$ K, by Maeda et al. [1]. In the meantime, much progress has been achieved, and the immediate goal of industrial fabrication is the manufacture of long lengths of superconducting tapes for energy cables, current limiters, and transformers. Both compounds mentioned above have been studied, but the main effort has been concentrated on the compound Bi-2223, which shows less sensitivity to magnetic fields at the temperature of liquid nitrogen (77 K).

Substantial progress has been made in the last few years in the understanding of both thermal processes and microstructure as well as in the fabrication of long multifilamentary tapes by means of appropriate deformation steps. The aim of this section is to review briefly the recent developments of short and long multifilamentary Bi-2223 tapes with high critical current densities because this material is promising for future applications.

2-3-2 Fabrication of Bi-2223 Tapes

Multifilamentary silver (Ag)-sheathed tapes based on lead (Pb)-stabilized Bi-2223 can be used in a wide temperature range, which extends from 77 to 4.2 K. The most applied

Table 2-7 The critical current of mono- and multifilamentary Bi,Pb (2223) tapes with their number of filaments, superconductor content, and references

Filaments	Superconductor content	Critical-current density (A/cm^2)	Length (m)	Reference
Thin films		1,000,000 at 70 K and 0 T		Yamasaki et al. [13]
1		69,000 at 77 K and 77 K	0.02	Li et al. [12]
1	≈0.40	66,000 at 77 K and 77 K	0.02	Yamada et al. [14]
1	≪	140,000 at 4.2 K and 20 T	≪	≪
1	≈0.40	43,000 at 77 K and 0 T	0.02	Grasso et al. [9]
1	≈0.40	35,000 at 77 K and 0 T	20	Grasso et al. [9]
1		35,000 at 70 K and 0 T		Zhou et al. [15]
85	0.27	54,600 at 77 K and 0 T	0.02	Fleshler et al. [6]
313		39,700 at 77 K and 0 T		Fleshler et al. [6]
multifilamentary	0.29	27,800 at 77 K and 0 T	114	Hayashi et al. [4]
≪	0.29	24,000 at 77 K and 0 T	479	≪
≪	0.29	17,700 at 77 K and 0 T	1,200	≪
55	0.25	33,000 at 77 K and 0 T	0.02	Leghissa et al. [7]
55	0.25	29,000 at 77 K and 0 T	10	≪
55	0.25	22,000 at 77 K and 0 T	400	≪
37		12,000 at 77 K and 0 T	1,260	Haldar et al. [5]
37	0.25	28,000 at 77 K and 0 T	14.5	Marti et al. [8]
37	0.25	200,000 at 4.2 K and 0 T	14.5	≪
37	0.25	80,000 at 4.2 K and 15 T	14.5	≪
34	0.27	30,000 at 77 K and 0 T	10	Grasso et al. [10]

technique for producing Ag-sheathed Bi-2223 tapes is the so-called powder-in-tube (PIT) method [2]. The highest reported values of j_c (77 K, 0 T), the critical-current densities at 77 K, and zero field for Bi-2223 tapes with lengths >10 m are listed in Table 2-7. (The values of j_c are defined for the superconducting cross section.) Strong efforts are being undertaken to fabricate tapes in kilometer lengths with critical current densities comparable to those of short tapes. The goal of these developments is not only to enhance the value of critical current density in the superconducting core (j_c) but also the engineering critical-current density (j_e) taken over the whole cross section. Actually, the content of superconductor is ≈25%, but values of 30–35% are envisaged.

At the end of 1996, the highest published value of j_c at 77 K, the temperature of liquid nitrogen, and at zero magnetic field (0 T) was around 40,000 A/cm^2 for long Bi-2223 tapes with 85 filaments [6]. For tapes with 37 filaments, a value of 28,500 A/cm^2 over 14.5 m has been reported [8]. Values as high as 55,000 A/cm^2 were reported for short lengths (<5 cm) of Bi-2223 tapes produced by industrial rolling procedures [2]. It can be expected that the highest value reported so far for short pressed Bi-2223 tapes, j_c (77 K, 0 T) = 69,000 A/cm^2 (see Table 2-7) will one day be reached for long industrial tapes.

The particular requirements for a sheath material for Bi-2223 or Bi-2212 tapes have so far only been satisfied by Ag, which is inert to oxygen as well as to the superconducting oxide and is permeable to oxygen. It is now commonly admitted that Ag has no "poisoning" effect on the formation of the bismuth-based superconductors.

0.2 mm

Figure 2-20 Typical transversal cross section of a multifilamentary Bi-2223 tape with 55 filaments (from Ref. [8]).

Nevertheless, the interaction between the Ag from the sheath and the precursor powders forming the core of the tape influences the formation of Bi-2223; Ag does not dissolve in the Bi-2223 phase but rather in the transient liquid and has thus to be regarded as an additional constituent of the complex Bi—Pb—Sr—Ca—Cu—O system [3].

Various powder types can be used for the fabrication of Bi-2223 tapes, but they all have a common point: the phase Bi-2223 must be formed by a reaction at the end of the tape deformation process [3]. Precursor mixtures of coprecipitated powders of cation ratio $Bi_{1.72}Pb_{0.34}Sr_{1.83}Ca_{1.97}Cu_{3.13}$ are calcined two times at a temperature of 800–820 °C for 24 h with an intermediate grinding step. Powders with average grain size of the order of 5–10 μm are filled into 6 × 4 mm (o.d. × i.d.) pure Ag tubes and compacted with a piston using a pressure of about 2 kbar. The tubes are properly sealed and then deformed by drawing them to an overall diameter of several millimeters after which they are drawn to a hexagonal shape. The hexagonal rods are bundled together and stacked into a Ag tube, which is deformed to final tape thicknesses of 200–250 μm, the width varying between 2.5 and 4 mm. A cross section of a multifilamentary tape after the deformation process is shown in Fig. 2-20. Particular attention has to be given to the deformation procedure to prevent cracks perpendicular to the longitudinal direction, which cause irreversible damage to the critical-current density.

Recently, a new deformation technique for multifilamentary tapes was introduced based on a motor-driven four-roll machine that permits the simultaneous reduction of thickness and width of the samples [10]. It was found that the rolling force on the tape is also more homogeneous than when using a conventional two-roll machine. Square monofilamentary wires of about 1- to 1.5-mm width were prepared by using the four-roll machine, the final dimensions being the same as for the usual tapes (i.e., 250-μm thickness and 3-mm width). The reaction conditions were the same in both types of Bi-2223 tapes. The advantages of the square symmetry are evident when comparing the cross sections of the multifilamentary tapes. In Fig. 2-21, two different cross sections are

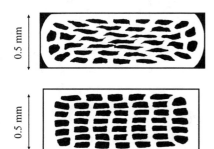

0.5 mm

0.5 mm

Figure 2-21 Transverse cross sections of two multifilamentary Bi-2223 tapes at an intermediate thickness of 500 mm. Upper cross section: standard tape, 37 filaments; lower cross section: four-rolled, 45 filaments (from Ref. [10]).

shown at an intermediate size of 500 μm $\times$ 2.0 mm. The upper cross section represents a standard multifilamentary tape with 37 filaments and a superconducting fraction of 20%. The lower cross section represents a four-rolled tape with 45 filaments and a superconducting fraction of about 35%. As shown in Fig. 2-20, the filaments near the center in standard tapes are more compressed than those at the sides, whereas the four-rolled ones show a homogeneous compression [10]. In addition, the distances between the single filaments show much higher fluctuations for the standard tape than for the four-rolled tape [10].

Once the final thickness is reached, the tapes have to be submitted to a reaction heat treatment, during which the original Bi-2212 phase first transforms to Bi,Pb-2212 and then to the final Bi-2223 phase. The empirically determined ideal reaction temperatures in air are 830 to 840 °C, the total reaction time being of the order of 200 h. A reduction of the oxygen partial pressure leads to a lowering of the reaction temperature to 820–825 °C and to shorter reaction times, thus allowing a more economical fabrication. In order to reach high critical-current densities, the reaction heat treatment has to be combined with one or more intermediate rolling steps. This thermomechanical treatment enhances the density inside the oxide core, thus creating the appropriate conditions for a large number of current-carrying grain boundaries.

The choice of the appropriate heat treatment and deformation parameters has a strong effect on the value of j_c. In air, a strong correlation between the value of j_c and the reaction temperature has been found [9]. In Fig. 2-22, the variation of j_c

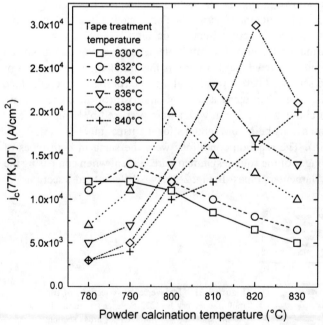

Figure 2-22 Variation of j_c with reaction temperature for a monofilamentary Bi-2223 tape. The reaction time was 200 at all temperatures (from Ref. [9]).

(77 K, 0 T) as a function of the reaction temperature for 200-h long heat treatments on rolled monofilamentary Bi,Pb(2223) tapes exhibits a sharp maximum. The value of j_c is lowered by 50% for reaction temperature differences as small as 1–2 °C. This effect can cause serious problems when reacting long tapes, a very high temperature homogeneity ($\Delta T < 1$ °C) being required over the whole furnace volume to achieve high j_c values reproducibly. It was found that the maximum shown in Fig. 2-22 is less marked when reacting in an atmosphere with reduced oxygen partial pressure. This explains why many manufacturers carry out their reactions in an atmosphere containing 7% oxygen, which has the additional advantage of a shorter reaction time.

At the end of the deformation process by cold rolling, the Bi-2212 grains in the unreacted tapes are already clearly oriented in the tape plane. A correlation was found between the texture in the Bi-2212 grains after rolling and the texture of the current-carrying Bi-2223 grains after reaction in monofilamentary as well as in monofilamentary tapes. The high degree of texturing of the Bi-2212 platelets after deformation is thus a necessary condition for high j_c values.

The rolling process between subsequent deformation heat treatments is strongly dependent on the forces acting during deformation. It has been shown [9] that on short tape lengths, the uniaxial pressure can be enhanced without damage up to 2 GPa, whereas for industrial tape lengths the deformation by rolling shows a sharp maximum at 0.6 GPa (see Fig. 2-23). This difference is easily explained by the fact that the rolling process induces a gliding of the grains, thus favoring the formation of cracks perpendicular to the tape length.

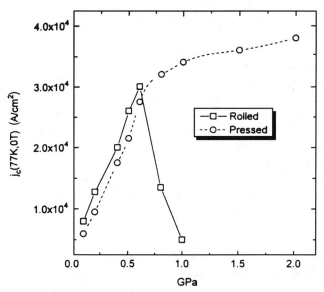

Figure 2-23 Critical-current density at 77 K and 0 T as a function of the pressure exerted on a Bi-2223 tape due to the deformation steps between the reaction heat treatments, either by pressing or by rolling (from Ref. [9]).

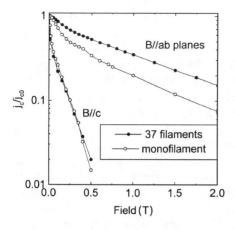

Figure 2-24 Normalized critical-current density of both mono- and multifilamentary Bi-2223 tapes as a function of applied field and field orientation at 77 K (from Ref. [8]).

2-3-3 Variation of j_c (B) for Multifilamentary Bi-2223 Tapes

Critical-current densities at $T = 77$ K. The variation of j_c as a function of applied field for a multifilamentary Bi-2223 tape with j_c (77 K, 0 T) = 28,000 A/cm^2 is represented in Fig. 2-24. The critical current density was measured over a total length of 14.5 m [8], the thickness was 200 μm, the width 3.5 mm, the superconducting cross section 20%, and the critical current $I_c = 37$ A. It is seen in Fig. 2-24 that the critical-current density decreases much more slowly when the magnetic fields are applied parallel to the surface ($B_{//}$). At 1 T, the value of j_c is 10,000 A/cm^2, which corresponds to an engineering value of $j_e = 6200$ A/cm^2. The value at 77 K and a field of 1 T can be considered as a reference for the quality of the tape: the values I_c (0)/I_c (0.5 T) = 3.8 and I_c (0 T)/I_c (1 T) = 3 in Fig. 2-24 are the lowest reported so far [6,8]. Figure 2-24 illustrates the anisotropy of the critical-current density in Bi-2223 tapes, the decrease of j_c versus B being very rapid when the field is applied perpendicularly to the tape surface ($B_\perp$), for the current falls to negligibly small values above $B \approx 0.5$ T.

As a consequence of the marked anisotropy of j_c, it follows that at 77 K all field components $B_\perp$ perpendicular to the tape surface have to be avoided. These perpendicular field components will limit the achievable magnetic field in a solenoid to 0.6–0.8 T at 77 K. If one takes into account that the field requirement for energy storage rings is of the order of 4–5 T, it is clear that it cannot be satisfied by the actual Bi-2223 material. On the other hand, this material is still envisaged for energy cables, transformers, and current limiters at 77 K, provided that the AC losses can be kept at a sufficiently low level. It follows that the reduction of the critical current anisotropy is one of the main goals of future developments of Bi-2223 tapes.

Critical current densities at intermediate temperatures (20–40 K). The critical current anisotropy can be strongly reduced when lowering the operating temperature to values of the order of 20–40 K. A further advantage is the simultaneously observed gradual enhancement of j_c with decreasing temperatures: The maximum value is obtained at 4.2 K, where the values of j_c are a factor ≈ 6 higher than the values of j_c at 77 K. Temperatures below 77 K can be produced by Gifford–McMahon cryocoolers, and the construction of prototype magnets producing fields of the order of 10 T in this

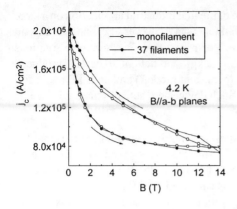

Figure 2-25 Critical current densities as a function of magnetic field and of its history at 4.2 K for mono- and multifilamentary Bi-2223 tapes (from Ref. [8]).

temperature range is actually under study in various companies. Nevertheless, economic arguments are still in favor of 77 K as an operating temperature.

Critical current densities at 4.2 K. The slow variation of j_c versus B for rolled Bi-2223 tapes at 4.2 K is of particular interest in view of their application for very high field magnets at temperatures ranging between 4.2 and 27 K, the boiling temperatures of helium and neon, respectively. Compounds Bi-2212 and Bi-2223 can be used at 4.2 K as an operating temperature, but Bi-2223 is mainly chosen. The variation of j_c versus $B_{//}$, the magnetic field applied parallel to the tape surface, for the same rolled tape as above with j_c (77 K, 0 T) = 28,000 A/cm² is shown in Fig. 2-25 up to $B = 15$ T [3]. The critical-current density values at 4.2 K in Fig. 2-25 are of the order of 220,000 A/cm² and 75–80,000 A/cm² at 0 and 14 T, respectively, the ratio I_c (0 T)/ I_c (14 T) being ≈2.5–2.7. The low anisotropy of j_c at 4.2 K can be illustrated by the low ratio j_c $(B_{//})/j_c$ $(B_\perp) \approx 1.4$–1.5 at $B = 14$ T.

It is interesting to compare these values with those of classical superconductors. From the behavior in Fig. 2-25, critical current density values of >75,000 A/cm² can be extrapolated for $B \approx 20$ T. Taking into account a superconducting cross section of 20–25%, this corresponds to an "overall" value of 15,000–18,000 A/cm². The classical systems Nb_3Sn, Nb_3Al, and $PbMo_6S_8$ are known to exhibit values of 20,000 A/cm² at 20 T but at a lower temperature, 2 K. At higher fields, however, the value for Bi-2223 remains quite constant, whereas the value for the classical systems decreases rapidly. Since the actual critical-current densities for long, rolled Bi-2223 tapes are a factor 2 below the highest reported ones on pressed tapes, it follows that without any doubt, Bi-2223 is an adequate material for the fabrication of very high field magnets at the operating temperature of 4.2 K.

Recently, a hybrid magnet of 40-mm diameter producing 1.5 T in a background field of 22.5 T was successfully tested in Japan, thus establishing the record value of 24 T at 4.2 K. From a comparison with the data plotted in Fig. 2-25, it follows that even higher fields can be produced using Bi-2223 tapes. It is noteworthy that the main problem arising when producing very high field magnets based on Bi,Pb(2223) tapes is not the critical current density but the mechanical strength necessary to withstand the important Lorentz forces at high fields. By alloying magnesium to the silver sheath, the mechanical properties of the tapes have been enhanced in the last years [11,18]. It is expected that the construction of high-field magnets will be one of the first industrial application on a large scale for HTC superconductors. From the available data, however, it cannot yet be said whether HTC magnets can be operated in the "persistent mode." Alternative solutions for high-field NMR have been proposed (e.g., a background field of 20 or 21 T produced by a classical Nb_3Sn magnet operated in the "persistent mode,") and an HTC insert coil controlled by a high-stability power supply. Such devices are actually planned, but it is too early to predict their impact on the market.

Reinforcement of Bi,Pb(2223) tapes by dispersion hardening. It is obvious that the problem of mechanical stability of Bi,Pb(2223) tapes has to be solved when envisaging magnets producing magnetic fields well above 20 T in a reproducible manner. It is known that the irreversible strain in Bi,Pb(2223) tapes is enhanced from 0.2 to 0.6% when going from the mono- to the multifilamentary configuration [11,18]. Several mechanisms have been proposed, all being based on dispersion hardening of Ag by alloying small quantities of other elements (e.g., Mg, Mn, or Sb). The tensile stress of reinforced multifilamentary Bi,Pb(2223) tapes increased from 80–100 MPa for pure Ag to 200–250 MPa for the dispersion-hardened Ag. The latter value is close to the value for multifilamentary Nb_3Sn wires, which is encouraging. However, a compromise must always be found between hardening of the Ag sheath and low reaction with the Bi,Pb(2223) phase, thus limiting the amount of additive to total contents of the order of 1 wt % [11,18].

Enhancement of the matrix resistivity. A second reason for the use of dispersion-hardened Ag is the very low electrical resistivity of the latter, which leads to high AC losses—a serious obstacle on the way to industrial applications (e.g., cables, transformers, current limiters, or motors). The problem is due to the fact that all alloyed elements mentioned above oxidize during the reaction heat treatment, either in air or in a 7% oxygen atmosphere. This leads in all cases to a "cleaning effect," the content of the additives in Ag being lowered, thus causing a lower electrical resistivity of Ag, which in turn causes higher AC losses. At present, the enhancement of the electrical resistivity of Ag at 77 K between neighboring filaments as a consequence of dispersion hardening has not exceeded a factor 2–3, which is insufficient. The only exception, Gold, has to be excluded for economic reasons. Another possibility to reduce AC losses is to twist the filaments, the twist pitch being of the order of 10 mm or less. Unfortunately, this technique is still unsatisfactory due to "bridging" between neighboring filaments. In our laboratory, a promising new technique has been introduced very recently [19] consisting of surrounding each filament in a multifilamentary tape by an "oxide barrier." This thin barrier consists of $BaZrO_3$, which leads to considerably enhanced electrical resistivities between the filaments and does not react with the superconducting core. Actually, this new "oxide barrier" technique has already been proven to lower the AC losses in multifilamentary Bi-2223 tapes [19], and major efforts are being placed on further development.

2-3-4 Conclusion

The highest possible critical current densities in industrial multifilamentary Bi-2223 tapes have not yet been reached, and a dynamic development is expected in the next years. The highest reported critical current values known to the author at the end 1996 have been listed in Table 2-7. However, even after having reached the highest short tape values [3–7,9] in long tapes, the "overall" or engineering critical-current density will not be sufficient for producing magnetic fields higher than 0.6–0.8 T at 77 K. As an example, energy storage devices should be operated at 4–5 T, which constitutes a goal that will be hard to reach with Bi,Pb(2223) tapes at the present level of development. For prototypes, it is actually envisaged to lower the operating temperature to 20–40 K by means of cryocoolers.

In view of the high level of technology of Bi-2223 tapes, it is worthwhile to continue the search for further enhancement of the current-carrying properties.

The most important reasons for a limitation of the engineering critical-current density j_e are the following:

1. Inhomogeneity of the precursors (composition, size, impurities).
2. Phase diagram and phase formation conditions (reaction heat treatment).
3. Homogeneity of the deformation process ("sausaging").
4. Microstructure and quality of grain boundaries.
5. Anisotropy of the critical-current density.

It is not the purpose of this section to discuss these points in detail, but it appears that all of them need further understanding and more experimental work. The most important improvements, however, could be obtained if it would be possible to introduce defects at an atomic level in order to enhance the pinning behavior of the grains and to get j_c values closer to the values reported in thin films, which are 20 to 50 times higher at 77 K (see Table 2-7). A second important requirement is the reduction of the observed anisotropy of the critical-current density at 77 K. Proton irradiation experiments have already shown that the decrease of j_c for $B_\perp$ tape surface can be reduced substantially [16]. The question is whether other processes can be found that introduce a partial disorder in the Bi,Pb(2223) structure.

The recent development of the competing Y(123) or R.E.(123) systems by deposition methods may be another alternative when envisaging industrial applications at the operating temperature of the liquid nitrogen [17]. The fabrication of such tapes requires the use of very sophisticated deposition techniques and yields not only good critical current densities at 77 K but also a reduced anisotropy compared with the one of Bi-2223. It appears, however, that it will be far more difficult to fabricate long multifilamentary tapes using these techniques than by using the powder-in-tube method, which is certainly the most economical one for tapes of kilometer lengths.

REFERENCES

1. Maeda, H., Tanaky, Y., Fukotomi, M., Asano, T., Togano, K., Kumakura, H., Uehara, M., Ikeda, S., Ogawa, K., Horiuchi, S., and Matsui, Y., *Japn. J. Appl. Phys.* 27 (1988):L209.
2. Flükiger, R., Graf, T., Decroux, M., Groth, C., and Yamada, Y., *IEEE Trans. Magn.* MAG-27 (1991):1258.
3. Flükiger, R., Grasso, G., Hensel, B., Däumling, M., Gladyshevskii, R., Jeremie, A., Grivel, J. C., and Perin, A., in *Bismuth Based High Temperature Superconductors*, H. Maeda and K. Togano, eds. (New York: Marcel Dekker, 1996), 319–356.
4. Hayashi, K., Hahakura, S., Saga, N., Kobayashi, S., Kato, T., Ueyama, M., Hikata, T., Ohkura, K., and

Sato, K., *IEEE Trans. Appl. Supercond.* 7 (1997):221.

5. Balachandran, U., Iyer, A. N., Jammy, R., Chudzik, M., Helovic, M., Krishanaraj, P., Eror, N. G., and Haldar, P., *IEEE Trans. Appl. Supercond.* 7 (1997).

6. Fleshler, S., Li, Q., Parrella, D., Walsh, P. J., Michels, W. J., Riley, G. N., Jr., Carter, W. L., and Kunz, B., in *Critical Currents in Superconductors.* Teruo Matsushita and Kaoru Yamafuji, eds. (Singapore: World Scientific, 1996), 81.

7. Leghissa, M., Fischer, B., Roas, B., Jenovelis, A., Wiezorek, J., Kautz, S., and Neumüller, H. W., *IEEE Trans. Appl. Supercond.* 7 (1997):357.

8. Marti, F., Grasso, G., Huang, Y., and Flükiger, R., *IEEE Trans. Appl. Supercond.* 7 (1997):2211.

9. Grasso, G., Jeremie, A., and Flükiger, R., *Supercond. Sci. Technol.* 8 (1995):827; and Grasso, G., Marti, F., Jeremie, A., and Flükiger R., in *Adv. Supercond.* VII (1966):855.

10. Grasso, G., and Flükiger R. (paper delivered at ISS 96, Sapporo, Japan, 21–24 October 1996).

11. Goldacker, W., Mossang, E., Quilitz, M., and Rikel, M., *IEEE Trans. Appl. Supercond.* 7 (1997):1407.

12. Li, Q., Broderson, K., Hjuler, H. A., and Freltoft, T., *Physica C* 217 (1993):360.

13. Yamasaki, H., Endo, K., Kosaka, S., Umeda, M., Yoshida, S., and Kajimura, K., *IEEE Trans. Appl. Supercond.* 3 (1993):1536.

14. Yamada, Y., Satou, M., Murase, S., Kitamura, T., and Kamisada, Y., in *Proc. 5th Int. Symp. Supercond. (ISS 92)*, Y. Bando and Y. Yamauchi, eds. (Tokyo: Springer–Verlag 1993), 717.

15. Zhou, R., Huilts, W. L., Sebring, R. J., Bingert, J. F., Coulter, J. Y., Willis, J. O., and Smith, J. L., *Physica C* 255 (1995):275.

16. Safar, H., Cho, J. H., Fleshler, S., Maley, M. P., Willis, J. O., Coulter, J. Y., Ulmann, J. L., Lisowski, P. W., Riley, G. N., Jr., Rupich, M. W., Thompson, J. R., and Krusin–Elbaum, L., *Appl. Phys. Lett.*, 67 (1995):130.

17. Hawsey, R., and Peterson, D., *Superconductor Industry* (Fall 1996):23.

18. Kessler, J., Blüm, S., Wildgruber, U., and Goldacker, W., *J. Alloys Comp.* 195 (1993):511.

19. Flükiger, R., Huang, Y., Grasso, G., Kwasnitza, K., Marti, F., Erb, A., and Clerc, S. (paper delivered at SPA 97, Xi'an, China, 6–8 March 1997).

2-4 MAGNETIC MATERIALS FOR CRYOGENIC REFRIGERATION

J. L. Hall

Jet Propulsion Laboratory, MS 157–316, 4800 Oak Grove Drive, Pasadena, CA 91109

J. A. Barclay

Cryofuel Systems—University of Victoria, P.O. Box 3055, Victoria, BC V8W 3P6, Canada

X. Y. Liu

Integrated Manufacturing Technologies Institute, National Research Council of Canada, 800 Collip Circle, London, Ontario, Canada N6G 4X8

2-4-1 Introduction

There are two ways in which magnetic materials are used in devices that refrigerate at cryogenic temperatures: (1) as an active substance that produces cooling due to the magnetocaloric effect and (2) as a high-heat capacity, passive regenerator material below

15 K. An example of the former is gadolinium gallium garnet (GGG) used in a 4-K Carnot cycle magnetic refrigerator [1]; an example of the latter is Er_3Ni used in the second-stage regenerator of a 4-K Gifford–McMahon cryocooler [2].

This section will focus on active refrigerant materials and briefly mention recent activity in passive magnetic regenerator materials [3]. Data for typical materials are presented in tabular and graphical form with references where additional information can be found. Note that the references and examples included in this article are not intended to be an exhaustive list. The reader is encouraged to check the latest literature because important new materials are being added frequently in this rapidly evolving field. This section also includes a short glossary of terms commonly used in magnetic refrigeration. More general discussions of terminology, magnetism, and magnetic properties of materials can be found in numerous books, including Refs. [4–7].

Magnetic refrigeration is based on the physics of the magnetocaloric effect. First discovered by Weiss and Piccard in 1918 [8], it is the physical process by which some magnetic materials experience a temperature change when subjected to a magnetic field under adiabatic conditions. Several thermodynamic cycles can be implemented using this effect typically involving magnetization and demagnetization processes coupled with heat transfer to and from the magnetic material. Magnetic analoges to the standard gas compression cycles exist (e.g., Carnot, Brayton, Ericcson) in addition to a unique cycle called active magnetic regenerative refrigeration (AMRR). Numerous references are available for both the basic physics of the magnetocaloric effect and its implementation in various types of magnetic refrigeration cycles [9–14]. We shall restrict ourselves here to a brief summary of the important material properties for the engineering designer.

The magnetocaloric effect of a particular magnetic material is a function of applied field and temperature. The effect increases monotonically with increasing field for most materials and has a maximum value at the magnetic phase transition temperature of the material. For simple ferromagnetic materials like gadolinium, the adiabatic temperature change (ΔT) as a function of temperature is caret-shaped and centered on the Curie temperature of 293 K, as illustrated in Fig. 2-26. The limited width of the temperature profile means that the designer must select a material that has a magnetic phase transition near the desired refrigeration temperature. For large temperature spans between source and sink, this often requires the layering of several materials to obtain adequate refrigeration over the span [12,13]. Of equal importance is the fact that the magnetocaloric effect is only of the order of 1 K per tesla of applied magnetic induction field for the best available materials based on rare-earth elements. This motivates the use of high-field superconducting magnets to provide sufficient heat pumping in most practical applications. The desire to provide refrigeration at all temperatures below 25 °C with as small a magnet (magnetic field) as possible has driven research into new materials that have a variety of transition temperatures and large magnetocaloric effects [15–27].

Additional design considerations arise when these magnetic solids are fabricated into porous regenerator geometries and coupled with a circulating fluid to facilitate heat transfer with the thermal load and environment. Ductile refrigerants are preferred to brittle materials that are difficult to fabricate into the desired form, whether they be particles, wire screens, or thin plates. Mechanical strength is a concern because of the necessity to withstand the large magnetic forces that can exist between regenerator and

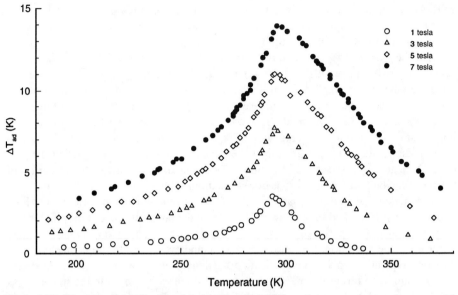

Figure 2-26 Magnetocaloric effect in gadolinium (from Ref. [20]).

magnet. Finally, eddy current generation in material exposed to time-varying magnetic fields can be a concern in higher-frequency refrigerators, leading to the use of low-electrical-conductivity material in highly discrete forms [28].

2-4-2 Classification of Magnetic Refrigerant Materials

The magnetic refrigerants can be grouped into five categories:

1. Rare-earth elements and their solid solution alloys.
2. Intermetallic compounds.
3. Nonmetallic (dielectric) compounds.
4. Amorphous materials and nanocomposites.
5. Exotic materials.

The rare-earth elements form the basis of virtually all practical magnetic refrigerants. This is due to their electronic structure in which unpaired electrons in the $4f$ orbitals generate high intrinsic magnetic moments for the atoms. The rare-earth elements and intra-rare-earth solid solution alloys tend to be ductile, have a relatively low electrical conductivity, and have large values of ΔT_{ad}. The physical and chemical properties of the rare-earths are documented extensively in the multivolume series by Gschneidner and Eyring [29].

Rare-earth elements can be combined with other metals to form intermetallic compounds like $GdNi_2$ and $GdPd$ [15]. These tend to be brittle materials that often have a reduced magnetocaloric effect due to the diluting effects of the non-rare-earth element.

There are a very large number of such materials, however, some of which offer superior performance in certain temperatures ranges [3,15,30].

A variety of nonmetallic elements can be combined with rare-earth elements to produce dielectric compounds. Gadolinium gallium garnet (GGG or $Gd_3Ga_5O_{12}$) is the most common example along with various dysprosium-oxygen-metal compounds [16]. These refrigerants have typically been used in their paramagnetic state for refrigeration below 20 K. This is in contrast to the rare-earth metals, alloys, and compounds in Categories 1 and 2 that are usually used at the transition point between paramagnetism and an ordered state (e.g., ferromagnetism).

Amorphous and nanocomposite materials based on rare-earth elements are a promising class of materials in the early stages of development at the time of this writing. Amorphous refrigerant materials are typically produced by extremely rapid cooling of molten alloy that is composed of a rare-earth metal with one or more alloying elements to facilitate glassification [31]. Potential advantages of amorphous materials over their crystalline counterparts include easily variable magnetic phase transition temperatures, reduced brittleness, and lower electrical conductivity [32]. Nanocomposites are materials with nanosized crystalline species dispersed in the matrix. The magnetic properties of these materials are currently under investigation [33].

Exotic materials are those magnetic refrigerants that do not fit into the other categories. A prime example is the iron–rhodium alloy $Fe_{49}Rh_{51}$ [34]. This material exhibits a very large adiabatic temperature change of −8 K at a field of only 2 T.

2-4-3 Representative Magnetic Refrigerant Data

Table 2-8 presents a list of some important magnetic refrigerants sorted by magnetic ordering temperature. It includes the peak ΔT_{ad} at high field and references for both the magnetocaloric effect data and any usage of the material in an experimental refrigeration device. Table 2-9 presents some selected property data for the key rare-earth elements, including density, room temperature, heat capacity, and yield strength.

Figure 2-26 presents the magnetocaloric effect data as a function of field for gadolinium. Figure 2-27 is a graph of ΔT_{ad} versus temperature at high field for five of the materials that have been used experimentally in a prototype refrigerator: Gd, Tb, Dy, $Gd_{0.2}Ho_{0.8}$, and $GdNi_2$. Figure 2-28 presents ΔT_{ad} versus temperature for GGG at moderate fields. Note that the relatively high value of ΔT_{ad} for GGG is partly the result of the very low heat capacity of the material below 20 K. This must be taken into account when designing GGG regenerators because of the potential problems associated with its low thermal mass compared with other components.

2-4-4 Passive Magnetic Regenerator Materials

Passive magnetic regenerator materials have been developed for use in gas-cycle cryocooler regenerators below 15 K [2,3]. The usefulness comes from magnetic materials that have a large zero-field heat capacity near their magnetic phase transition temperatures. Standard low-temperature regenerator materials like lead have a heat capacity that

Table 2-8 List of magnetic refrigerant materials

Material	Magnetocaloric effect reference	Ordering temperature (K)	$\Delta T_{ad}(K)$ @ field (T)	Application reference
Gd	Benford et al. 1981 [20]	293	13.8 K @ 7 T	[43,44,45,46]
$Gd_{0.8}Er_{0.2}$	Nikitin et al. 1985 [18]	267	8.6 K @ 6 T	
Tb	Green et al. 1988 [22]	233	10.5 K @ 7 T	[45]
Dy	Benford 1979 [21]	179	11.6 K @ 7 T	[42]
$Tb_{0.63}Y_{0.37}$	Kuz'man et al. 1993 [17]	177	5.5 K @ 6 T	
$Gd_{0.2}Ho_{0.8}$	Kuz'man et al. 1993 [17]	160	6.9 K @ 6 T	[42]
Ho	Kuz'man et al. 1993 [17]	132	6.1 K @ 7 T	
Er	Nikitin et al. 1985 [18]	85	3.2 K @ 6 T	
$HoCo_2$	Nikitin et al. 1990 [23]	82	5.1 K @ 6 T	
$GdNi_2$	Zimm et al. 1992 [15]	75	5.7 K @ 7 T	[40]
GdNi	Zimm et al. 1992 [15]	70	7.5 K @ 7 T	
Tm	Kuz'man et al. 1993 [17]	58	1.5 K @ 6 T	
$Dy_{0.5}Er_{0.5}Al_2$	Gschneidner et al. 1994 [30]	40	10.4 K @ 7.5 T	
GdPd	Zimm et al. 1992 [15]	38	8.7 K @ 7 T	
GGG	Hashimoto et al. 1982 [16]	24	18.2 K @ 4.6 T	[1,41,47,48,49]
$Dy_3Al_5O_{12}$	Hashimoto et al. 1982 [16]	23	18.1 K @ 4.6 T	
$Er_{0.86}Gd_{0.14}$	Zimm et al. 1992 [15]	23	8.8 K @ 7 T	
$Dy_2Ti_2O_7$	Hashimoto et al. 1982 [16]	21	17.3 K @ 4.6 T	
Nd	Zimm et al. 1990 [19]	10	2.5 K @ 7 T	
Er_3AlC	Pecharsky et al. 1995 [25]	5	12.5 K @ 7.5 T	

quickly drops toward zero below 15 K (see Fig. 2-29), which compromises their ability to absorb thermal energy from helium gas in a low-temperature cryocooler. Conversely, materials with magnetic phase transition temperatures below 15 K can retain adequate heat capacity for regeneration. The key achievement with these materials is the production of roughly 1 W of cooling power at 4 K in a Gifford–McMahon cryocooler [35]. This advance eliminates the need for liquid helium cooling in some applied superconductivity applications.

Table 2-9 Selected properties of rare-earth elements

Element	Atomic number	Density (kg/m^3)	Melting temperature (K)	Heat capacity @ 20 °C $(J/kg \cdot K)$	Thermal conductance @ 20 °C $(W/m \cdot K)$	Electrical resistivity @ 20 °C $(\Omega \cdot m)$	Yield stress @ 20 °C (MPa)	Young's modulus @ 20 °C (GPa)
Gd	64	7900	1586	230	10.5	1.34×10^{-6}	179	56.1
Tb	65	8229	1629	183	11.1	1.16×10^{-6}		57.5
Dy	66	8550	1685	173	10.7	0.91×10^{-6}	228	63.0
Ho	67	8795	1747	165	16.2	0.94×10^{-6}	221	67.1
Er	68	9066	1802	168	14.5	0.86×10^{-6}	292	73.3
Tm	69	9321	1818	160	16.9	0.79×10^{-6}		
Yb	70	6965	1092	145	35.0	0.29×10^{-6}		

Note: Data taken from Refs. [13] and [50].

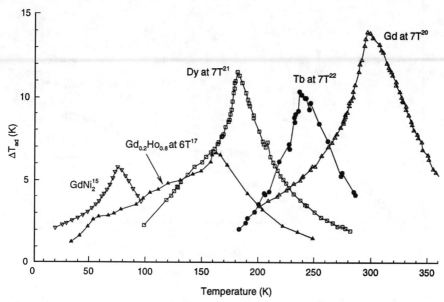

Figure 2-27 Magnetocaloric effect at high field.

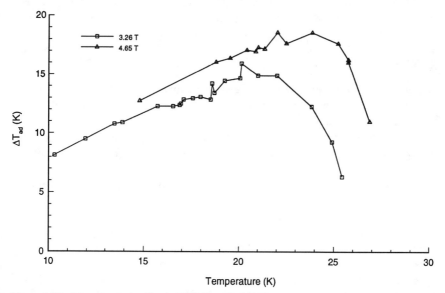

Figure 2-28 Magnetocaloric effect in GGG (from Ref. [16]).

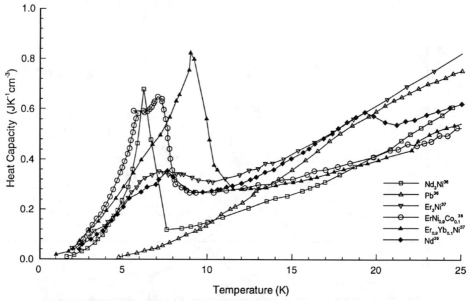

Figure 2-29 Heat capacity of low-temperature regenerator materials.

Figure 2-29 presents the zero-field heat capacity curves for lead [36], Er_3Ni [37], $Er_{0.9}Yb_{0.1}Ni$ [37], $ErNi_{0.9}Co_{0.1}$ [38], Nd_3Ni [36], and Nd [39]. Note that there is considerable activity in this field of research. The reader is therefore advised to consult the literature for the latest material developments.*

NOMENCLATURE

Active magnetic regenerator (AMR). A regenerator composed of magnetic material that performs both functions of regeneration (heat storage) and magnetic heat pumping (magnetocaloric effect).

Adiabatic temperature change (ΔT_{ad}). In this context ΔT_{ad} refers to the adiabatic temperature change of a material due to the magnetocaloric effect with SI units of Kelvin (K).

Curie temperature. The temperature above which a ferromagnetic material becomes paramagnetic.

Diamagnet. A material that has no intrinsic atomic moment (no permanent magnetic dipoles) and exhibits weak magnetization opposed to an applied induction field.

Eddy current. An electric current induced in a material due to time-dependent magnetic fields.

Ferrimagnet. A material whose magnetic domains are composed of antiparallel dipoles of unequal strength. Exhibits very strong macroscopic magnetization aligned with

---

*Additional information on small cryocoolers may be found in chapter 7 of this handbook.

an applied induction field; similar to ferromagnets. Antiferrimagnets are the same except that the antiparallel dipoles are of equal strength at zero applied field.

Ferromagnet. A material whose magnetic domains are composed of parallel magnetic dipoles. Domains can be easily aligned with weak induction fields. Exhibits very strong macroscopic magnetization in the direction of the applied field. Antiferromagnets are the same except that the antiparallel dipoles are of equal strength at zero applied field.

Magnetic dipole. A current loop with a dipole moment (m) defined by $m = I \int dS$, where I is the current and S is area enclosed by the loop. Can also refer to a single atom (atomic moment) where electron orbitals define the current loop. SI units of A-m^2.

Magnetic domain. Microscopically large region of a magnetic material containing a large number of permanent dipoles (atomic moments) of nearly identical orientation.

Magnetic field intensity (H). Defined by $H = B/\mu_0 - M$. Related to the free electrical current distribution (J) by Ampere's circuital law: $H = \nabla \times J$. SI units of A/m.

Magnetic induction field (B). Defined to be the field with which a charged particle interacts. $F_{\mathrm{mag}} = qv \times B$, where F_{mag} is the magnetic force, q is the electric charge, and v is the velocity of the particle. SI units of tesla (T).

Magnetocaloric effect. The temperature change occurring in a material when it is subjected to a change in magnetic field intensity.

Magnetization (M). Average dipole moment per unit volume of a material. SI units of A/m. (Sometimes defined as average dipole moment per unit mass with SI units of A-m^2/kg.)

Néel temperature. The temperature above which a ferrimagnetic material becomes paramagnetic.

Paramagnet. A material composed of randomly oriented permanent magnetic dipoles. Exhibits moderate magnetization that is aligned to an applied induction field.

Regenerator. A porous solid used for periodic heat transfer to and from a circulating fluid.

REFERENCES

1. Barclay, J. A., Stewart, W. F., Overton, W. C., Chandler, R. J., and Harkleroad, O. D., "Experimental Results on a Low-Temperature Magnetic Refrigerator," *Adv. Cryog. Eng.* 31 (1986):743–752.
2. Sahashi, M. Tokai, Y., Kuriyama, T., Nakagome, H., Li, R., Ogawa, M., and Hashimoto, T., "New Magnetic Material R$_3$T System with Extremely Large Heat Capacities Used as Heat Regenerators," *Adv. Cryog. Eng.* 35 (1990):1175–1182.
3. Barclay, J. A., "Active and Passive Magnetic Regenerators in Gas/Magnetic Refrigerators," *J. Alloy and Compounds* 207/208, (1994):955–961.
4. Crangle, J., *The Magnetic Properties of Solids*, vol. 6 of *The Structures and Properties of Solids*, Bryan R. Coles, ed. (London: Edward Arnold Publishers Ltd., 1977).
5. Cook, D. C., *The Electromagnetic Field* (Englewood Cliffs, NJ: Prentice-Hall, 1975).
6. Reed, R. P., and Clark, A. F., *Materials at Low Temperatures* (Metals Park, Ohio: American Society for Metals, 1983).
7. Jiles, D., *Introduction to Magnetism and Magnetic Materials* (London: Chapman & Hall, 1991).
8. Weiss, P., and Piccard, A., "Sur un nouveau phénomène magnétocalorique," *Compt. Rend.* 166 (1918): 325–354.

9. Hudson, R. P., *Principles and Application of Magnetic Cooling*, vol. 2 of the North-Holland series in Low-Temperature Physics, C. J. Gorter, R. De Bruyn Ouboter, and D. De Klerk, eds. (London: North Holland Publishing Co., 1972).

10. Kuz'min, M. D., and Tishin, A. M., "Magnetocaloric Effect. Part 1: An introduction to Various Aspects of Theory and Practice," *Cryog.* 32, no. 6 (1992):545–557.

11. Barclay, J. A., "Magnetic Refrigeration: A Review of Developing Technology," *Adv. Cryog. Eng.* 33 (1988):719–731.

12. Hall, J. L., Reid, C. E., Spearing, I. G., and Barclay, J. A., "Thermodynamic Considerations for the Design of Active Magnetic Regenerative Refrigerators," *Adv. Cryog. Eng.* 41 (1996).

13. Reid, C. E. J., *Development of Magnetic Refrigerants for Active Magnetic Regenerative Refrigerators*, M. A. Sc. thesis, Department of Mechanical Engineering, University of Victoria, Victoria, B.C., Canada (1995).

14. Barclay, J. A., and Steyert, W. A, U.S. Patent 4,332,135 (1982).

15. Zimm, C. B., Ludeman, E. M., Severson, M. C., and Henning, T. A., "Materials for Regenerative Magnetic Cooling Spanning 20 K to 80 K," *Adv. Cryog. Eng.* 37 (1992):883–890.

16. Hashimoto, T., Numazawa, T., Watanabe, Y., Sato, A., Nakagome, H., Horigami, O., Takayama, S., and Watanabe, M., "The Magnetic Refrigeration Characteristics of Several Magnetic Refrigerants Below 20 K: I Magnetocaloric Effect," in *Proc. ICEC 9* (Kobe, Japan: 1982).

17. Kuz'min, M. D., and Tishin, A. M., "Magnetocaloric Effect Part 2: Magnetocaloric Effect in Heavy Rare Earth Metals and Their Alloys and Application to Magnetic Refrigeration," *Cryog.* 33, no. 9 (1993): 868–882.

18. Nikitin, S. A., Andreyenko, A. S., Tishin, A. M., Arkharov, A. M., and Zherdev, A. A., "The Magnetocaloric Effect in Rare-Earth Alloys Gd-Ho and Gd-Er," *Phys. Met. Metall.* 59, no. 2 (1985):104–108.

19. Zimm, C. B., Ratzmann, P. M., Barclay, J. A., Green, G. F., and Chafe, J. N., "The Magnetocaloric Effect in Neodynium," *Adv. Cryog. Eng. Mat.*, 36 (1990):763–768.

20. Benford, S. M., and Brown, G. V., "T-S diagram for Gadolinium Near the Curie Temperature," *Appl. Phys.* 52, no. 3 (1981):2110–2112.

21. Benford, S. M., "The Magnetocaloric Effect in Dysprosium," *J. Appl. Phys.* 50, no. 3 (1979):1868–1870.

22. Green, G., Patton, W., and Stevens, J., "The Magnetocaloric Effect of Some Rare Earth Metals," *Adv. Cryog. Eng.* 33 (1988):777–783.

23. Nikitin, S. A., and Tishin, A. M., "Magnetocaloric Effect in $HoCo_2$ Compound," *Cryog.* 31, no. 3 (1990): 166–167.

24. Hashimoto, T., "Recent Progress in Magnetic Regenerator Materials and Their Application," in *Proceedings of the 18th International Conference of Refrigeraton* (1991).

25. Pecharsky, V. K., Gschneidner, K. A., and Zimm, C. B., "New Er-based Materials for Active Magnetic Refrigeration Below 20 K," *Adv. Cryog. Eng.* 42 (1996):451–455.

26. Hashimoto, T., U.S. Patent 5,213,630 (1993).

27. Gschneidner, K. A., and Takaja, H., U.S. Patent 5,435,137 (1995).

28. Kittel, P., "Eddy Current Heating in Magnetic Refrigerators," *Adv. Cryog. Eng.* 35 (1990):1141–1148.

29. Gschneidner, K. A., and Eyring, L. R., *Handbook of the Physics and Chemistry of Rare-Earths*, Vols. 1–13 (New York: North-Holland Publishing Co., 1978).

30. Gschneidner K. A., Jr., Pecharsky, V. K., and Malik, S. K., "The $(Dy_{1-x}Er_x)Al_2$ Alloys as Active Magnetic Regenerators for Magnetic Refrigeration," presented at the 1995 CEC/ICMC, Columbus, OH, 17–21, 1995.

31. Liu, X. Y., Barclay, J. A., Gopal, R. B., Földeàki, M., Chahine, R., Bose, T. K., Schurer, P. J., and LaCombe, J. L., "Thermomagnetic Properties of Amorphous Rare-Earth Alloys with Fe, Ni or Co.," *J. Appl. Phys.* 79 (1996):1630–1641.

32. Liu, X. Y., Barclay, J. A., Földeàki, M., Gopal, B. R., Chahine, R., and Bose, T. K., "Magnetic Properties of Amorphous $Gd_{70}(Fe,Ni)_{30}$ and $Dy_{70}(Fe,Ni)_{30}$ Alloys," presented at the 1995 CEC/ICMC, Columbus, OH, 17–21, 1995.

33. Shull, R. D., McMichael, R. D., Ritter, J. J., Swartzendruber, L. J., and Bennett, L. H., "Magnetic Nanocomposites as Magnetic Refrigerants," in *Proceedings of the 7th International Cryocoolers Conference* (1992), 1133–1144.

34. Annaorazov, M. P., Nikitin, S. A., Tyurin, A. L., Asatryan, K. A., and Dovletov, A. Kh., "Anomalously High Entropy Change in FeRh Alloy" *J. Appl. Phys.* 79, no. 3 (1996):1689–1695.

35. Hashimoto, T., Yabuki, M., Eda, T., Kuriyama, T., and Nakagome, H., "Effect of High Entropy Magnetic Regenerator Materials on Power of the GM Refrigerator," *Adv. Cryog. Eng.* 40 (1994):655-661.
36. Gschneidner, K. A., Jr., Pecharsky, V. K., and Gailloux, M., "New Ternary Magnetic Lanthanide Regenerator Materials for the Low-Temperature Stage of a Gifford—McMahon (G—M) Cryocooler," in *Cryocoolers* 8, R. G. Ross, ed. (New York: Plenum Press, 1995):685–694.
37. Kuriyama, T., Ohtani, Y., Takahashi, M., Nakagome, H., Nitta, H., Tsukagoshi, T., Yoshida, A., and Hashimoto, T., "Optimization of Operational Parameters for a 4 K GM Refrigerator," in *Proceedings of the 1995 CEC/ICMC* (1995).
38. Satoh, T., Onishi, A., Li, R., Asami, H., and Kanazawa, Y., "Development of 1.5 W 4 K G-M Cryocooler with Magnetic Regenerator Material," *Adv. Cryog. Eng.* (1995):1631–1637.
39. Osborne, M. G., Anderson, I. E., Gschneidner, K. A., Jr., Gailloux, M. J., and Ellis, T. W., "Centrifugal Atomization of Neodynium and Er₃Ni Regenerator Particulate," *Adv. Cryog. Eng.* 40 (1994):631–638.
40. Wang, A. A., Johnson, J. W., Niemi, R. W., Sternberg, A. A., and Zimm, C. B., "Experimental Results of an Efficient Active Magnetic Regenerator Refrigerator," in *Cryocoolers* 8 (New York: Plenum Press, 1994):665–676.
41. Seyfert, P., Brédy, P., and Claudet, G., "Construction and Testing of a Magnetic Refrigeration Device for the Temperature Range of 5 to 15 K," in *Proceedings of ICEC* 12 (1988).
42. Hall, J. L., and Barclay, J. A., "A Prototype Active Magnetic Regenerative Liquefier for Natural Gas, Part 1: Design and Construction," manuscript in preparation (1998).
43. Patton, G., Green, G., Stevens, J., and Humphrey, J., "Reciprocating Magnetic Refrigerator," in *Proceedings of the 4th International Cryocoolers Conference* (1986).
44. Kirol, L. D., and Dacus, M. W., "Rotary Recuperative Magnetic Heat Pump," *Adv. Cryog. Eng.* 33 (1988):757–766.
45. Green, G., Chafe, J., Stevens, J., and Humphrey, J., "A Gadolinium–Terbium Active Regenerator," *Adv. Cryog. Eng.* 35 (1990):1165–1174.
46. Rosenblum, S. S., Steyert, W. A., and Pratt, W. P., Jr., "A Continuous Magnetic Refrigerator Operating Near Room Temperature," Los Alamos Report LA-6581 (Los Alamos: Los Alamos Scientific Laboratory, 1977).
47. Nakagome, H., Kuriyama, T., Ogiwara, H., Fujita, T., Yazawa, T., and Hashimoto, T., "Reciprocating Magnetic Refrigerator for Helium Liquefaction," *Adv. Cryog. Eng.* 31 (1987):753–760.
48. Prenger, F. C., Hill, D. D., Trueblood, J., Servais, T., Laatsch, J., and Barclay, J. A., "Performance Tests of a Conductive Magnetic Refrigerator Using a 4.5 K Heat Sink," *Adv. Cryog. Eng.* 35 (1990):1105–1113.
49. Taussig, C. P., Gallagher, G. R., Smith, J. L. Jr., and Iwasa, Y., "Magnetic Refrigeration Based on Magnetically Active Regeneration," in *Proceedings of the 4th International Cryocoolers Conference* (1986).
50. Weast, R. C., and Astle, M. J., eds., *CRC Handbook of Chemistry and Physics*, 61st ed. (Boca Raton, Florida: CRC Press, 1980).

2-5 CRYOGENIC PROPERTIES OF POLYMERS

G. Hartwig

Forschungszentrum Karlsruhe, IMF II Postfach 3640, 76021 Karlsruhe, Germany

2-5-1 Introduction

Low-temperature applications of polymers are increasing, and data at cryogenic temperatures are required for most designs. Mechanical, thermal, dielectric, and gas permeability data will be presented and discussed. The physical background of each property will be discussed briefly, and a compilation of the data will be given in the Appendix. It will be shown that a study of cryogenic properties helps in the understanding of room temperature properties.

For many applications, the resistance of a polymer to environmental effects (e.g., moisture or ionizing radiation) is an important design parameter. The limited data available will be presented.

An important question is the accuracy of the data. The errors from measurements usually are small compared with the deviations caused by processing, treatments, or insufficiently known polymer configurations or conformations. Therefore, those parameters will be considered first before going into details.

2-5-2 Accuracy of Data

Materials data are anything but exact values of universal character. They can be used as a guideline for characterizing materials with the same nominal chemical composition and structure. For most polymers, the exact composition, production methods, and additives are not well known or are a trade secret. Even the crystalline content is not well defined or is a matter of thermal treatment and processing. For example, extruded PEEK is rather low in crystallization and sensitive to moisture. This is not true for compression-molded PEEK, where the cooling rate during processing is small enough to allow a crystallization of up to 40 vol %.

Material properties of several polymers are influenced by the environment. Water absorbed at high temperatures might influence properties even at cryogenic temperatures (see Fig. 2-30). The cooling media might influence the fracture mechanical properties. For PE and PC, the critical stress concentration factor (K_{IC}) and the energy release rate (G_{IC}) are much higher with nitrogen cooling than in a helium environment at the same temperature. Nitrogen (liquid and gaseous) enhances the formation of crazes at the crack tip.

Most deviations of data originate in a different and not well-defined sample history. The measuring methods themselves usually allow an accuracy of a few percent to

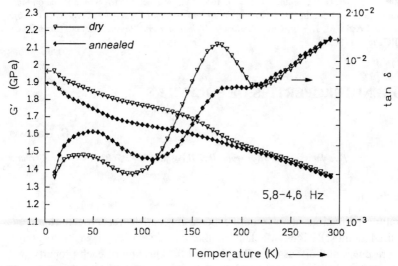

Figure 2-30 Mechanical loss factor tan δ and shear modulus G for dry and annealed PEI.

be achieved. The errors in measurement in most cases are negligible compared with the deviations resulting from production method, sample treatment, or environment. As a rule of thumb, the uncertainties of the data presented are about 10 to 15%.

2-5-3 Sample Treatments and Their Influence on Cryogenic Properties

Thermal cycling between 300 and 77 K does not influence the properties of polymers more then ≈3 to 5%. Most of the effects occur during the first ten cycles. Brittle polymers, such as PS, show the largest effect since microcracks are induced. Semicrystalline and cross-linked polymers are less sensitive. If polymers are bonded to materials having different thermal expansions (e.g., fiber composites), properties are much more influenced by thermal cycling.

Annealing influences several parameters that may slightly change the properties. These effects are

- Increase of crystalline content (for semicrystalline polymers)
- Desorbtion of water content
- Relaxation of orientation effects or internal stresses from manufacturing (e.g., extrusion) or sample preparation (machining).

Annealing just below the glass transition temperature leads to water desorbtion and relaxation. Many polymers such as PC, PS, PMMA, PE, PI, polycyanates, and epoxies are less sensitive to moisture, and the effect of annealing is less than 5% for most properties. There are, however, polymers such as PEI and PESU whose mechanical damping and modulus are influenced by dissolved water molecules. It is astonishing that water dissolved at room temperature changes low-temperature properties. At about 160 to 180 K, a damping peak is induced and certain molecular mobilities are hindered by dissolved water molecules. Figure 2-30 compares the damping spectrum and shear modulus for dry and annealed PEI. The dry specimen exhibits a "water peak," and a low-temperature peak at 40 K is suppressed. The shear modulus of annealed PEI is reduced by 8% below 150 K.

For most of the polymers, thermal expansion is reduced by less than 5% after annealing. Fracture properties (e.g., fracture stress and strain) are slightly improved by annealing because internal stresses are relaxed. Usually, the data presented apply to annealed specimens.

2-5-4 Cryogenic Applications of Polymers

Cryogenic applications of polymers concentrate on superconductivity, fusion technology, and hydrogen technology. Electrical and thermal insulation are major topics. When polymers are used for liquid hydrogen storage, their gas permeability is another important property. At low temperatures, polymers become brittle and sensitive to the formation of microcracks, which may increase permeability even at low temperatures.

When superconducting magnets are used in accelerators or fusion reactors, irradiation will be a problem for polymeric components. Most polymers are not resistant to radiation. Their mechanical properties degrade at a dose of 10^6 to 10^8 Gy.

Many polymers are used as matrices in fiber composites [1]. Their applications in cryogenics are of great importance in structural supports, nonmetallic cryostats, and

Table 2-10 Applicability of polymer bulk properties

Property	Bulk property	Restrictions
Specific heat	Yes	
Thermal conductivity	Yes	Boundary effects below 5 K
Thermal expansion	Yes	–
Permittivity	Yes	–
Mechanical and dieletric damping	Yes	Microcracks may increase the values
Relaxation	No	Multiaxial stresses and steric hindrances by the fibers
Moduli	Yes	–
Fracture properties	No	Multiaxial and internal stresses, stress concentrations

electrical as well as thermal insulation.* Some cryogenic properties of composites can be predicted from the properties of their components. Polymers in composites, however, may exhibit a behavior different from that of the bulk material. In Table 2-10, the applicability of bulk properties of polymers to composites is compiled.

Inorganic particulate fillers are used to reinforce polymers or reduce their thermal expansion. Polymers filled with very small-sized particles can be used as excellent thermal insulating materials. The additional thermal resistance (inverse thermal conductivity) arises from phonon scattering at the bounderies of particles (Kapitza resistance). It increases drastically with decreasing temperature and decreasing particle size. The thermal conductivity (e.g, of PI at 2 K) can be lowered by a factor of 50 when filled by 50 vol % with particles of about 1 μm in diameter. In addition, this particulate composite exhibits a rather high compressive strength (about 600 MPa at 2 K) and thus can be used for strong thermal insulating support elements.

For transmission of electromagnetic waves, a material with very low dielectric damping is required. Lowest loss factors are achieved with polymers at low temperatures (e.g., $\tan \delta_e \approx 5 \times 10^{-7}$ for MDPE at 4 K and 5 GHz) [2].

2-5-5 Scientific Aspects of Low-Temperature Polymer Investigations

There are several scientific aspects to studying cryogenic properties of polymers. At low temperatures, the following properties or features can be investigated:

- Basic properties
- Universal low-temperature properties
- Weak van der Waals potential
- Molecular motions of singular segments
- Features of long-wavelength phonons
- Tunneling processes

*Additional details on composite materials may be found in section 2-2 of this chapter.

Basic properties. At low temperatures most molecular mobilities are frozen, and polymer properties obey the principles of solid-state physics. These properties are called "basic properties." At higher temperatures (>120 K) properties are changed by secondary and primary glass transitions. Secondary or tertiary transitions refer to those occurring in the backbone or the sidegroups, respectively, of a polymer. The properties of polymers above about 120 K are determined mainly by glass transitions. The great differences in polymer properties are caused by glass transition that occur at different temperatures.

Universal low-temperature properties. A striking feature of polymers at low temperatures (<10 K) is that most of their thermal, elastic, and mechanical damping properties are rather similar, irrespective of their chemical compositions. Differences, however, exist between amorphous and semicrystalline polymers and between different crystalline contents. Below 10 K several properties approach a narrow band of values:

- $\tan \delta_e \approx 10^{-3}$ for amorphous polymers
- Shear modulus $\quad G \approx$ 2–3 GPa (amorphous)
  $G \approx$ 2.5–4.5 GPa (semicrystalline; 60 vol %)
- Young's modulus $\quad E \approx$ 5–8 GPa (amorphous)
  $E \approx$ 7–9 GPa (semicrystalline or cross-linked)
- Specfic heat is rather independent of chemical composition below 80 K.

Amorphous polymers exhibit higher values than semicrystalline ones. There are, however, parameters that influence cryogenic properties:

- Thermal conductivity of semicrystalline polymers depends on the size of the crystallites (boundary resistance at very low temperatures).
- Dielectric properties depend on the polarity of the monomers and therefore on the chemical composition.

Binding potential. It is a feature specific to polymers that different binding forces act within a polymer chain (intrachain binding) and between chains (interchain binding).

- Intrachain binding is caused by the strong covalent potential.
- Interchain binding is caused by the weak van der Waals potential (for several polymers the hydrogen bond also contributes).

At low temperatures most properties are determined mainly by the weak interchain binding (van der Waals). The chains are frozen; deformations are controlled by the interchain potential. Weak van der Waals forces can therefore be studied at low temperatures.

Molecular motions of singular segments. Van der Waals forces indirectly control molecular mobilities at low temperatues. Most mobilities are due to small rotations of chain segments or side groups. An example will be given for the end monomer of a polyethylene chain. The CH_3 group would be able to rotate freely if there were

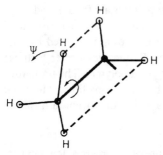

Figure 2-31 Rotation of CH_3 against a CH_2 monomer. Van der Walls interactions between neighboring side substituents are marked by dashed lines.

no barrier. A barrier arises from van der Waals interactions of neighboring hydrogen substitutes, as shown in Fig. 2-31 (dashed lines). These barriers are small and can be activated at rather low temperatures.

Rotations within a chain are possible for a collective motion of a segment of 4 to 5 monomers having a common axis. A sketch of the so-called crankshaft motion is given in Fig. 2-32. A small barrier against free rotation again arises from van der Waals interactions of side substitutes. These interactions increase with the size and polarity of side substituents (see section 2-5-7). The crankshaft rotations can be activated at 140 K. This leads to increased flexibility of chains. These low-temperature processes influence properties at higher temperatures. At low temperatures, the mobility of singular segments or side groups can be studied separately. At high temperatures many molecular mobilities are overlapped.

Features of long-wavelength phonons. At low temperatures (<50 K) only long wavelength phonons are activated, which propagate in all directions of a polymer. The force constant of these vibrations arises mainly from van der Waals forces. Above 50 K, however, phonon wavelengths are too small for propagating between polymer chains (mean chain distance ≈ 0.4–0.5 nm). Most thermal properties at higher temperatures are therefore determined by intrachain phonons. The behavior of long-wavelength phonons can only be studied at low temperatures.

Tunneling processes. At very low temperatures (<1 K) most thermal and damping properties of amorphous polymers are dominated by tunneling processes [3]. The temperature dependencies of specific heat and thermal conductivity are very different from those of crystals.

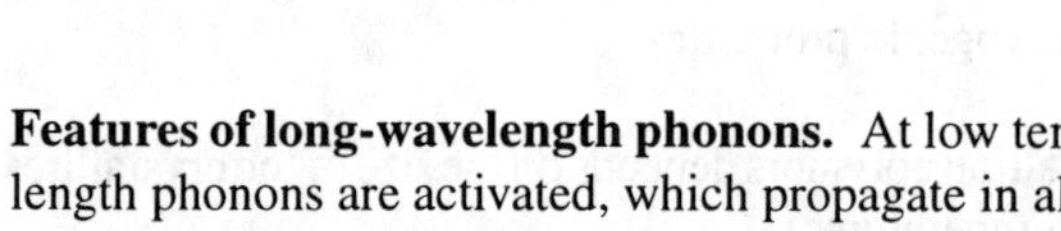

Figure 2-32 Crankshaft motion. The van der Waals interactions are marked by dashed lines.

2-5-6 Glass Transitions and Properties

Glass transitions influence most of the properties of polymers. However, at low temperatures they are frozen, and the so-called basic properties dominate. Glass transitions are characterized by the unfreezing of mobilities of specific molecular segments or side groups. An important mobility is the crankshaft motion shown in Fig. 2-32. Unfreezing (around 140 K) makes the chains more flexible. Side-group motions, such as the wagging of neighboring phenylrings of PS, induce small glass transitions at ≈ 40 K. Side-group motions, however, do not greatly influence the mechanical properties.

Equilibrium is usually determined by the minimum of the binding potential. Because of the loose polymer structure, a second neighboring potential minimum exists in some cases that is separated by a barrier. At a sufficiently high temperature and under load, specific molecular segments are able to surpass this barrier. These statistical and thermally activated jumping processes are dissipative and can be characterized by a damping maximum that occurs at a temperature T_{gs}, the glass transition temperature. The position of T_{gs} depends on the frequency or deformation rate of loading. For cryogenic properties, only secondary glass transitions are of interest.

Tunneling processes become dominant at very low temperatures at which jumping processes are no longer possible [3]. This results from a quantum mechanical process that allows the barrier to be penetrated by violation of energy or momentum conservation laws over a short distance or period of time (uncertainty principle).

The influences of tunneling and jumping processes on properties are shown in Fig 2-33. The broken line symbolizes the basic properties without glass transitions. Below 10 K the mechanical and electrical damping behaviors are dominated by tunneling processes; the specific heat and thermal conductivity, below 1 K.

For jumping processes, a drop of moduli and an increase in the dielectric permittivity are correlated to the glass transition at T_{gs} and the corresponding damping peak. For the mechanical cases, chains become more flexible and moduli drop. For the dielectric case, more polar groups become more mobile and better oriented by the electrical field.

Thermal expansion is strongly increased by glass transitions because more free volume is created above the transition temperature by mobile segments.

2-5-7 Damping Behavior

Jumping processes of singular molecular segments over the barrier take some time (the so-called relaxation time) $\tau(T)$, which is a function of temperature. Relaxation time can be determined from the damping peak specific to this mobility and occurring at the transition temperature (T_{gs}). For the case of sinusoidal loading with an angular frequency ω, relaxation time holds at the peak:

$$\tau(T)\omega = 1 \qquad (2\text{-}9)$$

The barrier $\Delta\Phi$ controlling the statistical jumping process can be calculated by the Arrhenius equation:

$$\tau(T_{gs}) = v_0^{-1}\exp\left(\frac{\Delta\Phi}{RT_{gs}}\right) \qquad (2\text{-}10)$$

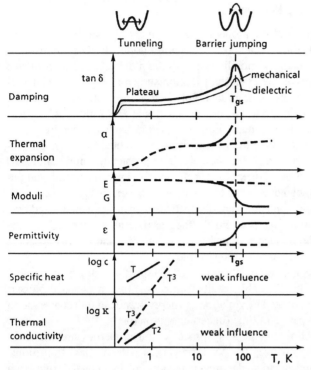

Figure 2-33 Effect of tunneling and jumping processes on physical properties. The expression T_{gs} is a secondary glass transition. The basic properties are marked by dashed lines.

with the gas constant $R = 8.3\,\mathrm{J\,mol^{-1}\,K^{-1}}$ and $\nu_0 \approx 10^{12}$ to 10^{13} Hz. For crankshaft motions of PE, for example, $\Delta\Phi \approx 40\,\mathrm{kJ/mol}$. The damping behavior is usually expressed as a loss factor ($\tan\delta$), which can be detected by several methods as follows:

Mechanical damping. The mechanical loss factor can be determined from hysteresis effects (forced oscillations) or the logarithmic decrement Λ of damped free vibrations (torsion pendulum): $\tan\delta = \Lambda/\pi$. Several examples of damping spectra are shown in Fig. 2-34. The damping peaks are shifted to higher temperatures for side substitutes with higher polarities and larger sizes. The largest barrier for place changes occurs for chloride side substituents in this presentation (e.g for PVC). It already has been mentioned that at about 4 K. The mechanical loss factor of most amorphous polymers ($\tan\delta_m \approx 10^{-3}$) is independent of the chemical composition. Semicrystalline polymers (e.g., HDPE) exhibit lower values because damping occurs only for the amorphous phase.

Dielectric damping. Damping can also be activated by an oscillating electrical field. The dielectric loss factor $\tan\delta_e$ of amorphous polymers depends strongly on the polarity of mobile monomers or segments. There exists an interesting correlation between the

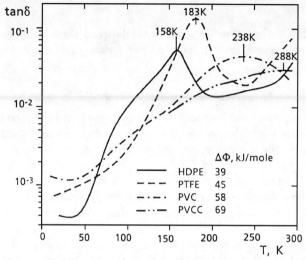

Figure 2-34 Mechanical damping spectra versus temperature for linear polymers with different side substituents.

mechanical and dielectric loss factors both activated at the same frequency [4]:

$$\frac{\tan \delta_e}{\tan \delta_m} = f = \bar{\mu}^{2.4} \tag{2-11}$$

This ratio is independent of temperature (<350 K) and only a function of the mean polarity ($\bar{\mu}$) of the specfic polymer. For PE, which is rather nonpolar, $f \approx 5 \times 10^{-3}$, PVC is rather polar, and $f \approx 1$.

The dielectric loss factor at 4 K ranges from $\tan \delta_e \approx 5 \times 10^{-6}$ (middle density PE) to $\tan \delta_e \approx 5 \times 10^{-4}$ (PVC) at 6.5 GHz [2] (see Fig. 2-35).

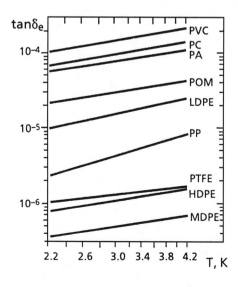

Figure 2-35 Dielectric loss factor at 6.5 GHz of several polymers.

2-5-8 Deformation Behavior

External forces cause both fast deformations of electron orbitals and slow deformations (change of places) of molecular segments. For polymers, mainly three types of deformations are fundamental:

- *Elastic deformations* at very low temperatures or extremely high deformation rates. They are reversible, nondissipative, and independent of temperature and time (deformation rate). The forces are controlled by fast deformations of electron orbitals. Mainly weak van der Waals binding forces are involved, which are responsible for the low moduli of elasticity.
- *Viscoelastic deformations* in the region of a glass transition. They are reversible, dissipative, and dependent on temperature and time. Their response results from time-consuming changes of place of molecular segments or side groups. This deformation is linear for small loads only.
- *Viscous deformations* at higher temperatures or high loads. They are irreversible, dissipative, and time-and temperature-dependent. Their response results from molecular slipping while surpassing several potential barriers.

The deformation behavior of polymers is usually described by a combination of elastic springs F and damping elements η. An example is given in Fig. 2-36. At very low temperatures, the damping elements are frozen, and the elastic spring F_0 remains; the polymers become linear elastic.

Tensile moduli. Depending on the type of loading, different moduli are defined to describe deformation behavior as follows:

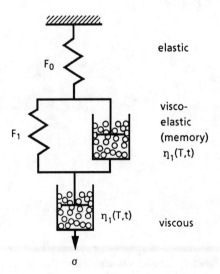

elastic

F_0

visco-
elastic
(memory)
$\eta_1(T,t)$

F_1

$\eta_1(T,t)$

viscous

σ

Figure 2-36 Model showing elastic, viscoelastic, and viscous components.

- Step function with a constant load → creep modulus $E(T, t)$ or relaxation compliance $F(T, t)$
- Deformation at a constant load rate ε → Initial modulus E or secant modulus
- Cyclic loading with frequency ω → complex modulus $E^* = E' + iE''$

E': storage modulus
E'': damping modulus

The creep modulus $E(T, t)$ (defined by a strain step) is nearly the inverse relaxation compliance at low temperature. The latter is easier to measure.

The relaxation compliance $F(T, t)$ can be determined by applying a load step σ_0 and waiting for the strain to reach a constant (relaxed) state. The time-dependence of F is given by [5]:

$$F(t, T) = F_u + [F_R(T) - F_u](1 - e^{-t/\tau}) \qquad (2\text{-}12)$$

where F_u is the start compliance, which is assumed to be unrelaxed and τ is the time constant defined by $(F_u - F_R)$ being reduced by the factor $1/e$. If several relaxation processes are involved, a summation has to be performed. In Fig. 2-37 the creep compliance F is plotted versus time for several polymers at 77 K. When plotting the curves of Fig. 2-37 in a log–log scale, straight lines result. The slope m chracterizes the relaxation or creep behavior. It holds for the complience F or the modulus E as follows:

$$\frac{d \ln F}{d \ln t} = m(T) \quad \text{or} \quad \frac{d \ln E}{d \ln t} = -m(T) \qquad (2\text{-}13)$$

The parameter m is a function of temperature; some values are given in Table 2-11 It is worth mentioning that HDPE creeps up to 3% even at 4 K.

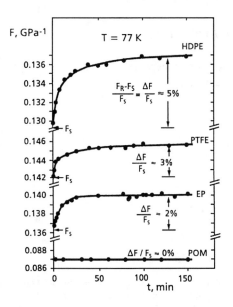

Figure 2-37 Relaxation compliance F at 77 K versus relaxation time.

Table 2-11 Relaxation parameter m (T)

Polymer	T (K)	m (T)
HDPE	158	0.043
	124	0.020
	77	0.006
	4	0.002
PC	187	0.018
	77	0.005
EP	151	0.017
	77	0.003

The **initial modulus** E (Young's modulus) is determined from stress–strain diagrams. A schematic presentation is given in Fig. 2-38 for diagrams at different temperatures and deformation rates (e.g., strain rate $\dot{\varepsilon}$). At very low temperatures, a linear elastic relation exists without any dependence on $\dot{\varepsilon}$. The largest dependence on $\dot{\varepsilon}$ as well as hysteresis effects exist in the region of a glass transition. At higher temperatures, irreversible deformations are overlapped.

The **complex modulus** E^* is usually applied under sine-wave loading, where hysteresis effects and phase shifts (δ) occur. In Fig. 2-39 the real and imaginary components are defined in a vector diagram. The absolute value E_D is determined by the maximum values of stress σ_0 and strain ε_0 of a sine-wave loading: $E_D(\omega, T) = \sigma_0/\varepsilon_0$. At low temperatures, damping and hysteresis effects are small and E'' is negligible. Then the complex modulus E_D and the storage modulus E' are approximately equal to the Young's modulus. At the same time scale of loading,

$$E_D (\omega, T) \approx E'(\omega, T) \approx E(t, T) \tag{2-14}$$

The dependence of E' on frequency is maximum in the vicinity of a glass transition and a little above. Figure 2-40 presents two examples.

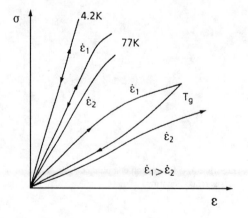

Figure 2-38 Schematic stress–strain diagrams at different temperatures and deformation rates ($\dot{\varepsilon}$).

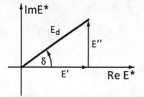

Figure 2-39 Vector diagram.

Shear moduli. The treatment given for the tensile (E) moduli also applies to the shear modulus G. Data are given in the appendix. The correlation between E and G is given by

$$G = \frac{E}{2(1 + \mu)} \tag{2-15}$$

where μ is Poisson's ratio:

$$\mu_{xy} = -\frac{\varepsilon_y}{\varepsilon_x} \tag{2-16}$$

and where ε_y is the (negative) transverse strain resulting from a strain ε_x. Poisson's ratio is somewhat dependent on the deformation rate. Some data at low deformation rates are plotted in Fig. 2-41.

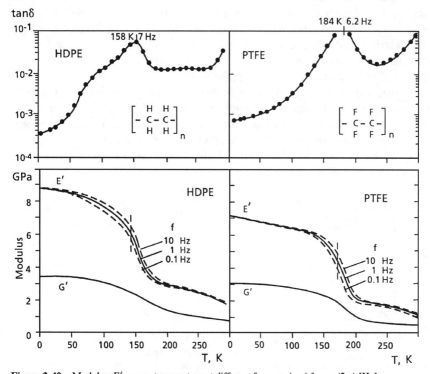

Figure 2-40 Modulus E' versus temperature at different frequencies ($f = \omega/2\pi$) [Hz].

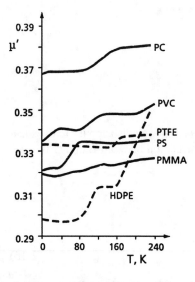

Figure 2-41 Poisson's ratio versus temperature.

2-5-9 Dielectric Permittivity

Permittivity has a time- and temperature-independent component that arises from electron polarization. This component dominates at very low temperatures or very high frequencies. The magnitude of the cryogenic permittivity is $\varepsilon_e \approx 2$. There is a slow component overlap arising from polar groups that are somewhat oriented by a low-frequency electrical field. This component is called orientation polarization and depends on the time (frequency) and temperature. At low frequencies or high temperatures, permittivity of polymers can reach $\varepsilon_e \approx 5$ (e.g., for PVC).

There exists a great similarity between the permittivity and the mechanical compliance F' (inverse modulus). Like the permittivity, there is a fast electronic component for the compliance that is time- and temperature-independent. It is the elastic component arising from electron deformations. At a glass transition, chain segments become flexible, and F' increases. This is the slow viscoelastic component. Figure 2-42 illustrates the analogous behavior of F' and ε'_e.

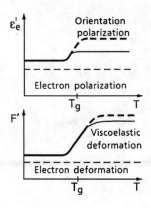

Figure 2-42 Analogous behavior of dielectric permittivity ε_e and mechanical compliance F'. The dashed line represents the real part of the complex modulus, permittivity, and compliance.

2-5-10 Fracture Behavior

From a microscopic point of view, it is astonishing that isotropic polymers exhibit a poor fracture behavior. Despite the fact that polymer chains are extremely strong (up to 15 GPa), entangled isotropic polymers exhibit a tensile strength in the range of 30–200 MPa only. The upper value applies to low temperatures (4 K). The observed low strength is due to inhomogeneities, internal stress, stress concentrations at microcracks, and surface cracks.

Isotropic polymers have high compressive strength, low shear strength, and intermediate tensile strength. By contrast, in aligned polymers, the high strength of the chains is concentrated in the alignment direction, and the tensile strength becomes rather high. Kevlar fibers, which are aligned aramid molecules, have a tensile strength of ≈ 2 GPa.

At very low temperatures, isotropic polymers are brittle but have a higher fracture strength than at warmer temperatures. The reason is a higher binding strength due to the more compact packing that results from thermal contraction. At higher temperatures several processes are induced by loading, which counteracts brittle formation—especially for thermoplastic polymers. The main processes are yielding, necking, and the formation of crazes. These processes, however, increase mainly the fracture strain. Cross-linked polymers, such as epoxy resins do not exhibit these processes, and they have a low fracture strain even at higher temperatures. Several thermoplastics (PC, PMMA, PESU, PS) tend to form crazes at a crack tip that resist crack propagation. Perpindicular to the crack direction, fibrils are pulled out of the bulk material [6]. The fibrils are mechanically strong. A schematic of this situation is shown in Fig. 2-43.

Stress intensity factor. Stress concentrations in the vicinity of crack tips can be described by stress intensity factors (K) which depend on the mode of loading. The expression K_I represents tensile loads, K_{II} and K_{III} represent shear loads, and K_{Ic} is the critical value that characterizes the onset of crack propagation. Figure 2-44 shows a specimen for the measuring of K_{Ic}, which is a function of the critical stress required to fracture σ_c, the crack length a, the temperature T, the deformation rate $\dot{\delta}$, and a factor Y that describes the sample geometry (for a rectangular compact tension specimen $Y = (2\pi)^{1/2}$). Linear elastic fracture mechanics yields [7]

$$K_{Ic}(T, \dot{\delta}) = \sigma_c(T, \dot{\delta})a^{0.5}Y \qquad (2\text{-}17)$$

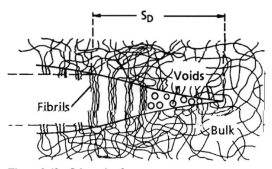

Figure 2-43 Schematic of crazes.

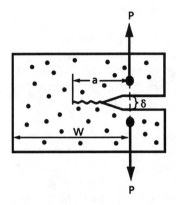

Figure 2-44 Specimen for the measurement of crack propagation. (P is the force and δ the crack opening displacement [COD]).

At low temperatures K_{Ic} ranges from 2 to 10 MPa m$^{1/2}$. It is not very sensitive to deformation rate.

Energy release rate. Although the stress intensity factor describes the crack initation, the energy release rate G_I describes the crack propagation. When a load is applied, elastic energy is stored in the specimen. During crack propagation, this energy is consumed by chain scissions, plasticization of the crack tip, and acceleration of the crack propagation. The critical value is defined by

$$G_{Ic}(T, \dot{\delta}) = \frac{-\Delta E_{el}}{\Delta A} \ [\text{J/m}^2] \tag{2-18}$$

where ΔE_{el} is the released energy and ΔA is the area created by the crack. The expression G_{Ic} is also a function of temperature and deformation rate. It can be determined by a force–crack opening diagram (COD) like that shown in Fig. 2-45. At low temperatures, unstable crack propagation with crack arrests takes place. In Fig. 2-45 the dashed area is the released elastic energy, and the newly created area can be detected by the "arrest lines" between crack stops. The cause of intrinsic crack arrest is adiabatic heating and plasticization of the crack tip. The size of the plasticization zones can be estimated by

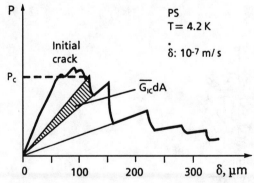

Figure 2-45 Force–COD diagram for unstable crack propagation.

the Irwin or Dugdale models [7]. The local temperature rise from adiabatic heating is on the order of 50 to 80 K for tests carried out at 77 K. The value of G_{Ic} ranges from 0.16 to 9.8 kJ/m^2 at low temperatures (see Table A-4 in the appendix).

There is an additional complication for several polymers (e.g., PC, PE). In LN$_2$-cooled systems, G_{Ic} is much larger than in helium environments at the same temperature. Nitrogen enhances craze formation, which consumes energy during crack propagation.

Adiabatic heating at the crack tip occurs not only during unstable crack propagation but also at very fast deformation rates [8]. Microcracks exist in every polymer and any one may form the nucleus of a macroscopic crack during loading. At very fast deformation rates, adiabatic heating and plasticization occur at the crack tips and increase fracture strength and strain significantly. These processes are especially enhanced at low temperatures, where specific heat is small and fracture energy by internal friction or chain scissioning causes large temperature rises.

2-5-11 Fatigue Behavior

At cyclic loading, damage accumulates until fracture occurs. The fatigue behavior depends on the load amplitude (stress or strain), the mean load σ_m, and the frequency. The loading is generally characterized by the ratio

R = minimum load/maximum load.

Two important types of uniaxial loading are

- Tensile threshold ($R \approx 0$)
- Alternative tension–compression ($R \approx -1$). The load-time profiles are shown in Fig. 2-46. An aspect of fatigue loading is the internal heating of the specimen, which is affected by the frequency, the sample size, and the cooling conditions. The heat produced in a specimen is given by

$$W \sim \pi (\tan \delta) E^{-1} f \sigma_a^2 \qquad (2\text{-}19)$$

where $\tan \delta$ is the loss factor (small at these temperatures), σ_a is the stress amplitude, f is the frequency, and E is the Young's modulus.

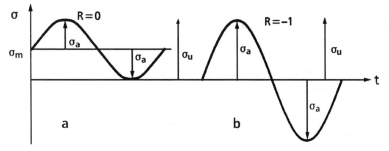

Figure 2-46 (a) Tensile threshold cycling and (b) tension compression cycling.

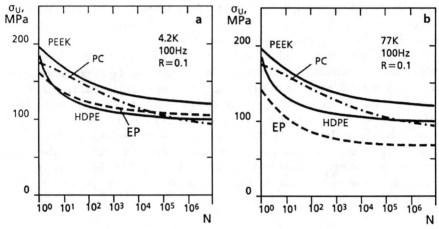

Figure 2-47 Tensile threshold loading versus load cycles N (S–N curves); σ_u is the upper load.

In the case of surface cooling, much of the heat is removed, but the center of the specimen is heated [6]. For LN_2-cooling of an 8-mm-diameter rod, a frequency up to 100 Hz can be applied for $R \approx 0$, but for $R \approx -1$, only a quarter of this frequency (25 Hz) is possible without significant heating. The reason is that at the same σ_u for $R \approx -1$, σ_a is twice that of $R \approx 0$ (see Fig. 2-46), and the internal heat depends quadratically on σ_a. Fatigue curves at 4.2 and 77 K are shown in Figs. 2-47(a,b). As can be seen, there is no large difference in fatigue behavior at these two temperatures [9].

For $R \approx -1$, the fatigue curves are very similar to $R \approx 0$ curves if a sufficiently low frequency is applied. In Fig. 2-48 shear fatigue curves are shown. The static shear strength is higher in PEEK, but degradation is similar for both polymers [10].

2-5-12 Thermal Vibrations of Polymers

The thermal properties of polymers are determined by thermal vibrations more generally known as phonons. The term phonon comprises energy, momentum, velocity, and polarization. The loose structure of polymers gives rise to several vibrational modes [11]:

1. Longitudinal vibrations along the chain (intrachain vibrations)
   - Driven by covalent binding forces
   - Significant above 50 K
2. Transverse vibrations along the chains
   - Result from the intrinsic bending stiffness
   - Significant above 80 K
3. Stretching vibration between chains (interchain vibrations)
   - Driven by van der Waals forces
   - Dominate below 50 K

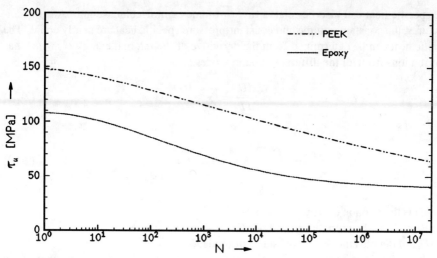

Figure 2-48 Shear threshold loading versus load cycles N for PEEK and EP (E162, E113, Shell) at 77 K.

4. Tunneling vibrations (nonpropagating vibration or localized mode)
  • Dominant below 1 K

A more general phonon theory defines the vibrational modes according to the force constants. The most important modes are stretching vibrations (change of distance) and bending vibrations (change of valence angle).

Stretching phonons that are driven mainly by van der Waals forces are long-wavelength vibrations that propagate in three dimensions. Thus, they propagate in a continuum.

Stretching phonons that are driven by covalent binding are short-wavelength vibrations and are bound to the polymer chain; they are longitudinal vibrations in linear chains.

Bending phonons result from the intrinsic bending stiffness of the chains. Below 10 K, wavelengths are large and the valence angles are not stressed. Bending phonons become significant above 10 K and propagate in all three dimensions up to $T \approx 80$ K. Above 80 K the wavelength is small, and the propagation is bound to the chain (transverse vibrations of stiff chains).

The different vibration modes lead to different features of phonon density and propagation. The density D and probability of their activation P obey certain temperature dependencies, which for D are specific to the mode. The probability of activation of the phonon modes are given by Bose–Einstein statistics. The thermal properties of polymers are determined by the specific mixtures of the phonon modes.

2-5-13 Specific Heat

The specific heat C relates the heat input Q with the temperature rise ΔT in a mass m.

$$Q = C(T)\, m\, \Delta T \tag{2-20}$$

The specific heat can also be related to the volume or molecular weight. At low temperatures, the constant volume and constant-pressure specific heat are nearly equal. The specific heat can be determined from the derivitive of the internal energy U, which has contributions from all the different phonon modes i:

$$C = \frac{dU}{dT} = \sum_i \frac{dU_i}{dT} \tag{2-21}$$

$$U_i = \int_0^{\omega\,\text{max}} \hbar\omega D_i(\omega) P(\omega, T)\, d\omega \tag{2-22}$$

where
   $\hbar\omega$ is the phonon energy
   $P(\omega, T)$ is the probability of states (Bose–Einstein statistics)
   $D_i(\omega)$ denotes the density of states of mode i

$D = $ constant for tunneling modes and linear chains.
$D \approx \omega^2$ for continuum modes
$D \approx \omega^{1/2}$ for stiff bending continuum modes
$D \approx \omega^{-1/2}$ for bending stiff linear chains
$D = $ constant for linear chains

The maximum frequency, ω_{max}, is determined by each mode's specific Debye temperature, θ_i, which is on the order of 80 K for van der Waals–dominated vibrations; for vibrations driven by strong covalent binding forces, θ_i is less than 400 K. For each mode there exists a specific Debeye temperature. The temperature dependence of the specific heat can be determined by the exponent n of the frequency dependence of D.

$$C(T) \approx T^{n+1} \quad \text{if } D(\omega) \approx \omega^n \tag{2-23}$$

The well-known Debye law ($C \approx T^3$) is thus true for the continuum modes where $n = 2$ since $D \approx \omega^2$. For the specific heat of tunneling modes and, at much higher temperatures, of linear chains, $D \approx \omega^0$ and $C \approx T$.

Figure 2-49 illustrates the temperature dependence of C. This behavior is different for amorphous and crystalline polymers. Amorphous polymers have higher values and show contributions from tunneling behavior. The lower values of crystalline polymers come from their higher mean phonon velocities $\bar{v}$. It can be shown that $c \approx \bar{v}^{-2}$. The Debye law is valid for crystalline polymers below 80 K and for amorphous ones below 10 K. Semicrystalline polymers have values between amorphous and crystalline ones.

As shown in Figure 2-50, at higher temperatures, the specific heat shows a temperature dependence of between $C \approx T^{0.7}$ and $C \approx T^{0.9}$. This result is expected for a linear chain when taking into account the bending stiffness. The component of bending phonons only would give $C \approx T^{0.5}$.

At a main glass transition the specific heat increases sharply. This effect is less significant at secondary glass transitions.

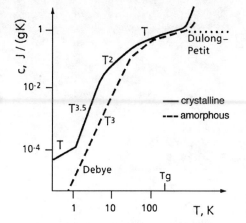

Figure 2-49 Schematic representation of the temperature dependence of the specific heat.

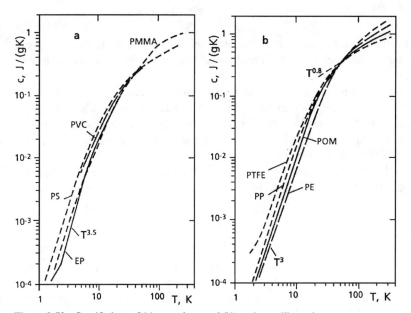

Figure 2-50 Specific heat of (a) amorphous and (b) semicrystalline polymers versus temperature.

2-5-14 Thermal Expansion

The different phonon modes contribute to the thermal expansion in different ways. Stretching vibrations contribute to the thermal expansion if the driving potential is asymmetric. This is true for the case of covalent and van der Waals potentials, as shown in Fig. 2-51. The mean distance of the vibrations increases with temperature. Below 50 K, the highest contributions to the thermal expansion arise from stretching vibrations driven by van der Waals potentials. Above 50 K, the stretching vibrations are driven by the

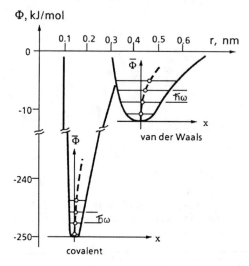

Figure 2-51 Covalent and van der Waals potentials as a function of the relative distance r of vibrations.

more symmetric covalent potential. In this case the coefficient of thermal expansion (α) rises weakly with temperature. Contributions to α from stretching vibrations are always positive.

Transverse bending vibrations reduce the amount of thermal expansion. As shown in Fig. 2-52, the mean length of an aligned polymer chain decreases when the amplitude A increases with temperature. Thus, transverse vibrations cause a negative thermal expansion in the chain direction. Perpendicular to the chains bending vibrations, however, cause a large positive thermal expansion.

If a fully aligned polymer is assumed, the coefficient of thermal expansion in the chain direction $\alpha_{//}$ and the coefficient perpendicular to the chain direction $\alpha_\perp$ may be written as

$$\alpha_{//} = \alpha_{//c} + \alpha_{//b} \tag{2-24}$$

$$\alpha_\perp = \alpha_{\perp w} + \alpha_{\perp b} \tag{2-25}$$

In the chain direction, the transverse bending vibration $\alpha_{//b}$ usually dominates the longitudinal covalent component $\alpha_{//c}$, and a negative expansion coefficient results. The components perpendicular to the orientation of molecular chains yield very large positive values, both from the van der Waals vibration $\alpha_{\perp w}$ and from the transverse component $\alpha_{\perp b}$.

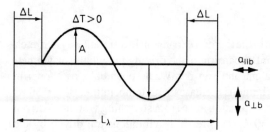

Figure 2-52 Transverse vibrations of an aligned piece of a polymer chain.

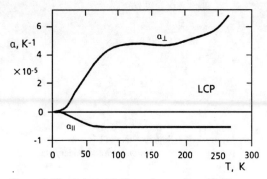

Figure 2-53   Anisotropic thermal expansion of LCP.

An example of the expansion behavior for a fully aligned polymer (LCP) is given in Fig. 2-53. The direction of orientation α_{ll} is small but negative, whereas $\alpha_{\perp}$ is positive and large.

Isotropic polymers are entangled, and the main contributions arise from $\alpha_{\perp}$. This represents interchain vibrations in the van der Waals potential $\alpha_{\perp w}$ below about 50 K and transverse bending vibrations $\alpha_{\perp b}$. Above about 70 K, the wavelengths are small and restricted to propagation in the chain direction; only small components of α_{llb} and α_{llc} contribute. This is shown for real data in Fig. 2-54 and schematically in Fig. 2-55.

The dashed line in Fig. 2-55 illustrates the so-called basic property. For polymers, however, thermal expansion is strongly increased by secondary and tertiary glass

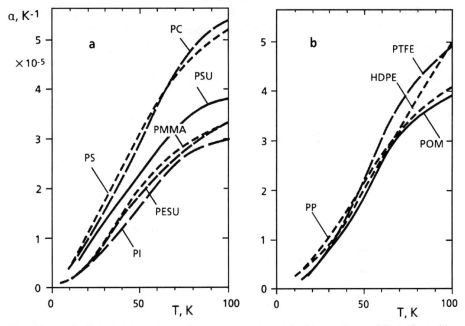

Figure 2-54   Coefficient of thermal expansion α versus temperature for (a) amorphous and (b) semicrystalline polymers.

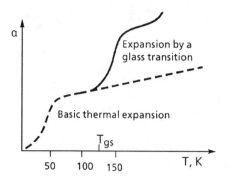

Figure 2-55 Superposition of basic thermal expansion and a contribution from a secondary glass transition at T_{gs}.

transitions. When the temperature increases above a glass transition, more free volume is created by the unfreezing of molecular mobilities. The high coefficient of thermal expansions found for polymers at elevated temperatures results from glass transitions.

Grüneisen relation. The Grüneisen relation relates the thermal expansion α, specific heat C, bulk modulus K, and density ρ of a solid:

$$\gamma = \frac{3\alpha}{C\rho} K \qquad (2\text{-}26)$$

The Grüneisen parameter γ is constant for most solids but not for polymers. This results from the fact that each vibration mode contributes to Eq. (2-26). The modes have partial Grüneisen parameters γ_i of different magnitudes that dominate at different temperatures. Thus, for polymers, γ is strongly temperature-dependent. Examples of this are shown in Fig. 2-56 for several amophorous and semicrystalline polymers.

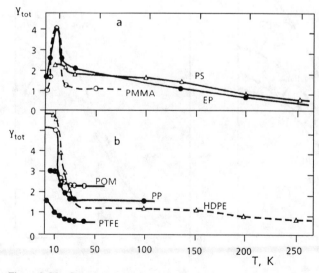

Figure 2-56 Grüneisen parameter γ of several (a) amorphous and (b) semicrystalline polymers.

The Grüneisen parameter for a polymer is a measure of the asymmetry of the binding potential. At very low temperatures, the very asymmetric van der Waals potential dominates and causes much higher γ values than the covalent potential at higher temperatures. The drop of γ for amorphous polymers below 10 K comes from a tunneling contribution to the specific heat (the value of α is not influenced).

At first, it is surprising that γ is not affected by glass transitions. The reason is that at the same the product of the thermal expansion and bulk modulus (αK) is fairly constant at glass transitions. The expansion coefficient increases at glass transition, and the bulk modulus decreases.

The Grüneisen parameter can also be used to calculate the pressure dependence of several properties. For example, the change in thermal conductivity κ with pressure P can be obtained by

$$\gamma = K\frac{d\kappa}{dP} - \frac{1}{3} \tag{2-27}$$

where K is the bulk modulus.

2-5-15 Thermal Conductivity

Heat is transferred within a polymer by lattice vibrations (phonons) that are thermalized by various scattering processes. This leads to the establishment of "local" thermal equilibrium at each point of the heat flux. Scattering occurs at tunneling systems at very low temperatures, at boundaries of crystallites below 20 K or cross-link points of thermoset polymers. At higher temperatures mainly defect or structural scattering takes place.

The thermal conductivity κ is a measure of the efficiency of this heat transfer and is given by the relation

$$\dot{Q} = -\kappa A \frac{\Delta T}{\Delta l}[\mathrm{W}] \tag{2-28}$$

where $\dot{Q}$ is the power transferred through the cross-sectional area A and length l.

An approximation for calculating thermal conductivity from the specific heat C, the density ρ, the mean phonon velocity $\bar{v}$, and the mean free phonon path $\bar{l}$ is:

$$\chi(T) \approx \frac{\rho}{3}C(T)\bar{l}(T)\bar{v}(T) \ [\mathrm{W/g\,K}] \tag{2-29}$$

The temperature dependences of χ and the dominant phonon scattering processes are summarized in Table 2-12. The thermal conductivity of amorphous polymers is constant between about 4 to 15 K and has a T^2 dependence below 1 K (due to tunneling effects) [3]. Semicrystalline polymers have a higher thermal conductivity than amorphous ones at higher temperatures. Below 15 K the situation is reversed where boundary scattering of crystallites drastically reduces thermal conductivity. Figure 2-57 is a schematic presentation of the temperature dependence of thermal conductivity in amorphous, crystalline and semicrystalline polymers.

The impact of boundary scattering on the thermal conductivity increases strongly with decreasing temperature and depends on the size of the crystallites. For the same crystalline volume, more scattering surfaces exist for smaller-sized crystallites. (This is

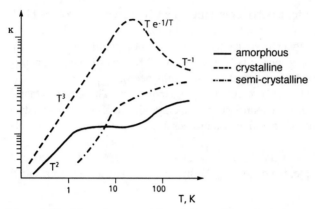

Figure 2-57 Schematic representation of the temperature dependence of thermal conductivity.

also true for polymers filled with small-size particles.) An example is given in Fig. 2-58 for amorphous and semicrystalline polymers. The smaller the crystallite size, the higher the boundary scattering and the lower the thermal conductivity.

Thermal diffusivity. The thermal diffusivity a is given by

$$a = \frac{\chi}{\rho C} \ [\text{m}^2/\text{s}] \tag{2-30}$$

The temperature dependence of a for two polymers is given in Fig. 2-59. The thermal relaxation time ξ_t is inversely proportional to a. For a rod of diameter d the thermal relaxation time is

$$\xi_t \approx 1.1 \frac{d^2}{a} \tag{2-31}$$

At very low temperatures, ξ_t is very short compared with its value at room temperature.

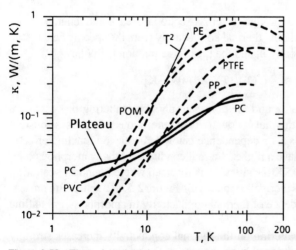

Figure 2-58 Thermal conductivity versus temperature for several polymers (full lines–amorphous; dashed lines–semicrystalline).

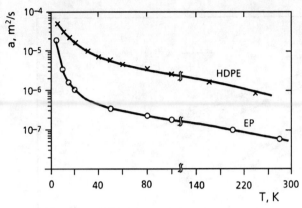

Figure 2-59 Thermal diffusivity versus temperature.

Table 2-12 Temperature dependence of thermal conductivity

Temperature range	T dependence	Assumed scattering process
Amorphous polymers		
$T \leq 1\,\text{K}$	$K_a \propto T^2$	Scattering at tunneling systems
$T \approx 4\text{–}10\,\text{K}$	$K_a \propto$ constant	Rayleigh scattering
$T > 30\,\text{K}$	$K_a \propto T^m$	Defect and structure scattering
	m: 0.3–0.5	
Semicrystalline polymers		
$T < 20\,\text{K}$	$K_{semi} \propto T^2$	Interface scattering at crystallites
$T > 30\,\text{K}$	K_{semi} is determined mainly by K_a	

2-5-16 Gas Permeability

The loose structures of polymers give rise to a relatively high gas permeability. The highest values have been observed for amorphous polymers. Semicrystalline polymers are less permeable. The permeability also depends on the type of gas. Helium and hydrogen exhibit a similar behavior, whereas methane, which is a larger molecule, has a lower permeation capability.

The gas leakage rate Q through a material of thickness a, with an area A, driven by a pressure difference ΔP, is given by [12,13]

$$Q = P(T)\frac{A}{d}\,\Delta P \ [\text{bar} \cdot \text{m}^3/\text{s}] \tag{2-32}$$

where $P(T)$ is the temperature-dependent permeatation coefficient given by

$$P(T) = P_0 \exp(E_p/RT) \ [\text{m}^2/\text{s}] \tag{2-33}$$

Here R is the gas constant and P_0 is a constant specific to each material. If the permeation barrier (or activation energy) E_p is known, an extrapolation to any temperature is possible using Eq. (2-33). Typical Arrhenius plots are shown in Figs. 2-60 and 2-61. The slopes are proportional to E_p. It can be seen that the permeability of helium and hydrogen is similar, with helium having a slightly higher E_p for a given material.

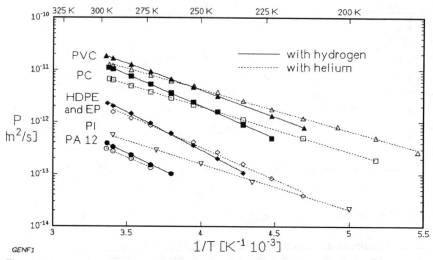

Figure 2-60 Arrhenius plots of the permeability P versus $1/T$ for several polymers and H_2 and He gas.

The amorphous polymers (PVC and PC) exhibit higher permeabilities than the semicrystalline ones (HDPE, PA12) or cross-linked ones. Epoxy resins (EP) and HDPE exhibit nearly the same behavior. The polymers PA12 and PI (Vespel) have almost the same permeability at room temperature, but the slopes are different [14,15]. It should be mentioned that PA12 has a rather low permeability and can be used as a barrier material for vessels [14,16]. It is obvious from Fig. 2-61 that permeabilities with methane are much lower than with helium or hydrogen.

In Table 2-13 the permeabilities P at 293 K and the permeation barriers E_p are compiled.

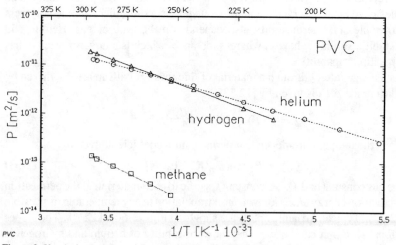

Figure 2-61 Arrhenius plots of the permeability P versus $1/T$ for several gases.

Table 2-13 Permeation barriers E_p and permeabilities P at room temperature (293 K)

Polymer	Density (g/cm^3)	Helium P (m^2/s)	E_p (kJ/mol)	Hydrogen P (m^2/s)	E_p (kJ/mol)	Methane P (m^2/s)	E_p (kJ/mol)
PVC (amorphous)	1.08	1.2×10^{-11}	16	1.7×10^{-11}	20	1×10^{-13}	28
PC (amorphous)	1.19	6.4×10^{-12}	17	1.0×10^{-11}	23		
Epoxy (amorphous)	1.2	1.9×10^{-12}	22	1.4×10^{-12}	28		
HDPE (semicrystalline)	0.98	1.6×10^{-12}	22	2.0×10^{-12}	27	3.0×10^{-13}	42
PI (Vespel)	1.4	5.6×10^{-13}	17				
PAI (Torlon)	1.3	3.9×10^{-13}	17				
PA 12 (semicrystalline)	1.36	2.8×10^{-13}	23	3.4×10^{-13}	26		

Solubility and diffusivity. Gas permeation is thought to occur in three steps:

1. Solution of the gas at the pressure-side surface.
2. Diffusion through the material.
3. Desorption at the low-pressure side.

For an isotropic and homogeneous material, the permeability P is given by the solubility S and the diffusivity D [13]:

$$P = SD \qquad (2\text{-}34)$$

Typical values of S are shown in Fig. 2-62. It can be seen that the solubility is nearly independent of temperature [14,15,17]. The solubility of hydrogen is much greater than that of helium. For the diffusivity D the reverse is true, as shown in Figure 2-63.

The diffusivity is temperature-dependent and obeys an Arrhenius equation. In Fig. 2-63, Arrhenius plots are presented. It is seen that D is highest for helium and lowest for methane. The permeativity is mainly dominated by the diffusivity.

A compilation of data on D and S at room temperature is given in Table 2-14.

Table 2-14 Diffusivity D and solubility S at room temperature (293 K)

Polymer	Helium D (m^2/s)	S	Hydrogen D (m^2/s)	S	Methane D (m^2/s)	S
PVC	9.8×10^{-10}	1.2×10^{-2}	3.2×10^{-10}	5.3×10^{-2}		
PC	5.0×10^{-10}	1.3×10^{-2}	1.4×10^{-10}	7.1×10^{-2}	6.6×10^{-12}	4.2×10^{-2}
HDPE	4.5×10^{-10}	3.6×10^{-3}	1.8×10^{-10}	1.1×10^{-2}		
PA12	4.7×10^{-11}	6.0×10^{-3}	3.0×10^{-11}	4.4×10^{-2}		
Epoxy	2.1×10^{-10}	9.0×10^{-3}	3.2×10^{-11}			
PI (Vespel)	1.8×10^{-10}	3.1×10^{-3}				
PAI	1.1×10^{-10}	3.0×10^{-3}				

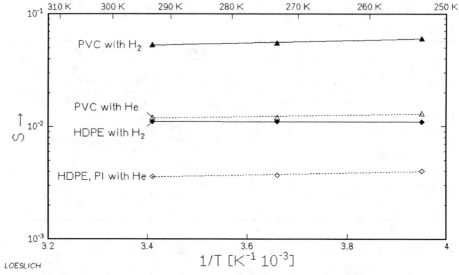

Figure 2-62   Solubility of helium and hydrogen (HDPE and PVC [10], PI (Vespel) [11]).

PUR foam. Polyurethane foam combines good thermal insulation with a reasonable mechanical stability. It is used, for instance, as insulation in liquid natural gas (LNG) storage vessels. The permeability depends strongly on the density of the foam. Some room temperature values of the permeability of this material are given in Table 2-15 [14].

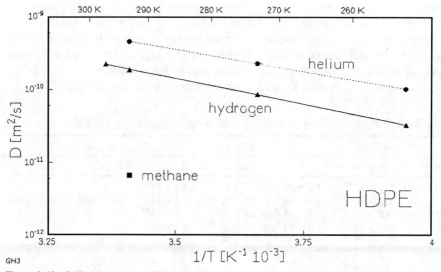

Figure 2-63   Diffusivity versus $1/T$ for several gases.

Table 2-15 Permeability P at room temperature of PUR foam with different densities

Density (Kg/m^3)	P (m^2/s)
450	2.5×10^{-10}
200	4.7×10^{-10}
50	21.0×10^{-10}
33	25.0×10^{-10}

2-5-17 Radiation Damage

In some applications, polymers are exposed to ionizing radiation. The mechanisms are different for γ, e^-, or neutron irradiation. In all cases, the irradiation leads to direct or indirect ionization of the electronic orbitals and gives rise to free radicals, chain scission, or changes in the covalent binding structure. Changes in the molecular composition occur when hydrogen ions are removed from the polymer skeleton [18,19].

Neutron irradiation initiates additional nuclear processes involving high-energy depositions:

- Hydrogen (H) knock off
- High cross section of relatively heavy atoms in polymers containing halogens, such as, PVC, and PTFE (Teflon). Thus, polymers having high densities of hydrogen or halogens are less favorable for use in fusion technology and particle accelerators.

The radiation damage depends somewhat on the temperature of irradiation and on warm-up before measurement. Degradation processes that occur during warm-up after irradiation include the following:

- Free radicals, which are immobile at cryogenic temperatures, may regenerate or produce cross-linking or less favorable compositions.
- Formation of H_2 gas (or other low-molecular gases) by neutron knock-off processes and ionization by gamma rays. The dilatation of gas causes a foam-like structure and is an important process of degradation.

The admissible dose is defined as that at which a property is degraded to half of its previous value. For most polymers, degradation of mechanical properties occurs first followed by dielectric and thermal properties. The dose of different radiation sources (gamma, electron, neutron) is intercalibrated and expressed in grays (1 Gy $\approx$ 100 rad) [19,20].

General conclusions. Polymers are resistant to radiation if their structure has

- A low hydrogen density (otherwise formation of H_2 gas results)
- Strong molecular units such as aromatic rings (not always true)
- Few ether bonds
- Few tertiary or quarternary C atoms
- Many double bonds or cycloaliphatic units

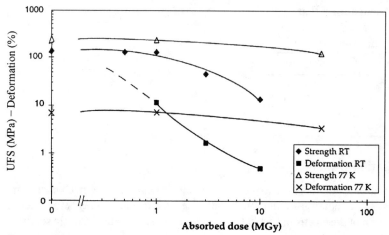

Figure 2-64 Ultimate flexural strength and deformation of PESU versus absorbed dose (from Ref. [16]).

- Few possibilities for radiation-induced cross-linking (e.g., PE is very susceptible to this effect)
- No heavy elements with large neutron cross-sections, such as polymers with halogen (PVC, PTFE, etc.)
- For epoxy resins, the following resistances hold:
  best: aromatic amines
  medium: cycloaliphatic components
  worst: aliphatic or acid anhydride components

The highest resistance has been found for PI, especially the cross-linked PI (Kerimide). The lowest admissible dose is found for PTFE (Teflon) [21–23].

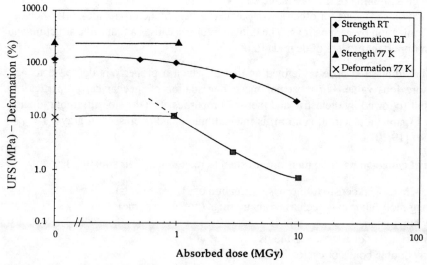

Figure 2-65 Ultimate flexural strength and deformation of PSU versus absorbed dose (from Ref. [16]).

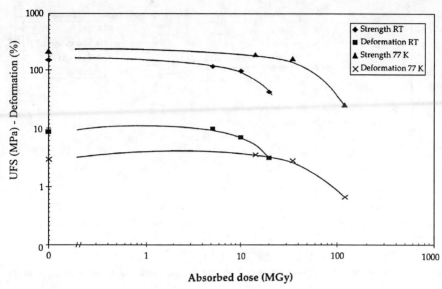

Figure 2-66 Ultimate flexural strength and deformation of epoxy (MY745 + HY906 Ciba–Geigy) versus absorbed dose.

Degradation of Properties

Mechanical properties. Some results of irradiation on flexural strength and deformation (strain) properties are shown in Figs. 2-64 to 2-66 and Table 2-16 [20]. The impact of irradiation on tensile strength and elongation is shown in Figs. 2-67 and 2-68 [20]. The figures show that the radiation resistance is higher at 77 K than at room temperature. The impact is greater on the deformation properties than the strength properties.

Dielectric properties. The dielectric loss factor tan δ is not seriously influenced by irradiation. A dose of 10^6 Gy causes a degradation of 30% for epoxies [24].

Table 2-16 Impact of ionizing radiation on flexural and compressive strength

Material	Admissible dose (Gy)	Reference
PI (Kapton foil)	8 to 10×10^7	16,18
PI (Vespel, Bulk)	1×10^7	16
PI (Kerimide, duropl.)	10 to 20×10^7	18
Epoxies unfilled:		
with aromatic amine	5×10^7	16,19
with acid anhydride	1×10^7	17
with aliphatic amine	0.7×10^7	
Thermoplastic polymers:		
PEEK	5×10^7	16
PC	0.2×10^7	17
HDPE	0.2 to 0.5×10^7	17

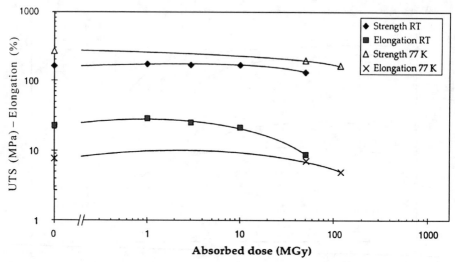

Figure 2-67   Ultimate tensile strength and elongation of Kapton H film versus absorbed dose (from Ref. [16]).

The dielectric constant (permittivity) of epoxies is more influenced, especially by gamma rays. A dose of 10^7 Gy degrades ε_l from 3.4 to 1.8 at 100 K [24]. Similar results have been observed in PI [25].

The dielectric strength is less sensitive to irradiation. Even a dose of more than 10^8 Gy does not reduce the initial breakdown voltage remarkably (see Table 2-17). Dielectric strength is defined by the breakdown voltage per thickness. It should be mentioned that

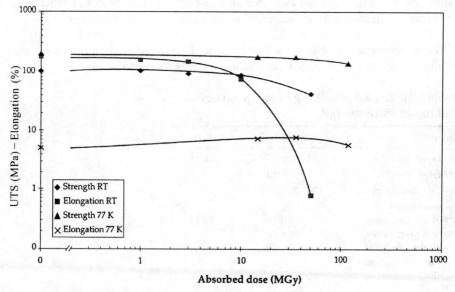

Figure 2-68   Ultimate tensile strength and elongation of PEEK film versus absorbed dose (from Ref. [16]).

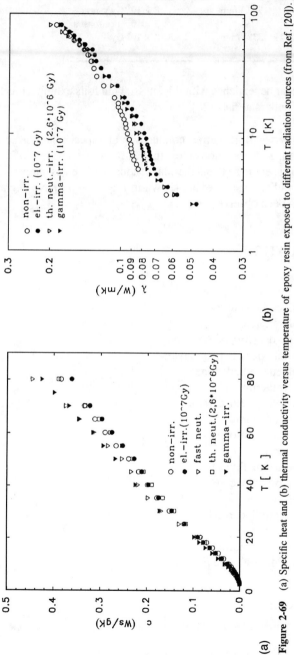

Figure 2-69 (a) Specific heat and (b) thermal conductivity versus temperature of epoxy resin exposed to different radiation sources (from Ref. [20]).

155

Table 2-17 Dielectric strength and irradiation

Material	Dielectric strength	Admissible dose
Kapton–H film (125 μm)	70 kV/mm	8×10^7 Gy γ rays + 3×10^{22} neutrons/m^2
Epoxy; Epon 828 (2-mm thick)	33kV/mm	2×10^8 Gy

there is no linear dependence with thickness. Thin foils exhibit a much higher dielectric strength than bulk materials [26].

Thermal properties Both thermal conductivity and specific heat do not degrade seriously with irradiation. A degradation of less than 30% has been observed for epoxy at doses up to 10^7 Gy. The specific heat and thermal conductivity versus temperature for epoxyresin and different radiation sources are shown in Fig. 2-69(a,b). No degradation of thermal expansion has been observed.

NOMENCLATURE

EP	Epoxy resin
PA	Polyamide
PC	Polycarbonate
PE	Polyethylene
HDPE	High-density polyethylene
MDPE	Middle-density polyethylene
PEEK	Polyetheretherketone
PEI	Polyetherimide
PEMA	Polyethermethacrylate
PMMA	Polymethylmethacrylate
PESU	Polyethersulfone
PI	Polyimide
POM	Polyoxymethylene
PP	Polypropylene
PS	Polystyrene
PTFE	Polytetrafluorethylene
PUR	Polyurethane
PVC	Polyvinylchloride
LCP	Liquid crystalline polymers

REFERENCES

1. Hartwig, G., "Status and Future of Fiber Composites at Low Temperatures," *Adv. Cryog. Eng.* (Mat.) 40B (1994):961.
2. Meyer, W., *Solid State Commun.* 22 (1977):285.
3. Hunklinger, S., "Phonon Scattering in Condensed Matter," *Solid State Sci.* (1984):384.

4. Hartwig, G., and Schwarz, G., "Correlation of Dielectric and Mechanical Damping at Low Temperatures," *Adv. Cryog. Eng.* 30 (1984):61.
5. Hartwig, G., *Polymer Propertiers at Room and Cryogenic Temperatures* (New York: Plenum Press, 1994):146.
6. Döll, W., *Adv. Polym. Sci.*, 52/53 (1983):108.
7. Hartwig, G., and Christoph, G., "Crack Properties in Polymers at Low Temperatures," *Adv. Cryog. Eng.* (Mat.) 42 A (1997):42.
8. Hartwig, G., Kneifel, B., and Pöhlmam, P., "Fracture Properties of Polymers and Composites at Low Temperatures," *Adv. Cryog. Eng.* 32 (1986):169
9. Hartwig, G., and Knaak, S., "Fatigue Behavior of Polymers," *Cryog.* 31 (1991):231.
10. Hübner, R., thesis, University of Karlsruhe, Germany (1996).
11. Hartwig, G., *Polymer Properties at Room and Cryogenic Temperatures* (New York: Plenum Press, 1994), 17.
12. Viety, W. R., *Diffusion In and Through Polymers* (Munich: Carl Hansen Press, 1991).
13. Barrer, R. H., "Diffusion and Solution of Gases in Organic Polymers," *Trans. Faraday Soc.*, 35 (1939):628–643.
14. Humpenoder, J., "Gas Permeation Through Polymers and Fiber Composites at Low Temperatures," *Cryog.* (1997) (in press).
15. Schmidtchen, U., Gradt, T., Borner, H., and Behrend, E., "Temperature Behavior of Permeation of Helium Through Vespel and Torlon," *Cryog.* 34 (1994):105.
16. Evans, D., and Morgan, J. T. "The Permeability of Composite Materials to Hydrogen and Helium Gas," *Adv. Cryog. Eng.* (Mat.) 34 (1987):11.
17. Disdier, S., Roy, J. M., Pallier, and P., and Bunsell, and A. R., "Helium Permeation in Composite Materials for Cryogenic Applications," *Cryog.* (1997) (in press).
18. Evans, D., Reed, R. P., and Hazelton, C. S., "Fundamental Aspects of Plastic Materials at Low Temperatures," *Cryog.* 35 (1995):755.
19. Takamura, S., and Kato, T., "Effect of Low Temperature Irradiation on the Mechanical Strength of Organic Insulators for Superconducting Magnets," *Cryog.* 20 (1980):441.
20. Humer, H., Schöbacher, H., Szeless, B., Tarlet, M., and Weber, H. W., CERN Report 96-05, 4 July 1996.
21. Evans, D., and Morgan, J. T., "A Review of the Effect of Ionizing Radiation on Plastic Materials," *Adv. Cryog. Eng.* 28 (1982):147.
22. Coltman, R. R., Jr., "Organic Insulators and Copper Stabilizers for Fusion Reactors," *J. Nucl. Mat.*, 108/109 (1982):559–571.
23. Hurley, G. F., and Coltman, R. R., Jr., "Organic Materials for Fusion Reactors," *J. Nucl. Mat.*, 123 (1984):1327.
24. Jäckel, M., Leucke, U., Jahn, K., Fitzke, F., and Hegenbarth, E., "Thermal and Dielectric Properties of Epoxy Resins at Low Temperatures After Irradiation," *Adv. Cryog. Eng.* (Mat.) 40 (1994):1153.
25. Wright, W. W., ed., *Polyimides* (New York: Plenum Press, 1987):147.
26. Schutz, J. B., Fabian, P. E., Hazelton, C. S., Bauer-Macdonald, T. S., and Reed, R. P., "Effect of Cryogenic Irradiation on Electrical Strength of Candidate ITER Insulation Materials," *Cryog.* 35 (1995):759.

BIBLIOGRAPHY

Hartwig, G., *Polymer Propertiers at Room and Cryogenic Temperatures* (New York: Plenum Press, 1994).
Kausch, H. H., *Polymer Fracture* (Berlin: Springer–Verlag, 1987).
Kinlock, A. J., and Young, R. J., *Fracture Behavior of Polymers* (Applied Science Publishers, 1983).
Strobl, S., *Polymer Structure* (Berlin: Springer–Verlag, 1996).

APPENDIX A

Table A-1 Integral thermal expansion

Polymer	$-\Delta L/L_0$, % 293–77 K	$-\Delta L/L_0$, % 293–4.2 K
PEEK	0.9	1.0
PESU	0.9	1.1
PETFE	1.4	1.6
PETP	1.1	1.3
PC	1.2	1.4
	–	–
PSU	1.0	1.1
PMMA	0.9	1.0
PS	1.3	1.5
PVC (gray)	1.0	1.1
(red)	1.1	1.3
PVDF	1.4	1.5
PI (Kerimid)	0.8	0.9
PI (Vespel)	0.8	0.9
PI	–	–
PEI	0.8	1.0
PAI	0.7	0.8
PA 12	1.5	1.6
Epoxy (Cy221/Hy979)	1.0	1.1
Epoxy (DGEBA diam.)	0.9	1.1
Epoxy (rigid)	1.0	1.1
(semiflexible)	1.3	1.5
HDPE	2.0	2.1
PE	–	–
PE	–	–
PE	–	–
PE	–	–
PTFE	1.7	1.8
POM	1.4	1.5
PP	1.2	1.3

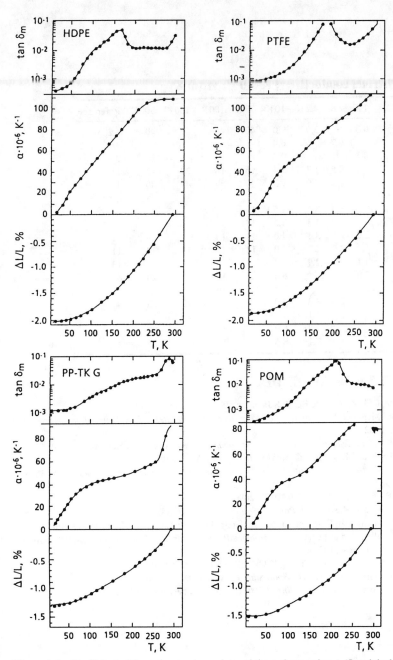

Figure A-1 Coefficient of thermal expansion α; integral thermal expansion Δ/L and the loss factor $\tan\delta$.

Table A-2 Thermal conductivity; $K \cdot 10^{-2}$; W/(m,K)

Polymer	1 K	2 K	4.2 K	10 K	70 K	100 K	150 K	300 K	Reference
HDPE	0.3		2.9	9.0	40	45		40	1,2
MDPE		0.7		6.0					3
PTFE	0.3			9.5				25	3
PP		0.5	1.2	3.4	16	18	20	22	11
POM		1.2	3.0	9.3	49	50	49	40	11
PETP									4,10
(amorphous)		3.0	3.5	4.5	15				
(crystalline 25%)		0.7	1.3	3.0	17				
PC	2.0	2.5	3.1	4.0	13	15			11
PVC		2.0	2.7	4.0	12	13	13	14	11
PS	1.1		2.9	3.0		5			13
PMMA	2.0			6.0		16		20	8
	3.0			7.5		20			7
PI (Kerimid)		2.5	3.8	4.0		9	12	23	9
(Vespel)			1.1						
Epoxies			4.8[1]	6.0		13		22	
			7.1[2]	8.5		16		25	

REFERENCES FOR APPENDIX

1. Van de Voorde, CERN 77-8 ISR-BOM, 8 January; 1977.
2. Engeln, J., and Meissner, M., *Nonmetallic Materials and Composites at Low Temperatures* (New York: Plenum Press, 1982), 4.
3. Perepechko, I. I., *Low-Temperature Properties of Polymers* (New York: Pergamon Press, 1980), 57.
4. Greig, D. and Sahota, M., *J. Phys. C. Solid State Phys.* 16 (1983):105.
5. Rosenberg, H. M., *Nonmetallic Materials and Composites at Low Temperatures 2* (New York: Plenum Press, 1980), 181.
6. Stephens, R. B., *Phys. Rev.* B 8., no. 6 (1973):2896.
7. Finnlayson, D. M. and Mason, P., *J. Phys. C. Solid State Phys.* (1984).
8. Finnlayson, D. M., Mason, P., Rogers, J. N., and Greig; D., *J. Phys. C. Solid State Phys.* 13 (1980):13.
9. Claudet, G., Disdier, F., and Locatelli, M., *Nonmetallic Materials and Composites at Low Temperatures* (New York: Plenum Press, 1978).
10. Choy, C. L., Salinger, G. L., and Chiang Y. C., NBS Spec. Publ. 301 (1961):567.
11. Choy, C. L., and Greig, D., *J. Phys C. Solid State Phys.* 10 (1977):169.
12. Evans, D., and Morgan, J. T., *Proceedings ICMC* (London: Butterworths, 1982), 286.
13. Hager, N. E., Jr., *Rev. Sci. Instr.* 31 (1960):177.

Table A-3 Moduli and fracture data

Polymers	4.2 K E' (GPa)	G' (GPa)	σ_{UT} (MPa)	ε_{UT} (%)	77 K E' (GPa)	G' (GPa)	σ_{UT} (MPa)	ε_{UT} %	150 K E' (GPa)	G' (GPa)	250 K E' (GPa)	G' (GPa)	290 K E' (GPa)	G' (GPa)
HDPE	9.8	3.8	196	3.0	8.3	3.7	153	4.0	6.0	2.3	2.5	1.2	2.0	1.0
POM	13.3	5.0			12.4	4.6			10.8	4.3	4.5	1.8	3.8	1.5
PTFE	7.2	2.9	87	1.5	6.7	2.7	77	1.6	5.9	2.1	1.7	0.5	1.3	0.4
PP	7.7	2.8			6.8	2.6			6.4	2.3		1.7		0.9
PEEK	6.9	2.6	197	3.3	6.1	2.5	192	5.5		2.0		1.7	3.6	1.4
PS	5.6	2.2	79	1.6	4.5	1.7	57	2.0	4.3	1.6	3.9	1.4	3.6	1.3
PSU	5.2	1.8			4.3	1.5	130	7.0	3.8	1.2	3.1	1.0	2.9	0.9
PC	5.6	2.2	177	3.3	4.9	1.9	156	6.0	3.8	1.5	2.6	1.0	2.5	1.0
PMMA	8.2	2.9			8.0	2.7			7.5	2.6	7.2	2.1		1.7
PI (Vespel)	5.8	2.1	157	3.0		1.9				1.7		1.4		1.3
PI (Kerimid)		2.3				2.2				2.1		1.8		1.5
PEI	5.9	1.7	166	3.4	4.9	1.5	157	5.2		1.5		1.3	3.0	1.2
PAI	5.9	2.3	147	2.6	5.6	2.2	150	3.2		2.0		1.6		1.5
EP I	7.1		150	2.4	6.1	3.1	150	3.1						
II	7.8	3.1	180	2.0	7.2	3.0	150	3.1	6.2	2.5	4.2	1.6	3.1	1.3

Note: Dynamic moduli E' at 10 Hz and G' between 5 and 10 Hz; Epoxies: EP(1): LY 556/Hy 917 EP(11): Cy221/Hy 979(Ciba–Geigy). From Perepechko, j, *Low temperature Properties of Polymers* (New York: Pergamon Press, 1977), 243.
E' = Young's modulus, G' = shear modulus, σ_{UT} = fracture strength, ε_{UT} = fracture strain.

Table A-4 Fracture mechanical data

Material	Temperature (K)	G_{IC} (kJ/m^2)	K_{IC} (MPa,m$^{1/2}$)	E' (GPa)	σ_{UT} (MPa)	ε_{UT} (%)
PS	4.2	0.16	1.0	5.6	80	1.5
	77.0	7.1[a]	6.1[a]	4.4	55	2.0
EP II	4.2	0.16	1.3	7.1	170	
	77.0		1.9[a]	6.1	150	1.9
PC	4.2	1.3	2.9	5.6	175	3.7
	77.0	4.8[a]	5.2[a]	4.8	155	6.6
		1.5[b]	4.7[b]			
HDPE	4.2	5.8	7.8	9.8	195	3.0
	77.0	9.8[a]	9.6[a]	8.0	155	4.0
		5.8[c]	6.0[c]		153	
PMMA	77.0	0.3[a]	2.2[a]	8.0		
PEEK	4.2			6.9	197	3.3
	77.0		3.4	6.2	190	5.2

Note: G_{IC} = Critical energy release rate, K_{IC} = critical strength concentration factor (both in mode I).
[a] At LN$_2$ environment and a COD rate of $3 \cdot 10^{-5}$ m/s.
[b] At He environment and a COD rate of $5 \cdot 10^{-7}$ m/s.
[c] Stable crack propagation at a COD rate of $7 \cdot 10^{-6}$ m/s.

THREE

CRYOGENIC HEAT TRANSFER

P. Kittel

*NASA Ames Research Center, MS 234-1,
Moffett Field, CA 94035-1000*

L. J. Salerno

*NASA Ames Research Center, MS 234-1,
Moffett Field, CA 94035-1000*

T. Nast

*Lockheed Martin Missiles and Space, 3251 Hanover
Street, Orgn. H121, Building 205,
Palo Alto, CA 94304*

M. Shiotsu

*Kyoto University, Dept. of Energy Science and
Technology, Gokasho, Uji, Kyoto 611, Japan*

J. G. Weisend II

*MKS, DESY Laboratory, Notkestrasse 85,
22607 Hamburg, Germany*

3-1 INTRODUCTION

This chapter is not meant as a general review of heat transfer but as a discussion of those aspects of heat transfer that are particularly important in cryogenics. Some general heat transfer texts are Refs. [1–3], whereas Refs. [4] and [5] are books devoted to cryogenic heat transfer. The study of heat transfer is generally divided up into the topics of heat transfer by conduction, convection, and radiation. This chapter follows a similar approach. The conduction section discusses thermal conductivity integrals and thermal contact conductance. The convection section covers convective heat transfer correlations for cryogenic fluids and boiling limits. The radiation section discusses the use of multilayer insulation (MLI) to reduce radiation heat transfer. The unique aspects of heat transfer in helium II (including Kapitza conductance) are covered in chapter 10 of this handbook.

3-2 CONDUCTION HEAT TRANSFER

3-2-1 Thermal Conductivity Integrals

J. G. Weisend II

MKS, DESY Laboratory, Notkestrasse 85, 22607 Hamburg, Germany

Conduction heat transfer in cryogenic systems frequently involves large temperature differences (e.g., 300–77 K). The thermal conductivity of solids is strongly temperature-dependent, and this dependence can not be neglected in the heat transfer calculations. Thermal conductivity integrals provide a way to allow for this dependence.

Recall that the general equation for steady-state, one-dimensional conduction heat transfer between temperatures T_2 and T_1 is

$$Q = \frac{-1}{\int_{x_1}^{x_2} \frac{dx}{A(x)}} \left[\int_{T_1}^{T_2} K(T) \, dT \right] \tag{3-1}$$

where $K(T)$ is the thermal conductivity, $A(x)$ is the cross-sectional area, T_2 is the higher temperature, and T_1 is the lower temperature. The minus sign is present due to the definition of heat flowing opposite the temperature gradient. Equation (3-1) may be expanded to

$$Q = \frac{-1}{\int_{x_1}^{x_2} \frac{dx}{A(x)}} \left[\int_{0}^{T_2} K(T) \, dT - \int_{0}^{T_1} K(T) \, dT \right] \tag{3-2}$$

or

$$Q = -G(\theta_2 - \theta_1) \tag{3-3}$$

where the geometry factor G is defined by

$$G = \frac{1}{\int_{x_1}^{x_2} \frac{dx}{A(x)}} \tag{3-4}$$

Note that in the frequent case of uniform cross section of length L, $G = A/L$.

The terms θ_1 and θ_2 are known as the thermal conductivity integrals and are defined as

$$\theta_i = \int_{0}^{T_i} K(T) \, dT \tag{3-5}$$

Figures 3-1 and 3-2 show the thermal conductivity integrals of a number of technically useful materials. These figures were created by D. S. Holmes of Lakeshore Cryotronics [6]. The value of the thermal conductivity integrals and Eq. (3-3) is that they permit a straightforward calculation of the conduction heat transfer while allowing for the temperature dependence of the thermal conductivity.

3-2-2 Thermal Contact Conductance

L. J. Salerno and P. Kittel

NASA Ames Research Center, MS 234-1,
Moffett Field, CA 94035-1000

Introduction. The performance of cryogenic instruments is often a function of their operating temperature. For example, the sensitivity of infrared bolometers is a function of $T^{-5/3}$; similarly the performance of photoconductive detectors deteriorates rapidly

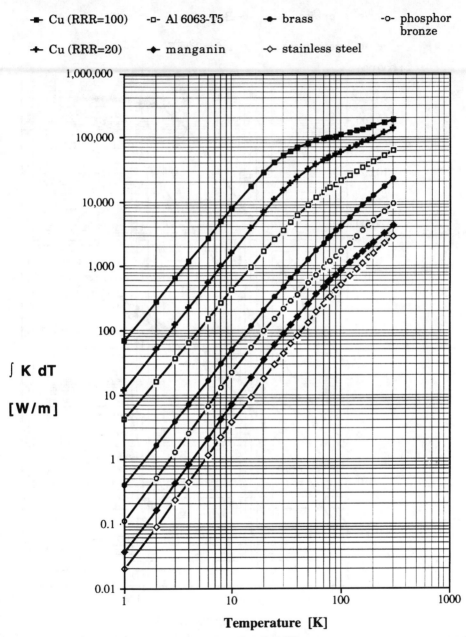

- ▪ Cu (RRR=100)
- ❏ Al 6063-T5
- ● brass
- ○ phosphor bronze
- ✛ Cu (RRR=20)
- ✦ manganin
- ◇ stainless steel

$\int$ **K dT**

[W/m]

Temperature [K]

Figure 3-1 Thermal conductivity integrals of metals (from Ref. [6]).

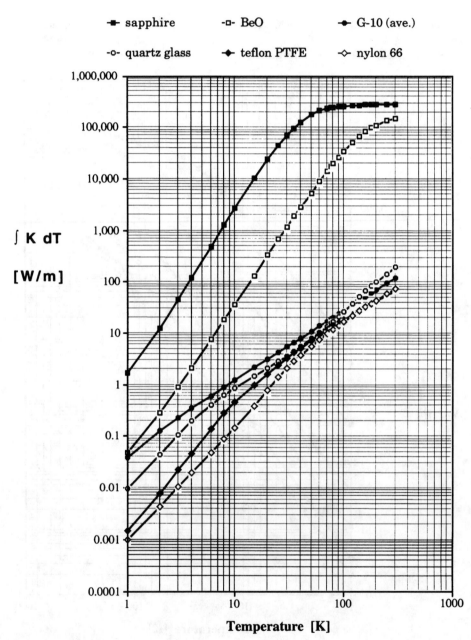

Figure 3-2 Thermal conductivity integrals of insulators (from Ref. [6]). D. S. Holmes, Lakeshore Cryotronics.

when the temperature reaches or exceeds their band gap and superconducting components must operate below their transition temperatures. Thus, designers of cryogenic instruments often are required to predict the operating temperature of each instrument they design. This requires accurate thermal models of cryogenic components that include the properties of the materials and assembly techniques used. When components are bolted or otherwise pressed together, a knowledge of the thermal performance of such joints is also needed. In some cases, the temperature drop across these joints represents a significant fraction of the total temperature difference between the instrument and its cooler. Although extensive databases exist on the thermal properties of bulk materials, similar databases for pressed contacts do not. This has often led to instrument designs that avoid pressed contacts or to the overdesign of such joints at unnecessary expense. These are not always viable options. Although many people have made measurements of contact conductances at cryogenic temperatures, these data are often very narrow in scope and even more often have not been published in an easily retrievable fashion, if published at all. This section presents a summary of the limited pressed contact data available in the literature.

Theory of thermal contact conductance and review of work. Thermal contact resistance is attributable to several factors, the most notable being that contact between two surfaces is made only at a few discrete locations rather than over the entire surface area. A close examination of even the smoothest surfaces reveals an asperity that limits the actual area of contact to as few as three discrete locations irrespective of the dimensions of the sample. This is supported empirically by findings that the thermal conductance of pressed contacts is dependent on the applied force and not on the area of contact or on the apparent contact pressure [7].

As the applied force is increased, surface deformation of the material occurs. The initial area of contact increases and, as the material deforms further, contact occurs at new locations. The heat flow is constricted in the vicinity of the contact locations because of the narrowness of the effective areas of contact, as represented in Fig. 3-3. This constriction is, in large part, responsible for contact resistance.

Additionally, the presence of surface films or oxides contributes to the phenomenon. The thickness of these layers adds an additional variable to the conductance. In the case of oxides, because the oxide layer generally has high thermal resistance, it must be penetrated to obtain a consistent measure of the thermal resistance of the actual contacts. At low temperatures, each oxide layer acts as an additional boundary resistance, and the problem is compounded because of the acoustic mismatch between the layers (Kapitza resistance). Further, the thickness of the oxide layer is often a function of time.

Estimates of the constriction resistance have been made for specific assumed contact geometries by modeling the contacts as individual elements. By arranging the elements in groups of varying heights, the asperity can be accounted for as well. Although contact pressure and material hardness can be used to determine the ratio of the sample surface area to the actual contact area, the equivalent radius of the contact spot must be well known, and a probability distribution of the spots must be calculated. Because each sample represents a new problem, estimation of the contact resistance from theoretical models

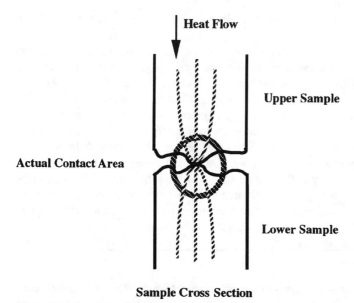

Sample Cross Section

Figure 3-3 Heat flow constriction.

is not a trivial task [8,9], and most data in the field are empirical. Table 3-1 presents a summary of low-temperature thermal contact data available in the literature. [7,10–25]

Experimental data have shown [11,17–19] that the thermal conductance of metallic pressed contacts increases according to a simple power law function of temperature and can be described by the relation

$$k(T) = \alpha T^n \qquad (3\text{-}5)$$

where n typically ranges from 0.75 to 2.5.

Thermal conductance also increases asymptotically with increasing applied force. As the applied force increases, the actual area of contact approaches the apparent area. For uncoated samples of aluminum, brass, copper, and stainless steel at liquid helium temperature, it has also been found that thermal conductance is related to the surface finish of the samples. Except in the case of aluminum, for lapped sample pairs with finishes of 0.1, 0.2, 0.4, 0.8, and 1.6 μm, the maximum observed contact conductance at 4.2 K was exhibited by the 0.4-μm surface finish: For aluminum samples, the conductance was lowest for the 0.4-μm surface finish and peaked at 0.2 μm. Although several mechanisms have been postulated to account for this effect, no causal relationship has been established, and the possibility of a systematic anomaly in sample pair preparation cannot be excluded.

Because constriction resistance plays a major role in limiting thermal transfer, increasing the effective contact area by applying a conforming coating can significantly enhance contact conductance, even if the coating material is of relatively low thermal conductivity. The reason for this is that, ideally, a conforming coating allows the entire contact surface to transfer heat, rather than a few narrow areas. In reality, although the ideal condition is unattainable, considerable improvement in thermal contact

Table 3-1 Summary of thermal contact literature

Researcher (Ref.)	Year	Material	Temperature (K)	Applied force (lbs)[a]	Conductance (W/K)
Berman [7]	1956	Copper	4.2	50	5.5×10^{-3}
		Copper	4.2	100	1.02×10^{-2}
		Copper	4.2	150	1.46×10^{-2}
		Copper	4.2	200	1.9×10^{-2}
		Copper	4.2	250	2.3×10^{-2}
Deutsch [10]	1979	Copper	4.2	225	0.34
Kittel et al. [11,14]	1992	Gold-plated: aluminum brass copper stainless steel	1.6–4.2	5–150	1.3×10^{-4} to 3.3×10^{-2}
Kittel et al. [12,21]	1994	Bimetallic: aluminum/ stainless steel	77	2–60	9×10^{-3} to 2.1×10^{-2}
Manninen and Zimmerman [13]	1977	Copper	4.2	225	0.34
Mian et al. [14]	1979	Mild steel	300	220	0.825^b 1.25^c
Nilles and Van Sciver [15] (at 4.2 K)	1988	Copper -oxidation treatment -normal	4–290	29	4×10^{-3} 1.4×10^{-2} 2.0×10^{-2} 8.0×10^{-2} 1.3×10^{-1} 1.4×10^{-1}
Radebaugh et al. [16]	1977	Copper	4.2	110	10^{-2}
		Polished silver	4.2	110	1.1
		Stainless steel	300	110	10^{-2}
Salerno et al. [17,18,19,20]	1984 1985 1986 1988	Aluminum brass copper stainless steel	1.6–4.2	5–150	1×10^{-4} to 2.0×10^{-2}
Salerno et al. [21,22]	1993 1994	Augmented: aluminum brass copper stainless steel	1.6–4.2	5–150	3.6×10^{-5} to 1.0×10^{-2} (aluminum-plated washer)
	1994				5.0×10^{-4} to 0.28 (In, Ap)
Suomi et al. [23]	1968	Copper	0.02–0.2	?	10^{-2}
Thomas and Probert [24]	1970	Stainless steel	88–95	100 200	0.36 0.5

(Continues)

Table 3-1 (*Continued*)

Researcher (Ref.)	Year	Material	Temperature (K)	Applied force (lbs)[a]	Conductance (W/K)
Wanner [25]	1981	Aluminum	1–4	1050	0.2[d]
				2100	0.6[d]
				2800	1.5[d]

[a] To convert applied force to newtons, multiply pounds by 4.4482.
[b] Optically flat.
[c] Roughness < 3 μm.
[d] At 4.2 K.

conductance is possible by applying conforming coatings. Several methods have been reported [15,21,22] such as gold plating the contact surfaces, coating the surfaces with low-temperature grease, or inserting a thin sheet of indium metal between the contact surfaces. Of the methods reported, a thin layer of low-temperature grease appears to offer the best enhancement of thermal conductance.

In practice, measuring such enhanced contacts is not as straightforward as it might appear. Ordinarily, the contribution of the bulk material thermal conductivity to the thermal contact conductance is negligible; however, the high thermal conductance of indium- or Apiezon-coated contacts requires that a correction be made to the experimental data to account for the bulk thermal conductivity of the sample material between the thermometers and the contact interfaces. Figure 3-4 represents the situation schematically. The upper sample temperature T_U and lower sample temperature T_L are measured 3.17 mm from the interface, resulting in a ΔT across the bulk material of the samples. These are denoted by ΔT_U and ΔT_L in the figure. The ΔT of interest across the interface ΔT_c is

$$\Delta T_c = (T_U - \Delta T_U) - (T_L + \Delta T_L) \tag{3-6}$$

The ΔT_U and ΔT_L are found for each data point from

$$Q = A_U/L \int_{T_U - \Delta T_U}^{T_U} k\, dT \tag{3-7}$$

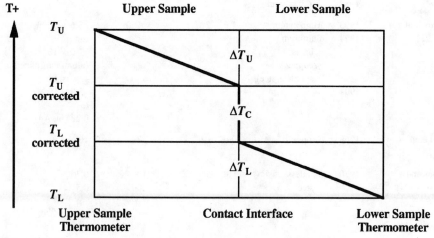

Figure 3-4 Schematic representation of temperature drop across samples and contact area.

and

$$Q = A_L/L \int_{T_L}^{T_L + \Delta T_L} k \, dT \qquad (3\text{-}8)$$

where the quantities A_U and A_L denote the areas of the upper and lower samples, respectively, and L denotes the length from the thermometer to the contact interface.

Summary of experimental data. Data are shown in Fig. 3-5 for thermal conductance versus temperature at 670-N applied force for uncoated contact surfaces, gold-coated contact surfaces, contacts with a gold-coated aluminum washer placed between the surfaces, contacts having a thin sheet of indium foil between the surfaces, and contact surfaces coated with a layer of Apiezon-N grease. Although only copper is shown for clarity, similar trends are observed for aluminum, brass, and stainless steel. Depending on the sample bulk material and the thickness of the coating, improvement of thermal conductance ranges from a factor of 2 for gold coating to an order of magnitude for indium foil. The improvement gained by insertion of the gold-coated aluminum washer between the contact surfaces was essentially offset by the addition of two extra contact interfaces.

In Fig. 3-6, thermal conductance of copper contact pairs at 4.2 K is plotted versus applied force for several of the references in Table 3-1. Nilles and Van Sciver [15] prepared both rigorously cleaned copper samples and oxidized copper samples that were heated in laboratory air. Deutsch [10] and Manninen and Zimmerman [13] derived thermal conductance from measurements of the electrical conductance using the Weidemann–Franz

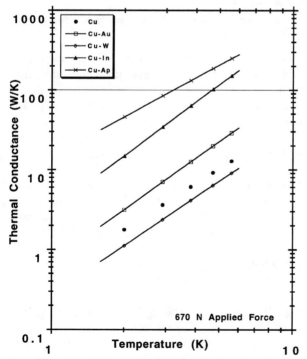

Figure 3-5 Surface coating comparison (Au–gold-plated; W–aluminum washer; In–indium foil; Ap–Apiezon grease).

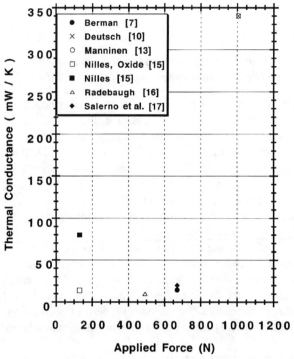

Figure 3-6 Thermal conductance of copper sample pairs at 4.2 K versus applied force (references from Table 3-1).

law. It appears that the room temperature Lorentz number was used. At low temperatures, the Lorentz number is known to decrease by an order of magnitude [26]. If their data are corrected for this effect, they then lie within the range of the other data plotted.

In Figs. 3-7 through 3-10, thermal conductance at an applied force of 670 N is plotted against temperature with surface finish as a parameter for uncoated aluminum, brass, and copper sample pairs. For stainless steel, only results for the 0.8-μm finish are presented. Both the aluminum and copper sample pairs exhibit a temperature-dependent crossover of specific finishes.

Figures 3-11 through 3-14 present thermal conductance versus applied force for several 0.8-μm finish sample pairs, with surface coating as a parameter. In Fig. 3-15, thermal conductance of bimetallic contact pairs (5052 aluminum/304L stainless steel; 5083 aluminum/304L stainless steel) is plotted against applied force at 77 K [12].

Discussion. It is apparent that conforming coatings offer significant enhancement to the thermal contact conductance and that indium and Apiezon exhibit the most significant enhancement.

In principle, the same result should be realizable with any conforming coating. Previous work with gold coating showed that, although the conductances were improved as the result of gold coating the surfaces, the improvement was nowhere near the magnitude of that realized with indium. There are two reasons for this. Firstly, gold, although soft

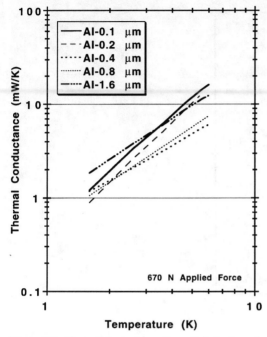

Figure 3-7   Thermal conductance of uncoated aluminum for various surface finishes.

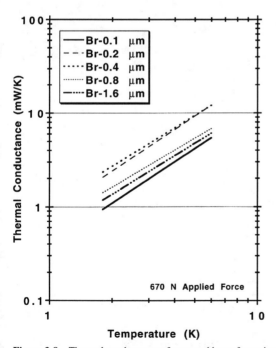

Figure 3-8   Thermal conductance of uncoated brass for various surface finishes.

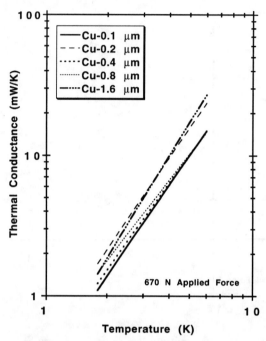

Figure 3-9 Thermal conductance of uncoated copper for various surface finishes.

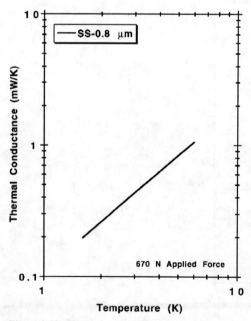

Figure 3-10 Thermal conductance of uncoated stainless steel for 0.8-μm surface finish.

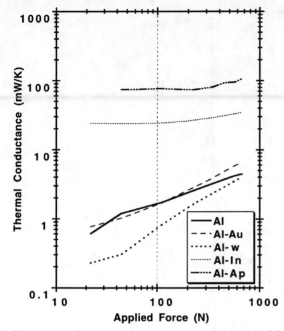

Figure 3-11   Thermal conductance versus applied force for 0.8-μm aluminum at 4.2 K.

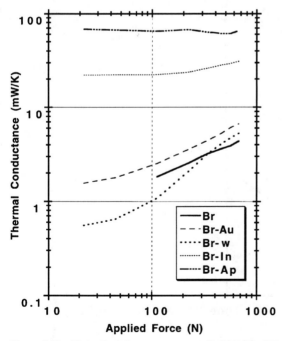

Figure 3-12   Thermal conductance versus applied force for 0.8-μm brass at 4.2 K.

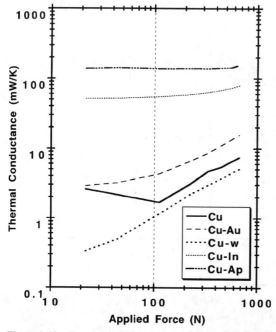

Figure 3-13 Thermal conductance versus applied force for 0.8-μm copper at 4.2 K.

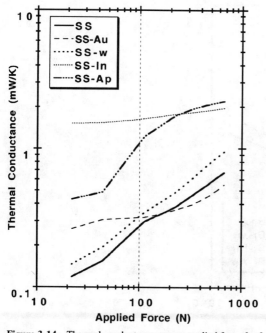

Figure 3-14 Thermal conductance versus applied force for 0.8-μm stainless steel at 4.2 K.

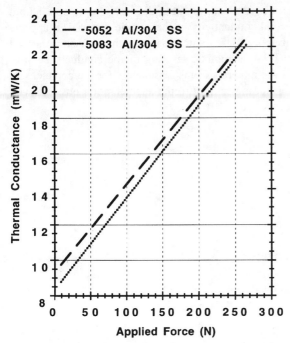

Figure 3-15 Thermal conductance versus applied force for aluminum/stainless steel at 77 K.

compared with the sample materials, is still much harder than indium, especially at low temperatures, where indium remains pliable. Secondly, the thickness of the gold coating was 2 μm per sample, a total of 4 μm. The thickness of indium was 0.13 mm, over thirty times that of the gold. As a side note, although the superconducting transition temperature of indium is 3.4 K, no measurable effects of the transition on the thermal conductance were noted.

Although the insertion of indium foil between the contact surfaces greatly improved the conductance, a significant improvement over indium was realized with Apiezon in the cases of aluminum, brass, and copper. Early data taken where only a moderate contact force was applied at room temperature before cooling of the sample pair were problematic and, in many cases, impossible to analyze. This can be attributed to the fact that, unlike indium foil, which flows, the Apiezon grease becomes rigid at cryogenic temperatures. If good contact is not made at room temperature, the resultant thick, nondeforming layer of Apiezon separates from the contact surfaces at liquid helium temperatures, and the thermal resistance across the contact area actually increases. To be effective, a large force must be applied at room temperature. This also assures that the layer of grease is thin, providing minimum contribution to the resistance.

It can be seen from Fig. 3-5 that the improvement in conductance at 670 N and 6 K is far greater for aluminum, brass, and copper, being over an order of magnitude, than for stainless steel, which improves by roughly a factor of three. This suggests that the thermal conductivity of the bulk material may play a role. If the improvement in thermal conductance over uncoated surfaces by the addition of Apiezon-N grease and indium foil is plotted versus the bulk thermal conductivity of the sample material, it appears that conductance increases in a roughly logarithmic manner with increasing thermal conductivity of the bulk material. The asymptotic leveling of the conductance with increasing thermal conductivity of the material seems reasonable, for the conductivity of the bulk material would serve as an upper limit to the augmentation possible with enhancement of the contact surfaces.

NOMENCLATURE

α Proportionality constant
A Overall contact surface area
A_L Area of lower sample
A_U Area of upper sample
d Sample diameter
dT Incremental temperature difference
F Applied force
k Effective thermal contact conductance
L Length from thermometer to contact interface
n Exponent
Q Applied heater power
Q_0 Offset (parasitic) heater power
T_L Lower sample temperature
T_U Upper sample temperature
ΔT Temperature difference across boundary
ΔT_L Temperature drop across bulk material of lower sample
ΔT_U Temperature drop across bulk material of upper sample

3-3 CONVECTION HEAT TRANSFER

3-3-1 Correlations for Forced Convection Heat Transfer

J. G. Weisend II

MKS, DESY Laboratory, Notkestrasse 85, 22607 Hamburg, Germany

Introduction. As with other fluids, the heat transfer from a heated surface to a moving cryogenic fluid may be described by Newton's law of cooling

$$Q = hA(T_w - T_b) \tag{3-9}$$

where Q is the heat transferred, A is the surface area, T_w is the wall temperature, T_b is the bulk fluid temperature, and h is the heat transfer coefficient. The heat transfer coefficient is determined empirically and is typically a function of fluid properties (thermal conductivity, viscosity, specific heat), flow velocity, and channel geometry. The determination of h is the most challenging part of using Eq. 3-9 to predict heat transfer from a surface into moving cryogenic fluid.

The correlations for h are generally given in terms of nondimensional groups. The most important groups for this analysis are the following:

Nusselt number

$$Nu = \frac{h D_h}{k} \tag{3-10}$$

Reynolds number

$$Re = \frac{\rho v D_h}{\mu} \tag{3-11}$$

Prandtl number

$$Pr = \frac{C_p \mu}{k} \tag{3-12}$$

These nondimensional groups are not completely arbitrary but in fact can be thought of as ratios of physical processes in the fluid. The Nusselt (Nu) number compares the surface heat transfer into the fluid with the conduction heat transfer in the fluid. The Reynolds (Re) number compares the inertial and viscous forces in the fluid, and the Prandtl (Pr) number compares the momentum transport with the thermal transport in the fluid.

The general form of the convective heat transfer correlation is then given by

$$Nu = f(Re, Pr) \tag{3-13}$$

With the exception of heat transfer in He II (see chapter 10) convective heat transfer into cryogenic fluids is not a priori any different than that for room temperature fluids. Thus, one can frequently use the same correlations that were developed for noncryogenic fluids. However, care must be taken to ensure that the correlation is valid for the flow conditions being examined and that the fluid properties are evaluated at the pressure and temperature of the cryogenic fluid.

Another issue is the state of the fluid. In this section, we will consider three different possibilities: single-phase liquid, single-phase gas (which includes supercritical fluids), and fluids near the critical point.

Liquid flows In the case of heat transfer to a turbulent, fully developed cryogenic liquid flow the Dittus–Boelter correlation can be used [27] as follows:

$$Nu = 0.023 Re^{4/5} Pr^{2/5} \tag{3-14}$$

Here the properties are evaluated at the film temperature T_f:

$$T_f = \frac{(T_b + T_w)}{2} \tag{3-15}$$

Gas flows In the case of heat transfer to a turbulent, fully developed cryogenic gas flow the following correlation has been shown to be useful [4]:

$$Nu = 0.023 Re_b^{4/5} Pr_b^{2/5} \left(\frac{T_w}{T_b} \right)^{-0.57 - (1.59/x/D)} \tag{3-16}$$

Here the fluid properties are evaluated at the bulk temperature, D is the hydraulic diameter of the channel, and x is the axial position at which Nu is evaluated. Note that this correlation will give results close to that of Eq. (3-14). In the particular case of heat transfer to supercritical helium, studies have shown that the best predictions are given by [28] as follows:

$$Nu = 0.0259 Re_b^{4/5} Pr_b^{2/5} \left(\frac{T_w}{T_b} \right)^{-0.716} \tag{3-17}$$

Flows near the critical point As discussed in chapter 1, fluid properties can vary significantly near the critical point. The behavior of forced-convection heat transfer into flows near the critical point is also quite complex. For the purposes of this discussion, the near critical region can be defined as a system in which $0.8 < P/P_c < 3$ and $T_{sat} < T < T^*$ [4], where P_c is the critical pressure, T_{sat} is the saturation temperature, and T^* is the transposed critical temperature. Reference [4] has a very good discussion of the problems in modeling forced convection heat transfer in this region. Researchers have noted both maximums and minimums of the heat transfer coefficient in the near critical region. Readers should view skeptically any convective heat transfer predictions in the near critical region and avoid working in this region if at all possible. With this warning in mind, the following correlations may be of occasional use.

An altered version of Eq. (3-14) has been shown to work for oxygen and carbon dioxide [29] in the form

$$Nu = 0.023 Re^{4/5} Pr_{min}^{2/5} \tag{3-18}$$

where Pr_{min} is the minimum of the Prandtl numbers evaluated at the wall and at the bulk fluid temperatures. Equation (3-18) does not work for hydrogen and also does not allow for temperature spikes that have been observed in oxygen in this region.

For the special case of hydrogen in which the bulk temperature of the hydrogen is above the transposed critical temperature, the following correlation can be used [4]:

$$Nu = 0.0208 Re^{4/5} Pr^{2/5} [1 + 0.0146(v_w/vb)] \tag{3-19}$$

NOMENCLATURE

A Area (m^2)
C_p Specific heat (J/kg · K)
D_h Hydraulic diameter (m)
h Heat transfer coefficient (WK/m^2)
k Thermal conductivity (W/mK)
μ Viscosity (Pa s)

Q Heat (W)
ρ Density (kg/m^3)
T_b Bulk fluid temperature (K)
T_w Wall temperature (K)

3-3-2 Predicting the Critical Heat Flux for a Horizontal Cylinder in Saturated Liquid He I

M. Shiotsu

Kyoto University, Dept. of Energy Science and Technology, Gokasho, Uji, Kyoto 611, Japan

Introduction. The critical heat flux (CHF) is the heat flux at which boiling changes from nucleate boiling to film boiling. Knowledge of the critical heat flux in liquid He I is important as a basis for designing liquid-helium-cooled superconducting magnets. Another advantage of studying CHF in liquid He I is that we can obtain detailed CHF data near the critical pressure, which is rather difficult to do with ordinary liquids such as water owing to their high saturation pressure and temperature at the critical point.

Experimental CHF data for a horizontal cylinder in liquid He I have been measured by Frederking [30] with very thin 16- and 32-μm-diameter wires under pressures ranging from 5.7 to 97 kPa. Recently, Shiotsu et al. [31] measured the CHF for 0.3-, 0.5-, and 1.2-mm-diameter horizontal cylinders under saturated conditions at pressures ranging from 24.4 kPa ($P/P_{cr} = 0.11$) to 198.6 kPa ($P/P_{cr} = 0.87$).

Figure 3-16 shows the CHF data [31], q_{cr}, plotted against system pressure together with Frederking's data [30] and Schmidt's data [32] on a 52-μm-diameter wire. As shown in the figure, the CHF at a constant pressure decreases with an increase in wire diameter, but this decrease is almost saturated for diameters larger than 0.3 mm. The CHF value for each diameter reaches a maximum at around 80 kPa and decreases when the pressure is changed from this value. The ratio of P/P_{cr} at this maximum point is about 0.4, which is similar to that for noncryogenic liquids.

CHF correlation The critical heat flux correlation for saturated pool boiling on a horizontal flat plate was presented by Kutateladze [33] and Zuber [34] for noncryogenic liquids as

$$q_{cr} = K L \rho_v \left[\sigma g (\rho_l - \rho_v)/\rho_v^2 \right]^{1/4} \tag{3-20}$$

The coefficient K for a horizontal cylinder was given by Kutateladze et al. [35] as a curve against the nondimensional diameter D', and by Lienhard and Dhir [36] as a function of D'. The predicted values of K given by Kutateladze and by Lienhard and Dhir are shown in Fig. 3-17 as a solid line and dashed line, respectively. The values of K calculated from Eq. (3-20) by using the experimental data for horizontal wires in He I are shown in the figure for comparison. The values of K based on the experimental data are significantly different from the solid curve given by Kutateladze in the lower D' range. The values

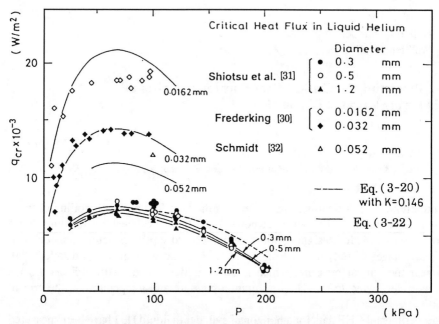

Figure 3-16 Critical heat flux versus pressure for horizontal cylinders in liquid helium.

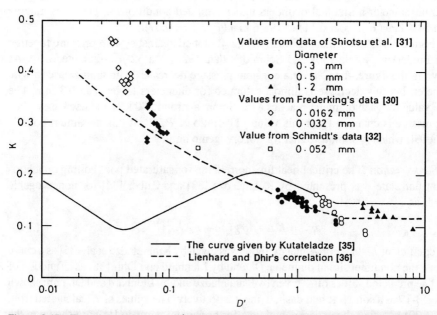

Figure 3-17 The values of K versus D' for liquid helium compared with Kutateladze's correlation and Lienhard and Dhir's correlation.

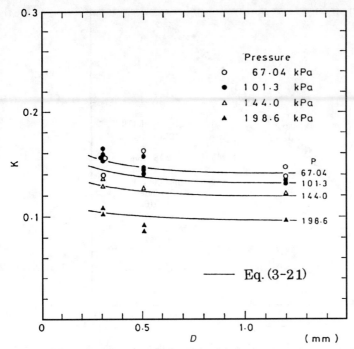

Figure 3-18 Effect of pressure and cylinder diameter on critical heat flux in liquid helium.

of K for D' larger than around 2 for the diameters of 0.5 and 1.2 mm decrease with an increase of D' (owing to an increase in pressure), although they are predicted to be constant.

Figure 3-18 shows the values of K in the range of large D' versus cylinder diameter with the system pressure as a parameter. The effect of cylinder diameter at each pressure is slight as expected, but the value of K for each diameter significantly decreases with the increase in pressure, especially near the critical pressure. Thus, the effect of pressure cannot be expressed through the variation of D' caused by pressure, although it appears as if it were expressed in the D'-dependent region of K in Fig. 3-17. Shiotsu et al. [31] presented the following correlation of K based on their data, referring to Frederking's data for horizontal wires of 16.2- and 32-μm diameter:

$$K = 0.155(1 + 0.035/D)[\rho_l/(\rho_l + \rho_v)]^{3/2} \tag{3-21}$$

The correlation for the critical heat flux in saturated pool boiling for a horizontal cylinder in liquid He I is then a combination of Eqs. (3-20) and (3-21) as follows:

$$q_{cr}/L\rho_v = 0.155(1 + 0.035/D)[\rho_l/(\rho_l + \rho_v)]^{3/2}[\sigma g(\rho_l - \rho_v)/\rho_v^2]^{1/4} \tag{3-22}$$

Figure 3-19 shows the comparison of the existing data with the correlation. It can be seen that these data for pressures from that near the λ point to that near the critical point and for cylinder diameters from 16.2 μm to 1.2 mm are within $\pm15\%$ of the values given

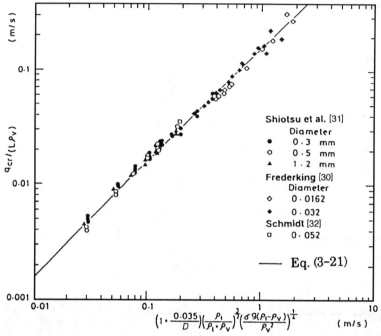

Figure 3-19 Comparison of critical heat flux data for a horizontal cylinder in liquid helium with the CHF correlation given by Eq. (3-22).

by the correlation. The CHF curves for the diameters derived from Eq. (3-22) are also shown in Fig. 3-16 for comparison.

Shiotsu et al. [31] showed that Eq. (3-22) with $D \rightarrow \infty$ would also be applicable for horizontal plates: the CHF data for He I ($P/P_{cr} = 0.027 - 0.95$) by Lyon [37], those for ethanol ($P/P_{cr} = 0.016 - 0.92$) by Chichelli and Bonilla [38], and those for water ($P/P_{cr} = 0.046 - 0.85$) by Kazakova [39] on horizontal flat surfaces facing upwards are compared in Fig. 3-20 with the values derived from Eq. (3-22) in which D is taken to be infinity. These data for helium, ethanol, and water were almost in agreement with the values given by Kutateladze's correlation for horizontal plates in the lower pressure range, but they became lower than the predicted values with increasing pressure and reached about 50 to 60% of the predicted values at the highest pressure for each liquid. However, as shown in Fig. 3-20, almost all the data are within ±25% of the new correlation throughout the pressure range.

Sakurai et al. [40] studied the mechanism for nucleate boiling in He I and suggested that the CHF values for lower pressure that are almost in agreement with Kutateladze's correlation with a constant coefficient would be due to hydrodynamic instability, and the CHF values for high pressure becoming lower than predicted values would be those affected by explosive heterogeneous spontaneous nucleation in originally flooded cavities. The suggestion is based on the analysis of heat transfer processes on a graph of heat flux versus liquid superheat close to the wire surface ($\Delta T_{sat,1}$) in comparison with the superheat corresponding to the homogeneous spontaneous nucleation temperature. The $\Delta T_{sat,1}$ was evaluated from the wire surface superheat, taking off the temperature drop

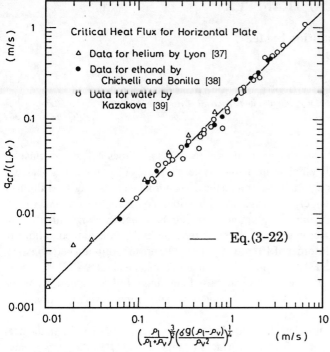

Figure 3-20 Comparison of critical heat flux data for a horizontal flat surface facing upward in liquid helium with the CHF correlation given by Eq. (3-22).

caused by Kapitza resistance, and estimated from the Kapitza resistance results from the same surface in He II [41, 42].

NOMENCLATURE

D	Diameter of cylinder heater (mm)
D'	$D[g(\rho_1 - \rho_v)/\sigma]^{1/2}$ nondimensional cylinder diameter
g	Acceleration due to gravity (m/s^2)
L	Latent heat of vaporization (J/kg)
P	System pressure (kPa)
P_{cr}	Critical pressure (kPa)
q_{cr}	Critical heat flux (W/m^2)
$\Delta T_{sat,1}$	Liquid superheat close to the wire surface (K)
ρ	Density (kg/m^3)
σ	Surface tension (N/m)

Subscripts

l	Liquid
v	Vapor

3-4 RADIATION HEAT TRANSFER

3-4-1 Multilayer Insulation Systems

T. Nast

Lockheed Martin Missiles and Space, 3251 Hanover Street, Orgn. H121, Building 205,
Palo Alto, CA 94304

Introduction/Overview. Multilayer insulation (MLI), sometimes called superinsulation, is the most thermally efficient insulation system known, achieving a heat leak approximately an order of magnitude lower than the best alternative techniques. Multilayer insulation systems, used widely in cryogenic applications, consist of low-emittance radiation shields (commonly using pure aluminum coatings) often alternating with a spacer material such as silk or Dacron netting. These systems depend on vacuum conditions in the interstitial spaces on the order of 10^{-5} to 10^{-7} torr pressure for optimum performance.

The original work on MLI systems is attributed to Sir James Dewar [43].

In early work on MLI systems, Kropshot used aluminum foil for radiation shields and originated the approach of using low-conductivity spacer materials in combination with the radiation shields [44].

In addition to the ultralow heat leak, MLI has other unique properties. First, the heat transfer parallel to the layers (along the surface) is approximately 1,000 times greater than the normal heat transfer (through the blanket). This is a result of the relatively high thermal conductivity of the aluminum coating. This highly anisotropic property leads to great difficulty in the successful application of the system because thermal coupling between penetrations (supports, vent lines, etc.) and blanket edges can have an overwhelming effect on the applied system heat rate. Proper treatment and termination of the edges does not yield to intuitive approaches because of this extreme anisotropy. Second, the heat rate of these systems is very sensitive to layer density. A single local compression or poorly made edge can affect the temperature profile over the entire blanket, substantially increasing the heat leak (in some cases by several times), as shown by analysis and test data.

These considerable difficulties also create problems in the reporting of data from various types of apparatus—if the ends and penetrations are not perfectly treated and the layer density not completely controlled, the apparatus will yield data on a "system" performance relating to installation imperfections or to unique features of the test apparatus rather than comparative data on MLI systems alone. It is believed that many disagreements in data on what are thought to be identical MLI blankets are largely due to these problems (different edge effects, etc.). Additional problems that can arise in testing include residual gas effects caused by faulty vacuum systems that increase gas conduction, insufficient test time to reach thermal equilibrium (particularly under the influence of a varying barometric pressure, which changes boil-off rates with time), and, for systems using helium, neon, or hydrogen as the cryogen, the presence of thermal acoustic oscillations (TAOs).

The resulting testing is relatively costly and time consuming, which partially explains the many unresolved issues and the very large variation in the heat leak to cryogen tanks and equipment developed by different sources.

At the Lockheed Martin Advanced Technology Center, we have been investigating various types of MLI systems for approximately 25 years, principally for spaceborne operation. Because of the high premium on minimizing system weight and maximizing lifetime, every possible means is used to reduce heat load for the system to a minimum. By far the most difficult obstacle has been the MLI blanket, which normally is the largest contributor to the heat load and the most difficult to predict and control. Because of this we have had an extensive research program to produce the best systems attainable.

Much of our work has been focused on optimizing the system for various sets of boundary conditions, with warm boundaries substantially below room temperature. Many of our systems have multiple cryogen stages with separate blankets for each. For example, we may use solid methane ($T = 60$ K) in combination with solid ammonia ($T = 145$ K) as coolants so that one blanket operates between 145 and 60 K and the other between 200 (radiation-cooled boundary in space) and 145 K. The optimum blankets for these two conditions are different because of the relatively low radiation component at a hot boundary of 145 K. The use of multiple vapor-cooled shields on hydrogen or helium systems also results in various sets of boundary temperatures, each with an optimum MLI.

Much of the information presented here is directed at systems in which the cost of the MLI systems (materials and installation) is a small fraction of the total, and therefore little effort is spent in cost effectiveness. For some laboratory systems, the cost is an important factor, and approaches that reduce cost and give "good enough" performance are selected.

The present effort and cost of the maximum-performance systems are quite high because they are applied a layer at a time. Techniques and approaches to reduce the labor involved but yet achieve a blanket with optimum performance are still needed.

The optimum application of MLI to a system is still rather obscure for many practitioners of the art, and many of the complexities and subtleties are not appreciated or understood, leading to a large variation in performance of applied systems.

Description of multilayer insulation (MLI) systems Present-day MLI systems are generally made up of radiation shields such as aluminized Mylar alternating with low-conductivity spacers such as silk or Dacron netting. There are also numerous systems that have been tested or are in use that have integral spacers, such as "crinkled" aluminized Mylar or "Dimplar," in which the shields are treated to provide bumps that prevent intimate contact and resultant thermal shorting between shields. The benefit of the integral shield spacer approach is quicker installation time; the disadvantage is reduced thermal performance.

Development of governing equations Our approach in developing the governing equations for an MLI system is based on a combination of theoretical analysis and empirical data. The empirical data are principally associated with the heat transfer through the spacer material, which is very complex because of the thermal resistance at the boundary between the spacer and the radiation shield.

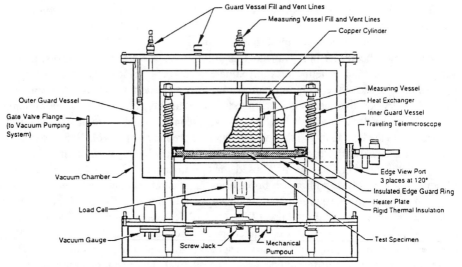

Figure 3-21 Flat-plate calorimeter schematic.

Of the various apparatuses used for MLI testing, we believe the most ideal (unperturbed) is the double-guarded flat-plate apparatus (Fig. 3-21). This apparatus consists essentially of a calorimeter and two guard cryogen reservoirs, a hot-boundary surface plate, a vacuum chamber and pumping system, and a means for remotely changing and measuring the specimen thickness [45]. An edge guard ring is provided to control the radiative environment viewed by the circumferential edge of the specimen. Suitable decoupling between the MLI edge and the guard ring is verified in the calibration procedure, in which the effect of variations in the guard-ring temperature profile on the measured heat flux is shown to be negligible over the range of variation experienced during the test.

This apparatus has a lower limit for the layer density because of the self-weighting of the layers, unlike some other approaches (for example, vertical shields or tanks) in which lower layer densities are possible. During the tests, the layer density is varied by a movable boundary to permit layer density effects to be measured. The boundary temperatures are also varied by using various cryogens and appropriate heaters. Testing was conducted on a wide variety of systems over a wide range of conditions so that semiempirical equations could be developed to predict the performance of the MLI. In developing these models, the radiation was modeled theoretically (with experimentally verified values of the shield emissivity), and the conduction through the spacers was determined empirically as a function of layer density for each material. We believe this testing provides the basis for the thermal performance of an ideally applied blanket. Whether this value could be attained or approached on real hardware is discussed in the following paragraphs.

Some of the data on the emissivity of the shields, obtained on an emittance calorimeter [45], are presented in Figs. 3-22 and 3-23 for goldized Mylar and aluminized Mylar, both vacuum metallized. Note that the emittance for gold is lower than that for aluminum

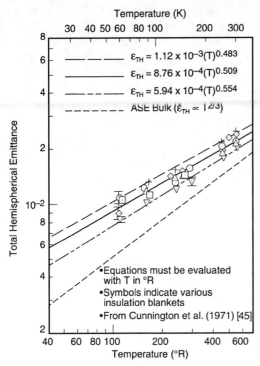

Temperature (K)

$\varepsilon_{TH} = 1.12 \times 10^{-3}(T)^{0.483}$

$\varepsilon_{TH} = 8.76 \times 10^{-4}(T)^{0.509}$

$\varepsilon_{TH} = 5.94 \times 10^{-4}(T)^{0.554}$

ASE Bulk ($\varepsilon_{TH} \propto T^{2/3}$)

•Equations must be evaluated
with T in °R
•Symbols indicate various
insulation blankets
•From Cunnington et al. (1971) [45]

Temperature (°R)

Figure 3-22 Total hemispherical emittance of double-goldized 1/4-mil Mylar as a function of temperature.

at room temperature but higher at the cryogenic temperatures. The value of the total hemispherical emittance for bulk material as a function of temperature as predicted by the anomalous skin effect theory (ASE) [46] is shown for gold (Fig. 3-22) and for an aluminum thickness of 400 Å (Fig. 3-23). Data on various coatings at various thicknesses at 300 K are shown in Fig. 3-24 [47]. Note that the coating thickness must be on the order of 800 Å at 300 K in order to attain the asymptotic value. Although little data on the effect of thickness on the emittance at lower temperatures are available, the ASE theory can be used to predict this effect. Figure 3-25 [48], shows these predictions, which indicate that about the same thickness is required, regardless of temperature. Although we assume that a thin aluminum oxide surface film forms, which we believe to be transparent to the radiation wavelengths of interest, this matter has not been resolved to our knowledge. Vacuum-metallized Mylar may have a widely varying thickness as received and must be carefully controlled and checked to ensure acceptable values.

Some typical thermal performance data for gold and aluminized shields using double layers of silk net are shown in Figs. 3-26 and 3-27. These results are for a warm-boundary temperature of 278 K and cold boundaries of 20 and 77 K. The test data for the four systems studied for a 77-K cold boundary are summarized and compared in Fig. 3-28.

The equation describing the heat flux for a system commonly used at Lockheed Martin—double-aluminized Mylar (DAM) with double silk net (DSN), which is referred

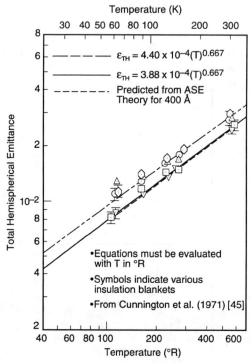

Figure 3-23   Total hemispherical emittance of double-aluminized 1/4-mil Mylar as a function of temperature.

to in this paper as DAM/DSN—is presented below. (DAM has an aluminum coating on each side of the Mylar. DSN has two layers of net between each radiation shield.)

$$q = \frac{C_s(\bar{N})^{2.56} T_m}{N_s + 1}(T_H - T_C) + \frac{C_r \varepsilon_{RT}}{N_s}\left(T_H^{4.67} - T_C^{4.67}\right) \qquad (3\text{-}23)$$

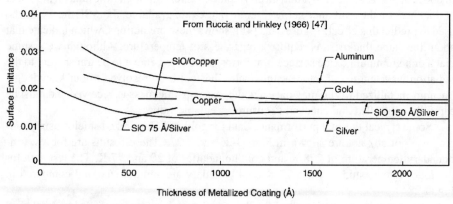

Figure 3-24   Emittance of vacuum-metalized polyester film at 300 K for various metal coating materials and thicknesses.

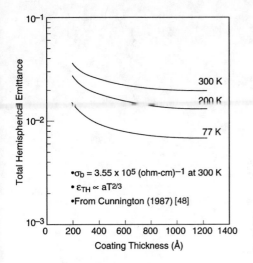

Figure 3-25 Prediction of total hemispherical emittance of thin aluminum films on Mylar based on ASE theory.

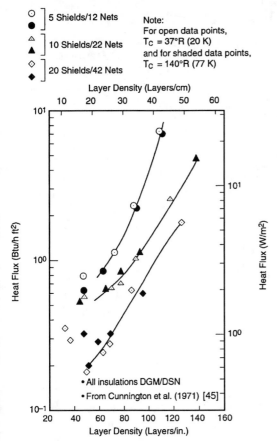

Figure 3-26 Heat flux as a function of layer density for double-goldized Mylar/silk net with $T_H = 500\,°R$ (278 K).

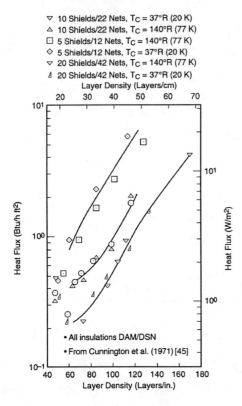

∇ 10 Shields/22 Nets, $T_C = 37°R$ (20 K)
△ 10 Shields/22 Nets, $T_C = 140°R$ (77 K)
▢ 5 Shields/12 Nets, $T_C = 140°R$ (77 K)
◇ 5 Shields/12 Nets, $T_C = 37°R$ (20 K)
▽ 20 Shields/42 Nets, $T_C = 140°R$ (77 K)
◢ 20 Shields/42 Nets, $T_C = 37°R$ (20 K)

• All insulations DAM/DSN
• From Cunnington et al. (1971) [45]

Figure 3-27 Heat flux as a function of layer density for double-aluminized Mylar/silk net with $T_H = 500°R$ (278 K).

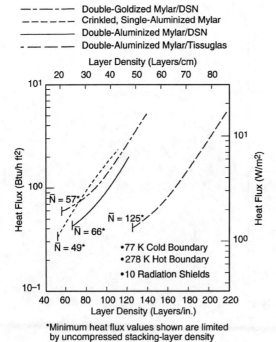

— - — - — Double-Goldized Mylar/DSN
— — — — — Crinkled, Single-Aluminized Mylar
—————— Double-Aluminized Mylar/DSN
- — — — — Double-Aluminized Mylar/Tissuglas

$\bar{N} = 57*$
$\bar{N} = 125*$
$\bar{N} = 66*$
$\bar{N} = 49*$

• 77 K Cold Boundary
• 278 K Hot Boundary
• 10 Radiation Shields

*Minimum heat flux values shown are limited by uncompressed stacking-layer density values derived for each system.

Figure 3-28 Heat flux as a function of layer density for four MLIs.

192

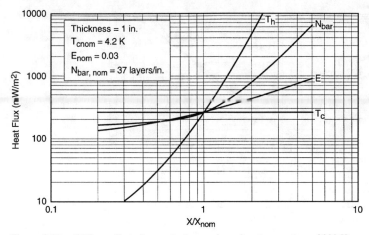

Figure 3-29 X / X_{nom} effects for nominal warm boundary temperature of 300 K.

This equation has been shown to be very useful in predicting the performance of various systems. It provides a basis for predicting the minimum heat load to an MLI system, and when used with various factors based on tank testing (referred to as degradation factors here), can be of substantial value in predicting and optimizing the performance of MLI systems.

Parametric curves describing performance for "ideal" insulation blanket The following parametric data present plots of the MLI blanket heat rate per unit area (mW/m^2) as a function of the major variables. These data are based on Eq. 3-23 and therefore are representative of a perfect installation of the best blanket materials we have found.

Real installation effects, which can have considerable effect on the heat rate, are described below.

Figures 3-29 through 3-31 show the heat flux as a function of the room temperature total hemispherical emittance (E), the boundary temperatures (hot boundary, T_H) and

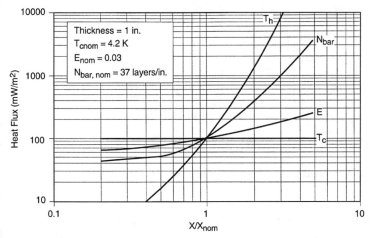

Figure 3-30 X / X_{nom} effects for nominal warm boundary temperature of 225 K.

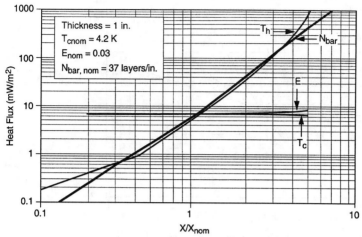

Figure 3-31 X/X_{nom} effects for nominal warm boundary temperature of 77 K.

(cold boundary, T_C), and the layer density. These results are for a 1-in.-thick blanket at three hot boundary temperatures: 300, 225, and 77 K. The X/X_{nom} coordinate of 1 represents the reference values of the parameters ($E = 0.03$, $N_{bar} = 37$ layers/in., $T_C = 4.2$ K, and $T_H = 300, 225$, or 77 K, depending on the figure).

The heat flux for various conditions can be calculated using Fig. 3-29, which is for a 300-K hot boundary. For example, if the radiation shield emissivity were 0.06, double the reference value, the heat flux would change from 270 to 410 mW/m². If the layer density were doubled from 37 to 74 layers/in., the heat flux would increase from 270 to 780 mW/m², thus showing the high sensitivity to compressions.

Figures 3-32 through 3-36 provide information on the heat flux for specific variables rather than in normalized form.

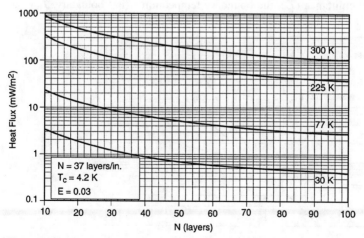

Figure 3-32 Heat flux versus MLI thickness for different warm boundary temperatures.

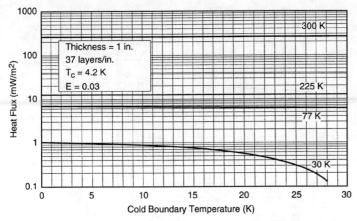

Figure 3-33   Heat flux versus cold boundary temperature for different warm boundary temperatures.

Thermal performance associated with practical installations   The thermal performance of an installed system is typically not as good as that presented in the previous family of curves. Although this latter level of performance can be attained or approached, it requires painstaking attention to detail and very precise installation techniques with the optimum materials. Unfortunately, the effects of local compressions, gaps, and so on are not intuitively obvious and are normally mastered only after years of research, both in test apparatus and detailed analytical models. These models typically incorporate several hundred nodes and are two-dimensional so that parallel heat transfer in the MLI blanket to the supports and penetrations is accounted for.

At Lockheed Martin, we have conducted an extensive series of testing on "tank colorimeters." These are tanks of various sizes that have been carefully designed and constructed so that the heat losses from penetrations such as fill lines and supports are

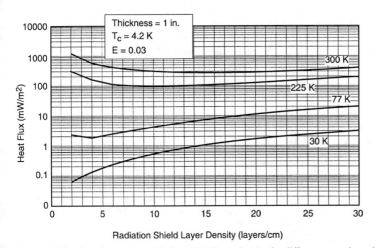

Figure 3-34   Heat flux versus radiation shield layer density for different warm boundary temperatures.

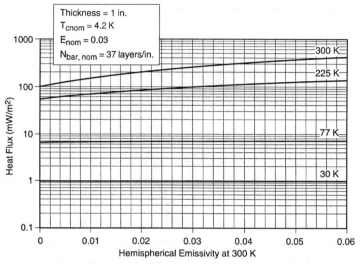

Figure 3-35 Heat flux versus room temperature emissivity for different warm boundary temperatures.

negligible compared with the MLI heat leak. We have found from these tests that we can achieve values very close to the ideal given in Eq. (3-23). For complete tankage systems, which include numerous penetrations such as vent and fill lines, instrumentation, supports, and so forth, our experience indicates we can achieve systems that vary in the range of 1.2 to 1.6 times that given by Eq. (3-23), providing proper care is utilized.

Effect of vacuum pressure on performance The calculation of gas conduction in the blanket is relatively straightforward, provided the gas is noncondensable for the blanket

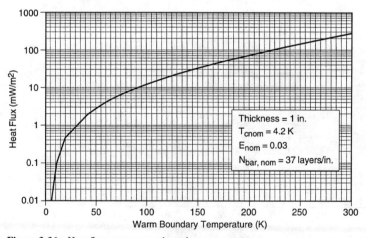

Figure 3-36 Heat flux versus warm boundary temperature.

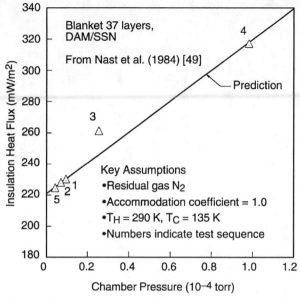

Figure 3-37 Correlation of experimental and predicted gas conduction effects.

operating temperatures and that it operates in the free molecular regime, which is usually the case. A relatively simple expression that has been used successfully is based on the average pressure and temperature in the blanket and includes the thermal transpiration effects. The result can easily be related to the vacuum chamber pressure. This equation, from Ref. [49], is

$$q = \frac{(\gamma + 1)}{2(\gamma - 1)} \left(\frac{R}{2MT_{ins}} \right)^{1/2} \frac{\bar{P}_{ins}(T_H - T_C)}{\bar{N}} \tag{3-24}$$

where

$$\bar{P}_{ins} = P_{CH} \left(\frac{\bar{T}_{ins}}{T_{CH}} \right)^{1/2} \quad \text{and} \quad \bar{T}_{ins} = \frac{1}{2}(T_H + T_C)$$

Figure 3-37 shows the predicted heat flux as a function of the chamber pressure along with test data from the large-tank calorimeter. (The numbers indicate the sequence of the measurements so that any effects of hysterisis due to gas condensation can be considered.) The blanket tested was 1-in. thick and used DAM/single SN. The cold boundary was 135 K, and the hot boundary 290 K. The data show excellent agreement with predictions and no hysteresis is apparent. Numerous investigations of the effects of residual gas have been made on a range of MLI systems. Figure 3-38 shows a broad summary of some of these results.

Figures 3-39 through 3-41 provide working curves to calculate the gas conduction contribution to the heat load for a wide range of parameters.

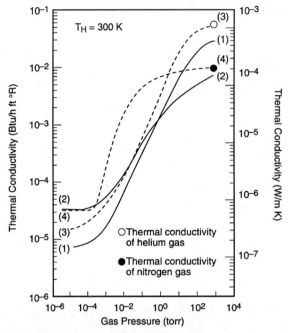

Figure 3-38 Thermal conductivity of multilayer composites as a function of gas pressure.
(1) AL Foil + Fiberglass Paper (helium filled). $T_c = 20$ K (from Arthur D. Little, Inc., Report 65008-00-03, July 1963, p. 36.)
(2) Al Foil + Fiberglas Paper (nitrogen filled), $T_c = 77$ K (from *Themophysical properties of Thermal Insulating Materials*, p. 150)
(3) DAM + Dexiglas (helium filled), $T_c = 77$ K, (from Lockheed Missiles & Space Co., Inc., unpublished data, Thermophysics Laboratory, 1964–65.)
(4) Crinkled Mylar (NRC-2) (nitrogen filled), $T_c = 79$ K, (from Lockheed-California Co., Progress Report II; "Storage of Cryogenic Fluids for Long Duration Spacecraft Missions," J.E. Boderg, Report 17410, 25 Mar 1964, p. 21.)

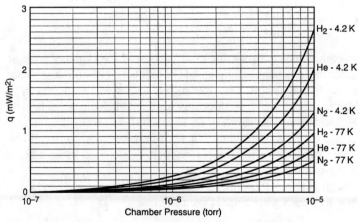

Figure 3-39 Gas conduction versus chamber pressure for various interstitial gases and cold boundaries (hot boundary = 300 K, 1 in., 37 layers/in.).

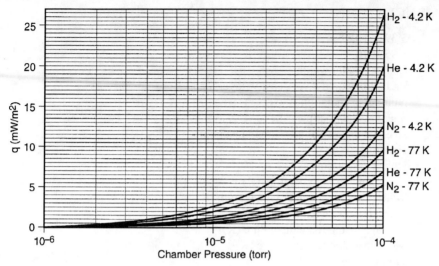

Figure 3-40 Gas conduction versus chamber pressure for various interstitial gases and cold boundaries (hot boundary = 300 K, 1 in., 37 layers / in.).

Summary. It is hoped that this brief summary will be useful to those designing cryogenic equipment. The difficulty of achieving optimum values in insulating equipment should not be underestimated. Unfortunately there is not sufficient space available to cover the many other facets of this technology, such as appropriate treatment of the edges of the blankets, where they may come into contact with penetrations and local compressions that may be caused by special geometry or packaging requirements. Our experience indicates that these are among the most important installation features. References 50–58 give additional details on MLI systems.

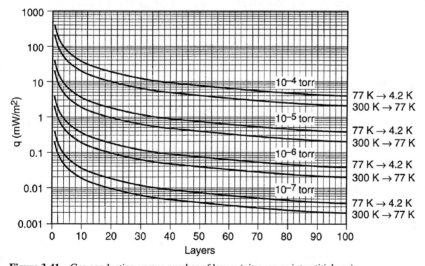

Figure 3-41 Gas conduction versus number of layers (nitrogen as interstitial gas).

NOMENCLATURE

C_R	5.39×10^{-10}
C_S	8.95×10^{-8}
M	Gas molecular weight
N	Radiation shield layer density (layers / cm)
$\bar{N}_s$	Number of radiation shields
P_c, P_{CH}	Vacuum chamber pressure
P_{ins}	Average interstitial pressure in insulation
q	Heat flux (W/m^2)
R	Universal gas constant
T_c	Cold boundary temperature (K)
T_{CH}	Warm vacuum chamber temperature (K)
T_H	Warm boundary temperature (K)
T_{ins}	Average insulation temperature (K)
T_m	Mean insulation temperature (K)
t	Time
γ	Specific heat ratio
ε_{RT}	Room temperature (300 K) emissivity
ε_{TH}	Total hemispherical emissivity
σ_b	Bulk electrical conductivity

ACKNOWLEDGMENTS

The author wishes to acknowledge some of the major contributors to this work: I. E. Spradley, who made major contributions in both testing and analysis; G. A. Bell, who largely developed the small calorimeter and made substantial contributions to the testing and also to the large calorimeter set-up; and G. R. Cunnington, who did much of the pioneering experimental and analytical work on the systems. This work was supported by both U.S. Government contracts and company-supported research funds.

REFERENCES

1. Eckert, E. R. G., and Drake, R. M., *Analysis of Heat and Mass Transfer* (New York: McGraw–Hill, 1973).
2. Bird, R. B., Steward, W. E., and Lightfoot, E. N., *Transport Phenomena* (New York: John Wiley & Sons, 1996).
3. El-Wakil, M. M., *Nuclear Heat Transport* (La Grange Park, IL: American Nuclear Society, 1978).
4. Frost, W., *Heat Transfer at Low Temperature* (New York: Plenum Press, 1975).
5. Barron, R., *Cryogenic Heat Transfer* (Washington, D.C.: Taylor & Francis, in press).
6. Holmes, D. S., Personal communication. Letter May 96.
7. Berman, R., "Some Experiments on Thermal Contact at Low Temperatures," *J. Appl. Phys.* 27, no. 4 (1956).
8. Kittel, P., "Modeling Thermal Contact Resistance," in *Cryocoolers* 8 (New York: Plenum Press, 1995).
9. Yovanovich, M. M., "General Expression for Circular Constriction Resistances for Arbitrary Flux Distributions," *Prog. Aeronaut. Astronaut.* 49 (1976).
10. Deutsch, M., "Thermal Conductance in Screw-Fastened Joints at Helium Temperatures," *Cryog.* 18 (1978).

11. Kittel, P., Spivak, A. L., and Salerno, L. J., "Thermal Conductance of Gold Plated Metallic Contacts at Liquid Helium Temperatures," *Adv. Cryog. Eng.* 37, Pt. A (1992).
12. Kittel, P., Salerno, L. J., and Spivak, A. L., "Thermal Conductance of Pressed Bimetallic Contacts at Liquid Nitrogen Temperatures," *Cryog.* 34 (ICEC Supplement) (1994).
13. Manninen, M., and Zimmerman, N., "On the Use of Screw-Fastened Joints for Thermal Contact at Low Temperatures," *Rev. Sci. Instrum.* 48, no. 12 (1977).
14. Mian, M. N., Al-Asuabadi, F. R., O'Callaghan, P W. and Probert, S. D., "Thermal Resistance of Pressed Contacts Between Steel Surfaces: Influence of Oxide Films," *J. Mech. Eng. Sci.* 21, no. 3 (1979).
15. Nilles, M., and Van Sciver, S., "Effects of Oxidation and Roughness on Cu Contact Resistance from 4 K to 290 K," *Adv. Cryog. Eng.* (Mat.) 34 (1988).
16. Radebaugh, R., Siegwarth, J. D., Lawlless, W. N., and Morrow, A. J., *Electrocaloric Refrigeration for Superconductors*, NBS Report No. NBSIR 76-847 (February 1977).
17. Salerno, L. J., Kittel, P., and Spivak, A. L., "Thermal Conductance of Pressed Copper Contacts at Liquid Helium Temperatures," *AIAA J.* 22 (1984).
18. Salerno, L. J., Kittel, P., and Spivak, A. L., "Thermal Conductance of Pressed OFHC Copper Contacts at Liquid Helium Temperatures," in *Thermal Conductivity 18* (New York: Plenum Press, 1985).
19. Salerno, L. J., Kittel, P., Brooks, W. F., Spivak, A. L., and Marks, W. F., "Thermal Conductance of Pressed Brass Contacts at Liquid Helium Temperatures," *Cryog.* 26 (1986).
20. Salerno, L. J., Kittel, P., and Scherkenbach, F. E., "Thermal Conductance of Pressed Aluminum and Stainless Steel Contacts at Liquid Helium Temperatures," in *Thermal Conductivity* 19 (New York: Plenum Press, 1988).
21. Salerno, L. J., Kittel, P., and Spivak, A. L., "Thermal Conductance of Augmented Pressed Metallic Contacts at Liquid Helium Temperatures," *Cryog.* 33 (1993).
22. Salerno, L. J., Kittel, P., and Spivak, A. L., "Thermal Conductance of Pressed Metallic Contacts Augmented with Indium Foil or Apiezon Grease at Liquid Helium Temperatures," *Cryog.* 34 (1994).
23. Suomi, M., Anderson, A. C., and Holmstrom, B., "Heat Transfer Below 0.2 K," *Physica* 38 (1968).
24. Thomas, T. R., and Probert, S. D., "Thermal Contact Resistance; the Directional Effect and Other Problems," *Int. J. Heat and Mass Transfer* 13 (1970).
25. Wanner, M., "Thermal Conductance of a Pressed Al-Al Contact," *Cryog.* 21 (1981).
26. Kittel, C., *Introduction to Solid State Physics*, 5th ed. (New York: John Wiley & Sons, 1976).
27. Dittus, F., and Boelter, L., *UC–Berkeley Publ. Eng.* 2 (1930):443.
28. Taylor, M., NASA-TND-4332 (1968).
29. Miropolski, Z. L., Picus, V. J., and Shitsman, M. E., *Proc. 3rd Int. Heat Trans. Conf.* 2 (1966):95.
30. Frederking, T. H., "Warmeübergang bei der Verdampfung der Verflussigten Gase Helium und Stickstoff," *Forschung Gebiete Ingenieur* 27 (1961):17–30.
31. Shiotsu, M., Hata, K., and Sakurai, A., "Effects of Diameter and System Pressure on Critical Heat Flux for Horizontal Cylinder in Saturated Liquid Helium I," *Cryog.* 29 (1989):593–596.
32. Schmidt, C., "Transient Heat Transfer and Recovery Behavior of Superconductors," *IEEE Trans. Mag.*, Mag-17 (1981):738–741.
33. Kutateladze, S. S., "Heat Transfer in Condensation and Boiling," AEC-tr-3770 (1959).
34. Zuber, N., "Hydrodynamic Aspects of Boiling Heat Transfer," AECU-4439 (1959).
35. Kutateladze, S. S., Valukina, N. V., and Gogonin, I. I., "The Dependence of the Critical Hreat Flux on the Heater Dimensions During Pool Boiling of Saturated Liquids" (in Russian), *Inzhenerno-fizicheskii Zhurnal* 12, no. 5 (1967).
36. Lienhard, J. H., and Dhir, V. K., "Hydrodynamic Prediction of Peak Pool Boiling Heat Fluxes from Finite Bodies," *ASME J. Heat Transfer* 95 (1973):152–158.
37. Lyon, D. N., "Boiling Heat Transfer and Peak Nucleate Boiling Fluxes in Saturated Liquid Helium Between λ and Critical Temperatures," *Adv. Cryog. Eng.* 10 (1965):371–379.
38. Chichelli, M. T., and Bonilla, C. F., "Heat Transfer to Liquid Helium Under Pressure," *Trans. AICHE* 41 (1945):757–787.
39. Kazakova, E. A., AAEC-tr-3405 (1953):86–94.
40. Sakurai, A., Shiotsu, M., and Hata, K., "Incipient Boiling Superheats and Critical Heat Fluxes Due to Increasing Heat Inputs in Subcooled He I at Various Pressures," *Adv. Cryog. Eng.* 41 (1996):203–210.

41. Shiotsu, M., Hata, K., Takeuchi, Y., Hama, K., and Sakurai, A., "Estimation of Kapitza Conductance Effects on Steady and Transient Boiling Heat Transfer in He I Based on Kapitza Conductance Results in He II," *Cryog*. 36, no. 3 (1996):197–202.
42. Sakurai, A., Shiotsu, M., and Hata, K., "Boiling Phenomena Due to Quasi-steady and Rapidly Increasing Heat Inputs in LN_2 and LHe I," *Cryog*. 36, no. 3 (1996):189–196.
43. *Collected Papers of Sir James Dewar*, ed. Lady Dewar, 2 vols. (Cambridge: Cambridge University Press, 1927).
44. Kropshot, R. H., "Cryogenic Insulation," *ASRAE J*. Sept. (1959).
45. Cunnington, G. R., Keller, C. W., and Bell, G.A., "Thermal Performance of Multilayer Insulations," NASA-CR72605 (1971).
46. Armaly, B. F., and Tien, C. L., "Emissivities of Metals at Cryogenic Temperatures," in *Heat Transfer 1970* (Amsterdam: EL Servier Publishing, 1970).
47. Ruccia, F. E., and Hinckley, R. B., "The Surface Emittance of Vacuum-Metalized Polyester Films," *Adv. Cryog. Eng*. 12 (1966):300.
48. Cunnington, G. R., "Analysis of DAM Emittance Thickness and Temperature Effects," unpublished (1987).
49. Nast, T. C., Naes, L., and Stevens, J., "Thermal Performance of Tank Applied Multilayer Insulation at Low Boundary Temperatures," in *Proc. ICEC 10* (1984).
50. Androukalis, J. G., and Kosson, R. L., "Effective Thermal Conductivity Parallel to the Laminations and Total Conductance of Multilayer Insulation," *J. Spacecraft* 6, no. 7 (1969).
51. Bell, G. A., Nast, T. C., and Wedel, R. K., "Thermal Performance of Multilayer Insulation Applied to Small Cryogenic Tankage," *Adv. Cryog. Eng*. 22 (1977):272.
52. Caren, R. P., Gilcrest, A. S., and Zierman, C.A., "Thermal Absorptions of Cryodeposits for Solar and 290 K Blackbody Sources," *Adv. Cryog. Eng*. 9 (1963):457.
53. Glassford, A.P.M., "Outgassing of Multilayer Insulation Materials," *J. Spacecr. Rockets* 7, 12 (1970):1464.
54. Glassford, A. P. M., Osiecki, R. A., and Lin, C. K., "Effect of Temperature and Preconditioning on the Outgassing Rate of Double Aluminized Mylar and Dacron Net," *J. Vac. Sci. Tech*. A2, no. 3 (1984).
55. Leung, E. M. W., Fast, R. W., Hart, H. L., and Hiem, J. R., "Techniques for Reducing Radiation Heat Transfer Between 77 and 4.2 K," *Adv. Cryog. Eng*. 25 (1980):489.
56. Nast, T. C., and Coston, R. M., "Investigations of the Gas Flow Within Multilayer Insulations and Its Effect on Cryogenic Space Vehicle Design," *Chem. Eng. Prog. Symp. Ser*. 62, no. 61 (1966).
57. Pogson, J. T., and MacGregor, Rk. K., "A Method of Increasing the Lateral Thermal Resistance of Multilayer Insulation," (Paper No. 70-15 presented at the 8th AIAA Aerospace Sciences Meeting, 1970).
58. Spadley, I. E., Nast, T. C., and Frank, D. J., "Experimental Studies of MLI Systems at Very Low Temperature Boundaries," *Adv. Cryog. Eng*. 35 (1990):477.

FOUR

CRYOGENIC INSTRUMENTATION

D. S. Holmes and S. S. Courts

Lake Shore Cryotronics, 575 McCorkle Boulevard, Westerville, OH 43802

4-1 MEASUREMENT SYSTEMS

Making measurements at cryogenic temperatures requires far greater care than the making of similar measurements near room temperature. Just finding sensors and signal conditioners capable of working at cryogenic temperatures can be a challenge. Cryogenic measurement systems commonly operate with many of their components at room temperature to avoid problems with operation at low temperatures. Additional problems are created as the distance increases between the measurement location and the instrumentation.

This review chapter can cover little material not specific to cryogenic instrumentation. The reader is referred to other general sources on the subjects of measurement and instrumentation [1–3]. The chapter is organized with general cryogenic measurement system considerations followed by separate sections on specific measurements (temperature, strain, pressure, flow, liquid level, magnetic, and other).

4-1-1 Balanced Design of a Measurement System

A system to measure a physical quantity is typically made up of interacting components, as shown in Fig. 4-1. The sensor responds to the quantity of interest and produces an electrical or optical output that can be measured by the instrumentation. The system is shown with the sensor inside and the instrumentation outside the cryogenic environment, but all combinations are possible.

The performance of a measurement system depends on the performance of each of the components. The sensor often requires the greatest attention in a cryogenic measurement system, but the entire system must still be considered. The process of designing a measurement system can be described with the following steps:

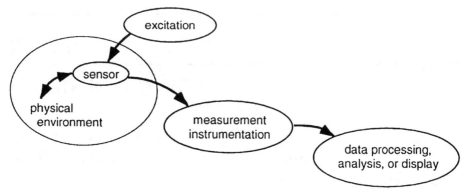

Figure 4-1 Typical measurement system components and interactions.

1. Decide what is to be measured.
2. Find sensors that will work in the environment.
3. Design measurement systems around the sensors.
4. Select the best sensor and measurement system combination.

Sometimes no sensors will work in an environment, or only one sensor will work, and the measurement system must be designed around that sensor. More commonly, more than one sensor will work and trade-offs must be made between cost, size, accuracy, ease of use, or other considerations to select the best sensor and overall measurement system.

4-1-2 Defining the Measurement

The physical property to be measured is frequently given, whether it is temperature, pressure, liquid level, strain, or some other quantity. In some cases the required measurement can be inferred from other measurements that are more convenient to make.

Also important is the choice of resolution, precision, or accuracy as the important statistical feature of the measurement. Good resolution is easiest to achieve, and good accuracy is hardest to achieve. Selecting an inappropriate statistical measure either adds cost to, or decreases the value of, a measurement.

Resolution. The resolution of a measurement system is the smallest change that can be detected in the measured property. Resolution is the most important statistical measure if, for example, small temperature changes must be measured, but the absolute temperature either is not important or can be measured independently. Other examples are the measurement of pressure variations or strain changes.

Measurement resolution often is not affected by offsets such as thermoelectric voltages or self-heating of the sensor. The unimportance of offsets also allows resolution to be improved by using filtered or bridge measurement schemes that eliminate the large, unchanging portion of the sensor's output and allow the instrumentation to concentrate on the smaller, changing portion of the signal.

Precision. The precision (or reproducibility or stability) is a measure of how closely the measured values are grouped. Good precision requires good resolution. Precision is important when successive measurements must return the same value, but the true value of the quantity is not required. An example might be a temperature control system that must run successive samples through identical temperature cycles, but the actual temperatures are less important than the repeatability of the cycles.

Accuracy. Accuracy is the closeness of the agreement between the result of a measurement and the true value of the measurand. The accuracy of a single measurement can be no better than the resolution but is degraded by calibration and measurement uncertainties.

4-1-3 Selecting a Sensor

Look to the sections at the end of this chapter for information about cryogenic sensors for making particular measurements. The selection of a sensor for an application usually requires prioritizing the most important attributes necessary for the application and compromising on the less important attributes. The most stable and accurate sensors tend to be very large, slow in response, fragile, and expensive. Sensors with the highest sensitivity and resolution have the smallest dynamic range. Choices must be made. Several important sensor characteristics to consider are listed in Table 4-1.

Next, develop measurement systems around the acceptable sensors and then compare the complete systems. For systems of comparable cost, size, reliability, or ease of use, the measurement uncertainty can be used to select the best system. Measurement systems not comparable on the basis of measurement uncertainty alone require development of additional selection criteria by the system designer.

Table 4-1 Important sensor characteristics

Operating range
Excitation
Output signal
Sensitivity (or span)
Offset
Stability
Interchangeability
Ease of use
Simplicity
Effect on its environment
Size
Environmental compatibility:
  Robustness
  Response time
  Magnetic field effects
  Radiation resistance
  Electromagnetic noise effects

4-1-4 Measurement Uncertainty

The probable resolution, precision, or accuracy of a temperature measurement can be evaluated using uncertainty analysis. The expected uncertainty of a measurement is expressed in statistical terms. As stated in the *Guide to the Expression of Uncertainty in Measurement* [4],

> The exact values of the contributions to the error of the measurement arising from the dispersion of the observations, the unavoidable imperfect nature of the corrections, and incomplete knowledge are unknown and unknowable, whereas the uncertainties associated with these random and systematic effects can be evaluated.... the uncertainty of a result of a measurement is not necessarily an indication of the likelihood that the measurement result is near the value of the measurand; it is simply an estimate of the likelihood of nearness to the best value that is consistent with presently available knowledge.

The uncertainty is given the symbol u and has the same units as the quantity measured. The combined uncertainty u_c arising from several independent uncertainty sources can be estimated by assuming a statistical distribution of uncertainties, in which case the uncertainties are summed in quadrature according to

$$u_c = \sqrt{u_1^2 + u_2^2 + \cdots + u_i^2 + \cdots + u_n^2} \qquad (4\text{-}1)$$

Note that both sides of Eq. (4-1) can be divided by the measurement quantity to express the measurement uncertainty in relative terms. Finding statistical data suitable for addition by quadrature can be a problem; instrument and sensor specifications frequently give maximum or typical values for uncertainties. Two approaches may be taken to dealing with maximum uncertainty specifications. The conservative approach is to use the specification limit value in the combined uncertainty calculation. The less conservative approach is to assume a statistical distribution within the specification limits and assume the limit is roughly three standard deviations, in which case one-third of the specification limit is used in uncertainty calculations. The manufacturer may be able to supply additional information to help improve uncertainty estimates. Practical recommendations and procedures for problems related to the estimation of measurement uncertainties are discussed in greater detail by Rabinovich [5].

Uncertainty conversions using dimensionless sensitivities. A sensor produces some output signal such as a voltage, frequency, resistance, or capacitance that is measured by the instrumentation. Uncertainties in the measured quantity are not in units of the physical quantity of interest and must be converted before use in Eq. (4-1). In the case of a temperature sensor with an output voltage V, the temperature uncertainty u_T is related to the voltage uncertainty u_V by the dimensionless formula

$$\frac{u_T}{T} = \frac{u_V/V}{(T/V)(dV/dT)} \equiv \frac{u_V/V}{S_T} \qquad (4\text{-}2)$$

The quantity in the denominator $S_T = (T/V)(dV/dT)$ is defined as the dimensionless temperature sensitivity of the sensor's output voltage, where V is the sensor output voltage at absolute temperature T. The dimensionless sensitivity is also equal to $(d \ln V / d \ln T)$, the slope of the voltage versus temperature on a log–log plot. Note that Eq. (4-2) can be made to apply to temperature sensors based on other temperature-dependent properties (capacitance, resistance, or pressure) by replacing V with C, R, or P as appropriate. Dimensionless sensitivities dependent on pressure, strain, or other physical quantities can be constructed similarly.

The dimensionless nature of Eq. (4-2) makes the comparison of sensors based on different property dependencies somewhat easier. A dimensionless sensitivity in the 0.1 to 10 range is usually best for property measurements over a wide range, although other factors such as physical size or sensitivity to environmental conditions can be much more important. A large dimensionless sensitivity allows good relative temperature resolution, but the temperature range becomes limited if the value of the property measured becomes too large or small to be determined accurately with the measurement system.

4-1-5 Sources of Measurement Uncertainty

The following subsections discuss specific sources of temperature measurement uncertainty and how to estimate their magnitudes. Sources of uncertainty include (1) sensor excitation, (2) sensor self-heating, (3) sensor output measurement instrumentation, (4) thermoelectric voltages and zero drift, (5) thermal and shot noise, (6) electromagnetic noise, (7) sensor calibration, and (8) interpolation and fitting to the calibration data. Example measurement uncertainty calculations are summarized in Table 4-2. Environmental effects (e.g., magnetic fields, ionizing radiation, pressure, strain, heat leaks, etc.) are also important and should be included in uncertainty estimates but will be discussed later in the sections on specific sensor types.

Instrumentation measurement uncertainty. The accuracy of the instrumentation measuring the output of the temperature sensor is normally specified by the manufacturer.

Analog meter accuracy is typically given as a percentage of full scale. An accuracy of $\pm 1\%$ on a 1-V full-scale range thus equals a voltage uncertainty u_V of ± 10 mV. The resulting temperature measurement uncertainty can be calculated using the actual temperature sensor output voltage V in Eq. (4-2). A major consideration with analog meters is that the accuracy of the temperature measurement decreases as the sensor output voltage drops below full scale.

The accuracy of a digital meter is usually specified as a percentage of reading plus a number of counts of the least significant digit. The percent accuracy is calculated as a function of the actual reading, not full scale. For example, a digital accuracy specification of $\pm(0.05\% + 1$ count) for a 4-1/2-digit meter reading 3.000 mV on a 20-mV range equals a voltage uncertainty u_V of $\pm(0.0015 + 0.001)$ mV $= \pm 2.5\,\mu$V. Equation (4-2) is again used to translate to temperature uncertainty.

Sensor self-heating. Any difference between the temperature of the sensor and the environment the sensor is intended to measure produces a temperature measurement error or uncertainty. Dissipation of power in the temperature sensor will cause its temperature to rise above that of the surrounding environment. Power dissipation in the sensor is

Table 4-2 Example temperature measurement uncertainty calculations

Sensor		Silicon diode		Cernox	
Temperature sensor model (Lake Shore)		DT-470-SD-11		CX-1050-AA	
Temperature, T		80 K		4.2K	
Mounting environment (N-greased to block)		Vacuum		Liquid helium	
Electrical resistance, R_e		1000 Ω (dynamic $R_d = dV/dI$)		4920 Ω	
Excitation current, I		10 μA		1 μA	
Output voltage, V		1.01525 V		4.92 mV	
Dimensionless temperature sensitivity, S_T		-0.1521		-1.71	

Uncertainties due to	Eq.	Value used	u_T/T (ppm)	Value used	u_T/T (ppm)
1. Measurement instrumentation (Keithley Instruments 2000 DVM)					
• Meter range full-scale (FS)		10.00000 V		100.0000 mV	
• Voltage accuracy specification (ppm)	(4-2)	$\pm(30 + 5$ FS/V)	521	$\pm(50 + 35$ FS/V)	761
2. Sensor self-heating					
• Thermal resistance	(4-8)	$R_t = 1000$ K/W[a]	127	$R_t = 3500$ K/W	4.1
3. Excitation uncertainty (Lake Shore Model 120CS)					
• Current accuracy specification	(4-3)	$u_I/I = 0.05\%$	3290	$u_I/I = 0.1\%$	585
4. Thermal and shot noise			0.01		0.3
5. Thermal voltages and zero drift	(4-4)	10 μV	65	0[b]	0
6. Electromagnetic noise	(4-7)	2 mV[c]	1040	0[b]	0
7. Calibration uncertainty		0.25 K[e]	3130	4 mK	952
8. Interpolation uncertainty [d]			313		95.2
Combined uncertainties	(4-1)		4700		1355

Note: Uncertainties are given in parts per million (ppm).

[a] Estimated from data for CX-type sensors in a similar SD package at 10 K in vacuum.

[b] Eliminated by current reversal and use of Eq. (4-4).

[c] Assuming an AC voltage of 2 mV is read across the voltmeter terminals.

[d] Assumed to be one-tenth the calibration uncertainty.

[e] Standard curve tolerance.

also necessary to make a temperature measurement. Minimization of the temperature measurement uncertainty thus requires balancing the uncertainties due to self-heating and output signal measurement.

Attempting to correct for self-heating errors by calculation or extrapolation is not considered good practice. An estimate of the self-heating error should be included in the total uncertainty calculation instead. Self-heating is particularly a problem for temperature sensors and is discussed in detail in that section.

Excitation uncertainty. The temperature measurement uncertainty due to an uncertainty in the excitation current can be calculated using Eq. (4-2) by replacing the quantity u_V/V by the relative voltage change due to the current uncertainty u_I. The resulting expression is

$$\frac{u_T}{T} = \frac{(u_I/I)(R_d/R_s)}{S_{T/V}} \qquad (4\text{-}3)$$

where $R_d = dV/dI$ and $R_s = V/I$ are the dynamic and static resistances of the temperature sensor, respectively. Note that the dynamic and static resistances of an ohmic sensor are equal. Typical dynamic resistances of a Lake Shore DT-470 silicon diode are $3000\ \Omega$ at 300 K, $1000\ \Omega$ at 77 K, and $2800\ \Omega$ at 4.2 K, whereas the static resistances are, respectively, $51.9\ k\Omega$, $102\ k\Omega$, and $163\ k\Omega$. As an example, the accuracy of a Lake Shore Model 120CS current source is specified as $\pm0.05\%$ at 10 μA. For a DT-470 diode at 4.2 K, the resulting relative temperature measurement uncertainty would be

$$\frac{u_T}{T} = \frac{(\pm0.0005)(2800\ \Omega/163{,}000\ \Omega)}{-0.087} = \pm9.9 \times 10^{-5} = \pm99\ \text{ppm}$$

or a temperature uncertainty of 416 μK.

Thermal (Johnson) noise. Thermal energy produces random motions of the charged particles within a body, giving rise to electrical noise. The minimum root-mean-square (rms) noise power available is given by $P_n = 4kT\Delta f_n$, where k is the Boltzmann constant and Δf_n is the noise bandwidth. Peak-to-peak noise is approximately five times greater than the rms noise. Metallic resistors approach this fundamental minimum, but other materials produce somewhat greater thermal noise. The noise power is related to current or voltage noise by the relations $I = (P_n/R)^{0.5}$ and $V = (P_n R)^{0.5}$. The noise bandwidth is not necessarily the same as the signal bandwidth but is approximately equal to the smallest of the following [6]:

- $\pi/2$ times the upper 3-db frequency limit of the analog DC measuring circuitry, which is given as approximately $1/(4R_{eff}C_{in})$, where R_{eff} is the effective resistance across the measuring instrument (including the instrument's input impedance in parallel with the sensor resistance and wiring) and C_{in} is the total capacitance shunting the input;
- $0.55/t_r$ where t_r is the instrument's 10–90% rise time;
- 1 Hz if an analog panel meter is used for readout; or
- One-half the conversion rate (readings per second) of an integrating digital voltmeter.

Thermoelectric and zero offset voltages. Voltages develop in electrical conductors with temperature gradients when no current is allowed to flow (Seebeck effect). Thermoelectric voltages appear when dissimilar metals are joined and joints are held at different temperatures. Typical thermoelectric voltages in cryogenic measurement systems are on the order of microvolts.

A zero offset is the signal value measured with no input to the measuring instrument. The zero offset can drift with time or temperature and is usually included in the instrument specifications.

Thermoelectric voltages and zero offsets can be eliminated from voltage measurements on ohmic resistors by reversal of the excitation current and use of the formula

$$V = (V_+ - V_-)/2 \qquad (4\text{-}4)$$

where V_+ and V_- are the voltages with respectively positive and negative excitation currents. Alternating current (AC) excitation can also be used with ohmic sensors to eliminate zero offsets.

Measurements made in rapid succession might not allow time for current switching and the required settling times. The uncertainty can be reduced by measuring the offset before and after a series of rapid measurements and subtracting the offset voltage from the measured voltages. The sum of the thermoelectric voltages and zero offset can be calculated as

$$V_0 = (V_+ + V_-)/2 \qquad (4\text{-}5)$$

Note that the resolution of V_0 is practically limited by the resolution of the measurement system. The value of V_0 can be expected to vary little in a static system but may change during a thermal transient under study. The value of V_0 should be rechecked as often as practical.

The offset voltage V_0 is best measured by reversing the current through a resistor. Measurement of V_0 with zero excitation current is also possible, but large resistances can produce excessive time constants for discharge of any capacitances in the circuit, requiring long waiting times before V_0 can be measured accurately.

Diode measurements do not allow current reversal. The value of V_0 can be estimated by shorting the leads at the diode and measuring the offset voltage with zero excitation current at operating temperature.

Ground loops and electromagnetic noise. Improper grounding of instruments or grounding at multiple points can allow current flows that result in small voltage offsets. One common problem is the grounding of cable shields at both ends. The current flow through ground loops is not necessarily constant, resulting in a fluctuating voltage. Books on grounding and shielding can help to identify and eliminate both ground loops and electromagnetic noise.

Electromagnetic pickup is a source of additional noise. Alternating current noise is a serious problem in sensors with nonlinear current–voltage characteristics. Measurement of the AC noise across the terminals of the reading instrument can give a quick indication of the magnitude of this noise source (thermal noise will be included in this measurement). Electromagnetic pickup can be reduced by twisting wire pairs, using coaxial cables, adding shielding, or shortening the wires.

Calibration uncertainty. Commercially calibrated sensors should have calibrations traceable to international standards. About the best accuracy attainable is represented by the abilities of national standards laboratories [7]. Many laboratories provide calibrations for a fee [8,9]. The calibration uncertainty typically increases by a factor of 3 to 10 between successive devices used to transfer a calibration. An algorithm for selecting the number and spacing of calibration points is given by Nara et al. [10].

Calibration fit interpolation uncertainty. Once a calibration has been performed, an interpolation function is required for temperatures that lie between calibration points. The interpolation method must be chosen with care, since some fitting functions can be much worse than others [11]. Common interpolation methods include linear interpolation, cubic splines, and Chebyshev polynomials. Formulas based on the physics of the sensor material may give the best fits when few fit parameters are used.

Use of an interpolation function adds to the measurement uncertainty. The additional uncertainty due to an interpolation function can be gauged by the ability of the interpolation function to reproduce the calibration points. Each calibration can be broken up into several ranges to decrease the fitting uncertainties. Typical uncertainties introduced by the interpolation function are on the order of one-tenth the calibration uncertainty.

4-1-6 Other Measurement System Considerations

Wiring. Wiring for cryogenic instrumentation requires attention, especially when carrying low-voltage or high-frequency signals. Considerations for cabling at ambient temperature between the instruments and the Dewar or cryogenic enclosure include (1) physical robustness; (2) low resistance; (3) coaxial, triaxial, or twisted and shielded pairs to reduce noise; (4) use of separate conductor pairs for excitation current and voltage sensing; and (5) markings that will last the life of the cable. Pen on masking tape is not adequate! Connectors are frequently a weak link; consider (1) the ability of the connector to make the required number of matings, (2) strain relief for the cabling, (3) potential for generating thermoelectric voltages, (4) resistances of the contacts, (5) noise generated by the contacts, and (6) ease of repair or rewiring. Feed-throughs or bulkhead connectors are frequently required at interfaces to the cryogenic or vacuum environment. Vacuum-tight (hermetic) feed-throughs capable of operating at low temperatures are often expensive, available in limited variety, and prone to failure on thermal cycling. Locate vacuum-tight feed-throughs at ambient temperature when possible. Junction-type feed-throughs should be kept isothermal to reduce thermoelectric voltages. An alternative is to use continuous wire feed-throughs in regions with temperature gradients.

One of the first steps is to determine the number and type of wires required. Most resistance measurements require four leads to eliminate errors due to the resistance of the current-carrying leads. Two wires sometimes can be used if the sensor has high sensitivity and the lead resistance is small relative to the active sensor resistance. Use Eq. (4-2) to determine if the additional error due to the resistance of lead wires is tolerable. Three wire measurements are sometimes used at room temperature, but the saving of one wire is usually not worth the additional uncertainty or effort for cryogenic measurements. Another trick is to connect sensors in series or parallel, depending on the excitation mode, but the increased risk of losing several sensors due to some break or failure in the circuit must be considered carefully.

Wiring can provide a significant heat conduction path from the ambient environment to a sensor at cryogenic temperatures. The heat conducted to the cryogenic environment wastes expensive cooling power and can affect the operation of the sensor. The heat conducted to the cryogenic environment can be reduced by the following means:

1. Use wires of low thermal conductivity materials, such as manganin, constantan, phosphor bronze, nichrome, stainless steel, or Evan-ohm. The thermal conductivity and electrical resistivity of a metal are inversely related, and thus lower thermal conductivities come at the expense of increased electrical resistivity.
2. Use wires with smaller cross section.
3. Make the wires longer.
4. Reduce the number of wires.
5. Heat sink the wires at a temperature near the sensor operating temperature to intercept the heat leak.
6. Reduce the insulation thickness to improve contact with the heat sink. Thin enamel is better than thicker Teflon.

The arrangement used to analyze wire heat-sinking requirements is shown in Fig. 4-2. The required heat-sinking length is a function of the wire material, wire cross section, temperature difference between the ends of the wire, and the tolerable temperature rise at the sensor. Hust [12] devised a procedure for calculating the heat-sinking length given as follows with some modifications to allow for the now common ability to calculate inverse hyperbolic sines with ease:

1. Compute

$$m = (K_c d_e / K_w A_w t)^{0.5}$$

where K_c is the thermal conductivity of the adhesive at temperature $\bar{T} = (T_2 + T_3)/2$, K_w is the thermal conductivity of the wire at $\bar{T}$, A_w is the cross-sectional area of the wire, and d_e and t are the effective width and thickness of the adhesive bond.

2. Compute

$$\frac{B}{2} = \frac{\xi(T_1) - \xi(T_2)}{L_1 K_w(T_2) T_s f m}$$

where $\xi(T_1)$ and $\xi(T_2)$ are thermal conductivity integrals for the wire material at the indicated temperatures, $K_w(T_2)$ is the thermal conductivity of the wire at T_2, L_1 is the

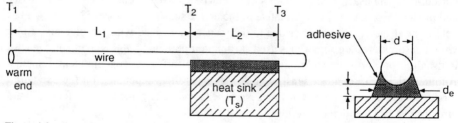

Figure 4-2   Arrangement for heat-sinking wires. The two schematic views are not to the same scale.

Table 4-3 Wire heat-sinking lengths required to thermally anchor to a heat sink at temperature T to bring the temperature of the wire to within 1 mK of T

Material	T_1 [K]	T_s [K]	Heat-sinking length, L_2 (mm) for wire sizes			
			0.21 mm² (24 AWG)	0.032 mm² (32 AWG)	0.013 mm² (36 AWG)	0.005 mm² (40 AWG)
Copper	300	80	160	57	33	19
	300	4	688	233	138	80
Phosphor-	300	80	32	11	6	4
Bronze	300	4	38	13	7	4
Manganin	300	80	21	4	4	2
	300	4	20	7	4	2
304 ss	300	80	17	6	3	2
	300	4	14	5	3	2

Note: Values are calculated assuming wires are in a vacuum environment, and the thermal conductivity of the adhesive is given by the fit to the thermal conductivity of GE 7031 varnish.

length of the wire before the heat-sink station, T_s is the temperature of the heat sink, and $f = (T_3 - T_s)/T_s$, the fraction of temperature T_s that is allowed as a temperature differential after the heat-sink station. Note that Hust used a fixed-temperature differential, but temperature errors are relative (1 mK is much more significant at 1 K than at 1000 K), and thus a means of expressing the allowable temperature difference as a fraction of T_s is more appropriate. Hust also used the mean thermal conductivity of the wire multiplied by the temperature difference $(T_1 - T_2)$ rather than the difference of the thermal conductivity integrals.

3. Set $T_2 = T_s$ as a first approximation.
4. Calculate the required heat-sinking length as $L_2 = \frac{1}{m}\sinh^{-1}(\frac{B}{2})$.
5. Calculate $T_2 = T_s(1 + fB/2)$. Repeat steps 4 and 5 until T_2 converges.

Typical values calculated with this procedure are given in Table 4-3 using the polynomial fits to $K(T)$ and $\xi(T)$ given in Tables 4-4 and 4-5. The heat Q conducted down a wire of cross-sectional area A_w and length L can be calculated as

$$Q = \frac{A_w}{L}[\xi(T_1) - \xi(T_2)] \tag{4-6}$$

using the thermal conductivity integral polynomials.

Low-loss wiring for high-frequency signals can require the presence of some low-resistivity electrical conductor, with the amount required depending on the signal frequency, wire geometry, and allowable attenuation [13].

DC measurement instrumentation. Potentiometric four-wire resistance measurement instrumentation is shown in Fig. 4-3. Offset voltages and noise in DC measurement circuits are typically on the order of microvolts. The noise floor can be lowered an order of magnitude or more by reversing the excitation current polarity and combining the two measurements. Some measurement systems place a reference resistor in series with the sensor and provide switching of the voltmeter to allow measurement of the voltage across either the sensor or reference resistor. The additional switching and data

Table 4-4 Thermal conductivities k (W/m · K) as a function of temperature T(K) for some wire and adhesive materials

n	Phosphor bronze[a]	Manganin[b]	304 ss[c]	Cu[d] (RRR = 100)	Adhesive[e] (GE varnish)
0	-1.51470×10^0	-2.61774×10^0	-3.21922×10^0	4.92877×10^0	-3.71479×10^0
1	2.05381×10^0	5.21160×10^{-1}	1.12634×10^0	-2.09010×10^0	5.02559×10^{-1}
2	-1.99187×10^0	2.34033×10^0	4.95025×10^{-1}	1.07864×10^1	–
3	2.21730×10^0	-2.47410×10^0	-3.33933×10^{-1}	-1.39205×10^1	–
4	-1.19306×10^0	1.31338×10^0	4.68700×10^{-2}	8.97033×10^0	–
5	3.39998×10^{-1}	-3.80896×10^{-1}	3.16436×10^{-2}	-3.15031×10^0	–
6	-5.31001×10^{-2}	6.06708×10^{-2}	-1.39767×10^{-2}	6.08560×10^{-1}	–
7	4.27246×10^{-3}	-4.99540×10^{-3}	2.06039×10^{-3}	-6.07406×10^{-2}	–
8	-1.37001×10^{-4}	1.66975×10^{-4}	-1.05984×10^{-4}	2.44937×10^{-3}	–

Note: Polynomial log–log fits are given in the form $\ln k = \Sigma\{A_n^*(\ln T)^n\}$, where the sum is over n terms, and the coefficients A_n are given in the table.

[a] Childs, G. E., Ericks, L. J., and Powell, R. L., *Thermal Conductivity of Solids at Room Temperature and Below*, NBS Monograph 131 (1973), p. 291, Fig. 43a, curve: Z.Z.-P-Bronze.
[b] Ibid., p. 291, Fig. 43a, curves: Z.Z.-Manganin, L.-Manganin.
[c] Ibid., p. 257, Fig. 40a, Curve: B.-Stainless.
[d] Reed, R. P., and Clark, A. F., eds., *Materials at Low Temperatures*, American Society for Metals. Ohio (1983), p. 150, Fig. 4.25.
[e] Ibid., p. 517, Table 14.2, GE 7031 Varnish.

manipulation are often well worth the improvements in measurement accuracy. Averaging many readings obtained with high-stability instruments can push the noise floor down towards 1 nV.

Resistance bridges are also used for cryogenic measurements, but the lead resistances must be fully compensated to make accurate measurements if the entire bridge is not in the cryogenic environment. The Kelvin and Mueller bridges accomplish this [14,15,16].

AC measurement instrumentation. Offset voltages can be eliminated by using AC measurements without requiring switching of the excitation and extra data manipulation. Phase-sensitive detectors (or lock-in amplifiers, as they are commonly known) provide further noise rejection, allowing the possibility of measurements with subnanovolt

Table 4-5 Thermal conductivity integrals ξ (W/m) as a function of temperature T(K) for some wire and adhesive materials

n	Phosphor Bronze	Manganin	304 ss	Cu (RRR = 100)
0	-2.20748×10^0	-3.31049×10^0	-3.91204×10^0	4.23453×10^0
1	2.09234×10^0	1.82014×10^0	2.00718×10^0	1.33420×10^0
2	3.63836×10^{-1}	8.04489×10^{-1}	2.89596×10^{-1}	2.28628×10^0
3	-4.59520×10^{-1}	-5.87260×10^{-1}	-4.71671×10^{-2}	-2.78065×10^0
4	3.80748×10^{-1}	2.15398×10^{-1}	-7.23868×10^{-2}	1.68865×10^0
5	-1.69769×10^{-1}	-3.48585×10^{-2}	4.61190×10^{-2}	-5.51670×10^{-1}
6	3.92451×10^{-2}	4.10190×10^{-3}	-1.15073×10^{-2}	9.70723×10^{-2}
7	-4.51372×10^{-3}	4.64626×10^{-4}	1.31212×10^{-3}	-8.66608×10^{-3}
8	2.05250×10^{-4}	-3.46385×10^{-5}	-5.66671×10^{-5}	3.07554×10^{-4}

Note: Polynomial log–log fits are given in the form $\ln \xi = \Sigma\{A_n^*(\ln T)^n\}$, where the sum is over n terms and the coefficients A_n are given in the table. The fitted thermal conductivity integral data were produced from thermal conductivities taken from the sources noted for Table 4-4.

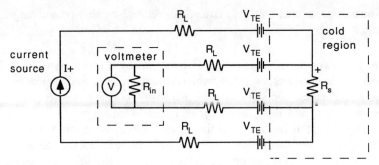

Figure 4-3   Instrumentation for four-wire resistance measurements.

sensitivities. The ability to detect small signals allows the use of smaller excitation pow-ers, which are often important in cryogenic measurements where even a small heat input can disturb the system. Note that because a phase-sensitive detector produces no even harmonics in its output, an exact even submultiple frequency output synchronized to the line frequency (e.g., 30, 15, or 10 Hz with a 60-Hz line frequency) provides automatic rejection of noise at line and higher harmonic frequencies.

AC instrumentation is more complex than DC instrumentation, but can be employed economically on a large scale [18].

Pulse measurement techniques.   Difficulties in measuring low-voltage DC signals also can be overcome by using pulse techniques. In one application at Fermilab [19] 50-μs pulses of 2.5 mA were used to measure carbon composition and platinum resistance thermometers at a repetition rate of 1 Hz. The average power dissipation was thus reduced by a factor of 20,000.

Control circuits.   The properties of materials can change rapidly at low temperatures. Temperature control circuits especially must be able to adapt to a wide range of charac-teristic system response times [20]. Selection of PID (proportional, integral, derivative) control parameters is especially difficult in a system cooled by a mechanical refrigerator operating near its minimum temperature.

Cold electronics.   Ideally, electronic readout circuits should be located as close to the sensor as possible. Operation of excitation sources, multiplexers, amplifiers and analog-to-digital converters at cryogenic temperatures could greatly reduce the noise, number of feed-throughs, and heat leak. Unfortunately, many common semiconductor components do not operate below about 100 K. Currently available operational amplifiers use bipolar transistors that undergo carrier freeze-out and become inoperable at low temperatures. There are some exceptions, mostly FETs [21–25], but operation of the readout electronics at room temperature continues to predominate.

Superconducting devices and circuits can be used below about 80 K and have some unique advantages [26]. One of the best known is the superconducting quan-tum interference device (SQUID) capable of detecting extremely small changes in electromagnetic quantities such as voltage, current, magnetic susceptibility, and magnetic field.

Communications bus bars. Communications bus bars can cause problems with instruments at cryogenic temperatures, especially when the instrument is used to measure temperatures below 1 K. In these applications, noise picked up from the computer can be transmitted to the instrument and along the sensor excitation to the temperature sensor. The noise current produces resistive heating in the sensor, yielding erroneous temperature measurements if the power dissipation is significant. In these cases, the computer should be optically isolated from the instrument. Many companies now sell inexpensive optical isolation kits.

4-2 TEMPERATURE MEASUREMENT

Cryogenic temperature sensors have been developed using a variety of temperature-dependent properties. Common, commercially available temperature sensors include resistors, capacitors, thermocouples, and semiconductor junction devices such as diodes or transistors. Such sensors, suitable for use as secondary or tertiary temperature standards, are of greatest concern here. Primary standards-grade sensors are very sensitive to thermal and mechanical shock and are therefore not suitable for ordinary laboratory or industrial temperature measurements. Other temperature measurement techniques such as gas, vapor pressure, acoustic, noise, and magnetic susceptibility thermometry, are not covered here, for they require much greater effort to implement or severely constrain system design.

Requirements most often placed on temperature sensors include the temperature range, reproducibility, accuracy, sensitivity, physical size, thermal response time, interchangeability, and ease of instrumentation. In addition, the sensors are often used in harsh environments (e.g., high mechanical shock, ionizing radiation, or magnetic fields) and must be relatively immune to calibration shifts from these environmental factors. Important characteristics are summarized in Table 4-6. More detailed information is provided on temperature-dependent characteristics in Table 4-7, on thermal response times in Table 4-8, on temperature errors in magnetic fields in Tables 4-9, and on effects of ionizing radiation in Tables 4-10 through 4-12. Dimensionless temperature sensitivities of some representative cryogenic temperature sensors are plotted in Fig. 4-4. Relative temperature measurement resolutions are plotted in Fig. 4-5 for given excitations and measurement system resolutions.

A large variety of resistance temperature sensors (RTDs) are commercially available. Measurement with a four-wire potentiometric circuit (see Fig. 4-3) is most common. Measurement with an AC bridge has advantages at lower temperatures, especially below 1 K. Measurement systems for many similar RTDs have been built [18,19].

The variety of cryogenic temperature sensors in use reflects the difficulty in satisfying all requirements with a single sensor. Many sources are available with more specific information than can be covered in this general overview [27–31].

Table 4-6 Overview of cryogenic temperature sensors

Sensor	Measurement technique	Range [K]	Sensitivity	Stability	Size	Magneto-resistance	Radiation effect	Cost [$]
Carbon	Resistance	0.01–300	Good	Poor	Moderate	Moderate	–	0.1
Carbon-glass	Resistance	1.4–325	Very high	Moderate	Moderate	Moderate	–	195
Capacitance	Capacitance	0.2–250	Moderate	Poor	Moderate	None	–	300
Cernox	Resistance	0.3–325	Good	Good	Small to moderate	Small	Low	125
CLTS	Resistance	4–300	Very low	Good	Large	–	Small	–
CMN	Susceptibility	0.001–10	–	–	–	<0.02 T	–	DIY
GaAs or GaAlAs diode	Voltage	1.4–475	Low	Good	Moderate	Moderate	–	–
Germanium	Resistance	0.05–100	Good to low	Very good	Moderate	Large	–	150–2000
^{3}He melting curve	Pressure	0.001–0.32	–	–	–	Small	–	DIY
Mössbauer	Gamma detector	0.002–0.02	–	–	–	–	–	DIY
NMR	NMR	μK–mK	–	Moderate	Very large	Moderate	–	DIY
Noise	Voltage (SQUID)	μK–300	–	Moderate	–	–	–	DIY
Nuclear orientation	Gamma detector	0.004–4	–	Moderate	–	Small	–	680
Platinum	Resistance	10–800	Low to good	Very good	Moderate	Large	Small	75
Rhodium–iron	Resistance	0.1–600	Low to good	Very good	Small to large	Large	Small	360
Ruthenium oxide	Resistance	0.05–20	Good to low	Moderate	Moderate	Small	–	90
Si diode	Voltage	1.4–475	Low	Moderate	Moderate	Very large	Large	100
Superconducting fixed points	Susceptibility	0.015–7	–	Very good	Moderate	Zero field required	–	3500
Thermistor	Resistance	77–300	Very high	Good	Small	Small	–	–
Thermocouple, Au–Fe	Voltage	2–300	Low	Moderate	Small	Moderate	–	10

Note: DIY in the cost column stands for Do It Yourself and can be quite expensive.

Table 4-7 Temperature-dependent properties of some commercially available cryogenic temperature sensors

Sensor type (manufacturer) model	Tabulated quantity	$T(K)$				
		1.4	4.2	20	80	300
Capacitor (LS) CS–401	C (nF)	—	5.000	5.776	6.942	—
	S_T	—	0.0485	0.1488	−0.1939	—
Capacitor (LS) CS–501	C (nF)	—	6.11034	6.62276	9.4614	104.109
	S_T	—	0.0194	0.1082	0.4628	−4.455
Carbon–glass (LS) CGR-1-1000	R (Ω)	23270.0	837.8	38.86	14.08	8.323
	S_T	−7.347	−3.352	−1.066	−0.500	−0.339
Cernox (LS) CX–1030	R (Ω)	1613.1	513.78	185.66	79.26	28.99
	S_T	−1.320	−0.820	−0.566	−0.680	−0.793
Cernox (LS) CX–1050	R (Ω)	63049.0	4919.7	755.7	198.1	50.38
	S_T	−2.295	−1.710	−0.958	−0.997	−1.003
CLTS (MM) CLTS	R (Ω)	—	220.70	224.00	238.38	291.46
	S_T	—	0.0034	0.018	0.085	0.257
GaAlAs diode (LS) TG–120P	V (V)	5.04512	4.45595	2.29734	1.40646	0.90574
	S_T	−0.043	−0.200	−0.677	−0.068	−0.910
Germainium (LS) GR-200A-1000	R (Ω)	28949.0	1290.5	42.03	2.984	—
	S_T	−3.708	−2.144	−2.273	−1.159	—
Platinum (LS) PT–103	R (Ω)	1.47	1.48	2.115	21.35	110.38
	S_T	0.0003	0.008	0.795	1.591	1.0545
Rhodium–iron (LS) RF-800-4	R (Ω)	1.51	1.94	3.13	7.10	29.72
	S_T	0.157	0.290	0.291	1.105	1.011
Ruthenium oxide (SI) RO-600	R (Ω)	1602.7	1234.9	1052.0	1016.6	—
	S_T	−0.311	−0.172	−0.049	−0.0131	—
Silicon diode (LS) DT–470	V (V)	1.69812	1.62602	1.21440	1.01525	0.51892
	S_T	−0.0108	−0.0868	−0.2899	−0.1521	−1.3875

Note: Manufacturers are LS = Lake Shore, MM = Micro Measurements, SI = Scientific Instruments.

Table 4-8 Thermal response times of various cryogenic temperature sensors in a liquid helium bath (4.2 K), a liquid nitrogen bath (77 K), and an ice bath (273 K)

Sensor type	Packaging/construction	Response time at temperature		
		4.2 K	77 K	273 K
Silicon diode	Eutectically bonded to metallized sapphire substrate with hermetic seal	<10 ms	100 ms	200 ms
Silicon diode	Mounted on platinum disk with stycast epoxy dome	<10 ms	50 ms	NA
GaAlAs diode	Mounted on platinum disk with stycast epoxy dome	100 ms	250 ms	3 s
Cernox	Bare chip/gold leads	1.5 ms	50 ms	135 ms
Cernox	Epoxy bonded to metallized sapphire substrate with hermetic seal	15 ms	250 ms	0.8 s
Cernox	Epoxied to beryllium oxide slug and stycast epoxy sealed into gold-plated copper can	0.4 s	1 s	1 s
Carbon glass	Strain-free mounted and stycast epoxy sealed into gold-plated copper can	1 s	1.5 s	NA
Germanium	Strain-free mounted and stycast epoxy sealed into gold-plated copper can	200 ms	3 s	NA
RhFe	Bare chip/gold leads	2 ms	12 ms	35 ms
RhFe	Epoxied to beryllium oxide slug and stycast epoxy sealed into gold-plated copper can	0.8 s	3.6 s	14.5 s
RhFe	Ceramic encapsulated	NA	NA	10 s
RuOx	Epoxy bonded to sapphire slug and stycast epoxied into gold-plated copper can	500 ms	1.3 s	NA
Platinum	Ceramic encapsulated	NA	1.75 s	12.5 s
Platinum	Glass encapsulated	NA	2.5 s	20 s

4-2-1 Metallic Resistors

Positive temperature coefficient (PTC) resistors are metallic. The resistance versus temperature characteristic is nearly linear at higher temperatures and bottoms out at low temperatures, where the electrical resistance is dominated by temperature-independent scattering by impurities and defects in the metal. Constant current excitation results in decreasing power dissipation with decreasing temperature, as required to prevent self-heating. A single excitation current can be used for a wide temperature range, which simplifies the instrumentation requirements. The most common metallic temperature sensors are made from platinum or rhodium–iron.

Table 4-9 Magnetic-field-induced temperature errors $\Delta T/T$ (%) for various cryogenic temperature sensors

Sensor type (manufacturer) Model no.	$T(K)$	Relative temperature error $\Delta T/T$ (%) at magnetic field B (T)				Notes
		1	2.5	8	19	
Carbon glass (Lake Shore)	4.2		−0.5	−2.3	−6.6	
CGR-1-1000	10		−0.2	−1.1	−3.8	
	25		0.02	0.22	0.79	
	45		0.07	0.48	2.2	
	88		0.05	0.45	2.3	
Carbon resistors	4.2		<1	5	−	
47, 100, 220 Ω	10		<1	3	−	
(Allen Bradley)	20		<1	1	−	
Capacitance		<0.5 from 2 to 300 K				
CS-401, 501 (Lake Shore)						
Cernox	0.47		8.1	12.9	29.1	16, not 19 T
CX-1030 (Lake Shore)	1.2		1.7	5.1	7.6	
	4.8		0.9	0.7	0.5	
Cernox	1.4		2.1	3.9	6.3	
CX-1070 (Lake Shore)	3.5		0.3	−0.1	−1.0	
Diode, GaAlAs	4.2	2.9	3.8	−	−	J perp.,
TG-120 (Lake Shore)	30	0.2	0.3	−	−	little
	78	<0.1	0.15	−	−	orient.
	300	<0.1	<0.1	−	−	depend.
Diode, Si	4.2	−8	−10	−	−	J perp.,
DT-470 (Lake Shore)	20	−4	−5	−	−	strong
	80	−0.1	−0.4	−	−	orient.
	300	<0.1	0.3	−	−	depend.
Germanium	2.0		−8	−60	−	
resistors	4.2		−5 to −20	−30 to −50	−	
	10		−4 to −15	−25 to −60	−	
	20		−3 to −20	−15 to −35	−	
Platinum	20		20	100	−	
resistors	40		0.5	3	8.8	
	87		0.04	0.4	1.7	
	300		<0.01	0.02	0.13	
Rhodium–iron	4.2		11	40	−	6, not 8 T
resistors	40		1.5	12	47	
	87		0.2	1.5	6	
	300		<0.01	0.1	−	
Thermocouple,	10		1	3	−	
type E	20		<1	2	−	
	455		<1	<1	−	
Thermocouple, KP	10		3	20	−	
versus Au–0.7% Fe	45		1	5	−	
	100		0.1	0.8	−	

Table 4-10 Gamma-radiation-induced calibration offsets as a function of temperature for several types of cryogenic temperature sensors

Sensor type	Model	Radiation-induced offset (mK) at temperature				
		4.2 K	20 K	77 K	200 K	300 K
Platinum[a]	PT-103	NA	−15	−10[c]	10[c]	10[c]
Rhodium iron[a]	RF-100-AA	2[c]	15[c]	15[c]	5[c]	5[c]
Cernox[a]	CX-1050-SD	−10	−10[c]	−5[c]	25[c]	25[c]
Carbon glass[a]	CGR-1-1000	−30	−140	−700	−1,300	−3,400
Germanium[a]	GR-200A-1000	−5	−20	−25	NA	NA
Ruthenium oxide[a]	RO600	20	150	[c]	[c]	NA
GaAlAs diode[a]	TG-120P	−15	−25	2,200	2,500	400
Silicon diode[a]	DT-470-SD	25	1,000	1,300	1,000	2,700
Silicon diode[a]	DT-500P-GR-M	350	50	20	250	300
Silicon diode[a]	SI-410-NN	600	2,000	300	450	1,400
Platinum[b]	PT-103	NA	−50	5[c]	50	75
Rhodium iron[b]	RF-800-4	5[c]	15[c]	25	10[c]	−15[c]
Rhodium iron[b]	RF-100-AA	−5[c]	−5[c]	5[c]	−10[c]	5[c]
Carbon glass[b]	CGR-1-1000	−25	−175	−1,400	−4,200	−6,500
Germanium[b]	GR-200A-1000	2[c]	2[c]	5[c]	NA	NA
GaAlAs diode[b]	TG-120P	−50	−75	700	600	−250
Silicon diode[b]	DT-470-SD	+20	−200	1,500	11,000	18,000
Silicon diode[b]	DT-500P-GR-M	10[c]	10[c]	−5[c]	−5[c]	−100

[a] Sensors were irradiated in situ at 4.2 K with a cobalt-60 gamma source at a dose rate of 3,000 gray/hour to a total dose of 10,000 gray (1 Mrad).

[b] Sensors were irradiated at room temperature with a cesium-137 gamma source at a dose of 30 gray/hour to a total dose of 10,000 gray (1×10^6 rad).

[c] Deviations smaller than calibration accuracy.

Platinum RTDs. Platinum RTDs are the most accurate and reproducible thermometers available over a wide range of temperature. Measurements in the range from 15 to 725 K are made routinely with a high degree of accuracy using platinum RTDs available from several commercial sources. According to IEC-751, the industry standard for class B accuracy is specified as ±0.3 K at 273.16 K and ±0.75% variation in the specified 0.00385 K^{-1} temperature coefficient of resistance ($S_T = 1.052$). Class A accuracy is better by a factor of 2. Individual calibration is required for accurate temperature measurement below 100 K. Magnetoresistive temperature errors of platinum RTDs above 65 K are shown in Fig. 4-6 [32,33]. The magnetoresistance is orientation-dependent and continues to increase below 65 K. A new type of platinum RTD with the

Table 4-11 Gamma-radiation-induced calibration offsets as a function of temperature for several types of cryogenic temperature sensors

Sensor type	Model	Radiation-induced offset (mK) at temperature				
		4.2 K	20 K	77 K	200 K	300 K
Rhodium iron	RF-100-AA	5[a]	−5[a]	−25	−25	−35
Cernox	CX-1070-SD	10[a]	10[a]	25[a]	5[a]	10[a]

Note: Sensors were irradiated in situ at 4.2 K in a nuclear pool reactor to a total fluence of 2×10^{12} neutrons/cm^2 at a flux of 7.5×10^7 neutrons/cm^2/s.

[a] Deviations smaller than calibration accuracy.

Table 4-12 Neutron-radiation-induced calibration offsets as a function of temperature for several types of cryogenic temperature sensors

Sensor type	Model	Radiation-induced offset (mK) at temperature				
		4.2 K	20 K	77 K	200 K	300 K
Platinum	PT-103	NA	−40	−20	−20	−20[a]
Rhodium iron	RF-800-4	−3[a]	−7[a]	−3[a]	−3[a]	−5[a]
Carbon Glass[b]	CGR-1-1000	−15		−350		−1,100
Germanium	GR-200A-1000	−1[a]	−4[a]	−8[a]	NA	NA
GaAlAs diode	TG-120P	−125	−50	750	1,000	250
Silicon diode[b]	DT-470-SD	800		−6,700		−10,500

Note: Sensors were irradiated at room temperature in a nuclear pool reactor to a total fluence of 2.5×10^{12} neutrons/cm^2 at a flux of 3.8×10^7 neutrons/s cm^2.
[a] Deviations smaller than calibration accuracy.
[b] Total fluence for this device was 7.8×10^{12} neutrons/s cm^2.

sensing wire wound at optimal pitch angles reduces the magnetoresistance anisotropy from 35 to about 4% [34].

Rhodium-iron RTDs. Rhodium–iron RTDs are useful down to at least 1 K owing to the presence of temperature-dependent spin fluctuation effects contributed by the dilute iron alloy, typically 0.5 at %. The wide temperature range and excellent stability have made this a valuable thermometer for certain demanding applications. The magnetoresistance is large and somewhat higher than that of platinum.

Cryogenic linear temperature sensors (CLTS). Cryogenic linear temperature sensors (CLTS) are made by Vishay Micro-Measurements from thin-foil sensing grids laminated into fiberglass–epoxy. The two alloys are special grades of nickel and Manganin processed to produce a combined resistance that is very nearly linear in temperature from 4 to 300 K. The resistance rises from 220 Ω at 4 K to 290 Ω at 297 K with a temperature sensitivity of 0.2389 Ω/K. The maximum deviation from linearity is about ±3 K. Also available are matching networks designed for direct readout with strain gauge instrumentation [35]. The magnetoresistance at 4–6 K is sufficiently large that the CLTS has been used to measure magnetic fields [36,37]. The CLTS is a useful temperature indicator where high accuracy is not necessary and requires only a 100-μA current source and a voltmeter for instrumentation.

4-2-2 Semiconducting Resistors

Semiconducting resistors typically have negative temperature coefficients (NTC). The temperature sensitivity is often small near 300 K but increases with decreasing temperature. The resistance can change by five orders of magnitude over the sensor's useful temperature range. Semiconductors are typically piezoresistive, and thus bulk sensing elements must be mounted strain free, which reduces the thermal connection to the sample whose temperature is to be measured. Consequently, self-heating can be significant unless measurement power to the device is kept extremely small. The large

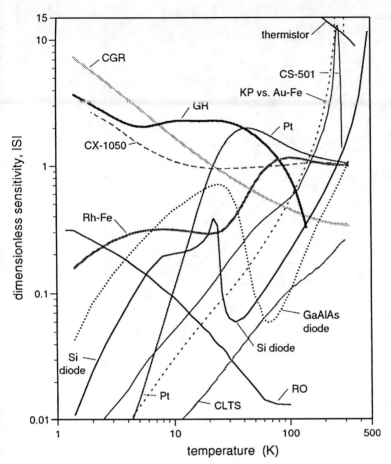

Figure 4-4 Dimensionless temperature sensitivities (absolute values) of representative commercial cryogenic temperature sensors. Model numbers refer to Lake Shore sensors except where noted. **CGR**: CGR-1-1000 carbon-glass resistor; **CLTS**: Vishay Micro-Measurements CLTS-2 metal foil gauge; **CS-501**: CS-501 capacitor; **CX-1050**: Cernox 1050 resistor; **GaAlAs diode**: TG-120P gallium-aluminum-arsenide @ 10 μA; **GR**: GR-200A-1000 germanium resistor; **KP versus Au–Fe**: KP chromel versus Au–0.07% Fe thermocouple referenced to 273.15 K; **Pt**: PT-103 platinum resistor; **Rh–Fe**: RF-800-4 rhodium–iron resistor; **RO**: Scientific Instruments RO-600 ruthenium oxide thick film resistor; **Si diode**: DT-470 @ 10 μA; **thermistor**: Yellow Springs Instruments 44003A.

resistance change coupled with thermal considerations results in a requirement for a variable current source for measurement in which the current must be varied from about 0.01 μA to 1 mA or more as well as a voltmeter capable of measuring voltages as small as 1 μV. The most common NTC temperature sensors are made from carbon, carbon–glass, germanium, Cernox™, and ruthenium oxide.

Carbon RTDs. Carbon RTDs are made from common radio resistors. Of the models in common cryogenic use, only the Allen–Bradley 1/8 W and 1/4 W models are still

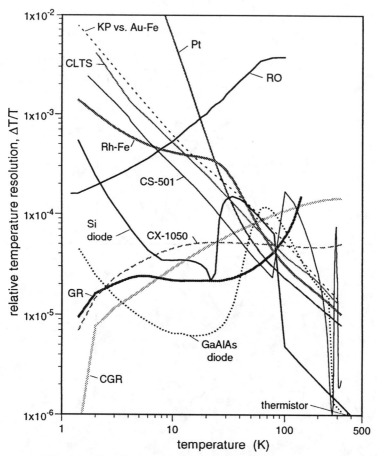

Figure 4-5 Relative temperature resolutions of representative commercial cryogenic temperature sensors under example operating conditions: **CGR**: 2 mV or $I = 0.1$ μA minimum; **CLTS**: 10 μA; **CS- 501**: 5-kHz excitation; **CX-1050**: 2 mV or $I = 0.1$ μA minimum; **GaAlAs diode**: 10 μA; **GR**: 2 mV or $I = 0.1$ μA minimum; **KP versis Au–Fe**: KP chromel versis Au–0.07% Fe thermocouple referenced to 273.15 K; **Pt**: 100 μA; **Rh–Fe**: 300 μA; **RO**: 10 μA; **Si diode**: 10 μA; **thermistor**: 1 μW. Measurement system resolution: **capacitance**: 0.1 pF or one part in 10^5; **voltage**: 0.1 μV or one part in 10^6, whichever is larger. Refer to Fig. 4-3 for sensor identification.

being manufactured [27]. Resistors with nominal values between 22 and 470 Ω are most commonly used. These resistors are cheap (less than one dollar) but labor intensive to use. The outer casing reduces thermal contact with the environment and is frequently abraded away or sanded through on two sides. The large lead wires should be cut down to prevent straining and to localize the region in good thermal contact with the carbon sensor. Baking removes moisture and improves stability. In general, these are medium-accuracy devices with only moderate stability on thermal cycling or aging. The frequent need to recalibrate carbon resistors in situ has led to schemes for calibrating carbon resistors with a minimum number of calibration points [38]. On the plus side, they are physically small with low heat capacity, have fast time response, are very sensitive to

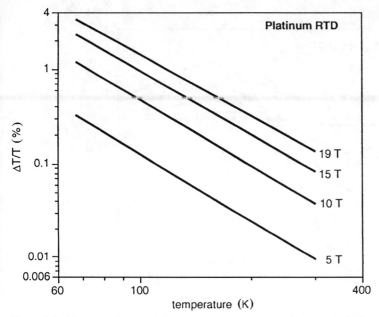

Figure 4-6 Magnetoresistance of platinum temperature sensors with magnetic field parallel to the long axis of the sensor. The lines shown are log–log linear fits to the data from several sensors and do not reflect scatter in the original data.

temperatures below about 20 K, and are only moderately affected by magnetic fields [39–41].

Carbon–glass RTDs. Carbon–glass RTDs are bulk devices manufactured from carbon-impregnated glass. The resistance–temperature characteristic is monotonic over the 1 to 325 K temperature range and very reproducible below 100 K. Such RTDs have a very high sensitivity below 10 K and can be used for submillikelvin control in this range. These devices behave very well in magnetic fields in fields up to 19 T, and accurate corrections can be made to their field-induced temperature errors [42] (see Fig. 4-7). Strain-free mounting in a canister is required. The contacts to the carbon–glass are a weak point and are prone to failure after repeated thermal cyclings.

Cernox RTDs. Cernox RTDs are ceramic oxynitride thin films sputtered onto a sapphire substrate. The devices have a monotonic response curve, and a single device can be used over the 0.3 to 330 K range with acceptable dimensionless temperature sensitivity. Other models are available that cover various temperature ranges with higher sensitivity in those ranges. Cernox sensors have lower magnetic-field-induced temperature errors than carbon glass, are highly resistant to ionizing radiation, and are repeatable to about ±3 mK at 4.2 K. The magnetoresistance becomes large below about 4.2 K, is complex, and is still not completely characterized (see Fig. 4-8). These devices are available in chip form (0.75 mm wide by 1 mm long by 0.05 to 0.38 mm thick) or packaged in a gold-plated

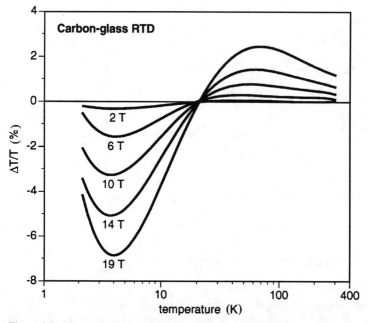

Figure 4-7 Magnetoresistance of carbon–glass temperature sensors.

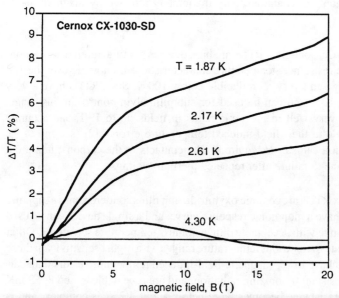

Figure 4-8 Magnetoresistance of a Cernox temperature sensor at liquid helium temperatures. The magnetoresistance changes with Cernox model.

copper can or hermetically sealed flat-mount package. Their small size yields a much faster thermal response time than traditional bulk devices.

Germanium RTDs. Germanium RTDs have been recognized as a "Secondary Standard Thermometer" and employed in the measurement of temperatures from 0.05 to 30 K for more than 30 years. They were used in the international intercomparisons, resulting in the development of the low-temperature scale (0.5 to 30 K) EPT-76 and leading to ITS-90. Germanium sensors are bulk devices available with different doping levels to meet the needed temperature range. A single device typically has a useful temperature range of about two orders of magnitude (e.g., 0.05 to 5 K or 1 to 100 K) and can normally be used to submillikelvin control in the lower portion of its range. These devices have extremely good stability (about ± 0.5 mK at 4.2 K) and are probably the best choice for high-accuracy work under 30 K when magnetic fields are not present. As with the carbon glass RTD, these devices are fragile and normally packaged in a gold-plated copper can. The magnetoresistance of ordinary germanium RTDs is large and orientation-dependent, although there is a report on a correction method applicable in the 1.5 to 10 K range up to 2.5 T [43]. Alternate doping techniques have yielded a germanium RTD with lower magnetoresistance [44].

Ruthenium oxide RTDs. Ruthenium oxide RTDs are typically thick-film sensors fabricated from ruthenium oxide or bismuth ruthenate pastes. Thick-film resistors made for the electronics industry are intended to have near-zero temperature dependence at ambient temperatures, and the exact composition of the paste is often a proprietary secret. Microcracks form in the thick film during initial thermal cycles, and thus 20 or more thermal cycles to 77 K are recommended before calibration. Depending on the model and manufacturer, ruthenium oxide RTDs can have low magnetoresistance below 20 K [45,46]. Currently, these devices have the lowest magnetoresistance below 1 K of any commercially available RTD capable of holding a calibration on thermal cycling. Some commercial thick-film RTDs are interchangeable within the same manufacturing lot. Thin-film ruthenium oxide RTDs can be deposited but are not yet common. The primary application is in the presence of magnetic fields at temperatures below 1 K, but the thermal resistance is large at such temperatures, and thus low excitation power is required to avoid heating the temperature sensor [47].

Thermistors. Thermistors are typically made of sintered metallic oxides. Important characteristics include large temperature sensitivity, small size, and low sensitivity to magnetic fields or ionizing radiation. The large temperature sensitivity reduces the useful temperature range for a given sensor. Most commercially available thermistors are designed for use above liquid nitrogen temperature.

4-2-3 Semiconductor Diodes

Diode temperature sensors have several advantages over resistance temperature sensors. Diodes tend to come in the smallest packages (both physical size and thermal mass) and as such have faster response times. When properly packaged, diodes are very robust and are suitable for temperature measurements from 1 to about 500 K. Diodes are relatively easy to use, and the instrumentation is fairly straightforward for these types of devices. Only a fixed-current source (typically at 10 μA) and a voltmeter with a range of 0.1 to 6 V are required for instrumentation. Their large voltage signal allows thermoelectric voltages to be ignored in most cases.

An important feature of diodes is interchangeability. A single diode series from a given manufacturer will have some degree of interchangeability defined in terms of tolerance bands about a standard voltage-temperature curve for that series. Interchangeability can be as good as ±0.1 K at 2 K and ±0.5 K at 300 K, and cost is directly dependent on the degree of interchangeability desired.

Diode measurements are no more difficult to perform but are typically less accurate. The reduced accuracy is a consequence of the nonlinear current–voltage characteristic and moderate dimensionless temperature sensitivities. The voltage across the diode can be measured only in the forward direction, and thus the voltmeter must now make an absolute measurement. Without current reversal, thermoelectric voltages and voltmeter offsets may be present, and these directly affect the achievable accuracy. The long-term accuracy and stability of the current source is also a factor. Fortunately, the small dynamic resistance reduces the uncertainty due to small current uncertainties by a factor of 100 to 1000 (see the discussion with Eq. (4-3).

Current noise through a diode produces a shift in the temperature reading caused by the nonlinear current–voltage characteristic of the diode. A model developed by Krause and Dodrill [48] predicts the temperature shift for temperatures above the knee in the voltage–temperature characteristic. Changes in the conduction mechanism typically produce a knee in the 20- to 30-K region for silicon diodes, and no model is available for conduction behavior below the knee. The calculated relative temperature shift is plotted in Fig. 4-9 using a diode ideality factor of 1.8 and the temperature sensitivities of a Lake Shore model DT-470 silicon diode. The temperature shifts increase with decreasing temperature to a maximum at around 30 K and then decrease. The following equation can be used to estimate the relative temperature shift for similar diodes in the range $0 < V_{rms} < 40$ mV and $30 < T < 300$ K:

$$\Delta T/T \ [\%] = 277.68T \ [\text{K}]^{-2.11953} V_{rms}^{2.01803} \ [\text{mV}] \tag{4-7}$$

where the units are shown in brackets. The presence of significant voltage noise can be determined by connecting a 10-μF or larger capacitor across the diode. A low-leakage capacitor must be used to avoid shunting DC current from the diode. If the temperature reading decreases measurably, then significant noise is present. An AC voltmeter can also be used to check for the presence of AC noise.

Magnetic fields strongly affect silicon diodes. Although, GaAs or GaAlAs diodes can be used to higher fields, these devices are not interchangeable and must be calibrated individually.

4-2-4 Capacitors

Capacitors are sometimes used for temperature measurement, but the largest application is in temperature control in high magnetic fields. The capacitance is usually measured

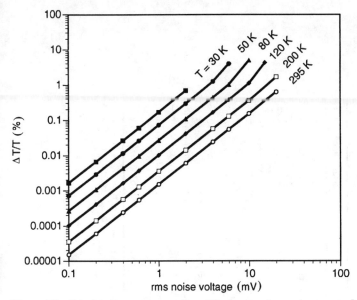

Figure 4-9 Calculated temperature reading shifts due to voltage noise across a Lake Shore Model DT-470 silicon diode temperature sensor.

with an AC capacitance bridge. Instrumentation for measuring capacitance is discussed in more detail in section 4-4-2. Some temperature controllers are designed to use a resistance temperature sensor to control temperature in zero magnetic field and then maintain the temperature in field with a capacitance sensor. The time response of capacitance sensors is usually limited by the physical size and low thermal diffusivity of the dielectric material.

Although $SrTiO_3$ capacitance temperature sensors are not detectably affected by magnetic fields, they commonly experience calibration shifts after thermal cycling and have been known to drift with time while at low temperatures [49,50]. Phase shifts in the ferroelectric materials are probably the cause of the thermal cycling shifts. Other commercially available capacitors have been investigated for use as cryogenic thermometers [51], but their use is not well established.

4-2-5 Thermocouples

Thermocouples are most useful where low-mass or differential temperature measurements are required. They must be calibrated in situ because the entire length of the wire contributes to the output voltage if it traverses a temperature gradient. Variations in wire composition, homogeneity, or even strain can affect the temperature readings. Many types of thermocouples are available for low-temperature use. Common types are copper versus constantan (Type T), nickel-10% chromium versus constantan (Type E), nickel-10% chromium versus nickel-5% aluminum and silicon (Type K), chromel versus Au–0.07% Fe, chromel versus Au–0.03% Fe, and chromel versus Cu–0.15% Fe. Polynomial fits for thermoelectric voltage versus temperature for several of these thermocouples are given in Table 4-13 [52,53]. Type E thermocouples are recommended for use in the

Table 4-13 Coefficients of reference equations giving the thermoelectric voltage, E, as a function of temperature

i	E	K	T	KP versus AuFe
0	2.731×10^2	2.7315×10^2	2.7315×10^2	2.7315×10^2
1	5.8665508708×10^1	3.9450128025×10^1	3.8748106364×10^1	$2.2272367466 \times 10^{-2}$
2	$4.5410977124 \times 10^{-2}$	$2.3622373598 \times 10^{-2}$	$4.4194434347 \times 10^{-2}$	$3.6406179664 \times 10^{-6}$
3	$-7.7998048686 \times 10^{-4}$	$-3.2858906784 \times 10^{-4}$	$1.1844323105 \times 10^{-4}$	$1.5967928202 \times 10^{-7}$
4	$-2.5800160843 \times 10^{-5}$	$-4.9904828777 \times 10^{-6}$	$2.0032973554 \times 10^{-5}$	$-4.5260169888 \times 10^{-9}$
5	$-5.9452583057 \times 10^{-7}$	$-6.7509059173 \times 10^{-8}$	$9.0138019559 \times 10^{-7}$	$4.0432555769 \times 10^{-11}$
6	$-9.3214058667 \times 10^{-9}$	$-5.7410327428 \times 10^{-10}$	$2.2651156593 \times 10^{-8}$	$4.9063035765 \times 10^{-12}$
7	$-1.0287605534 \times 10^{-10}$	$-3.1088872894 \times 10^{-12}$	$3.6071154205 \times 10^{-10}$	$1.2272348484 \times 10^{-13}$
8	$-8.0370123621 \times 10^{-13}$	$-1.0451609365 \times 10^{-14}$	$3.8493939883 \times 10^{-12}$	$1.6829773697 \times 10^{-15}$
9	$-4.3979497391 \times 10^{-15}$	$-1.9889266878 \times 10^{-17}$	$2.8213521925 \times 10^{-14}$	$1.4636450149 \times 10^{-17}$
10	$-1.6414776355 \times 10^{-17}$	$-1.6322697486 \times 10^{-20}$	$1.4251594779 \times 10^{-16}$	$8.4287909747 \times 10^{-20}$
11	$-3.9673619516 \times 10^{-20}$	—	$4.8768662286 \times 10^{-19}$	$3.2146639387 \times 10^{-22}$
12	$-5.5827328721 \times 10^{-23}$	—	$-1.0795539270 \times 10^{-21}$	$7.8225430483 \times 10^{-25}$
13	$-3.4657842013 \times 10^{-26}$	—	$1.3945027062 \times 10^{-24}$	$1.1010930596 \times 10^{-27}$
14			$7.9795153927 \times 10^{-28}$	$6.8263661580 \times 10^{-31}$

Note: The equations are of the form $E\ [\mu V] = \Sigma[C_i \cdot T^i]$ where the sum is over $i = 0$ to n terms; the temperature is in kelvins on the ITS-90 scale (set $C_0 = 0.0$ for temperatures in degrees Celsius); and the coefficients C_i are given in the table. AuFe refers to Au-0.07 at % Fe. The ranges of the fits are 3.15 to 273.15 K for E, K, T, and 0.15 to 280.15 K for AuFe.

temperature range from 3 to 1144 K in oxidizing or inert atmospheres. Aluminum–iron thermocouples are most commonly used for measurements below 10 K.

All but types E and K have one leg of a high-thermal-conductivity material, requiring small wire diameters, small temperature gradients, or heat sinking to prevent the measurement from being affected by heat conducted along the wire. The requirement for a reference junction is another disadvantage for many cryogenic temperature measurements.

Thermocouples are very difficult to use as low-temperature thermometers in the presence of magnetic fields because the thermoelectric power depends on both the temperature and magnetic field. Zero magnetic field effect is possible if the portion of the thermocouple exposed to magnetic field is isothermal, but this is difficult to achieve in practice. Type E thermocouples have a reproducible and relatively small magnetic field dependence but only marginal temperature sensitivity below 10 K.

4-2-6 Self-Heating of Temperature Sensors

Any difference between the temperature of the sensor and the environment the sensor is intended to measure produces a temperature measurement error or uncertainty. Dissipation of power in the temperature sensor will cause its temperature to rise above that of the surrounding environment. Power dissipation in the sensor is also necessary to make a temperature measurement. Minimization of the temperature measurement uncertainty thus requires balancing the uncertainties due to self-heating and output signal measurement.

Attempting to correct for self-heating errors by calculation or extrapolation is not considered good practice. An estimate of the self-heating error should be included in the total uncertainty calculation instead.

The following are two approaches to dealing with the problem of self-heating:

1. Choose an excitation that allows acceptable instrumentation measurement uncertainty and check to make sure self-heating is negligible at one or two points where it is likely to be most significant.

An easy way to check for self-heating is to increase the power dissipation and check for an indicated temperature rise. Unfortunately, this procedure will not work with nonlinear devices such as semiconductor diodes. An indication of the self-heating error can be made by reading the diode temperature in both a liquid bath and in a vacuum at the same temperature, as measured by a second thermometer not dissipating enough power to self-heat significantly.

2. Measure the thermal resistance in the temperature range of interest and calculate the optimum operating point.

Examination of Eq. (4-2) leads to the conclusion that an increase in the sensor output voltage will result in a decreasing temperature uncertainty, as long as the voltage uncertainty remains constant. This is possible with an ohmic sensor by increasing the excitation current. Unfortunately, a larger excitation will dissipate more power in the temperature sensor, raising its temperature above the surroundings.

The self-heating depends on the excitation power according to the equation

$$\Delta T_{sh} = P_s R_t = I^2 R_e R_t = V^2 R_t / R_e \qquad (4\text{-}8)$$

where ΔT_{sh} is the temperature rise due to self-heating, P_s is the power dissipated in the sensor, I is the excitation current, R_e is the electrical resistance, and R_t is the thermal resistance between the sensor and its environment. The thermal resistance is extremely difficult to calculate for all but the simplest cases and is best determined experimentally using the following procedure:

1. Mount the sensor as it will be used on a temperature-controlled block or directly in liquid.
2. Record the output voltage as a function of excitation current (I–V curve) until significant self-heating is observed (when $R_e = V/I$ is no longer constant).
3. Replot the data as sensor temperature reading versus power dissipated (T versus P).
4. Fit the data with a linear equation of the form $T = T_o + R_t P_s$ to find the thermal resistance, R_t.

Thermal resistance values determined from some commercial resistance temperature sensors in common mounting configurations are shown as a function of temperature in Fig. 4-10. The thermal resistance varies with the environment in and around the sensor package (vacuum, gas, liquid), sensor mounting (solder, grease, clamp pressure, epoxy, etc.), and details of sensor construction. The thermal resistances shown in the figure should be used only as a guide with reference to the source papers [47,54] and

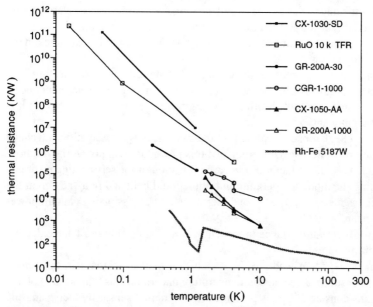

Figure 4-10 Thermal resistances for some cryogenic temperature sensors in typical mounting configurations. Models and manufacturers: CGR: carbon–glass resistor, Lake Shore; CX: Cernox, Lake Shore; GR: germanium resistor, Lake Shore; Rh–Fe: standards grade Rh-0.5 at % Fe, Tinsley; RuO: ruthenium oxide thin-film resistor, Siegert Elektronik.

preferably measurement on the actual sensor in the temperature range and environment of use.

The optimum operating point minimizes the combined temperature measurement uncertainty due to instrumentation and self-heating. The optimum is determined by (1) writing the instrument uncertainty (Eq. (4-2)) and the self-heating (Eq. (4-8)) in terms of sensor power, (2) including these two terms on the right-hand side of Eq. (4-1), (3) differentiating with respect to sensor power, (4) setting the result equal to zero, and (5) solving for the sensor power. The resulting expression for the optimum sensor power is

$$P_{s\,opt} = I^2 R_e = \frac{V^2}{R_e} = \frac{T(u_V/V)}{S_T R_t \sqrt{2}} + \left(\frac{u_V T}{S_T R_t \sqrt{2R_e}}\right)^{2/3} \tag{4-9}$$

where the first term on the right is for instrument uncertainties expressed as a fraction of sensor output signal and the second term on the right is for instrument uncertainties expressed in volts. Note that other experimental considerations might impose more stringent limitations on the power that can be dissipated in the temperature sensor.

As an example, consider a Cernox model CX-1050-SD temperature sensor attached to a copper block operating at 1.6 K and surrounded by vacuum. The voltmeter to be used to make the measurement is a Keithley Instruments Model 2000 with a one-year DC voltage accuracy specification of $\pm(50\ \text{ppm} + 3.5\ \mu\text{V})$. The sensor electrical resistance $R_e = 46,240\ \Omega$ and dimensionless sensitivity $S_T = 2.21$ are interpolated from Table 4-7 assuming linear relationships between $\log(R_e)$ or $\log|S_T|$ and $\log(T)$. The thermal resistance $R_t = 150,000\ \text{K/W}$ from Ref. [54] is about twice that of the CX-1050-AA model shown in Fig. 4-10. From the voltmeter accuracy specification, $u_{Vvm}/V = 50\ \text{ppm} = 5 \times 10^{-5}$ with an additional voltage uncertainty $u_V = 3.5\ \mu\text{V}$. The following values can be calculated:

$$P_{s\,opt} = \frac{(1.6\,\text{K})(5 \times 10^{-5})}{(2.21)(1.5 \times 10^5\ \text{K/W})\sqrt{2}} + \left[\frac{(3.5 \times 10^{-6}\ \text{V})(1.6\,\text{K})}{(2.21)(1.5 \times 10^5\ \text{K/W})\sqrt{2(46,240\,\Omega)}}\right]^{2/3}$$

$$= (0.17 + 1.46) \times 10^{-9}\ \text{W} = 1.63\ \text{nW}$$

$$I = \sqrt{\frac{P_{s\,opt}}{R_e}} = \sqrt{\frac{1.63 \times 10^{-9}\ \text{W}}{46,240\,\Omega}} = 1.9 \times 10^{-7}\text{A} = 0.19\ \mu\text{A}$$

$$V = I R_e = (1.9 \times 10^{-7}\text{A})(46,240\,\Omega) = 8.78 \times 10^{-3}\ \text{V} = 8.78\ \text{mV}$$

$$u_{T_{sh}} = \Delta T_{sh} = P_s R_t = (1.63 \times 10^{-9}\ \text{W})(1.5 \times 10^5\ \text{K/W}) = 245\ \mu\text{K}$$

$$u_{T_{vm}} = \left(\frac{T}{S_T}\right)\left(\frac{u_{Vvm}}{V}\right) = \left(\frac{1.6\,\text{K}}{2.21}\right)\left(5 \times 10^{-5} + \frac{3.5 \times 10^{-6}\ \text{V}}{8.78 \times 10^{-3}\ \text{V}}\right) = 325\ \mu\text{K}$$

$$u_T = \sqrt{u_{T_{sh}}^2 + u_{T_{vm}}^2} = \sqrt{(245\ \mu\text{K})^2 + (325\ \mu\text{K})^2} = 407\ \mu\text{K}$$

$$\frac{u_T}{T} = \frac{407\ \mu\text{K}}{1.6\,\text{K}} = 2.54 \times 10^{-4} = 254\ \text{ppm}$$

where $u_{T_{sh}}$ and $u_{T_{vm}}$ are the temperature measurement uncertainties due to self-heating and voltage measurement. Note that this combined uncertainty, u_T, does not contain all

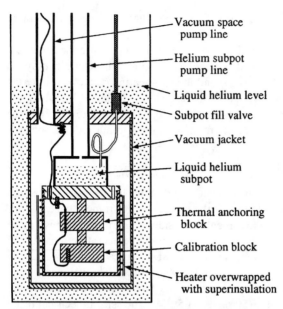

- Vacuum space pump line
- Helium subpot pump line
- Liquid helium level
- Subpot fill valve
- Vacuum jacket
- Liquid helium subpot
- Thermal anchoring block
- Calibration block
- Heater overwrapped with superinsulation

Figure 4-11 Temperature sensor calibration cryostat.

contributions to the total uncertainty. The optimal sensor excitation of nearly 9 mV is well above the 1–3 mV range conservatively recommended for this resistance sensor. Excitation of this sensor at 2 mV yields a combined relative uncertainty of 815 ppm, which is significantly worse than the optimum.

4-2-7 Temperature Sensor Calibration

Calibration cryostats and facilities are described by several authors [42,55,56,57,58]. Figure 4-11 shows a typical cryostat designed for temperature sensor calibrations in the 1.2- to 350-K range. The temperature sensors are calibrated against standard units mounted on the same temperature-controlled block.

4-3 STRAIN MEASUREMENT

Most measurements of strain are performed with bonded resistance strain gauges whose relative resistance changes according to the formula

$$\Delta R/R = F_s(\Delta L/L)$$

where F_s is the gauge factor or strain sensitivity factor and $\Delta L/L$ is the strain. Typical gauge factors are about 2 for most of the commonly used metallic alloys and up to 100 or more for semiconductors. Unfortunately, semiconductors are too strongly temperature-dependent for use at all but the highest and most stable cryogenic temperatures. The most common materials for cryogenic strain measurements are pure or modified nickel–chromium (Karma) alloys. The copper–nickel alloy most commonly used around 300 K has larger temperature and magnetic field effects and is seldom used for cryogenic temperatures. Typical resistances are 120 or 350 Ω, and the resistance change is linear with up to 1.5% strain at cryogenic temperatures.

Kelvin or Mueller resistance bridges are normally used to detect the small resistance changes in metal strain gauges while fully compensating for the lead resistances. Temperature also affects the strain gauge resistance through (1) temperature dependence of the gauge factor, (2) temperature dependence of the resistance, and (3) strains induced by differential thermal contractions between the gauge and the specimen. The gauge factor varies nearly linearly with temperature and is about 4–5% higher at 4 K than at 297 K for modified Ni–Cr gauges [59]. The resistance of a strain gauge typically decreases by 5% or less between ambient temperature and 4 K. Strains caused by differential thermal contractions can be lessened by heat treating the gauge alloy to more nearly match the substrate material properties. Look for a gauge matched to a material as similar as possible to the sample. These last two temperature effects represent a zero offset and are commonly combined into one apparent strain. Pavese [60] measured the apparent strain caused by differential thermal contraction between a variety of strain gauge and substrate material combinations (see Fig. 4-12). The curves are normalized at 280 K. The effect is seen to be significant even with the modified Ni–Cr gauges.

One way to compensate the apparent strain or thermal zero shift is to mount two gauges in the cryogenic environment with one active gauge at the strained location and the second in an unstrained location otherwise identical. The two gauges form one-half of a resistance bridge with the other half at ambient temperature.

Magnetic fields increase the gauge resistance, especially at very low temperatures, producing a strain error. For the nickel–chromium alloy, a strain error of $+160\,\mu\text{m/m}$ was found at 4.2 K in a magnetic field of 6 T, and the error increased approximately as the square of the field [61]. No magnetoresistance effect was detected at 77 or at 296 K with this alloy.

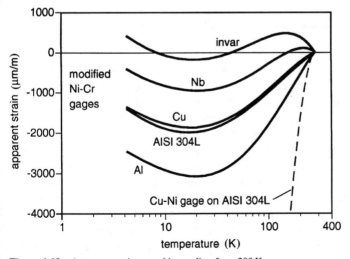

Figure 4-12 Apparent strain caused by cooling from 280 K.

Additional sources of information include the excellent book by Hannah and Reed [62] and, less extensive but specific to cryogenic applications, the chapter by Sparks [16].

4-4 PRESSURE MEASUREMENT

Pressure sensors for cryogenic applications are not nearly as well developed as temperature sensors. The reason is that the cryogenic pressure market is small, and therefore very few pressure sensors are actually designed for cryogenic applications. Construction details can strongly affect the performance of pressure sensors at cryogenic temperatures. All of the pressure sensors used at cryogenic temperatures require individual calibration—none are interchangeable.

The easiest method to measure pressure in a cryogenic environment can be connection by capillary tube to a pressure sensor at room temperature. Disadvantages of capillary tubes connected to room-temperature pressure sensors include the following:

1. Added complexity of the mechanical design and increased possibility of leaks.
2. Low frequency response of the capillary tube limits measurements to static or slowly varying pressures.
3. The thermomolecular pressure effect causes the pressure at the warm end of the capillary to be larger than at the cold end [58,63]. The correction for this effect becomes very significant below about 130 Pa.
4. Temperature gradients in capillary tubes can cause thermoacoustic oscillations in pressure [64,65]. The magnitude of the oscillations can exceed the pressure being measured. This is especially a problem with helium. Design to eliminate thermoacoustic oscillations further reduces the ability of the system to measure dynamically changing pressures. More information on thermoacoustic oscillations may be found in chapter 9 of this handbook.

Pressure sensors are made with absolute, differential, and gauge connection ports as follows:

1. An absolute port consists of one port connected to the pressure of interest. A pressure reference cavity is built into the sensor. A vacuum reference should be used for cryogenic measurements, or the reference pressure will change with temperature, especially if the reference atmosphere condenses and freezes.
2. A differential port consists of two ports connected to two pressure sources. Common applications include venturi flowmeters or measurement of pressure drops due to flows through piping. Differential ports are typically capable of measuring small pressure differences. Be careful to allow for the full range of pressure differentials to be encountered during cooldown and operation. These ports can be used to connect to a vacuum reference, if available.
3. A gauge port consists of one port connected to the pressure of interest. A hole in the pressure sensor body allows measurement of pressure relative to the ambient.

Discussions of specific types of pressure sensors follow.

4-4-1 Piezoresistive or Strain Gauge Pressure Sensors

A piezoresistive pressure sensor consists of strain-sensitive resistors (piezoresistors) on a diaphragm separating two pressure chambers. A pressure difference between the chambers causes the diaphragm to deflect, straining the piezoresistors and causing their resistance to change. Typically, four piezoresistors are arranged in a bridge. The output usually has a small zero offset at zero pressure differential and then rises nearly linearly with pressure.

$$V_{\text{out}} = V_0 + V_s (P/P_{\text{FS}}) = a\,I + b\,I\,P \qquad (4\text{-}10)$$

where V_0 is the zero offset voltage equal to a times the excitation current; V_s is the voltage span between zero pressure and P_{FS}, the full scale pressure; and b is the output voltage sensitivity to pressure and excitation current. Constant voltage excitation is commonly used with pressure sensors at room temperature, but large changes in sensor impedance and the need for high-resistance lead wires into a cryogenic environment usually make constant current excitation more reliable for cryogenic sensors. The calculated relative pressure measurement resolution for a representative pressure sensor is given in Fig. 4-13. Note that $100\,\mu\text{A}$ and 1 mA excitation currents yield the same resolution above 60 kPa. This is because the larger excitation produces an output signal large enough to cause the voltmeter to change to a less sensitive range.

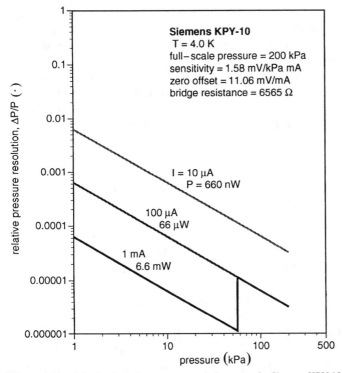

Figure 4-13 Calculated relative pressure resolution example. Siemens KPY-10 pressure sensor measured by a Keithley 2000 DVM with ranges of 0.1, 1, 10, 100, and 1000 V and 6-digit resolution (0.1 μV minimum).

Typical diaphragm materials include metal foils, sapphire, and silicon. Metal foil diaphragms have the greatest hysteresis but allow all-welded construction from compatible materials. The piezoresistors are deposited thin-film or bonded-metal-foil strain gauges. Sapphire diaphragms have low hysteresis but are difficult to make thin or seal to the package. They are most commonly found in high-pressure sensors. Silicon is an increasingly popular choice because silicon processing technology is well developed and silicon diaphragms are nearly hysteresis free. Miniature silicon pressure sensors can be made in small sizes, on the order of 1 mm^3, including an internal vacuum reference cavity. Small silicon diaphragms also have very high frequency responses. The excitation power is generated in a small region on the thin diaphragm, which can lead to problems at low temperatures or when the sensor is used to measure rapidly changing pressures of a gas [66].

Construction details can strongly affect the performance of pressure sensors at cryogenic temperatures. Commercial piezoresistive pressure sensors are often unsuitable for cryogenic applications for the following reasons:

1. The resistors frequently are made from a lightly doped semiconductor material that becomes too resistive at low temperatures. An ideal resistor material would have no temperature dependence or slightly metallic behavior so that the resistance would drop slightly with temperature and then remain constant.
2. Silicone sealant frequently is used as a protective coating or to attach the sensor chip to the package. The silicone contracts greatly on cooling, and the resulting pressure on the sensor element can distort the pressure reading or even damage the sensor. Protective silicone coatings also harden and screen the sensor from pressure changes in the fluid whose pressure is to be measured.
3. Seals to the silicon chip can break on thermal cycling or can be permeable to cryogenic gases such as helium. Epoxy or glass seals can be especially fragile. Some silicon chips are electrostatically bonded to a glass backing to reference cavities for absolute sensors. The glass backing might be permeable to helium gas, which could change the pressure in the reference cavity.
4. Compensation and linearization circuitry built into the package frequently does not work at cryogenic temperatures.
5. The reference cavity is filled with a gas, and thus the reference pressure changes with temperature.

Properties of some pressure sensors known to work at cryogenic temperatures are listed in Table 4-14. Siemens Model KPY pressure sensors were not designed for cryogenic applications but have been popular owing to their low cost and good operating characteristics. On the order of 20% fail during initial cooldown, but those that survive can be temperature-cycled repeatedly. The package style used for the older KPY-10 and -12 models is best for cryogenic use. Unfortunately, these models have been discontinued in favor of a new package-43 in which the silicon chip is mounted to the end of a long Kovar tube. Almost any plastic straining of the Kovar tube seems to shift the sensor calibration permanently. The characteristics of a KPY-10 sensor are shown in Fig. 4-14. These characteristics are very similar to those reported for the PSI sensor [67].

Table 4-14 Properties of some commercially available cryogenic pressure sensors

Type[a]	Manufacturer	Model	P range FS [kPa]	Style[b]	T range [K]	Excitation	Span [mV]	Linearity and hysteresis	Mass [g]	Cost [$]
BSG	Precise Sensors	111-3	1400 to 105 000	A	77–422	10 Vdc, 286 mW	20	±0.5%	170	770
BSG	Sensotec	Cryo Series	170 to 70 000	A, D	77–300[c]	10 Vdc, 286 mW	10–30	±0.25%	370	485
PE	Kistler	601B1	1000 to 100 000	Y	6–533	[d]	[d]	±1%	7	400
PE	PCB Piezotronics	102A	700 to 70 000	Y	20–373	2mA	5000	1%	11	660
PR Si	Endevco	8510B/C	7 to 14 000	D	219–394[c]	10 Vdc, 37 mW	300/220	±0.25%	2.3	610
PR Si	Endevco	8515C	100 to 34 000	A	219–394[c]	10 Vdc, 37 mW	200	±0.2%	0.08	590
PR Si	Kulite	CCQ-093	700 to 3500	A, D	77–393	10 Vdc, 125 mW	100	±0.1%	0.4	510
PR Si	Kulite	CT-190	350 to 14 000	A, D	77–393	10 Vdc, 125 mW	100	±0.1%	4	650
PR Si	Kulite	CT-375	350 to 14 000	A, D	77–393	10 Vdc, 125 mW	100	±0.1%	25	680
PR Si	Pressure Systems	4100,4200	7–3500	D, A	1.5–400	1 mA, 6 mW	150–350	±0.5%	75	695
PR Si	Siemens[e]	KPY-10,12	200	A, D	1.4–400	500 μA,1.5 mW	51	±0.7%	3	25
PR Si	Siemens[e]	KPY-14,16	1000	A, D	1.4–400	500 μA,1.5 mW	120	±0.7%	3	25
PR Si	Siemens	KPY-32R, 33R	5,10	D	1.4–400	500 μA,1.5 mW	21,24	±1.0%	5	25
PR Si	Siemens	KPY-43A, R	160	A, D	1.4–400	500 μA,1.5 mW	42	±0.4%	5	25
PR Si	Siemens	KPY-47A, R	6000	A, D	1.4–400	500 μA, 1.5 mW	120	±0.4%	5	25
PR Si	Toyoda Machine	PD116S	3000	G	4–300	100 μA, 8.5 μW	2	±2%		
PR ss	Omegadyne	PX1005	100 to 70 000	A	113–422[c]	10 Vdc, 250 mW	30	±0.25%	145	1500
PR SOS	Sensotron	SEN-202B-30	202	A	4–300	1 mA, 4.6 mW	15	±0.25%	170	225
VR	Validyne	DP10	0.5 to 22 000	D	1.4–390	5 Vac, 3 kHz	150	±0.7%	330	640

Note: Specifications are for operation at 298 K.

[a] BSG = bonded strain gage; PE = piezoelectric (dynamic pressure); PR Si = peizoresistive, Si diaphragm; PR ss = piezoresistive, stainless steel diaphragm; SOS = silicon on sapphire; VR = variable reluctance.

[b] A: absolute, D: differential, G: gauge, Y: dynamic.

[c] Operation possible at lower temperatures.

[d] Requires a charge amplifier for voltage output; prices vary from $400 to $1200.

[e] No longer in production.

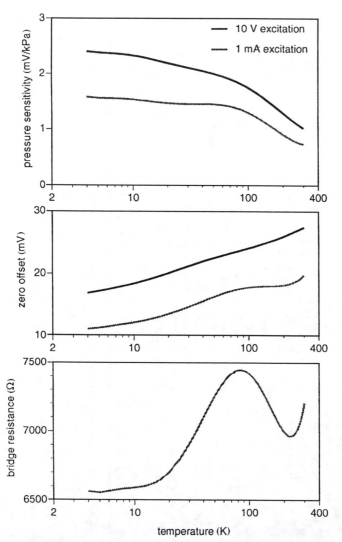

Figure 4-14 Characteristics of a Siemens KPY-10 pressure sensor (200 kPa absolute) as a function of temperature.

The Toyoda Model PD116S was tested in magnetic fields up to 8 T in the 6 to 41 K temperature range [68]. The pressure sensitivity changed by less than 1.5%, and the zero offset changed by less than 1% of full-scale output. Unfortunately, the packaging contains ferromagnetic Kovar metal, which will disturb the magnetic flux density nearby.

A multichannel differential pressure measurement module has been built from bare, piezoresistive pressure sensor die made by Omegadyne. The pressure sensor were tested over the range 77 to 273 K and -101 to $+241$ KPa [15]. A boron dopant density on the order of 10^{20} cm^{-3} in the silicon piezoresistors is described as one requirement for operation below 170 K.

4-4-2 Capacitance Pressure Sensors

A capacitance pressure sensor consists of two or more electrodes, one being a thin diaphragm that deforms under pressure, changing the gap between the electrodes and thus the capacitance. Several types have been built and used at cryogenic temperatures [69–72], but none are commercially available. A well-constructed capacitance pressure sensor has less than a 5% change in sensitivity when cooled from 300 to 4 K. The capacitance of these sensors is typically in the range of 20 to 50 pF. The change in capacitance is nonlinear with pressure, rising more rapidly as the electrodes come together.

The most common method for measuring the capacitance change is with a capacitance bridge. A three-lead bridge should be used to eliminate the effects of temperature-dependent lead capacitance. Coaxial leads are required, but the bridge operates at only a few kilohertz, and thus high-frequency performance is not required. The second common method of measuring capacitance changes is by incorporating the capacitor in a resonant circuit. A tunnel diode oscillator and inductor must be located very near the capacitor. Only one coaxial lead enters the cryogenic environment, but the lead must carry signals in the 10 to 100 MHz range. Resolutions of 1 part in 10^8 have been achieved with some capacitance pressure sensors, although 1 part in 10^5 would be more common without expensive electronics.

Capacitance sensors can be sensitive to impurity gases such as water vapor if they freeze to the diaphragm and change the capacitance.

4-4-3 Variable Reluctance Pressure Sensors

A variable reluctance sensor detects the position of a magnetically permeable diaphragm using induction coils on either side of the diaphragm. The two coils form one-half of a bridge circuit typically excited with an AC signal of 3 to 5 kHz. The power dissipated in the sensor is quite small, usually being on the order of 1 mW at temperatures of 77 K and below with conventional electronics and 5-V excitation.

Commercial variable reluctance pressure sensors with all-welded construction should be used for cryogenic use. Differential models with pressure ranges up to about 100 kPa have been found to remain linear at cryogenic temperatures [10]. The sensitivities decreased by about 13% from 300 to 77 K but then remained unchanged down to 4 K. Their size and mass are relatively large, but they are rugged and have been qualified for space applications [73]. Overpressurization had little effect on sensitivity. Linearity and repeatability of the sensors were within 1% after a few temperature cycles. Large deviations from linearity at 4 K have been observed in high-pressure models (5 MPa).

4-4-4 Piezoelectric Pressure Sensors

Dynamic (changing) pressures can be measured with some commercial piezoelectric pressure sensors. The pressure sensor is designed to strain the piezoelectric element, which generates a quantity of charge Δq proportional to the strain. No electrical power is required to generate the signal. The piezoelectric element has a capacitance C, and thus a voltage change $\Delta V = \Delta q / C$ is produced. Either the charge or the voltage can be amplified. The amplification circuit requires power. Location of the amplification circuit in the cryogenic region requires only a twisted pair of wires (two conductors), which can have moderate resistance to reduce the heat leak down the wires. Location of the amplification circuit at room temperature requires a low-noise coaxial cable with high resistance (10^{14} Ω) between the conductors to avoid shunting of the charge to the ground.

The output from piezoelectric pressure sensors is very linear with pressure. Typically, a single sensor can be used for dynamic pressure measurements from 100 kPa to 1 GPa with the pressure sensitivity over different ranges varying by less than 0.5%. The offset voltage and amplifier gain can be varied to optimize the output for a dynamic pressure range about a given static pressure.

4-5 FLOW MEASUREMENT

Many types of flowmeters have been used successfully at cryogenic temperatures. Several are commercially available, with some having been designed specifically for cryogenic applications.

Flowmeters typically measure either mass flow or volumetric flow. Conversion between the two requires measurement or knowledge of the fluid density. Mass flowmeters include the following types: angular momentum, Coriolis or gyroscopic, heat transfer rate, thermal or calorimetric, and dual turbine. Volumetric flowmeters include the following types: Doppler shift, fluidic, laminar flow, positive displacement, temperature pulse, turbine, vortex shedding, and weir.

Differential pressure flowmeters such as orifice plates or venturi flowmeters are not strictly mass or volumetric flowmeters because the square root of the density must be provided for either measurement. The advantages in reliability and lack of moving parts still make these among the most commonly used flowmeters.

Common considerations for cryogenic flowmeters include the following: (1) flow range or turndown ratio; (2) compatibility with the cryogen; (3) disruption of the flow; (4) heat load; (5) reliability, maintenance frequency, and ability to replace or repair the flowmeter; and (6) cost and availability.

Detailed descriptions of many types of flowmeters used in cryogenic service are given by Alspach et al. [74], Brennan et al. [75], Brennan and Takano [76], and Rivetti et al. [77]. Flowmeters specifically for use in He II have been reviewed by Van Sciver et al. [78] and in chapter 10 of this handbook.

4-5-1 Mass Flowmeters

Angular momentum flowmeters. Angular momentum flowmeters have a rotating member with vanes oriented parallel to the axis. The rotating member is driven by an electric motor through a constant-torque clutch (hysteresis drive). The liquid enters the meter through a flow straightener and passes the rotating vanes. The liquid tends to retard the rotational speed of the rotor by an amount inversely proportional to the mass-flow rate. Rotor speed is sensed by a magnetic pickup, and the resulting signal is treated electronically to indicate mass-flow rate. A flow range of 8 to 1 is typical with these meters. Maximum flow rates may vary from about 2 to 15 kg/s. Pressure drops of

20 to 50 kPa are typical at maximum flow. They have been tested with liquid hydrogen by Alspach et al. [25] and with liquid oxygen, nitrogen, and argon by Brennan et al. [26]. Flowmeters of this type are often used as custody transfer flowmeters on delivery vehicles. Uncertainties of ±2% or less are typical.

Heat transfer rate flowmeters. Heat transfer rate flowmeters are also called hot wire, hot film, or constant-temperature anemometers. A temperature-sensitive heater element is driven by feedback electronics to maintain the heater at a constant resistance automatically (temperature) as the flow rate varies [79]. The flow rate must be calibrated against the power dissipation using a standard flowmeter at ambient temperature. The heat transfer rate flowmeter is a true mass flowmeter for an ideal gas. Commercial hot wire anemometer probes have been used successfully for the measurement of helium gas flows at temperatures down to 77 K [80,81]. The calibration was found to change in a linear manner with, but not as a strong function of, the gas temperature. The probes were fabricated with a 3.8-μm-diameter tungsten wire about 2 mm long attached to the wire supports. The wire was heated to about 297 K to give high sensitivity and reproducible results. Because the power input with this high wire temperature was about 1 W, the hot wire anemometer was turned on only briefly when measurements were being made. The response time of the wire was measured to be less than 15 μs in zero flow. The response time becomes faster with increasing flow. The fast response time makes the hot wire anemometer useful for measuring turbulence, transient flow, or oscillating flow. Oscillating mass flow rates up to 30 Hz were measured in compressed helium gas at temperatures down to 77 K within a pulse tube refrigerator. The fine wire is somewhat fragile and can only be used in very clean gas flows.

Thermal or calorimetric flowmeters. Thermal or calorimetric flowmeters heat the flowing fluid with a constant power $\dot{Q}$, causing its temperature to rise by an amount ΔT. A thermocouple or thermopile measures this temperature difference between the fluid upstream and downstream from the heater. The mass flow rate is given by

$$\dot{m} = \frac{\dot{Q}}{C_p \Delta T} \tag{4-11}$$

where C_p is the specific heat of the fluid. This flowmeter is a true mass flowmeter. A commercial thermal flowmeter was used by Bugeat et al. [82] to measure mass flow rates around 10 mg/s of hydrogen and helium gas at temperatures between 100 and 300 K. They reported a nonlinearity of less than 2% and a response time of about 0.22 s at 158 K in hydrogen gas for a flow of 9 mg/s. Thermal flowmeters should work with flow in either direction.

4-5-2 Volumetric Flowmeters

Doppler shift flowmeters. Doppler shift flowmeters work by measuring the change in transit time of waves traveling with or against the flow. Waves of pressure, temperature (second sound in He II), and light have been used. When the speed of sound is temperature-dependent, measurements of the transit time both with and against the flow can be combined to eliminate the sound velocity. Ultrasonic flowmeters have been built by Lavocat [83] and by Hofmann and Vogeley [84]. Borner and coworkers [85] used the Doppler effect on both first and second sound in helium II to measure the circulation and flow velocities produced by a macroscopic vortex ring in He II. The signal processing required to determine a fluid velocity from a propagating sound pulse can be relatively complex. Laser Doppler velocimetry works by tracking neutral density particles suspended in the flow [86]. Laser beams can be focused to measure the velocity in a small region (≈ 1 mm^3). Disadvantages include the sophisticated and expensive equipment required and the need to introduce reflective particles.

Fluidic flowmeters. Fluidic flowmeters use hydrodynamic instabilities to generate oscillations in a flow stream, which are then detected. The oscillation frequency is proportional to fluid velocity in the turbulent flow regime. The amplitude of the oscillating pressure signal is also generally proportional to flow velocity, and thus use over a fairly wide range is possible. The major disadvantage is the large pressure drop compared with other devices. Operation of a Coanda-effect fluidic flowmeter made by Moore Products has been verified in liquid helium [78].

Positive displacement flowmeters. Positive displacement flowmeters work on the principle that the flowing liquid must displace or be displaced by some mechanical element. The volume flow is proportional to the movement of the mechanical element. Types of mechanical elements include pistons, rotating vanes, and gears. A detailed description of these various types of positive displacement flowmeters and an evaluation of them for cryogenic service is given by Brennan et al. [87]. These flowmeters are generally used with moderate flow rates (1 to 10 L/s) and are capable of being operated over a 5-to-1 flow range. A pressure drop of about 30 kPa is typical with these meters at maximum flow. With care, an uncertainty of $\pm 1\%$ is possible. Subcooling the liquid below the saturation curve is important to prevent the formation of vapor in the flowmeter. A disadvantage of positive displacement flowmeters is that they are subject to wear and must be recalibrated periodically.

Temperature pulse flowmeters. Temperature pulse flowmeters measure the transit time of a thermal disturbance within a moving fluid. The technique will not work if thermal diffusion or turbulence spreads the temperature pulse before it can travel to measurement locations. Circuitry is required to detect arrival of the thermal pulses. The transit time of a heat pulse can be determined more accurately using cross- or autocorrelation techniques [88,89], but many readings must be stored in a computer and manipulated to maximize the correlation function. The heat input can also disturb the fluid, especially in a fluid like He II with high thermal conductivity where large heat inputs are required.

Turbine flowmeters. Turbine flowmeters consist of a freely rotating bladed rotor supported by bearings inside a housing. An electrical transducer senses rotor speed, which is a direct function of flow velocity. Turbine flowmeters are used mostly for liquid flows and have a useful range of at least 10 to 1. Calibrations with liquid cryogens may differ from water calibrations by up to $\pm 2\%$ [90]. They are susceptible to errors caused by upstream swirl, and therefore some means of flow straightening is usually required for accurate measurements. An evaluation of several cryogenic turbine flowmeters was reported by Brennan et al. [91]. They ranged in size from 32 to 51 mm with maximum flow rates between 5 and 14 L/s. Maximum pressure drops ranged from 20 to 100 kPa. Flow measurement uncertainties were generally less than ±1%. A commercial turbine flowmeter with ball bearings and a bore diameter of 9.35 mm has even been used for measuring flow in normal and superfluid helium with flow rates between 0.01 and 0.3 L/s [92]. The meter output was about 0.5% higher for superfluid helium compared with normal helium. Avoidance of cavitation is important in superfluid helium. Kashani [93] used a Model MF20 Sponsler turbine flowmeter in He II, although it did not register a reading for low flows, a common problem with turbine flowmeters. A custom-made turbine flowmeter with magnetic bearings has also been used for liquid helium flow by Rivetti et al. [94]. Short-term repeatability of ±0.5% was reported for the magnetic-bearing flowmeter. Turbine flowmeters require low bearing friction for successful operation. To ensure this, the liquid must be free of solid particles such as frozen air or water. An upstream filter is often used. Like other flowmeters with moving parts, turbine flowmeters have a limited lifetime. Jewel bearings should be qualified for cryogenic service by dunking in liquid nitrogen—those with internal stresses or severe defects will fail under the thermal shock. Other models use austenitic stainless steel ball bearings. Turbine flowmeter response times in the range of 1 to 10 ms have been reported by Alspach and Flynn [90], depending on blade angle, flowmeter size, and flow rate. These authors also reported the successful use of turbine meters in reverse flow, allowing them to be used in oscillating flows with frequencies less than about 1 to 10 Hz.

4-5-3 Differential Pressure Flowmeters

The differential pressure flowmeter can be used with either gas or liquid flows. They operate on the principle that the pressure drop across some flow element is a function of the flow rate. These meters can be used at cryogenic temperatures if the pressure sensor is located at ambient temperature or if a cryogenic pressure sensor is used. They have no moving parts and can be highly reliable.

Orifice plate flowmeters. The most common type of flow element is the sharp-edged orifice plate. Usually the orifice plate is designed for flow in one direction with the sharp edge of the orifice on the entrance side. Symmetric orifice plates have been used by Radebaugh and Rawlins to measure oscillating flows [81].

The relation between the mass flow rate and the pressure drop ΔP across the orifice is given by

$$\dot{m} = C_0 A_0 [2\rho \, \Delta P / (1 - \beta^4)]^{1/2} \tag{4-12}$$

where C_0 is the orifice or discharge coefficient (≈ 0.6), A_0 is the cross sectional area of the orifice, ρ is the fluid density and β is the ratio of the orifice diameter to the tube inside diameter. Because the mass flow is proportional to the square root of ΔP, a range of 10 in ΔP yields a range of only 3 in mass flow. The resulting small range of operation is a disadvantage of the orifice meter. The orifice coefficient determined from a water calibration can be used for most liquid cryogens with ±2% uncertainty

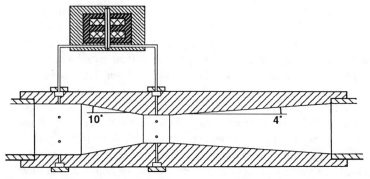

Figure 4-15 Venturi flowmeter diagram showing a variable reluctance pressure sensor connected across the differential pressure ports.

according to Brennan et al. [75]. The uncertainty for use with gas can be somewhat higher. Obtaining high accuracy with these meters requires a straight length of tube upstream of the orifice that is at least 20 times the tube diameter and a length of at least 5 tube diameters downstream. Alternatively, flow straighteners in the form of tube bundles can be used if length is restricted. The simple design of orifice plate flowmeters allows them to be scaled up or down to accommodate a very wide range of flow rates. Pressure drops can be made quite small, although for ΔP less than about 1% of the mean pressure, the signal-to-noise ratio may be too small to be easily measured. A disadvantage of the orifice meter is the large amount of turbulence created by the flow through the orifice.

Venturi flowmeters. Turbulence and pressure drop are reduced by using a venturi device as the flow element (see Fig. 4-15). The throat diameter is usually about one-half the tube diameter. The flow rate through the venturi meter is governed by the same relationship as for the orifice meter, but the discharge coefficient is near unity, thus reducing the pressure drop by about 60% for the same mass flow. Venturi meters have been used in many applications for measuring flow rates of normal, supercritical, and superfluid helium [92,95]. Short-term repeatability of ±0.5% was reported. Discharge coefficients varied by about 3% over a flow range of 10-to-1 and for temperatures between 1.7 and 4.2 K. The design requirements of the venturi flowmeter prevent it from being used for reverse flow.

Laminar flow elements. Laminar flow elements are a third type of differential pressure flowmeter. The laminar flow element gives rise to a linear relationship between mass-flow rate and pressure drop. As a result, it can be used over a wider range of flow rates than can the orifice meter and the venturi meter. The governing equation is

$$\dot{V} = \dot{m}/\rho = \Delta P/\mu Z_{\mathrm{f}} \tag{4-13}$$

where $\dot{V}$ is the volumetric flow rate, μ is the viscosity, and Z_{f} is the flow impedance of the laminar element. For laminar flow in a gap, the flow impedance is given by

$$Z_{\mathrm{f}} = 12L/wt^3 \tag{4-14}$$

where L is the length of the gap, w is the width of the gap, and t is the thickness of the gap. Eq. (4-13) shows that the laminar flow element is intrinsically a volumetric flowmeter. The gap thickness must be sufficiently small to prevent turbulent flow. As an example, for helium gas with a mass flow rate of 1 g/s, $P=2$ MPa, $L=1$ cm, and $\Delta P=20$ kPa, the gap thickness must be less than 34 μm at 80 K and less than 9.8 μm at 10 K. The gap width must be 116 mm at 80 K and 240 mm at 10 K. Even though the overall gap width can be achieved with many parallel gaps, the outside dimensions of the laminar flow element will be relatively large. The small gap thickness at cryogenic temperatures makes the laminar flow element difficult to fabricate. No commercial laminar flow elements are available for cryogenic use. A custom-made device has been used with some success by Radebuagh and Rawlins [80] to measure oscillating mass-flow rate at about 10 K in high-pressure helium gas.

4-6 LIQUID LEVEL MEASUREMENT

The quantity of interest for liquid level measurements can be either the position of the liquid surface or the total quantity of liquid present (mass or volume). Often one can be inferred from the other. The mass can be measured by weighing the entire container if (1) the empty weight is known accurately, (2) the mass of the liquid is a significant fraction of the total, and (3) the forces from pipes, cables, and other connections to the container are negligible.

Floats are only rarely used in cryogenic liquids because of low densities and problems with moving parts in cryogenic environments, especially where icing is possible.

The hydrostatic pressure difference between the bottom and top of a liquid is proportional to the liquid depth and is commonly used with large tanks or denser cryogens. Measurement of the hydrostatic pressure difference requires either two pressure sensors, one in the vapor and one at the bottom of the liquid, or a differential pressure sensor and some way to keep the pressure tap to the bottom filled with vapor. Bubblers work when a source of noncondensable gas is available, but using a source of heat to boil off some of the liquid is more common with cryogens. Capacitance level sensors are made with wire-in-tube or tube-in-tube geometries. The liquid and vapor have different dielectric properties, and thus the capacitance is proportional to the liquid level. One drawback is sensitivity to ice, which has a large dielectric constant. Commercially available capacitance level sensors can be used with most cryogenic liquids.

Detection of the presence or absence of liquid at a point is possible with a temperature-sensitive device excited to self-heat significantly. The temperature rise is higher in vapor, allowing detection of liquid. Diodes, transistors, or thermistors are frequently used with a comparator circuit. Several point sensors can be arrayed to provide a semicontinuous indication of level [96].

For continuous readings, a vertical wire of temperature-dependent material can be used with heat provided by the excitation current or by a parallel heater wire. These level sensors are sensitive to the temperature of the vapor and tend to be inaccurate with large temperature gradients found in containers with low thermal conductivity walls and during transients such as filling.

Superconductive level sensors consist of a wire or thin rod of material that is super-conducting at the liquid temperature. A small heat input either at the top end or along the length of the sensor warms any of the wire in vapor above the superconducting to normal transition temperature, making it electrically resistive. The sensitivity to variations in vapor temperature is greatly reduced. Several manufacturers make superconductive liquid helium level sensors using NbTi filaments, typically 30 to 100 μm in diameter. Operation is unaffected by magnetic fields to at least 5 T. The liquid temperature can vary from about 4.5 down to at least 1.2 K. Superconductive level sensors with an effective resistance greater than about 4.3 Ω/cm have a "blind spot" just above the lambda temperature (2.17 K) where the indicated liquid level suddenly drops to zero. The peak nucleate boiling heat flux is depressed in this region, and the liquid level will remain zero until the liquid temperature cools below 2.17 K or warms enough to reestablish nucleate boiling along the submerged portion of the filament. Superconductive level sensors for liquid nitrogen, oxygen, or argon could in principle be made using high-temperature superconductors, but technical problems and the availability of many workable alternatives have limited their usefulness.

Liquid level control systems of the following several types have been developed: (1) timer with no sensors, (2) on–off solenoid controlled by one or two point sensors [97], (3) on–off solenoid controlled by a continuous sensor, and (4) proportional control systems [98].

4-7 MAGNETIC MEASUREMENTS

Several magnetic field–dependent properties can be used to construct magnetic field sensors. Unfortunately, many of them are difficult to use in a cryogenic environment.

4-7-1 Hall Effect

Hall effect sensors are commercially available and are the most common way to measure magnetic fields. The sensors are based on the Hall effect in which charge carriers moving through a material are forced to one side or the other through their interaction with the magnetic field. The output voltage difference is directly proportional to the magnetic flux passing through the material perpendicular to the plane of the Hall plate. Care must be taken to orient the sensor properly, for the output voltage goes as the cosine of the angle between the magnetic field and the normal to the Hall plate. In practice, the Hall plates are fabricated as a thin sheet of semiconductor material to which four contacts are made. Commercial devices are available in relatively small packages for measuring either transverse or axial fields. Typical devices are operated at constant currents on the order of 1 to 100 mA with the output signal measured by a voltmeter. Sensitivity varies greatly with model, but the range is from about 10 to 1500 mV/T. The resistance varies from about 1 Ω to thousands of ohms, and the sensitivity is proportional to the resistance.

Hall sensors designed for cryogenic use have a finite lifetime measured in terms of the number of cycles to cryogenic temperatures. Hall sensors are delicate and easily damaged. Careful mounting is required to minimize mechanical strains during cool-down. A typical cryogenic Hall generator will last 50 to 100 thermal cycles. Two failure modes occur. The first is a catastrophic failure due to cracking in the Hall sensor itself. This is most likely to occur during the first few thermal cycles. The second failure mode is the result of continued microcracking upon each thermal cycle. The microcracking results in an increasing voltage offset, which eventually becomes too large to cancel out. The offset voltage for typical Hall generators will increase on the order of $1 \mu V$ per thermal cycle.

Commercially available Hall sensors are produced by F. W. Bell (BHT 921), Lake Shore Cryotronics (HGCA-3020 and HGCT-3020), and Siemens (RHY 17 and RHY 18). Temperature sensitivity is very low with slope changes on the order of $\pm 0.5\%$ between 4.2 and 300 K. All of these Hall sensors are slightly nonlinear, particularly at fields above 5 T and temperatures below 10 K, but should be accurate to within $\pm 1\%$. Requirements for higher accuracy necessitate calibration near the measurement temperature.

4-7-2 Induction Coils

Induction coils rely upon Faraday's induction law as their working principle. The major limitation with these coils is that the magnetic flux through the pickup coil must be changing with time to produce an output voltage. Their greatest application is in measuring pulsed or ramped fields. Rotating coils are required to measure DC magnetic fields. Thermal contraction can change the calibration at cryogenic temperatures. Specially shaped coils can be designed to respond preferentially to uniform fields or to higher-order components.

4-7-3 Magnetoresistance

Magnetoresistors made from high-purity copper wire have been widely used at low temperatures and in high magnetic fields. The sensor, typically made of coiled wire, must be designed and constructed with great care to minimize its size, temperature sensitivity, and mechanical strain. The large size of magnetoresistors often limits their usefulness. Semiconductors or bismuth crystals can also be used. The temperature dependence of the base resistivity is a problem unless the magnetoresistor is calibrated and used at the same temperature. The magnetoresistance increases quadratically at low magnetic fields, making measurement of small fields difficult. An accuracy of better than 0.1% is possible in magnetic fields greater than 3 T [99]. Magnetoresistance is not direction-dependent in most metals, and thus the sensor can not be used to determine field direction.

4-7-4 NMR

The use of nuclear magnetic resonance (NMR) magnetometers to measure magnetic fields is well established at room temperature. An atomic nucleus with nonzero spin quantum number and magnetic moment absorbs electromagnetic energy at a natural resonant frequency proportional to the magnetic field strength. One nucleus used at cryogenic temperatures is ^{27}Al with a gyromagnetic ratio relating resonance frequency and magnetic field of 11.094 MHz/T. Nuclear magnetic resonance magnetometers can be used for magnetic fields in about the 0.05 to 30 T range, which corresponds to resonance frequencies of roughly 0.1 to 100 MHz.

An NMR probe consists of a quantity of an appropriate material containing the desired nuclei, coils, and transmission line to the oscillator, typically at ambient temperature. The size of an NMR probe is typically on the order of 1 cm^3. Magnetic field uniformity on the order of 0.1% or better over the sample volume is needed. Nuclear magnetic resonance is the most accurate method available for measuring magnetic fields. Accuracies on the order of 0.001% are possible in very homogeneous fields.

Nuclear magnetic resonance's advantages of very high accuracy and orientation independence can also be exploited at cryogenic temperatures. Although there are not as yet any commercially available cryogenic NMR probes, several examples of custom probes have been published. Two of the earliest provide details of the probe construction and the electronic circuits. Maxfield and Merrill [100] describe a marginal oscillator design making use of ^{27}Al nuclei. Finely powdered aluminum is used to reduce eddy currents. Rupp [101] describes a crossed coil (transmitter–receiver) circuit used with a slurry containing ^{133}Cs and mentions that the water sample typically used in room-temperature NMR does not work when frozen.

4-7-5 SQUIDs

Superconducting quantum interference devices (SQUIDs) have the highest sensitivity of any magnetic flux sensor with a resolution on the order of a single flux quantum. The maximum measurable field is only about 1 μT. The active region is a small ring of superconductor broken by one or two weak links (Josephson junctions). The necessity of a superconducting material limits the upper temperature range of these devices to about 100 K. In addition, SQUIDs are extremely sensitive to noise and require sophisticated external electronics to operate properly.

4-8 OTHER MEASUREMENTS

Acceleration can be measured with a piezoelectric element. Commercial sources exist operational down to the liquid helium temperature range. Amplification is typically required and the instrumentation is similar to that described for piezoelectric pressure sensors. Extremely sensitive accelerometers can be designed using SQUIDs for signal readout [1].

Acoustic emission sensors are sometimes used to monitor cracking or other energy-releasing motions, particularly in superconducting magnets where small motions of the conductors can lead to quenches. Piezoelectric pressure or acceleration sensors are commonly used [2,3].

Chemical composition of cryogenic fluids is important in mixtures. Some examples include the relative fraction of ortho-to para-hydrogen [4] or of ^{3}He and ^{4}He in a dilution refrigerator.

Density is frequently inferred by measurement of the pressure and temperature or mass and volume, but other methods are commonly used [5,6].

Displacement or motion sensors of the resistive or strain gauge type can sometimes be operated at cryogenic temperatures [29]. Measurement of displacement with a warm sensor and a stiff connecting member can be complicated if the temperature along the length of the member varies with displacement and the thermal contraction is significant.

Flow visualization is sometimes used to get information about flowing liquids with minimal disturbance. Photography is possible in some cases [7]. Laser holography has been used to investigate shock waves in liquid helium [8]. Bubbles and turbulence can also be monitored by cheaper LED and photodiode circuits [9].

Heat capacity is measured by monitoring the temperature response to a known heat input [10,11,12]. The response time and heat capacity of the temperature sensor and heater are important.

Heat Flux is commonly measured with two temperature sensors on either side of a thermally resistive material. One application is measurement of thermal insulation effectiveness.

Leak detection can require special techniques at temperatures below 10 K. Hot cathode extractor gauges have been found to be reliable for very low pressure measurements at liquid helium temperatures [13].

Quench detection in superconducting magnets is commonly accomplished by measuring and comparing the voltages across various sections of the magnet winding [29]. Voltages from different sections are combined to eliminate the inductive component of the voltage and yield only the resistive voltage drop. The resistive voltage is zero when the winding is in the superconducting state but becomes finite and grows if a normal zone appears. Quick response is frequently required.

Void fraction in cryogenic fluids has been measured by using the difference between liquid and vapor dielectric constants. A concentric capacitance sensor has been used to measure quality of helium flows with an accuracy of 1% even though the liquid and vapor dielectric constants differ by only 4% [14].

REFERENCES FOR SECTION 4-8

1. Shirron, P. J., DiPirro, M. J., Moody, M. V., Canavan, E. R., and Paik, H. J., "Superconducting Angular Accelerometers for the Superconducting Gravity Gradiometer Experiment," *Adv. Cryog. Eng.* 41B (1996):1829–1835.

2. Pasztor, G., and Schmidt, C., "Acoustic Emission from NbTi Supweconductors During Flux Jump," *Cryog.* 19 (1979):608–610

3. Tsukamoto, O., and Iwasa, Y., "Acoustic Emission Diagnostic and Monitoring Techniques for Superconducting Magnets," *Adv. Cryog. Eng.* 31 (1986):259–268.

4. Clausen, J., Hofmann, A., and Wanner, M., "Novel Method for Measurement of the para-Content of a Hydrogen-Stream," *Adv. Cryog. Eng.* 41B (1996):1777–1782.

5. *Proc. Static Measurements of Refrigerated Liquids.* (London: Oyez Scientific & Technical Services Ltd., 1983).

6. Liu, F. F., and Chow, S. W. H., "Differential Dielectric-to-Density Measurement for Cryogenic Fluids," *Rev. Sci. Instrum.* 58 (1987):1917–1925.

7. Breon, S. R., and Van Sciver, S. W., "Boiling Phenomena in Pressurized He II Confined to a Channel," *Cryog.* 26 (1986):682–691.
8. Iida, T., Murakami, M., Shimazaki, T., and Nagai, H., "Visualization Study on the Thermo-Hydrodynamic Phenomena Induced by Pulsative Heating in He II by the Use of a Laser Holographic Interferometer," *Cryog.* 36 (1996):943–949.
9. Haruyama, T., "Optical Method for Measurement of Quality and Flow Patterns in Helium Two-Phase Flow," *Cryog.* 27 (1987):450–453.
10. Lawless, W. N., Clark, C. F., and Arenz, R. W., "Method for Measuring Specific Heats in Intense Magnetic Fields at Low Temperatures Using Capacitance Thermometry," *Rev. Sci. Instrum.* 53 (1982):1647–1652.
11. Stewart, G. R. "Measurement of Low-Temperature Specific Heat," *Rev. Sci. Instrum.* 54 (1983):1–11.
12. McMenamin, C. S., Bird, J. P., Brewer, D. F., Hussey, N. E., Moreno, C., Thomson, A. L., and Young, A. J., "Heat Pulse Measurement of Thermal Properties: An Improved Fitting Technique," *Cryog.* 33 (1993):941–946.
13. Rao, M. G., "Sensitive Helium Leak Detection in Cryogenic Vacuum Systems," *Adv. Cryog. Eng.* 41B (1996):1783–1788.
14. Hagedorn, D., Leroy, D., Dullenkopf, P., and Haas, W., "Monitor for the Quality Factor in Two-Phase Helium Flow Using a Low Temperature Oscillator," *Adv. Cryog. Eng.* 31 (1986):1299–1307.
15. Chapman, J. J., Hopson, P., Jr., and Jruse, N., "A Hybrid Electronically Scanned Pressure Module for Cryogenic Environments," NASA Technical Memorandum 110146 (1995).

4-9 COMMERCIAL SOURCES

(A: Acceleration, F: Flow, I: Instrumentation, L: Level, M: Magnetic field, P: Pressure, S: Strain, T: Temperature)

American Magnetics, Inc., Oak Ridge, Tennessee, USA (L, I)
Andeen–Hagerling, Inc., Chagrin Falls, Ohio, USA (I)
Arepoc, Bratislava, Slovak Republic (M)
ARi Industries, Inc., Franklin Park, Illinois, USA (T)
F. W. Bell, Inc., Orlando, Florida, USA (I, M)
Biomagnetic Technologies, Inc., San Diego, California, USA (I)
Conductus, Sunnyvale, California, USA (I, M, T)
Cryomagnetics, Inc., Oak Ridge, Tennessee, USA (I, L, M)
Degussa Corp., South Plainfield, New Jersey, USA (T)
Endevco Corp., San Juan Capistrano, California, USA (A, P)
Heraeus, Inc., Queens Village, New York, USA (T)
Hoffer Flow Controls, Inc., Elizabeth City, North Carolina, USA (F, P)
HY-CAL Engineering, El Monte, California, USA (T)
Keithley Instruments, Inc., Cleveland, Ohio, USA (I)
Kistler Instrument Corp., Amherst, New York, USA (P)
Kulite Semiconductor Products, Inc., Leonia, New Jersey, USA (P)
Lake Shore Cryotronics, Inc., Westerville, Ohio, USA (L, T, I)
Measurements Group, Inc. (Micro Measurements), Raleigh, North Carolina, USA (S, T)
Minco Products, Inc., Minneapolis, Minnesota, USA (T)
NIST, Gaithersburg, Maryland, USA (T)
Omegadyne, Inc. (acquired CEC), Sunbury, Ohio, USA (P)
Omega Engineering, Stamford, Connecticut, USA (T, I)

Oxford Instruments, Eynsham, Witney, Oxon, UK; Concord, Massachusetts, USA
   (L, T, I)
PCB Piezotronics, Inc., Depew, New York, USA (P)
Precise Sensors, Inc., Monrovia, California, USA (P)
Pressure Systems Inc., (KPSI), Hampton, Virginia, USA (P)
Rosemount, Inc., Minneapolis, Minnesota, USA (T)
RV-Elektroniikka Oy, Vantaa, Finland (I)
Sensotec, Columbus, Ohio, USA (P)
Sensotron, Huntington Beach, California, USA (P)
Scientific Instruments, Inc., West Palm Beach, Florida, USA (L, T, I)
Siemens AG, Semiconductor Division, Munich, Germany (P)
Sponsler Co., Westminster, South Carolina, USA (F)
Stanford Research Systems, Sunnyvale, California, USA (I)
Thermometrics (acquired Keystone), Edison, New Jersey, USA (T)
H. Tinsley & Co., New Addington, Croydon, Surrey, UK (T)
Toyoda Machine Works, Ltd., Aichi, Japan (P)
Validyne Engineering Corp., Northridge, California, USA (P)
Yellow Springs Instrument Co., Yellow Springs, Ohio, USA (T)

NOMENCLATURE

NIST	National Institute of Standards and Technology (formerly National Bureau of Standards, USA)
NTC	Negative temperature coefficient
PTC	Positive temperature coefficient
RTD	Resistance temperature detector
Sensor	Device that senses some physical quantity. See also transducer.
S_i	Dimensionless sensitivity of property i (e.g., $S_T = (T/R)(dR/dT)$)
SQUID	Superconducting quantum interference device
Transducer	Device that transforms a physical input into some signal output (e.g., a pressure transducer that transforms a pressure input into a voltage output).
u	Uncertainty

REFERENCES

1. Doebelin, E. O., *Measurement Systems*, 4th ed. (New York: McGraw–Hill, 1990); idem, *Engineering Experimentation: Planning, Execution, Reporting* (New York: McGraw–Hill, 1995).
2. Lipták, B., ed., *Instrumentation Engineer's Handbook*, 3rd ed., vol. 1, *Process Measurement and Analysis*; vol. 2, *Process Control* (Radnor, Pennsylvania: Chilton, 1995). —— *Analytical Instrumentation* (Chilton, 1994). —— *Flow Measurement* (Chilton, 1993); idem, *Temperature Measurement* (Chilton, 1993).
3. Fraden, J., *AIP Handbook of Modern Sensors* (New York: American Institute of Physics, 1993).
4. ISO, *Guide to the Expression of Uncertainty in Measurement*, ISO/TAG 4/WG 3 (Geneva, Switzerland: International Organization for Standardization, 1992).
5. Rabinovich, S., *Measurement Errors* (New York: American Institute of Physics, 1993).
6. "Low Level Measurements" (Cleveland: Keithley Instruments, Inc., 1993).

7. *Accuracy in Measurements and Calibrations*, National Bureau of Standards, NBS Technical Note no. 262 (Washington, D.C.: U.S. Government Printing Office, 1965). Old but still useful compilation of attainable limits of accuracy.

8. *A Directory of Standards Laboratories* (Boulder, Colorado: National Conference of Standards Laboratories, 1995–1996).

9. *NIST Calibration Services Users Guide*, NIST Special Publication 250 and pricing appendix, U.S. Department of Commerce (1998); (Fax: 301-869-3548).

10. Nara, K., Kato, H., and Okaji, M., "Derivation of Optimized Calibration Procedures for Practical Thermometers," *Cryog.* 35 (1995):291–295.

11. Hoge, H. J., "Useful Procedure in Least Squares, and Tests of Some Equations for Thermistors," *Rev. Sci. Instrum.* 59 (1988):975–979.

12. Hust, J. G., "Thermal Anchoring of Wires in Cryogenic Apparatus," *Rev. Sci. Instrum.* 41 (1970):622–624.

13. Hendricks, T. J., Bruns, M. W., and Hershberg, E. L., "Thermal Transport and Electrical Dissipation in Ultra-Low Thermal Load, Multi-Gigahertz I/O Cables for Superconducting Microelectronics," *Adv. Cryog. Eng.* Vol. 41B (1996):1761–1768.

14. Ekin, J. W., and Wagner, D. K., "A Simple AC Bridge Circuit for Use in Four-Terminal Resistance Thermometry," *Rev. Sci. Instrum.* 41 (1970):1109–1110.

15. Diamond, J. M., "A Mueller Bridge Set for Cryogenic Temperature Measurements," *J. Sci. Instrum.* 43 (1966):576–580.

16. Sparks, L. L., "Temperature, Strain, and Magnetic Field Measurements," in *Materials at Low Temperatures*, R. P. Reed and A. F. Clark, eds. (Metals City, Ohio: American Society for Metals, 1983), 515–571.

17. Ylöstalo, J., Berglund, P., Niinikosi, T. O., and Voutilainen, R., "Cryogenic Temperature Measurement for Large Applications," *Cryog.* 36 (1996):1033–1038.

18. Kuchnir, M., "Pulsed Current Resistance Thermometry," *Adv. Cryog. Eng.* 29 (1984):879–886.

19. Swartz, J. M., and Rubin, L. G., *Fundamentals for Usage of Cryogenic Temperature Controllers* (Westerville, Ohio: Lake Shore Cryotronics, Inc., 1985).

20. Lengeler, B., "Semiconductor Devices Suitable for Use in Cryogenic Environments," *Cryog.* 14 (1974):439–447.

21. Kirschman, R. K., "Cold Electronics: An Overview," *Cryog.* 25 (1985):115–122.

22. Rao, M. G., and Scurlock, R. G., "Cryogenic Instrumentation with Cold Electronics—A Review," *Adv. Cryog. Eng.* 31 (1986):1211–1220.

23. Kärner, J. F., Lorenzen, H. W., and Rehm, W., "Semiconductors at Low Temperature," 4th European Conf. on Power Electronics and Applications, *Proc. EPE 1991*, vol. 2 (1991):500–505.

24. Imai, J., and Flores, R., "Low Temperature Metal-Oxide Semiconductor Field-Effect Transistor Pre-amplifier," *Rev. Sci. Instrum.* 64 (1993):3024–3025.

25. Van Duzer, T., and Turner, C.W., *Principles of Superconductive Devices and Circuits* (New York: Elsevier, 1981).

26. Rubin, L. G., "Cryogenic Thermometry: A Review of Recent Progress," *Cryog.* 10 (1970):14–22.

27. Rubin, L. G., Brandt, B. L., and Sample, H. H., "Cryogenic Thermometry: A Review of Recent Progress, II," *Cryog.* 22 (1982):491–503.

28. Rubin, L. G., "Cryogenic Thermometry: A Review of Progress Since 1982," *Cryog.* 37 (1997):341–356.

29. Zichy, J. A., "Review of Instrumentation for Superconducting Magnets," *Adv. Cryog. Eng.* 33 (1988):1053–1062.

30. Courts, S. S., Holmes, D. S., Swinehart, P. R., and Dodrill, B. C., "Cryogenic Thermometry—An Overview," *Appl. Cryog. Technol.* 10 (1991):55–69.

31. Radebaugh, R., and Marquardt, E., *Cryogenic Instrumentation, Recent Advances in Cryogenic Engineering*, HTD-vol. 267 (New York: American Society of Mechanical Engineers, 1993), 13–27.

32. Rubin, L. G., Brandt, B. L., and Sample, H. H., "Some Practical Solutions to Measurement Problems Encountered at Low Temperatures and High Magnetic Fields," *Adv. Cryog. Eng.* 31 (1986):1221–1230.

33. Brandt, B. L., Rubin L. G., and Sample, H. H., "Low-Temperature Thermometry in High Magnetic Fields. VI. Industrial-Grade Pt Resistors Above 66 K; Rh–Fe and Au–Mn Resistors Above 40 K," *Rev. Sci. Instrum.* 59 (1988):642–645.

34. Nara, K., Kato H., and Okaji, M., "Development of Thin Wire Platinum Resistance Thermometer with Isotropic Magnetoresistance," *Cryog.* 33 (1993):931–935.
35. CLTS *Cryogenic Linear Temperature Sensor*, Micro-Measurements, Product Bulletin PB-104-3 (Raleigh, North Carolina: 1983).
36. McDonald, P. C., "Magnetoresistance of the Cryogenic Linear Temperature Sensor in the Range 4.2 to 300 K," *Cryog.* 13 (1973):367–368.
37. Jüngst, K. P., Kutschera, M., and Yan, L., "Magnetic Field Measurement Within Superconducting Windings by CLTS Temperature Sensors," *Cryog.* 25 (1985):23–25.
38. Lawless, W. N., Hampton, S. K., and Clark, C. F., "Calibration Scheme for Allen–Bradley Resistors, 4.1–100 K," *Rev. Sci. Instrum.* 59 (1988):2505–2507.
39. Neuringer, L. J., and Shapira, Y., "Low Temperature Thermometry in High Magnetic Fields. I. Carbon Resistors," *Rev. Sci. Instrum.* 40 (1969):1314–1321.
40. Schlosser, W. F., and Munnings, R. H., "A Method of Reducing the Effective Magnetoresistance of Carbon Resistor Thermometers," *Cryog.* 12 (1972):225–226.
41. Sample, H. H., Neuringer, L. J., and Rubin, L. G., "Low-Temperature Thermometry in High Magnetic Fields. III. Carbon Resistors (0.5–4.2 K); Thermocouples," *Rev. Sci. Instrum.* 45 (1974):64–73.
42. Sample, H. H., Brandt, B. L., and Rubin, L. G., "Low-Temperature Thermometry in High Magnetic Fields. V. Carbon-Glass Resistors," *Rev. Sci. Instrum.* 53 (1982):1129–1136.
43. Roy, A., Buchanan, D. S., and Ginsberg, D. M., "Method for Using Germanium Thermometers in Moderately High Magnetic Fields," *Rev. Sci. Instrum.* 56 (1985):483–485.
44. Zarubin, L. I., Nemish, I. Y., and Szmyrka–Grzebyk, A., "Germanium Resistance Thermometers with Low Magnetoresistance," *Cryog.* 30 (1990):533–537.
45. Briggs, A., "Characterization of Some Chip Resistors at Low Temperatures," *Cryog.* 31 (1991):932–935.
46. Uhlig, K., "Magnetoresistance of Thick-Film Chip Resistors at Millikelvin Temperatures," *Cryog.* 35 (1995):525–528.
47. Dötzer, R., and Schoepe, W., "Thermal Impedance Between Thick-Film Resistor and Liquid Helium Below 1 K," *Cryog.* 33 (1993):936–937.
48. Krause, J. K., and Dodrill, B. C., "Measurement System Induced Errors in Diode Thermometry," *Rev. Sci. Instrum.* 57 (1986):661–665.
49. Lawless, W. N., "Aging Phenomena in a Low-Temperature Glass-Ceramic Capacitance Thermometer," *Rev. Sci. Instrum.* 46 (1975):625–628.
50. Swenson, C. A., "Time-Dependent and Thermal History Effects in Low Temperature Glass-Ceramic Capacitance Thermometers," *Rev. Sci. Instrum.* 48 (1977):489–490.
51. Li, R. R., Berg, G. P., and Mast, D. B., "Ceramic Chip Capacitors as Low Temperature Thermometers," *Cryog.* 32 (1992):44–46.
52. Burns, G. W., Scroger, M. G., Strouse, G. F., Croarkin, M. C., and Guthrie, W. F., *Temperature-Electromotive Force Reference Functions and Tables for the Letter-Designated Thermocouple Types Based on the ITS-90*, U.S. Department of Commerce, NIST Monograph 175 (Washington, D.C.: U.S. Government Printing Office 1993).
53. ASTM Standard E1751-95, "Temperature-Electromotive Force (EMF) Tables for Non-Letter Designated Thermocouple Combinations," in *1996 Annual Book of ASTM Standards*, vol. 1403 ASTM (West Zonshohocken, Pennsylvania: American Society for Testing and Materials, 1996), 456–545.
54. Holmes, D. S., and Courts, S. S., "Thermal Resistances of Mounted Cryogenic Temperature Sensors," *Adv. Cryog. Eng.* 41B (1996):1699–1706.
55. Holmes D. S., and Courts, S. S., "Resolution and Accuracy of Cryogenic Temperature Measurements," in *Temperature: Its Measurement and Control in Science and Industry*, vol. 6, J. F. Schooley, ed. (New York: American Institute of Physics, 1992), 1225–1230.
56. Mangum, B. W., and Furukawa, G. T., *Guidelines for Realizing the International Temperature Scale of 1990 (ITS-90)*, U.S. Department of Commerce, NIST Technical Note 1265 (Washington, D.C.: U.S. Government Printing Office, 1990).
57. Pavese, F., Malyshev, V. M., Steur, P. P. M., Ferri, D., and Giraudi, D., "Routine Calibration of Cryogenic Thermometers in the Range 1.5–350 K with an Accuracy up to the Millikelvin Level," *Adv. Cryog. Eng.* 41B (1996):1683–1690.

58. Pavese, F., and Molinar, G., *Modern Gas-Based Temperature and Pressure Measurements* (New York: Plenum Press, 1992); see chapter 10 for the thermomolecular pressure difference effect and section 4-4 for cryogenic pressure sensors.

59. Starr, J. E., "Basic Strain Gage Characteristics," in *Strain Gage Users' Handbook*, R. L. Hannah and Reed, S. E., eds. (New York: Elsevier Applied Science, 1992), 1–77.

60. Pavese, F., "Investigation of Transducers for Large-Scale Cryogenic Systems in Italy," *Adv. Cryog. Eng.* 29 (1984):869–877.

61. Walstrom, P. L., "The Effect of High Magnetic Fields on Metal Foil Strain Gauges at 4.2 K," *Cryog.* 15 (1975):270–272.

62. Hannah, R. L., and Reed, S. E., *Strain Gage Users' Handbook* (New York: Elsevier Applied Science, 1992).

63. McConville, G. T., "The Effect of the Measuring Tube Surface on Thermomolecular Pressure Corrections in Vapor Pressure Thermometry," *Temperature* 4 (1972):159–165.

64. Tward, E., and Mason, P. V., "Damping of Thermoacoustic Oscillations," *Adv. Cryog. Eng.* 27 (1981):807–814.

65. Luck, H., and Trepp, Ch., "Thermoacoustic Oscillations in Cryogenics. Part 1: Basic Theory and Experimental Verification; Part 2: Applications; Part 3: Avoiding and Damping of Oscillations," *Cryog.* 32 (1992):690–706.

66. Hershberg, E. L., and Lyngdal, J. W., "Self-heating in Piezoresistive Pressure Sensors at Cryogenic Temperatures," *Adv. in Cryog. Eng.* 39B (1994):1123–1130.

67. Boyd, C., Juanarena, D., and Rao, M. G., "Cryogenic Pressure Sensor Calibration Facility," *Adv. Cryog. Eng.* 35B (1990):1573–1581.

68. Nara, K., Okaji, M., and Kato, H., "Piezo-Resistive Pressure Sensor Applicable for in situ Pressure Measurement at Cryogenic Temperatures Under Magnetic Fields," *Cryog.* 33 (1993):541–546.

69. Jacobs, R., "Cryogenic Applications of Capacitance-Type Pressure Sensors," *Adv. Cryog. Eng.* 31 (1986):1277–1284.

70. Adams, E. D., "High-Resolution Capacitive Pressure Gauges," *Rev. Sci. Instrum.* 64 (1993):601–611.

71. Miura, Y., Matsushima, N., Ando, T., Kuno, S., Inoue, S., Ito, K., and Mamiya, T., "Pressure Measurements with a Precision of 0.001 ppm in Magnetic Fields at Low Temperatures," *Rev. Sci. Instrum.* 64 (1993):3215–3218.

72. Echternach, P. M., Hahn, I., and Israelsson, U. E., "A Novel Silicon Micromachined Cryogenic Capacitive Pressure Transducer," *Adv. Cryog. Eng.* 41 (1996):1837–1842.

73. Kashani, A., Wilcox, R. A., Spivak, A., Daney, D. E., and Woodhouse, C. E., "SHOOT Flowmeter and Pressure Transducers," *Cryog.* 30 (1990):286–291.

74. Alspach, W. J., Miller, C. E., and Flynn, T. M., "Mass Flowmeters in Cryogenic Service," in *Flow Measurement Symposium* (New York American Society of Mechanical Engineers, 1966), 34–56.

75. Brennan, J. A., Stokes, R. W., Kneebone, C. H., and Mann, D. B., "An Evaluation of Selected Angular Momentum, Vortex Shedding, and Orifice Cryogenic Flowmeters, U.S. Department of Commerce, National Bureau of Standards Technical Note 650 (Washington, D.C.: U.S. Government Printing Office, 1974).

76. Brennan, J. A., and Takano, A., "A Preliminary Report on the Evaluation of Selected Ultrasonic and Gyroscopic Flowmeters at Cryogenic Temperatures," in *Proc. Ninth Intl. Cryog. Eng. Conf.*, K. Yasukochi and H. Nagano, eds. (Guildford: Butterworths, 1982), 655–638.

77. Rivetti, A., Martini, G., and Birello, G., "LHe Flowmeters: State of the Art and Future Developments," *Adv. Cryog. Eng.* 41B (1996):1789–1796.

78. Van Sciver, S. W., Holmes, D. S., Huang X., and Weisend II, J. G., "He II Flowmetering," *Cryog.* 31 (1991):75–86.

79. Williams, C. D. H., "An Appraisal of the Noise Performance of Constant Temperature Bolometric Detector Systems," *Meas. Sci. Technol.* 1 (1990):322–328.

80. Rawlins, W., Radebaugh, R., and Timmerhaus, K. D., "Thermal Anemometry for Mass Flow Measurement in Oscillating Cryogenic Gas Flows," *Rev. Sci. Instrum.* 64 (1993):3229–3235.

81. Radebaugh, R., and Rawlins, W., "Measurement of Oscillating Mass Flows at Low Temperatures," in *Devices for Flow Measurement and Control—1993* (New York: American Society of Mechanical Engineers, 1993), 25–32.

82. Bugeat, J. P., Petit, R., and Valentian, D., "Thermal Helium Mass Flowmeter for Space Cryostat," *Cryog.* 27 (1987):4–7.

83. Lavocat, P., "Ultrasonic Flow Measurement in Liquid Helium," in *Proc. ICEC 11* (Guildford: Butterworths, 1986), 577–581.

84. Hofmann, A., and Vogeley, B., "Acoustic Flowmeter for He I and He II Application," in *Proc. ICEC 10* (Guildford: Butterworths, 1984), 448–451.

85. Borner, H., Schmeling, T., and Schmidt, D. W., "Experiments on the Circulation and Propagation of Large-Scale Vortex Rings in He II," *Phys. Fluids* 26 (1983):1410–1416. ――――"Experimental Investigations on Fast Gold-Tin Metal Film Second Sound Detectors and Their Application," *J. Low Temp. Phys.* 50 (1983):405–426.

86. Murakami, M., Naki, H., Ichikawa, N., Hanada, M., and Yamazaki, T., "Application of Flow Visualization and Laser Doppler Velocimetry to Cryogenic Fluids," in *Proc. ICEC 11* (Guildford: Butterworths, 1986), 582–586.

87. Brennan, J. A., Dean, J. W., Mann, D. B., and Kneebone, C. H., "An Evaluation of Positive Displacement Cryogenic Volumetric Flowmeters," U.S. Department of Commerce, National Bureau of Standards Technical Note 605 (Washington, D.C.: U.S. Government Printing Office, 1971).

88. Beck, M. S., "Correlation in Instruments: Cross Correlation Flowmeters," *J. Phys. E: Sci. Instr.* 14 (1981):7–19.

89. Rivetti, A., Goria, R., Martini, G., and Lorefice, S., "Characterization of Anemometric-Type Flowmeters for Cryogenic Helium," *Adv. Cryog. Eng.* 29 (1984):895–902.

90. Alspach, W. J., and Flynn, T. M., "Considerations When Using Turbine-Type Flowmeters in Cryogenic Service," *Adv. Cryog. Eng.* 10 (1965):246–252.

91. Brennan, J. A., Mann, D. B., Dean, J. W., and Kneebone, C. H., "Performance of NBS Cryogenic Flow Research Facility," *Adv. Cryo. Eng.* 17 (1972):199–205.

92. Daney, D. E., "Behavior of Turbine and Venturi Flowmeters in Superfluid Helium," *Adv. Cryog. Eng.* 33 (1988):1071–1079.

93. Kashani, A., and Van Sciver, S. W., "Steady State Forced Convection Heat Transfer," in He II, *Adv. Cryog. Eng.* 31 (1986):489–497.

94. Rivetti, A., Martini, G., Gori, R., and Lorefice, S., "Turbine Flowmeter for Liquid Helium with the Rotor Magnetically Levitated," *Cryog.* 22 (1987):8–11.

95. Rivetti, A., Martini, G., and Birello, G., "Metrological Performances of Venturi Flowmeters in Normal, Supercritical and Superfluid Helium," *Adv. Cryog. Eng.* 39B (1994):1051–1058.

96. Shirron, P. J., DiPirro, M. J., and Tuttle, J. G., "Performance of Discrete Liquid Helium/Vapor and He-I/He-II Discriminators," *Adv. Cryog. Eng.* 39B (1994):1105–1112.

97. Chumbley, P. E., and Hulse, M. M., "Self-Pressurizing Liquid-Nitrogen Filler," *Rev. Sci. Instrum.* 56 (1985):1478–1479; Noijen, J. J., Baselmans, G. W. M., and Kopinga, K., "Simple and Reliable Liquid Nitrogen Refill System," *Cryog.* 28 (1988):185–187.

98. Christman, S. B., "Proportional Liquid-Nitrogen Valve and Control System," *Rev. Sci. Instrum.* 61 (1990):2452–2456.

99. Scott, G. B., Springford, M., and Stockton, J. R., "Use of a Magnetoresistor to Measure the Magnetic Field in a Superconducting Magnet," *J. Phys. E: Sci. Instr.* 1 (1968):925–928.

100. Maxfield, B. W., and Merrill, J. R., "NMR Calibration and Hysteresis Effects of Superconducting Magnets," *Rev. Sci. Instrum.* 36 (1965):1083–1085.

101. Rupp, Jr., L. W., "Nuclear Magnetic Resonance Probe for Calibrating Superconducting Solenoids," *Rev. Sci. Instrum.* 37 (1966):1039–1041.

FIVE

CRYOSTAT DESIGN

G. McIntosh

Cryogenic Technical Services, 164 Primrose Court, Longmont, CO 80501-6036

5-1 INTRODUCTION

A cryostat is a device in which something is to be done at a controlled low temperature. It may be as simple as a container (Dewar) to hold a liquid cryogen that surrounds a superconducting magnet or very complex assemblies for high-energy physics or multi-layer insulation (MLI) thermal conductivity measurements.

The initial design task is to determine just what function the cryostat is to perform and what are the driving factors (including the project budget). Typical considerations include the following:

1. Personnel and facility safety requirements and relevant codes.
2. Facility constraints.
3. Service conditions, including g loads and environmental exposure.
4. Required size and orientation of the cryostat.
5. Refrigeration source and temperature.
6. Requirements for periodic accessibility.
7. Lifetime (quick and dirty or for permanent service).
8. Necessary instrumentation and controls.
9. Special features such as bakeability, high-pressure containment, temperatures below 2.17 K, presence of high magnetic fields, vibration isolation, and provisions for combustible materials, including the cryogens themselves.
10. Level of usage ranging from continuous to infrequent.
11. Services required, including power, cryogens, air, and cooling water.

These typical guidelines may seem obvious, but some may be overlooked in the pressure to get a project started. To do so may be costly in time and money. The best approach is first to design the experiment or process and then build the cryostat around it.

5-2 MATERIALS

Present-day cryostat designers are fortunate in comparison with their predecessors in that there are more choices of materials to use, and better physical and thermal property values are available for them than previously. This improves design accuracy and equipment reliability. The following are properties of greatest interest for cryogenic structural applications:

- Warm and cold tensile and yield strengths
- Impact strength at design temperature
- Tensile and shear moduli
- Thermal conductivity
- Surface emissivity
- Vacuum characteristics
- Methods of fabrication and joining

Some of the most useful cryogenic structural materials are described in the sections that follow.

5-2-1 Austenitic Stainless Steels: Types 304, 304L, 304N, 316, 316L, and 321

Austenitic stainless steels are the workhorse materials for cryogenics over all temperature ranges. They are readily available in a variety of forms, have good impact strengths, are easily welded vacuum tight, and have a moderately high tensile modulus ($\approx$200 GPa), an ASME Code [1] design strength of 129.6 MPa at room temperature, and thermal conductivity [2] ranging from 14.7 W/mK at 300 K to 7.9 W/mK at 77 K to 0.28 W/mK at 4 K. These 300-series stainless steels are reasonably clean with respect to surface outgassing, are readily baked out, and have less diffused hydrogen than typical carbon steel. One caveat is that stainless steel bars sometime have axial inclusions that leak slowly or not at all at ambient temperature but may exhibit profuse vacuum leak rates at cryogenic temperatures. Also, very high tensile and yield strengths are obtained from cold-worked 300-series stainless steel machined parts and cables, but these improved properties are lost by the annealing effect of welding or brazing.

5-2-2 Nickel Steels: Primarily 9% Nickel Steel

Nickel steel is limited to uses at 77 K and higher temperatures. The ASME Code allowable stress for 9% nickel steel is 26.6% greater than for 304 stainless steel, and nickel steel is somewhat less expensive. Thus, it is widely used in large industrial gas containers in which the inner shell material is the largest cost. Nine-percent nickel steel is seldom used in laboratory-sized cryostats.

5-2-3 Aluminum Alloys: Alloys 1100, 3003, 6061, 6063, and 5083

Aluminum alloys are used for inner vessels (particularly 6061 and 5083), in heat-conducting baffles and shields (1100 and 3003), and in extrusions and piping (6063 and 6061). Aluminum is characterized by light weight ($2768 \, kg/m^3$), relatively high thermal conductivity (1100 and 6063), moderate allowable design stress (68 to 70 MPa for 6061 and 5083), and a low average modulus of 69 GPa. Aluminum alloys are clean in vacuum service and have a low rate of hydrogen diffusion. Clean aluminum has low thermal radiation emissivity, typically from 1 to 4 or 5%, depending on surface temperature and condition. This makes it effective for radiation shields and foil reflectors in MLI.

5-2-4 Copper: Commercial Alloys CDA 101 (OFHC), 110 (ETP), and 120 (Phosphorous Deoxidized)

High-purity copper alloys have high thermal conductivity and low radiation emissivity. Copper is typically fabricated by brazing or soldering, but it can be welded using the tungsten inert gas (TIG) process. However, only deoxidized copper should be welded to avoid cracking after the first cooldown to low temperature. Copper can also be TIG-welded to stainless steel by using Everdur (Cu-95%, Si-4%, and Mn-1%) filler rod. Annealed copper must be used in heat transfer applications because even mild cold work adversely impacts thermal conductivity.

5-2-5 Fiber–Epoxy Composites: NEMA Grades G-10-CR, G-11-CR, and Others

Fiber–epoxy composites are strong and light and have low thermal conductivity and good vacuum characteristics, although they cannot be baked out at high temperatures. Standard G-10-CR and G-11-CR (and other similar commercial products) have many uses as thermally insulating mechanical supports, and tubular forms are vacuum-tight to air and nitrogen vapor. (They diffuse helium gas at an unacceptable rate.) With proper radial clearance (0.1 to 0.2 mm), G-10 and G-11 make vacuum-tight epoxy joints with stainless steel that withstand cold cycling to 77 K and lower. However, like G-10/11 in layer-to-layer shear, the major problem of joining composites to metals is that the epoxy joints are much less strong than either material. This can be overcome by filament winding the composite into straps or trunnions that are mechanically locked into end spools or hubs. Filament winding offers other options in that a variety of fibers can be selected to enhance tensile and compressive strengths, improve fatigue life, and match the modulus or expansion coefficient of metals. The most common filament is E-glass followed by S-glass, which is considerably stronger. Kevlar fiber is widely used in body armor and has some cryogenic applications. Carbon fiber composites are very strong and can be formulated for tensile modulus values as high or higher than that of 304 stainless steel. Carbon fiber composites have lower thermal conductivity [3] than similar S-glass material below 60 K but substantially higher values at higher temperatures. Alumina fiber composite straps have been used as spacecraft cryogenic supports [4] based on superior fatigue life at high stress with strength and heat leak competitive with S-glass composite.*

5-2-6 Other Structural Materials: Titanium, Invar, Maraging Steels, Hastelloy Alloys

Although not commonly used in industry or for cryostat construction, there are several materials with special properties that are useful for aerospace and cryostat construction. These include titanium alloys, Invar, maraging steels, including 17-4PH, and the Hastelloy family of high-strength alloys. Titanium alloys, particularly Ti-6Al-4V and Ti-5Al-2.5Sn, are lighter than stainless steel and very strong. Extra low interstitials grades are recommended for cryogenic applications, and decreasing low-temperature fracture toughness below 125 K limits the range of use. However, machined and heat-treated Ti-5Al-2.5Sn rods have been in successful use as tension supports for helium Dewars for more than 30 years.

Invar, 64.5% Fe–35.5% Ni, is useful because it has a lower coefficient of expansion, α, than most metals. The integrated α from 300 to 70 K is approximately -40×10^{-5} m/m and essentially zero below 70 K. In comparison, the α for 304 stainless steel from 300 down to 20 K is -310×10^{-5} m/m. Low shrinkage of Invar gives rise to two useful applications. First, it is frequently used in transfer lines to reduce (but not eliminate) the number of expansion joints or bend loops required to keep shrinkage stress at an acceptable level. Second, Invar washers can be incorporated into bolted flange joints so as to make them *tighten* when cooled. This arrangement is illustrated in Fig. 5-1. As shown, an aluminum flange, $\alpha = -430 \times 10^{-5}$ m/m, is bolted to a 304 stainless steel flange with high strength stainless steel bolts using an Invar washer. To make the joint tighten when cooled from ambient temperature to 4 K, the bolt must shrink more than the sandwich of aluminum, stainless steel, and Invar. The basic equation for this situation is

$$L_A\alpha_A + L_S\alpha_S + X\alpha_I = (L_A + L_S + X)(\alpha_A - \varepsilon) \tag{5-1}$$

where

α_A = temperature expansion coefficient for aluminum
α_S = temperature expansion coefficient for stainless steel
α_I = temperature expansion coefficient for Invar
L_A = thickness of aluminum flange
L_S = thickness of stainless steel flange
X = required thickness of Invar washer
ε = unit strain of bolts due to cooldown (m/m)

This equation may be rearranged as follows to solve for the required Invar thickness X:

$$X = [L_A(\alpha_A - \alpha_S) + \varepsilon(L_A + L_S)]/(\alpha_S - \varepsilon - \alpha_I) \tag{5-2}$$

*Additional information on composite materials may be found in chapter 2 of this handbook.

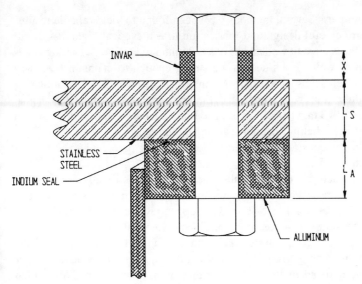

Figure 5-1 Flange joint with Invar washer.

For a strain value of 3×10^{-5} m/m and α values as listed above, thickness of the Invar washer is 0.472 unit for unit thickness aluminum and stainless steel flanges. The 3×10^{-5} m/m strain value is equivalent to a bolt stress *increase* of approximately 6 MPa (870 psi). For zero increase in strain, the Invar washer thickness is 0.444 unit.

Heat-treated maraging steels, particularly 17-4PH, are useful for cryogenic pins and bolts. Aside from having high strength at low temperature, the surface hardness of 17-4PH allows sliding contact with stainless steel and reduced chances of galling, especially if the rubbing surfaces are precoated with dry graphite film lubricant. The 17-4PH pins have been successfully used on 30,000-gal liquid oxygen Dewar supports where one end was fixed and the other was required to slide some 45 mm during cooldown.

High-alloy steels made by Haynes International, notably Hastelloy B and Haynes alloy No. 25, have excellent structural properties. Compared with 304 stainless steel, they are about 50% stronger and have high-impact strengths, good ductility, and 25% lower thermal conductivity. Mechanical properties are substantially enhanced by cold work. Low-loss Dewar neck tubes have been made in production quantities using 0.2-mm (0.008-in.) Hastelloy B, and improved units were made from thicker tubes that were cold reduced away from the ends. Leaving the ends without cold work improves weldability and lowers maximum bending stress in addition to reducing conduction heat leak in the center section.

5-3 COLD SEALS

It is frequently necessary to design cryostats with cold seals either because the use pattern may require frequent disassembly or because adjacent materials cannot be joined by conventional techniques. Several methods have been found to yield reliable results, but all of them require careful design and fabrication to achieve leak tightness. In all cases, the sealing surfaces must fit well and have a minimum of waviness. Bolting needs special consideration as well. Bolts need to be strong enough to maintain necessary clamping forces and be closely spaced to prevent intermediate gaps, and the quotient of stress divided by modulus must be low enough to limit bolt stretch. A typical design goal for total bolt stretch is 0.013 mm (0.0005 in.). (The Invar washer technique described in section 5-2-6 is particularly helpful in cold seal applications.)

Five successful techniques are discussed in the following paragraphs and four of them are illustrated in Fig. 5-2.

A number of manufacturers offer bakeable vacuum flanges utilizing a soft copper gasket that yields to sharp concentric rings machined into the mating stainless steel flanges. This seal is illustrated in Fig. 5-2(a). The copper gaskets can be replaced with other soft metals in some applications, particularly if bakeout is not required. These seals are satisfactory for low-temperature service but they must be made up carefully. Repeated high-torque tightening is required to yield the sealing rings fully on the copper gasket and to load the bolts adequately. Because they are primarily aimed at vacuum service, these joints are not reliable for high pressures.

Figure 5-2(b) shows a cold seal using indium metal as the sealing agent. As shown, a small 60° vee groove is overfilled with an indium wire having a cross-sectional area at least 50% greater than that of the groove. When compressed, the groove is completely filled with indium, and the excess extrudes on either side. Low bolting force is required to make the seal because the indium is very soft. However, strong, high-modulus bolts are required to maintain the seal under pressure because the compressed indium has little elasticity. Indium seals are particularly effective with soft flanges and materials that are not readily joined, such as quartz windows on aluminum ports. Invar washers are helpful in this application if high pressures are involved but are otherwise not needed because quartz has an even lower coefficient of thermal expansion than Invar.

Metal O-rings with a "C" cross section are commercially produced for low-temperature sealing. These typically are plated with silver or copper on the bearing surfaces to improve conformance with the mating flanges. As shown in Fig. 5-2(c), the open end of the "C" faces inward on these rings so that internal pressure increases the flange sealing forces. Metal O-rings are reportedly reusable if the mating surfaces are well finished.

An inexpensive cold seal shown in Fig. 5-2(d) was developed at the National Bureau of Standards Cryogenic Engineering Laboratory [5] (currently the National Institute of Science and Technology) in 1960. This simple seal requires a flat Mylar gasket 0.254 mm (0.010 in.) thick that is locally compressed by about 80% to a minimum thickness of 0.0508 mm by a raised ring machined in the mating flange. The raised ring has a generally circular profile with a height of 0.2032 mm and radial width of about 4 mm. (A smaller radial width of the raised ring decreases bolting force but increases the chance that the gasket will be cut when initially compressed.) This joint requires moderate bolting force but can tolerate bolt stretch of no more than 0.010 mm (0.0004 in.). These seals have been used in long-term service on 20-K, 7-bar manhole covers and to seal 20-bar quartz windows at 77 K.

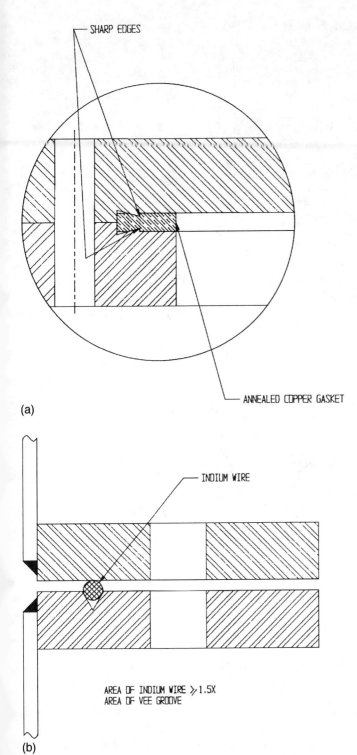

Figure 5-2 (a) Vacuum seal with copper gasket. (b) Indium cryogenic seal. (c) Metal C-ring seal. (d) High-squeeze cryogenic seal. (*Continues*)

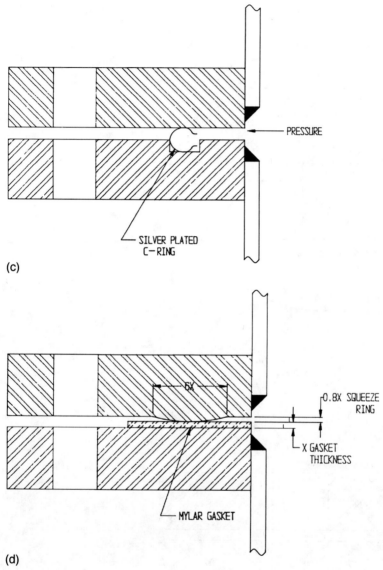

(c)

(d)

Figure 5-2 (*Continued*)

A variety of special seals have been fabricated based on volume compression of elastomers. This has typically been accomplished by using a tongue and groove arrangement to capture the glass-reinforced Teflon elastomer. Close-tolerance machining of the tongue with sharp outer edges to prevent elastomer extrusion out of the groove is the key to success with these joints. Unlike the high-squeeze gasket described above, only 1-to-5% volume compression is required to make the tongue and groove joints, but relatively high bolting forces are needed.

5-4 CRYOSTAT AND DEWAR SUPPORTS

Cryostat supports range from a single cryogen neck tube to an array of composite straps, depending on the service conditions. In almost every case, the objective is to support the cold inner assembly throughout the range of projected shipping and operating loads with an acceptable heat leak. Because of cost and handling considerations, acceptable heat leak is frequently a compromise and not the minimum attainable. Thus, any generalization about support designs is subject to specific case exceptions. With this in mind, the following support guidelines are suggested:

1. Use tension supports whenever they are feasible.
2. Factor shrinkage of the supports and internal structure into the design.
3. Use Belleville springs to accommodate shrinkage when possible.
4. Minimize multilayer insulation (MLI) penetrations.
5. Use simple welded assemblies of 304 stainless steel tubes or rods where possible.

Support materials can be ranked in order of cost and heat leak, which are generally parallel. Welded assemblies of stainless steel tubes or rods are usually low in cost and can be arranged for quite low heat leak if there is room for substantial thermal lengths. Higher performance with the same configurations can be achieved by using more expensive high-alloy steels or titanium alloy rods. Saddles, discs, and structural members made of G-10 or G-11 are also inexpensive and can be arranged for moderate heat leaks, particularly for large industrial gas containers.

Stainless steel cables are useful for supporting Dewars and cryostats. Cable heat leaks are lower than stainless steel rods or tubes because wires in the cables are cold-worked to ultimate stress levels about twice that of annealed material. Cable installation is convenient because assemblies can be purchased with commercial end fittings that do not require welding.

High-performance supports can be made of filament-wound composites formed into straps or trunnions. These have the highest strength-to-heat leak ratio and are generally most expensive. Straps can be made as strong as desired, but care must be taken to use a generous spool radius at each end to avoid stress concentrations [6]. Also, special winding procedures must be used to avoid uneven filament loads if heat-stationing copper foils are incorporated into the windings. Curing filament-wound straps under modest tension helps to distribute tension loads evenly. Trunnions [7] are an established method of supporting large Dewars or cryostats insulated with MLI. They can be filament-wound to support any size and mass of container or cryostat for static or mobile use. Trunnion heat leaks are low compared with metal supports, but costs are relatively high because large, rigid hubs are required at each end and special techniques must be utilized to lock the windings to them.

Heat stationing of supports is quite beneficial in reducing heat leaks. Heat stationing should be done at every temperature level where refrigeration is available and particularly at 77 K and colder. Two or three intercepts should be used for systems cooled by flow of helium vapor. Design of heat intercepts must reflect the thermal properties of the support to be effective. Thin metal supports need little more than a copper wire

soldered or brazed to the surface, but thick composite straps or trunnions need intercepts of substantial length to be really effective. Intercept lengths may range from four
to six times the composite thickness for cooling from one side. Finite-element heat
transfer calculations are a good way to evaluate support heat intercepts on composite
material.

5-5 HELIUM CRYOSTAT AND DEWAR DESIGN WITH VAPOR-COOLED SHIELDS

Because of helium's very high ratio of vapor enthalpy to latent heat of vaporization,
low-loss helium cryostats and Dewars can be designed that perform well without use
of auxiliary refrigerants. With a computer and suitable software, the procedure is sur-
prisingly easy. That the specific heat of helium vapor at low pressure is nearly constant
from 15 to 300 K makes these calculations possible without use of available [8] interactive helium data. The primary task is to assemble all of the requisite geometric data
between each shell and shield. These data include the insulation area and thickness on
each shield and the inner container surface and the cross-sectional area and length of the
supports and piping for each relevant temperature increment. In the conventional itera-
tive method, temperatures are assumed for each shield, and heat balances are written for
each of them and the inner container. Then, thermal conductivity integrals are applied
to each mode of heat transfer to see if balances are obtained. This labor can be avoided
if equations are written for the thermal conductivity integrals and each heat balance set
up with shield temperature as a variable. The following equations are representative
curve-fit relations for MLI, 304 stainless steel, and filament-wound glass–epoxy. Definite integrals of these equations between variable or fixed cold and warm temperatures
provide interactive values for solving heat balances in terms of the unknown shield
temperature.

MLI thermal conductivity (W/mK):

$$k = (1.2054 + (3.777 \times 10^{-2})T$$
$$+ (1.4438 \times 10^{-5})T^2 + (9.5682 \times 10^{-6})T^3) \times 10^{-6} \qquad (5\text{-}3)$$

304 stainless steel (W/mK):

$$k = [(1.3449 \times 10^{-1})T - (5.2208 \times 10^{-4})T^2 + (7.8902 \times 10^{-7})T^3] \times 10^{-6} \quad (5\text{-}4)$$

Filament-wound glass epoxy (in direction of filaments, W/mK):

$$k = [7.006 \times 10^{-7} + (3.2815 \times 10^{-3})T - (5.6717 \times 10^{-6})T^2$$
$$+ (3.4451 \times 10^{-9})T^3] \times 10^{-6} \qquad (5\text{-}5)$$

When set up properly, the heat balance equations will solve for the temperature of
each shield and the rate of cooling vapor flow, which is, of course, related to the helium
heat leak. The heat balance around the liquid helium container must be set up to allow
for retained vapor, which reduces the mass flow of vent gas available for cooling. This
fraction is 0.865 at 101.325 kPa and *decreases* as the helium reservoir pressure increases

above atmospheric. Although there are a number of computer software packages that will solve the related simultaneous equations, TK Solver provides an almost instant solution once the equations are correctly set up.

Spacing of vapor or liquid cooling lines on shields is frequently a matter of con- ·jecture. This design problem can be solved accurately using an analytically derived equation. Consider a shield of thickness t, temperature T, and thermal conductivity k at T on which the average heat transfer load is q W/m^2. The cooling tubes or passages are separated by a distance of $2L$ m so that the maximum heat conduction length is L m. The ΔT between any point in the shield and the cooling tube is given by

$$\Delta T = qL^2/2kt \qquad (5\text{-}6)$$

For a given acceptable ΔT value, Eq. (5-6) can be solved for the corresponding value of L, which is half of the maximum cooling passage spacing. Unsatisfactory combinations of L and ΔT can be altered by changing the shield thickness t and, in some instances, the shield material may be changed to obtain higher thermal conductivity k. The most common result of this calculation is that cooling tube spacing can be greater than generally assumed.

5-6 VACUUM-JACKETED TRANSFER LINE DESIGN

Vacuum-jacketed (VJ) transfer lines are a necessary utility for all aspects of cryogenics. Applications range from tonnage air separation plants to circulation of superfluid helium in orbiting satellites. In each case, the conceptual elements are the same:

1. A suitable pipe or passage is needed for the cryogen.
2. The cold pipe must have a highly reflective surface, be wrapped with MLI to limit heat leak, or both.
3. Low-heat-leak supports or spacers are needed to separate the cold pipe from the warm vacuum jacket.
4. There must be a vacuum-tight jacket around the inner assembly.
5. Expansion joints on either the inner or outer lines are required to compensate for differential thermal shrinkage.
6. Vacuum-jacketed pipe ends must be provided with low-heat-leak end pieces to join pipe sections together and to connect with Dewars.
7. Vacuum valves must be provided to evacuate line sections, sometimes in conjunction with vacuum gauge tubes.
8. Warm and cold getters are required to preserve the static vacuum in the line.

Conventional pressure drop and internal pressure requirements govern the size and thickness of the inner pipe, and it must be compatible with the cryogen being transferred. Pipe and tube made of 304 stainless steel is the most common material. In most cases, the flow work [W_f = (mass flow rate)(ΔP)/(density)] resulting from pressure drop is not significant, but, for pressure transfer, higher ΔP implies a higher supply Dewar pressure, which causes higher flash losses for initially saturated liquid. Therefore, within the constraints of cost, it is generally desirable to size the inner line for low-pressure drop transfer.

In a well-designed transfer line, most of the heat leak is by radiation or insulation conduction from the vacuum jacket to the inner pipe. Limiting this heat transfer is of primary importance. This can be accomplished with low emissivities on the facing surfaces or by imposing concentrically wrapped MLI on the inner pipe. Generally, using insulation is more economical than specially prepared surfaces unless very small radial clearances are necessary. The MLI must be put on one layer at a time because continuous wrapping results in a helical heat-flow path in the reflector material. This is especially damaging if aluminum foil is the reflector. Ten layers of MLI are usually sufficient for liquid nitrogen and other industrial gas lines. Twenty to forty layers may be cost-effective on hydrogen and helium lines.

Liquid helium lines that are in heavy or continuous use may employ traced construction. Traced lines have a copper or aluminum shield tube surrounding the helium line with a liquid nitrogen line running along its external surface or integral with it in the case of specially made aluminum extrusions. Typical copper trace lines are 6.35 to 9.53 mm (1/4 or 3/8 in.) outer diameter, which is sufficient for the small flow of liquid nitrogen required to maintain the shield tube at approximately 78 K. The trace tube is usually soft-soldered to the shield tube to assure good thermal contact. Spacers are required to keep the liquid helium line from touching the shield, but insulation is not normally used because radiation heat transfer between 4.2 and 78 K is comparable to that of typical MLI. The annular space between the shield and vacuum jacket is wrapped with MLI to limit the trace nitrogen heat load.

Transfer line spacers perform two essential tasks. On straight pipe runs they provide low-heat-leak separation between the cryogen line and vacuum jacket. Except for large lines, little strength and heat leak are required for this function. However, if lines have elbows and tees, as is frequently the case, spacers must react against substantial lateral loads to prevent cold shorts. These spacers must have substantial mechanical strength and low heat leak in a limited radial dimension. A great variety of materials and configurations have been used to meet these goals. These include G-10 and G-11 in sheet and tubular form, fiberglass-filled Teflon sheet, laced polyester cord "bicycle wheels," twisted strips of polyethylene, and simple polyester cord with closely spaced knots. Typical transfer line spacer configurations are shown in Fig. 5-3(a–d).

Selection criteria for transfer line vacuum jacket material are driven by cost, ease of fabrication, and the combination of low outgassing and low rate of hydrogen diffusion. The material of choice is 304 stainless steel because it ranks high in all three categories. Copper is a distant second choice because it has low emissivity and low outgassing. Carbon steel pipe is used occasionally, particularly with large, perlite-insulated lines that may be continuously evacuated.

On every transfer line cooldown cycle, the inner line tends to shrink to its unstrained length at the cryogen temperature whereas the vacuum jacket stays at substantially its ambient length. Aside from mechanical failure, three alternatives are presented:

1. The inner line can include bellows sections that allow shrinkage.
2. Expansion bellows can be placed on the vacuum jacket so that it can move with the inner line shrinkage.

3. The line can be formed with right-angle bends or combinations of bends to form expansion loops.

No single approach is right for all cases. Each has its advantages and disadvantages, as discussed in the following paragraphs.

Adding expansion bellows to the inner line is probably the least expensive solution. It minimizes end anchor and support problems because the line as a whole does not move. Vacuum-jacketed lines with internal bellows are durable because the expansion

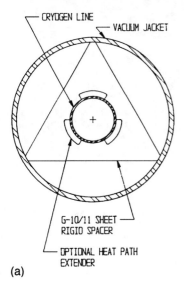

(a)

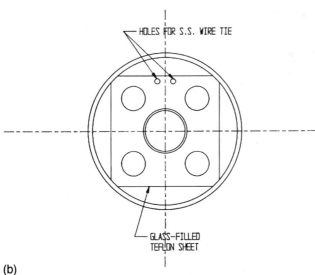

(b)

Figure 5-3 (a) G-10/11 transfer line spacer. (b) Teflon spacer. (c) G-10/11 tubular spacer. (d) "Bicycle wheel" spacer. (*Continues*)

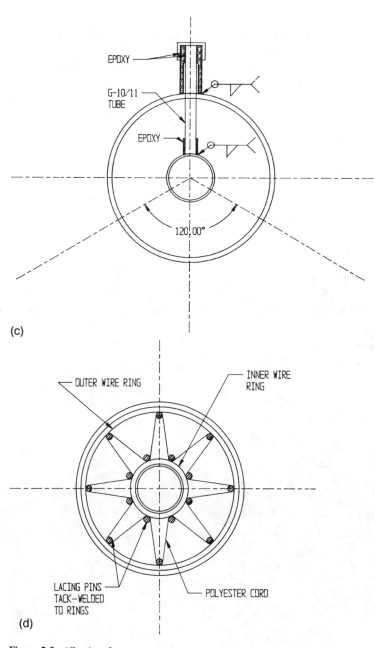

(c)

(d)

Figure 5-3 *(Continued)*

joints are not exposed to external damage or to internal corrosion if they are properly purged when not in use. The bad news is that highly flexible bellows sections can only tolerate limited internal pressure before failing by "squirm." A squirm-resistant internal expansion joint is shown in Fig. 5-4. As shown, the bellows section is almost completely guided by the inner flow pipe, and centering is maintained by support spacers on each end. Guide pipes inside the bellows have closely spaced bleed holes to allow solvent cleaning and thorough purging to prevent trapped contaminants.

Vacuum-jacketed lines with expansion bellows on the vacuum jacket are easily cleaned and can be designed for any appropriate working pressure. Negatives include possible high-end anchor loads and bellows exposed to mechanical damage and atmospheric corrosion. Both of these problems can be alleviated somewhat if low shrinkage Invar pipe is used on the inner line. This reduces the forces to be reacted against at the ends and requires fewer expansion joints.

Although frequently not convenient for cryostats, low-temperature contraction problems can be accommodated by incorporating a series of 90° bends and locating the support spacers to permit the pipe itself to flex. The vacuum jacket must also be designed with clearance to allow the inner pipe to move without causing thermal shorts. This approach results in durable, high-reliability lines that are particularly appropriate for Invar inner line material. Vacuum-jacketed lines for space shuttle launch facilities fall into this category.

Flex lines or rigid lines with flex sections are convenient for general-purpose use and for connections that must be taken apart with some regularity. Inner line and vacuum jacket sections made of annular corrugated stainless steel hose are most commonly used for low-pressure flex lines. For higher pressures and to protect from mechanical damage, the hose sections may be fitted with external stainless steel braid, which is pulled tight and permanently attached at each end. Braided hose is much less flexible than the same material without braid. Disadvantages of flex over rigid lines are higher cost, higher heat leak, and higher pressure drop for equivalent sizes. Higher cost stems mostly from more expensive material with a smaller fraction due to greater labor content.

Line spacers and insulation differences contribute to poorer heat leak of flex lines. Insulation heat leak is increased over rigid lines because it is partially compressed in bend regions and because the supports, helically counter-wrapped knotted polyester cord, also bear on the insulation. Pressure drop is much higher [9] in flex than smooth pipe or tube because each annular corrugation acts as an individual orifice. Insulation for flex lines and sections must be selected for mechanical durability as well as thermal performance. Polyester and polyolefin scrim and double-aluminized Mylar seem to survive this service and provide acceptable thermal performance. (These materials cannot be baked out at temperatures much above 125 °C.)

Vacuum-jacketed lines may be terminated by insertion probes, bayonets, and field joints. Vacuum-jacketed insertion probes (frequently of a U tube configuration) are typically used to transfer cryogens to or from small Dewars and cryostats. They consist of an elongated section of small diameter stainless steel tube that fits into the neck of the supply or receiving container. Sealing of the probe is done in a warm area of the vacuum jacket with an elastomer compression fitting. The preferred configuration of the

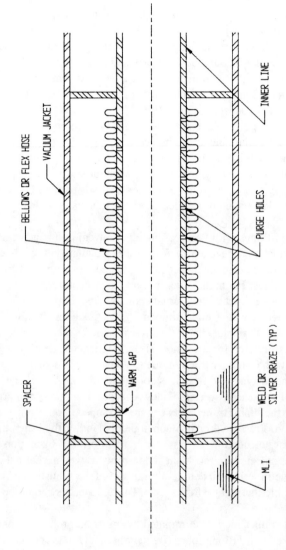

Figure 5-4 Internal expansion joint.

BELLOWS OR FLEX HOSE

VACUUM JACKET

INNER LINE

PURGE HOLES

SPACER

WARM GAP

WELD OR
SILVER BRAZE (TYP)

MLI

274

probe-receiving vessel is to locate a ball valve below the elastomer compression fitting. The ball valve allows the probe to pass when it is in the open position but maintains a gas-tight seal when closed after the probe is removed.

Bayonets are the most widely used method of low-heat-leak connection between VJ line sections and with liquid cryogen supply sources or receivers. As shown in Fig. 5-5, a bayonet pair consists of an interrupted cryogen line, two thermal isolation tubes, warm seal flanges incorporated into the vacuum jacket, and, in some designs, a cold nose seal. In concept, liquid cryogen flows through the inner line with minor impact where the line is interrupted. The male and female isolator tubes establish a thermal gradient to the warm flange with stratified gas in the annular space, which results in heat leak small enough to keep the O-ring from freezing. (One might ask, What could be simpler?) Actually, bayonets do perform substantially as described if they are oriented no more than 45° from vertical with the female half down, pressure is less than 400 to 500 kPa (60 to 75 psia), and the pressure is not pulsing.

Special design treatment is required to handle nonideal conditions. In particular, if the bayonet pair is oriented horizontally (*never* orient the male bayonet with its warm end down), gas in the annular space between the bayonets will not stratify but will, instead, set up a free-convection pattern. This will freeze the sealing O-ring and cause the bayonet joint to fail. A reasonably successful solution to this problem is to fabricate the bayonet pair so that the annular clearance is small enough, 0.02 to 0.05 mm, to inhibit free convection. Even bayonets of this design sometimes fail at higher pressure, especially when it is unsteady or pulsing. A backup for this problem is to design the bayonet flanges for high clamping forces and to use metal O-rings or other seals that can withstand low temperatures. In light of the preceding discussion, cold nose seals appear to have little redeeming value. They impede thorough purging of the transfer line system and contribute little to restraining free convection in the annular space between the isolator tubes.

Finally, for permanent VJ line installations, field joints are recommended. They combine the advantages of factory assembly of the major portion of each line and eliminate the functional problems of bayonets. Negatives include the necessity for field connections and the generally lower level of vacuum in the field joint volume. As shown in Fig. 5-6, the typical field joint includes a socket weld on the cryogen line between two factory-fabricated sections, insertion of a prepumped getter bag on the cold joint after leak testing, fitting of prepared insulation batts, positioning and welding of the VJ sleeve, and evacuation, which may include activation or insertion of hydrogen getter material. Heat leak of well-designed field joints is less than equivalent bayonet pairs, and fluid flow characteristics should be the same as other welded pipes.

Aside from the fundamental problems with bayonets, poor vacuum is the largest source of transfer line trouble. This stems from poor manufacturing vacuum technology in many cases and from inconvenient transfer line vacuum configuration. Consider that the typical transfer line has a high ratio of surface area to volume and a long pumping path with poor conductance, is filled with MLI that cannot properly be baked out, and is evacuated through a low-conductance valve and pumping line. Once these problems are recognized, positive actions can be taken to produce lines that maintain a good static vacuum for a period of several years. These actions should include the following:

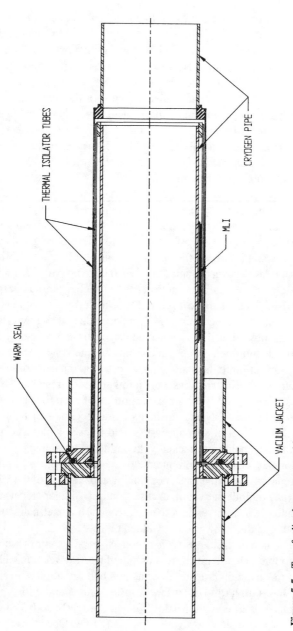

Figure 5-5 Transfer line bayonet assembly.

276

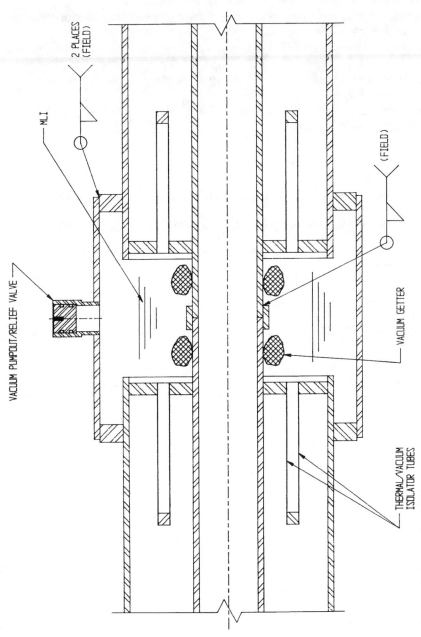

Figure 5-6 Transfer line field joint.

VACUUM PUMPOUT/RELIEF VALVE

MLI

2 PLACES (FIELD)

(FIELD)

VACUUM GETTER

THERMAL/VACUUM ISOLATOR TUBES

1. Use pumpout valves and lines with adequate vacuum conductance.
2. Throughout the pumping cycle, heat the inside and outside of the line to the highest temperature tolerated by the MLI and spacers (perhaps 125 °C).
3. Speed evacuation by periodically and slowly breaking the vacuum back to dry nitrogen gas to accelerate moisture removal.
4. Do not stop pumping until the liquid nitrogen cold trap shows no sign of ice or frost when taken apart for inspection and cleaning.
5. Pump the line to a dynamic vacuum in the 10^{-5} torr range or lower and a 1-hour hot static vacuum of no more than 10^{-3} torr.
6. Make sure that the cold and warm getters are sized for a 5-year life and that they are properly activated if required.

REFERENCES

1. *1995 ASME Boiler and Pressure Vessel Code*, Section VIII, Division 1 (New York: American Society for Mechanical Engineers, 1995),
2. Reed, R. P., and Clark, A. F., *Materials at Low Temperatures* (Metals Park, Ohio: American Society for Metals, 1983).
3. Takeno, M., Nishijima, S., and Okada, T., "Thermal and Mechanical Properties of Advanced Composite Materials," *Adv. Cryog. Eng.* 32 (1986):4.
4. Hopkins, R. A., and Payne, D. A., "Thermal Performance of the Cosmic Background Explorer Superfluid Helium Dewar, as Built and With Improved Support System," *Adv. Cryog. Eng.* 33 (1988):
5. Weitzel, D. H., Robbins, R. F., Bopp, G. R., and Bjorklund, W. R., "Elastomers for Static Seals at Cryogenic Temperatures," *Adv. Cryog. Eng.* 6 (1961):
6. Niemann, R. C., Gonczy, J. D., and Mataya, K. F., "An Epoxy Fiberglass Tension Member Support for Superconducting Magnets," *Adv. Cryog. Eng.* 24 (1978):
7. Holben, C. D., U. S. Patent 3,217,920 (1965).
8. HEPAK, Cryodata, Inc., Niwot, Colorado.
9. Kropschot, R., Birmingham, B., and Mann, D., *Technology of Liquid Helium*, U.S. Department of Commerce, National Bureau of Standards Monograph 111 (Washington, D.C.: U.S. Government Printing Office, 1968).

REFRIGERANTS FOR NORMAL REFRIGERATION

W. E. Kraus and M. Kauschke

Technische Universität Dresden, 01062 Dresden, Germany

6-1 INTRODUCTION

In the last few years, the public attention has turned to the field of normal refrigeration as a result of new discoveries about the environmental impact of the refrigerants currently in use. Normal refrigeration covers the fields of air conditioning, food preservation, and industrial refrigeration. For these applications, the temperature ranges from about 10 to $-100\,°C$ and in some cases down to $-180\,°C$ (cascade systems). This conventional usage is often realized by vapor compression systems.

In this chapter, we talk about refrigerants as the working fluid used in vapor compression refrigerating machines (VCRM). Generally, the name *refrigerant* is applied to all refrigerating systems or heat pumps. We want to distinguish clearly between refrigerants and cryogenic fluids. Table 6-1 compares the boiling points of refrigerants and cryogenic fluids.

6-2 CLASSIFICATION OF REFRIGERANTS

From the chemical point of view, the refrigerants that we treat in this chapter, can be divided into the following different groups:

1. Inorganic compounds
2. Halocarbon compounds
3. Hydrocarbons

6-2-1 General

Each of these substances is characterized by its molecular compound (formula, name) and also by a specific refrigerant number (R . . .). These numbers are generally used and

Table 6-1 Comparison of normal refrigerants and cryogenic fluid boiling points

Fluid	NBP[a] temperature, °C (range approximate)
Refrigerants (VCRM)	
Usual cycles	30[b] to −60
Cascade, second stage	−55 to −105
Cascade, third stage	−95 to −165
Cryogenic fluids	−160 to −269

[a] NBP-normal boiling point (101.3 kPa).
[b] An exception occurs with water at 100 °C

administrated by an American Society of Heating, Refrigerating and Air Conditioning Engineers (ASHRAE) committee.

For the chlorine–fluorine derivatives of hydrocarbons, the halogenated hydrocarbons, and the hydrocarbons from methane to propane, these numbers come with the structural formula in a special pattern. In Table 6-2 these assignments are given for 34 substances. A more detailed outline is contained in Refs. [1–3].

In order to cover all refrigerants with this nomenclature, some additional sets are designated.

6-2-2 Isomers

A small-letter suffix (a, b, ...) marks different isomers. For example, tetrafluoroethane:

$$C_2H_2F_4 \begin{cases} CHF_2CHF_2 & R134 \\ CF_3CH_2F & R134a \end{cases}$$

Two letters are used for propane derivatives, where the first letter characterizes the middle group: $c\text{-}CF_2$, $e\text{-}CHF$, $f\text{-}CH_2$. For example,

R245ca	$CHF_2\text{--}CF_2\text{--}CH_2F$
R245cb	$CF_3\text{--}CF_2\text{--}CH_3$
R245ea	$CHF_2\text{--}CHF\text{--}CHF_2$
R245eb	$CF_3\text{--}CHF\text{--}CH_2F$
R245fa	$CF_3\text{--}CH_2\text{--}CHF_2$

6-2-3 R4XX: Refrigerant Mixtures (Blends)

The current numbering indicates the components or single-fluid refrigerants that form the mixture.

For examples,

R404:	R125/R143a/R134a
R407:	R32/R125/R134a
R410:	R32/R125

Table 6-2 Thermophysical data of common refrigerants

Refrigerant number	Chemical formula	Molecular mass (kg/kmol)	Freezing point (°C)	Normal boiling point			Critical data		
				t (°C)	ρ^a (kg/m³)	r^b (kJ/kg)	t_c (°C)	p_c (MPa)	ρ_c (kg/m³)
R717	NH₃	17.03	−77.7	−33.3	682	1369	132.3	11.34	234
R718	H₂O	18.02	0.0	100.0	985.3	2258	374.4	22.12	314
R744	CO₂	44.01	−56.6	−78.5ᶜ	1563ᶜ	573.1ᶜ	31.05	7.38	465
R11	CCl₃F	137.38	−111	23.7	1479	182.2	198.0	4.40	554
R12	CCl₂F₂	120.91	−158	−29.8	1486	166.0	112.0	4.12	558
R13	CClF₃	104.46	−181	−81.4	1522	150	28.8	3.87	578
R13B1	CBrF₃	148.92	−168	−57.8	1992	118.2	67.0	3.97	745
R14	CF₄	88.01	−183.4	−128.0	1603	135.7	−45.7	3.74	630
R22	CHClF₂	86.47	−160	−40.8	1412	234.5	96.1	4.98	515
R23	CHF₃	70.01	−155	−82.1	1460	240	26	4.85	527
R32	CH₂F₂	52.02	−136	−51.8	1215	383	78.4	5.83	430
R116	C₂F₆	138.01	−100	−78.2	1605	117	19.7	2.98	610
R123	C₂HCl₂F₃	152.92	−107	27.6	1455	170	183.8	3.67	550
R124	C₂HClF₄	136.48	−200	−12.1	1474	163.1	122.5	3.64	554
R125	C₂HF₅	120.03	−103	−48.2	1516	165	66.3	3.63	572
R134a	C₂H₂F₄	102.03	−101	−26.1	1378	217	101.1	4.06	512
R141b	C₂H₃Cl₂F	116.95	−103.5	32.1	1220	225	208.4	4.55	464
R142b	C₂H₃ClF₂	100.50	−131	−9.2	1195	221	137.1	4.25	435
R143a	C₂H₃F₃	84.04	−111	−47.6	1166	230	73.1	3.76	434
R152a	C₂H₄F₂	66.05	−117	−24.7	1011	325	113.5	4.49	365
R218	C₃F₈	188.02	−150	−36.7	1603	104	71.9	2.68	629
R227ea	C₃HF₇	170.03	−131	−16.5	1535	131.8	101.8	2.93	582
R500	−	99.30	−159	−33.5	1332	201.3	105.5	4.43	497
R502	−	111.63	−160	−45.5	1481	172.6	82.2	4.07	561
R503	−	87.24	−160	−88	1474	180	19.4	4.34	562
R507	−	98.96	−118	−46.7	1326	200.1	70.9	3.79	500
R508A	−	100.10	−	−85.7	1556	163.1	23	4.06	565
R50	CH₄	16.04	−182.5	−161.5	423	510	−82.6	4.60	162
R170	C₂H₆	30.07	−183	−88.6	545	490	32.2	4.90	250
R290	C₃H₈	44.10	−188	−42	582	430	96.7	4.25	220
R600	n-C₄H₁₀	58.12	−138.5	−0.5	602	385	152.0	3.80	228
R600a	i-C₄H₁₀	58.12	−159.5	−11.8	595	367	135.0	3.65	222
R1150	C₂H₄	28.05	−170	−103.7	569	482	9.4	5.05	215
R1270	C₃H₆	42.08	−185	−47.7	611	439	91.7	4.60	225

ᵃ Saturated liquid density.
ᵇ Latent heat of vaporization.
ᶜ Sublimation.

In Tables 6-3 and 6-4, the capital letter suffix stands for a specified proportion of the components. The order of the components obeys the order of the temperature of the normal boiling point. The ratios in the tables are mass ratios.

Refrigerant mixtures are normally designed as substitute candidates because the CFC and HCFC phaseout has caused a lack of suitable single-fluid refrigerants. For practical uses, refrigerant mixtures should behave nearly as pure substances to be handled

Table 6-3 Examples of three-component refrigerant mixtures

	R32	R125	R134a	NBP/temperature glide
R407A	20%	40%	40%	$-45.6\,°C/6.6\,K$
R407B	10%	70%	20%	$-47.4\,°C/4.4\,K$
R407C	23%	25%	52%	$-44.0\,°C/7.2\,K$
R407D	15%	15%	70%	$-39.3\,°C \approx 6.5\,K$

and thought of in the traditional manner. The characteristic differences are shown in Fig. 6-1.

In refrigeration, the normal mixture (as opposed to azeotropes) are called *zeotropic mixtures*. For easy handling, a narrow boiling blend is the goal. The temperature glide in the phase transition should be less than about 10 K for a *narrow boiling mixture*. For a so-called *near-azeotropic mixture*, the temperature glide has to be less than about 1 K. Tables 6-3 and 6-4 also list the boiling temperature glides of commercial refrigerant mixtures.

6-2-4 R5XX: Azeotropic Refrigerant Mixtures

For the benefit of refrigeration applications azeotropic refrigerant mixtures have a minimum temperature at the azeotropic point combined with a maximum pressure for $T = $ constant. This is shown in Fig. 6-2. Examples of these mixtures are listed in Table 6-5. The numbers in brackets give the mass ratio of the components.

6-2-5 Butane Compounds

R600: normal butane $C_4H_{10}(CH_3CH_2CH_2CH_3)$
R600a: isobutane $C_4H_{10}(CH_3CHCH_3CH_3)$

6-2-6 R7XX: Inorganic Compounds

The last two digits represent the rounded molar mass of the compound. For example,

R717: NH_3
R718: H_2O
R744: CO_2

Table 6-4 Examples of two-component refrigerant mixtures

	R32	R125	NBP/temperature glide
R410A	50%	50%	$-51.8/0.1\,K$
R410B	45%	55%	$-51.7/0.1\,K$

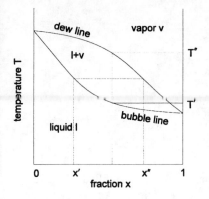

Figure 6-1 Refrigerant mixture showing temperature glide and composition difference. Temperature glide $\Delta T = T'' - T'$ for constant pressure p and constant composition x. Composition difference $\Delta x = x'' - x'$ for constant p and constant temperature T.

6-3 ENVIRONMENTAL IMPACT OF REFRIGERANTS

By the 1980s, scientists noticed the destruction of the stratospheric ozone layer, the protection shield of the Earth. This destruction is mainly caused by chlorine and bromine halocarbons. This discovery convinced the international community to ban the production, use, and trade of these chemicals in a special time schedule, which was first established in Montreal (Montreal Protocol, 1987) and concretized in following conferences. From the different atmospheric lifetime of the compounds, which may be especially high for fully halogenated compounds, and from different high ratios of chlorine, various ultimate dates for banning single components were declared. Nowadays it is common to split the halocarbons in groups and to give special abbreviations to these groups. In Table 6-6, the international agreements are presented; national regulations may be much stronger.

Besides the ozone depletion potential (ODP), some other environmental influences have to be named such as the global warming potential (GWP) and new categories like acidification potential (AP) and photochemical reactivity (PCR). Another new criterion for the valuation of refrigerants is (aquatic) ecotoxicity.

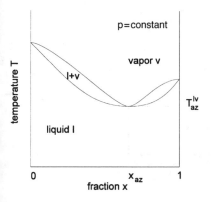

Figure 6-2 Illustration of an azeotropic mixture.

Table 6-5 Examples of azeotropic refrigerant mixtures

Refrigerant	Components	Mass ratio	NBP
R507	R125/R143a	(50/50)	−46.7 °C
R508A	R23/R116	(39/61)	−85.7 °C
R508B	R23/R116	(45/55)	−88.3 °C

6-4 SELECTION OF REFRIGERANTS

For the purpose of refrigeration, several requirements have to be fulfilled by the refrigerant that may be given by the working scheme or by the equipment of the refrigerating machine. Essential demands are as follows:

- Suitable vapor pressure–temperature behavior
- Zero ozone depletion potential
- Low global warming potential
- Nontoxicity
- Nonflammability
- Stability in the refrigerating circuit
- Compatibility with materials and lubricants
- High efficiency

Table 6-6 International regulations concerning normal refrigerants

Group	Chemistry	International regulations and remarks
CFC[a]	Fully halogenated chlorine and fluorine containing R11, 12, 13, 113, 114, 115, . . .	Banned since 1 January 1996
HCFC	Partly halogenated hydrogen, chlorine, and fluorine containing R21, 22, 123, 124, 141, 142, . . .	Banned at the latest 2030; from 2020 allowed only for maintenance work
HFC	Partly fluorinated R23, 32, 41, 125, 134, 143, 152, 227, 236, 245, . . .	Alternative refrigerants,[b]
FC (PFC)	Fully fluorinated (perfluorocarbons) R14, 116, 218, 31-10	Alternative refrigerants but high GWP

[a] Bromine is handled as chlorine. The ban is also valid for R12B1, 13B1, 114B2, etc. Also, mixtures, such as R 500(R12/152a), R502 (R22/115), and R503 (R23/R13) with these CFC compounds are banned if the ratio is higher than 1%.

[b] Note that flammability increases with decreasing GWP.

Because there is not an ideal refrigerant that fulfills all requirements, the engineer will have to choose the refrigerant that fulfills the most requirements in his special application. In Table 6-2 a summary of the main thermodynamic properties is given for some of the frequently used CFC (nowadays forbidden) and HCFC (soon to be forbidden) refrigerants, for some traditional inorganic refrigerants, and for some HFC, FC and HC representatives relevant for refrigeration. More refrigerants and their properties are introduced in the literature [4–9].

REFERENCES

1. Jungnickel, H., Agsten, R., and Kraus, W. E., *Grundlagen der Kältetechnik* (Berlin: Verlag Technik GmbH, 1990).
2. Kruse, H. et al., *Compression Cycles for Environmentally Acceptable Refrigeration, Air Conditioning and Heat Pump Systems*. (Paris: International Institute of Refrigeration, 1992).
3. *ASHRAE 1993 Handbook — Fundamentals* (Atlanta, Georgia: American Society of Heating, Refrigerating and Air Conditioning Engineers, 1993).
4. Deutscher Kälte- und Klimatechnischer Verein, *DKV-Arbeitsblätter für die Wärme- und Kältetechnik* (Heidelberg: Verlag C. F. Müller, Hüthig GmbH, 1991, currently being updated).
5. Reid, R. C., Prausnitz, J. M., and Poling, B. E., *The Properties of Gases and Liquids*, Int. ed. (New York: McGraw–Hill, 1988).
6. Japanese Association of Refrigeration, *Thermodynamic Table*, Vol. 1 (HCFCs and HFCs) (Tokyo, 1994).
7. Baehr, H. D., and Tillner-Roth, R., *Thermodynamische Eigenschaften Umweltverträglicher Kältemittel/ Thermodynamic Properties of Environmentally Acceptable Refrigerants* (Berlin and Heidelberg: Springer– Verlag, 1995).
8. Huber, M., Gallagher, J., McLinden, M., and Morrison, G., *NIST Thermodynamic Properties of Refrigerants and Refrigerant Mixtures Database (REFPROP)*, Version 5.0, Gaithersburg, Maryland: National Institute of Standards and Technology.
9. Wagner, W. et al., *Database FLUIDS* (Bochum: EMU, Ruhr Universität, 1996).
10. Cavallini, A., "CFC and HCFC Substitution," *Bull. IIR* 6 (1994):3–15.
11. Menzer, M., and Muir, E., "HCFC Substitutes: The US Experience with Air Conditioning and Refrigeration," *Bull. IIR* 3 (1996):3–12.
12. *FRIDOC—The Database of Refrigeration (Bibliographic Reference Database)*, Paris: International Institute of Refrigeration (IIR) version 5.0, 1995.

SEVEN

SMALL CRYOCOOLERS*

L. Duband and A. Ravex

Centre d'Etudes Nucleaires Grenoble, DRFMC/SBT, 17 Ave des Martyrs,
38054 Grenoble, Cédex 9, France

7-1 INTRODUCTION

Small mechanical cryocooler development has been strongly stimulated over the past years by the emergence of specific applications requiring low-temperature operation with relatively low cooling power.

Today the main applications for cryocoolers are

- Cryopumping for high and clean vacuum (semiconductor industry, space simulation chambers, particle accelerators).
- Cooling of detectors (for example, infrared detectors for Earth observation, night vision, and missile guidance as well as gamma ray detectors and bolometers for astrophysics).
- Cooling of electronic components (cold amplifiers) or of devices including Superconducting materials (SQUID, Josephson junctions, high-field magnets).
- Cooling of samples for physicists.
- Cooling of radiation thermal shields and recondensation of boil-off in cryogenic liquid storage tanks or large superconducting magnet cryostats for magnetic resonance imaging.

The typical cooling powers of the small cryocoolers devoted to these applications range from a few tenths of a watt at 4 K or less to about a few tens of watts at 80 K or more. These heat loads are small compared with the large duties required for industrial gas

---

*The majority of this work was previously published in *The Handbook of Applied Superconductivity*, Bernd Seeber, ed. (Bristol (UK) and Philadelphia: IOP Publishing, 1998). Used with permission.

liquefaction plants, which have driven the development of large refrigerators or liquefiers based on the Linde–Hampson or Claude processes. Large cold piston or centrifugal expanders are commonly used in the Brayton cycles (Claude processes) to achieve a good thermodynamical efficiency by isentropic expansion of the cycle fluid with external work extraction. These expanders undergo a drastic efficiency decrease when miniaturized. Thus, the small mechanical cryocoolers are developed on the basis of other cycles such as the Stirling, Ericsson (also known as Gifford–McMahon), Joule–Thomson, and, more recently, pulse-tube cycles that do not involve such isentropic expanders.

The thermodynamics of these cycles, their practical operation, their main applications, and present and future developments are discussed in the following sections.

7-2 THERMODYNAMIC CONSIDERATIONS OF CRYOCOOLERS

The purpose of a refrigerator is to extract an amount of heat Q_c at a cold temperature T_c. This heat load Q_c has two contributions: the intrinsic inefficiency of the refrigerator and either a parasitic heat input (conduction through mechanical structures, convection due to residual gas, thermal radiation from surrounding warm surfaces, etc.) or local heat dissipation (electronics, AC losses in a superconductor, etc.).

Thermodynamics tells us that for such an operation, some mechanical work W_c has to be transmitted to a fluid following a closed cycle during which the heat load Q_c is removed at the cold sink temperature T_c, and an amount of heat $Q_a = (Q_c + W_c)$ is dissipated at ambient temperature T_a to the surroundings.

The efficiency or the energy cost for this operation is commonly measured either by the coefficient of performance (COP $= Q_c/W_c$) or by the specific energy consumption (W_c/Q_c), which depends on the effective cycle followed by the fluid.

7-2-1 Theoretical Reversible Cycles

The maximum value of the COP is obtained in a reversible cycle such as the Carnot cycle, which is represented ($1 \rightarrow 2 \rightarrow 3 \rightarrow 4$) on a temperature–entropy (T–S) diagram in Fig. 7-1. In this cycle the heat transfers between the cycle fluid and the heat sinks at T_c and T_a are assumed to be reversible and isothermal. The compression and expansion of the fluid are supposed to be reversible and adiabatic (i.e., isentropic) transformations.

In the T–S diagram, the reversible specific heat exchanges ($q = \int T \, dS$) are represented by the area under the lines figuring the evolution of the fluid. For a reversible cyclic operation, the specific work w is represented by the area inside the closed loop of the cycle on the T–S diagram. Thus, the maximum COP of a refrigerator operating in a reversible way between heat sinks at temperatures T_c and T_a can be written as

$$\mathrm{COP}_{\mathrm{max}} = \frac{T_c}{T_a - T_c} \tag{7-1}$$

Typical values for the maximum achievable COP are given in Table 7-1 for cold sink temperatures corresponding approximately to the liquid nitrogen, hydrogen, or helium boiling temperatures under normal atmospheric pressure (1 atmosphere).

**Table 7-1 Maximum coefficient of
performance (COP) for reversible cycles
operating between cold temperature T_c
and ambient temperature ($T_a = 300$ K)**

T_c	80 K	20 K	4 K
COP_{max}	0.364	0.071	0.014

For mechanical coolers designed to operate at a cryogenic temperature ($T_c < 100$ K), it is practically impossible for them to operate following a Carnot cycle. In fact, the required pressure ratio would widely exceed the present technological and mechanical limitations in compressor technology. As shown in Fig. 7-2, some modifications of the basic Carnot cycle allow us to overcome these limitations and yet keep the COP of the cycle equal to that of a Carnot cycle, as described hereafter.

To bring the high pressure (point 4 on Fig. 7-1 for a Carnot cycle) back to a reasonable value, the isentropic compression and expansion in the Carnot cycle are substituted either by reversible isochoric evolution (Stirling cycle: $1 \rightarrow 2 \rightarrow 3' \rightarrow 4'$) or by reversible isobaric evolution (Ericsson cycle: $1 \rightarrow 2 \rightarrow 3'' \rightarrow 4''$).

It is obvious, in Fig. 7-2, that these new cycles allow the extraction at the cold sink T_c of the same amount of heat $\int_1^2 T\,dS =$ (area under the $1 \rightarrow 2$ line) as the original Carnot cycle with also the same mechanical work requirement (the area of the parallelepipeds representing the various cycles remains constant). Thus, these new cycles may theoretically obtain the maximum COP if reversible operation is achieved.

However, a new feature characterizes these cycles. During either the isochoric (Stirling) or the isobaric processes (Ericsson) a heat transfer at variable temperature between the fluid and the surroundings is required. This heat transfer ($\int T\,dS$) is represented on the T–S diagram in Fig. 7-2 by the area under the lines $2 \rightarrow 3'$ or $3''$ and $4'$ or $4'' \rightarrow 1$. The heat transfer corresponds to the variation of the energy of the fluid when it is transferred back and forth between the heat sinks at the temperatures T_a and T_c where

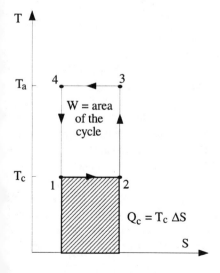

Figure 7-1 Carnot cycle (T–S diagram).

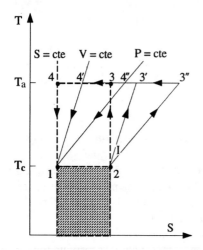

1-2-3-4: Carnot (isothermal–insentropic)
1-2-3'-4': Stirling (isothermal–isochoric)
1-2-3"-4": Ericsson (isothermal–isobaric)

Figure 7-2 Carnot, Stirling, and Ericsson cycles (T–S diagram).

isothermal heat exchange is accomplished. For a perfect gas we have

$$dh = c_p \qquad dT = T\,dS + v\,dP \quad \text{and} \quad du = c_v \qquad dT = T\,dS - P\,dv \qquad (7\text{-}2)$$

where u, h, S, and v are, respectively, the internal energy, enthalpy, entropy, and volume and c_p and c_v the isobaric and isochoric specific heat.

Consequently, we can write

$$\text{for an isobaric process } (dP = 0) \qquad \frac{dT}{T} = \frac{dS}{c_p} \qquad (7\text{-}3)$$

and

$$\text{for an isochoric process } (dv = 0) \qquad \frac{dT}{T} = -\frac{dS}{c_v} \qquad (7\text{-}4)$$

From these relations we deduce that in the T–S diagram the isobaric lines and the isochoric lines for a perfect gas are parallel lines with respective slopes T/c_p and T/c_v. This means that the amounts of heat transferred during the $2 \rightarrow 3'$ or $3''$ and $4'$ or $4'' \rightarrow 1$ processes, which are represented in the T–S diagram by $\int_2^{3' \text{ or } 3''} T\,dS$ and $\int_{4' \text{ or } 4''}^1 T\,dS$, are equal in magnitude and of opposite sign. Practically, when developing a cooler based either on the Stirling or Ericsson cycle, it will be possible to use either a counterflow heat exchanger (in the case of a continuous flow refrigerator) or a regenerator (in the case of an alternate flow refrigerator) to directly (counterflow heat exchanger) or indirectly (regenerator) exchange the energy between the fluid flowing from ambient temperature to low temperature and the fluid flowing back in the opposite direction.

The development of the small mechanical cryocoolers has been mainly based on the technology of the regenerative heat exchangers. These regenerators are generally constituted by a porous matrix (metal wire mesh or spheres) that acts like a thermal sponge by alternately storing or rejecting heat.

Gifford–McMahon-type cryocooler. A Gifford–McMahon (G–M) cryocooler is designed to allow the gas to follow an isobaric–isothermal Ericsson cycle. The high- and low-pressure sides of a compressor, in which the gas undergoes an isothermal compression, are alternately connected via an inlet and an outlet valve to a cylinder in which a displacer containing the regenerator can be moved. The valves[1] operation is synchronized with the position of the displacer, as shown schematically in Fig. 7-3, and the process theoretically operates as follows:

- Phase (1): The displacer is at its lowest position, the outlet valve is closed, and the inlet valve is opened. The high-pressure gas fills the regenerator and the space above the displacer at room temperature.

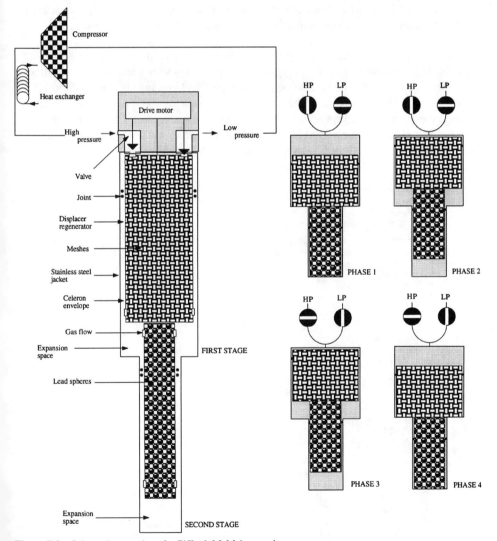

Figure 7-3 Schematic operation of a Gifford–McMahon cooler.

- Phase (2): The inlet valve is still open, and the displacer moves to its upper position. The high-pressure gas passes through the regenerator, is cooled down isobarically by the matrix, and fills the space below the displacer at low temperature.
- Phase (3): The displacer is at its upper position, the inlet valve is closed, and the outlet valve is opened. The gas in the regenerator and in the cold space undergoes expansion; the cooling effect achieved can be used for refrigeration theoretically assumed to occur at constant temperature.
- Phase (4): The outlet valve is still open, and the displacer moves back to its lowest position. The low-pressure gas passes through the regenerator, is warmed up isobarically by the matrix, and fills the space above the displacer at room temperature.

A heat exchanger at the exhaust of the compressor is used to reject heat at the ambient temperature and theoretically to achieve an isothermal compression.

Stirling-type cryocooler. A Stirling cryocooler is designed to allow the gas to follow an isochoric–isothermal cycle. A typical arrangement is shown in Fig. 7-4. A cylinder contains two pistons. The volume between the pistons (working volume) is divided into two parts by the regenerator. The compression piston can be moved in the compression volume, which is kept at ambient temperature by means of a heat exchanger; the expansion piston can be moved in the expansion volume, which remains at the cooling temperature. The ideal Stirling cycle can be described as follows:

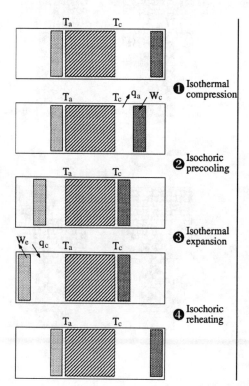

Figure 7-4 Schematic operation of a Stirling cooler.

- Phase (1)—Isothermal Compression: The expansion piston is kept close to the regenerator. The compression piston is moved to compress the gas isothermally in the compression volume. The compression work w_c is transmitted to the gas, and heat q_a is rejected at ambient temperature.
- Phase (2)—Isochoric Precooling: Both pistons are now moved simultaneously to transfer the compressed gas at constant volume through the regenerator from the compression volume to the expansion volume. The gas is cooled from the ambient temperature to the cooling temperature, transferring heat to the regenerator matrix.
- Phase (3)—Isothermal Expansion: The compression piston is kept close to the regenerator. The expansion piston is moved to expand the gas in the expansion volume. The expansion work w_e is extracted from the gas. The cooling effect q_c theoretically assumed to occur at constant temperature can be used for refrigeration.
- Phase (4)—Isochoric Reheating: Both pistons are now moved simultaneously to transfer the expanded gas at constant volume through the regenerator from the expansion volume back to the compression volume. The gas is heated from the cooling temperature to the ambient temperature. The heat transferred from the regenerator matrix to the gas theoretically equals the heat previously transferred from the gas to the regenerator.

7-2-2 Joule–Thomson Expansion

The expansion of a previously compressed gas through a calibrated orifice or an adjustable valve without heat (q) or work (w) exchange with the surroundings is an isenthalpic process. This results from the first principle of thermodynamics for an open system:

$$\Delta h = w + q = 0 \qquad (7\text{-}5)$$

Such an isenthalpic expansion process is referred as a Joule–Thomson (J–T) expansion.

From a basic expression for the enthalpy variation

$$dh = c_p\,dT + \left[v - T\left(\frac{\partial v}{\partial T}\right)_P \right] dP \qquad (7\text{-}6)$$

where c_p is the specific heat at constant pressure of the gas and v its specific volume, we can determine the ratio of the temperature variation (δT) to the pressure drop (δP) during a J–T expansion. This ratio is known as the Joule–Thomson effect coefficient μ

$$\mu = \left(\frac{\partial T}{\partial P}\right)_h = \frac{1}{c_p}\left[v - T\left(\frac{\partial v}{\partial T}\right)_P \right] \qquad (7\text{-}7)$$

Note that for an ideal gas we have a specific equation of state: $Pv = rT$. Thus, we can write $(\partial v/\partial T)_p = v/T$, and we get $\mu = 0$.

There is no temperature variation associated with an isenthalpic expansion for an ideal gas. On the contrary, for a real gas, the J–T coefficient μ can either be negative or positive. This fact is illustrated in Fig. 7-5 in which constant enthalpy lines for nonideal gas conditions are represented in a temperature versus pressure diagram.

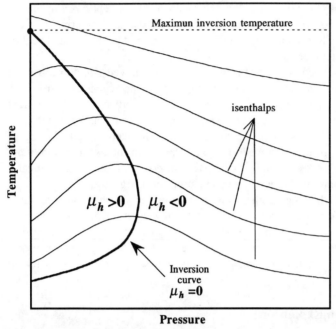

Figure 7-5 Joule–Thomson expansion inversion curve.

The full line, referred to as the inversion curve, corresponds to the condition $\mu = 0$. For an isenthalpic expansion, a cooling effect ($\mu > 0$) is observed inside the inversion curve, and a heating effect ($\mu < 0$) is noted outside. A temperature can also be defined above which no cooling effect can be achieved by any isenthalpic expansion. This temperature, referred as the maximum inversion temperature, is represented by a broken line in Fig. 7-5. Table 7-2 gives the maximum inversion temperatures for some cryogenic fluids.

The isenthalpic J–T expansion is basically an irreversible process, and therefore the associated theoretical COP is poor. Nevertheless this expansion is commonly used for cooling because of its simplicity and its capability for miniaturization owing to the absence of a need for any moving part at low temperature.

The representation of a typical refrigeration cycle, including a J–T. expansion process, is shown on a $T–S$ diagram in Fig. 7-6. The high-pressure gas is precooled ($1 \rightarrow 2$) by the low-pressure gas ($4 \rightarrow 5$) in a counterflow heat exchanger. If the counterflow heat exchanger is properly sized, the isenthalpic expansion of the precooled high-pressure gas leads to a two-phase mixture of liquid (3) in equilibrium with its vapor at the low

Table 7-2 Maximum Joule–Thomson inversion temperature for different cryogenic fluids

	Oxygen	Argon	Nitrogen	Air	Neon	Hydrogen	Helium
$T_{inversion}$ (K)	761	794	621	603	250	205	40

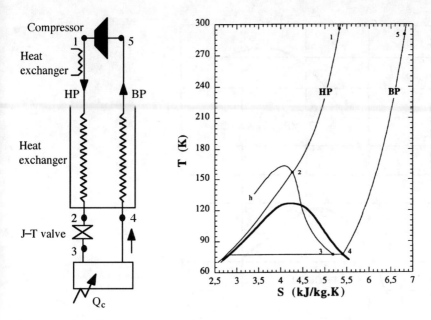

Figure 7-6 Joule–Thomson cycle (T–S diagram).

pressure. Thus, the cooling temperature T_c is determined by the low-pressure value (boiling temperature of the cycle fluid under the cycle low pressure). The heat load is removed at constant temperature (T_c) by evaporation of the liquid fraction in the mixture ($3 \rightarrow 4$).

If the counterflow heat exchanger operation is adiabatic, it can easily be shown that the specific cooling power ($q_c = \dot{Q}_c/\dot{m}$, where $\dot{m}$ is the fluid mass flow rate and $\dot{Q}_c$ the cooling power) is given by the specific enthalpy difference between the high- and low-pressure gas at the warm end of the heat exchanger ($q_c = h_1 - h_5$). For a perfect heat exchanger there is no temperature difference between the high- and low-pressure gas at the warm end (T_a). Then the maximum specific cooling power is available and is equal to the isothermal enthalpy variation:

$$q_{c.\mathrm{max}} = (\Delta h)_{T_a} \tag{7-8}$$

For a given low pressure (which is often the atmospheric pressure), the maximal specific cooling power is a function of the high pressure, and there is an optimal value for this high pressure that maximizes the specific cooling power. Figure 7-7 shows the variation of the specific cooling power with the high pressure for nitrogen and argon, which are commonly used for cooling around 80 K.

7-3 INEFFICIENCIES AND PARASITIC LOSSES IN REAL CRYOCOOLERS

Real cryocoolers operate practically in a markedly different way from the ideal description given in the previous section, and the resulting performances are strongly

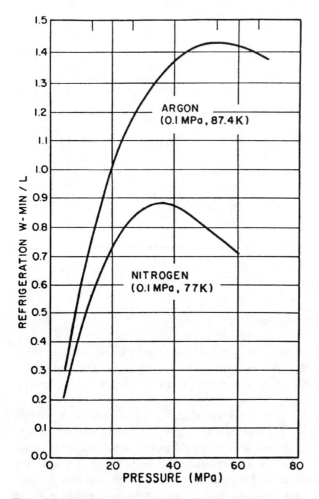

Figure 7-7 Joule–Thomson specific cooling power for nitrogen and argon.

degraded. Some of the reasons for inefficiency or parasitic losses are briefly discussed hereafter.

7-3-1 Piston Motion

In the ideal Stirling cycle description given in section 7-2-1 the compression and expansion piston motions are discontinuous to achieve a truly isochoric gas transfer between the compression and the expansion volumes. In practical Stirling cryocoolers these pistons move with continuous quasisinusoidal motions, the expansion piston leading the compression piston by a phase angle generally about 90° to approximate the theoretical figure. The resulting overlap in the motion of the compression and expansion pistons induces a deformation of the ideal work diagram and a loss in efficiency.

7-3-2 Dead Volumes

In the ideal regenerator cycles the gas is assumed to be totally expelled from the cold volume and the regenerator when it undergoes compression. In practice, the existing dead volumes waste part of the compression work. The reduction of void volumes is thus important but is practically restricted because, in the heat exchangers and regenerators, there is a competition between the efficiency of heat transfer and a low-pressure drop constraint. A similar parasitic effect occurs during the expansion process.

7-3-3 Pressure Drop

The pressure drop in the regenerator matrix and heat exchangers induces a reduction of the amplitude of the pressure variation in the expansion space compared with the pressure variation in the compression space, resulting in a decrease of the specific refrigeration effect and in a relative increase of the compression work.

7-3-4 Nonisothermal Operation

In the ideal regenerative cycles, reversible isothermal compression and expansion processes are assumed. In the real machines, large variations of the gas temperature are observed either in the compression or in the expansion volume owing to the limited surface area for heat transfer, resulting in a significant efficiency loss. When it is technically possible, heat exchangers are introduced on both sides of the regenerator to improve the heat transfer between the cycle working gas and the ambient or cold heat sinks.

7-3-5 Regenerator or Counterflow Heat Exchanger Inefficiency

In a regenerative cycle, the thermal efficiency of the regenerator is of major importance. This efficiency can be defined in a rough estimate as $\varepsilon = (T_a - T)/(T_a - T_c)$, where T_a and T_c are, respectively, the ambient and cold heat sinks temperature and T the average temperature of the gas after it has passed through the regenerator for precooling before entering the expansion volume. Thermal efficiencies larger than 0.99 are necessary to achieve reasonable overall efficiency of the cryocooler. The actual process of regenerator heating and cooling is very complicated because it involves periodic variation of the gas and matrix temperatures in space and time. A precise modeling of the regenerator operation is nevertheless necessary to obtain a realistic simulation of the regenerative cryocooler's operation for sizing and optimization. Extensive effort has been and is always devoted to theoretical analysis and numerical simulation of regenerators. Extensive information on cryocooler theoretical analysis and computer simulation status are given in two specialized books [1,2].

Similarly, for cycles based on the Joule–Thomson expansion, the efficiency of the counterflow heat exchanger is critical. For miniature J–T cryocoolers the heat exchanger is usually made of a cupro–nickel capillary tube, with copper fins soldered to its outside, wound around a cylindrical mandrel and inserted in a stainless steel or glass sheath (i.e., internal well of a Dewar). The compressed gas flows inside the coiled capillary tube. The expanded gas flows transversely over the coiled finned tube in the annular gap between the mandrel and the outer sheath. Such a heat exchanger is shown in Fig. 7-9 in section 7-4-1. The modeling and heat transfer analysis of this type of heat exchanger have been studied and compared with experience by Geist and Lashmet [3].

7-3-6 Thermal Losses

Thermal conduction along the walls of the regenerator sleeve, the expansion cylinder, or both, and through the porous matrix of the regenerator reduces the net cooling power of any practical cryocooler. To minimize these losses, a high-strength and low-thermal-conductivity material (such as stainless steel or titanium) is used for the cylinder walls. Epoxy–fiberglass material or plastic materials with low thermal conductivity are often used for the regenerator sleeve. The regenerator matrix itself is generally made from stacks of metallic wire mesh or balls. The axial heat conduction from one disk or ball to another is negligible compared with the radial heat conduction along the wire or in the ball.

Parasitic convective heat transfer is generally eliminated by using cryocoolers in high-vacuum Dewars. The radiative heat transfer from all surrounding surfaces at higher temperature than the cold heat sink temperature can be minimized by properly controlling the reflectivity and the emissivity (polishing, gold or silver coating) of these surfaces or by incorporating multilayer insulation (MLI) such as aluminized Mylar or Kapton sheets acting as thermal radiation screens between the cold and the warm surfaces.

For Stirling and G–M cryocoolers, specific thermal losses are linked to their dynamic operation. A temperature gradient exists along the cylinder and the expansion piston (or displacer) walls between the ambient and the cold tip temperature. When the expansion piston (or displacer) is moving in the cylinder, large differences in the temperature of the stationary surface may occur, resulting in a heat transfer from the ambient side to the cold tip. This process, generally called shuttle heat transfer, can be limited by reducing the stroke of the expansion piston.

Additional heat loss may occur from the gas mass flow circulating in the annular dead volume between the expansion piston and the cylinder wall.

7-3-7 Conclusion

Owing to various irreversibilities and parasitic losses occurring in real cryocoolers, their actual efficiency is quite far from the theoretical figure. To illustrate this point we report in Fig. 7-8 the result of a comprehensive compilation made at the National Bureau of Standards [4] about the performances of over 100 cryocoolers. The efficiency, in terms of percentage of Carnot value (actual COP/Carnot COP), is given as a function of the cooling capacity for various types of cryocoolers at various cooling temperatures.

For small cryocoolers (cooling capacity <100 W) we note that the actual COP ranges from 1 to 10% of the theoretical Carnot COP.

Another reference is given by the measured performances of the most efficient Stirling cryocoolers that have recently been developed for space application. Typically, for a cooling power of a few watts at 80 K, the specific energy consumption is about 30 W of electrical input power per watt of cooling power (about 10% of the Carnot COP).

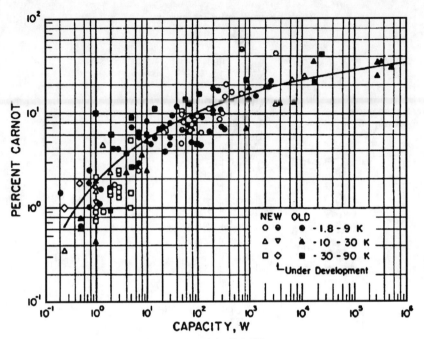

Figure 7-8 Actual efficiency of cryocoolers (from Ref. [4]).

7-4 CRYOCOOLERS: APPLICATIONS AND STATE OF THE ART

7-4-1 Joule–Thomson Expansion Cryocoolers

Miniature cryocoolers employing Joule–Thomson (i.e., isenthalpic) expansion have been developed in the mid-1950s almost simultaneously by Hymatic Engineering Company in England and Air Products, Inc., in the United States.

A well-established market for these coolers is the military infrared missile guidance systems that require cooling capacities of a few hundreds of milliwatts at liquid nitrogen temperature (about 80 K). Joule–Thomson expansion cryocoolers have been preferred for this application because of their capability for miniaturization, ability to withstand large accelerations (no moving part), and rapid cool-down times (few seconds). In these applications they are used in an open-cycle mode. High-pressure gas is supplied from a storage reservoir (rechargeable, if necessary, if subsequent cool-downs are expected).

A typical miniature J–T expansion cryocooler is represented in Fig. 7-9. The finned-type counterflow heat exchanger wound around an insulating mandrel is introduced in an evacuated Dewar.

High-purity compressed gas (air, nitrogen, or argon) is required for operation to avoid plugging of the expansion orifice by condensation of contaminants such as water, carbon dioxide, or hydrocarbons. A microporous filter is incorporated at the inlet to remove solid particles. After precooling by the low-pressure return flow in the counterflow heat exchanger, the high-pressure gas is expanded isenthalpically in an expansion orifice.

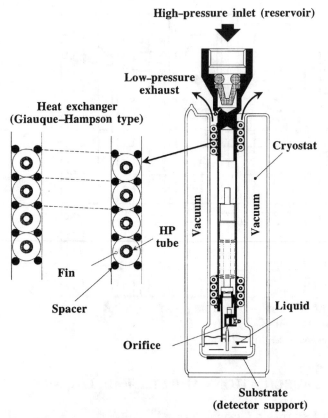

High–pressure inlet (reservoir)

Low-pressure exhaust

Heat exchanger (Giauque–Hampson type)

Cryostat

Vacuum

Vacuum

HP tube

Fin

Spacer

Liquid

Orifice

Substrate (detector support)

Figure 7-9   Schematic of a Joule–Thomson cooler.

The liquid–vapor mixture obtained after expansion is collected in a separation chamber on the bottom of which is attached the infrared detector to be cooled.

Two different types of expansion devices are commonly used. The simplest system is a fixed-area orifice that has the main advantage of being easy and cheap to manufacture. However, a fixed-area expansion orifice has a major disadvantage: the mass flow rate through the orifice increases continuously as the temperature decreases (because gas density increases and viscosities decrease). If the orifice is sized for high mass flow rate at room temperature to ensure a quick cool-down time, the mass flow rate at operating conditions will be largely excessive. On the other hand, if the orifice is sized for the proper mass flow rate at nominal operating conditions, the cool-down time will be very long owing to a very low mass flow rate at room temperature. To overcome these difficulties, variable area, temperature-sensitive expansion devices have been developed. A schematic of such a system is represented in Fig. 7-9. The area of the expansion orifice is adjusted by moving a needle in or out of it. The motion of the needle is controlled by a metallic bellow to which it is attached. The pressure inside the bellows is the J–T cooler's low pressure. A gas charge in a chamber surrounding the bellows squeezes it. The pressure in this chamber is controlled by a vapor pressure thermometer with its bulb immersed in the expanded gas. Thus, as the temperature of the expanded gas decreases, the pressure in the chamber and the force acting on the bellows decrease, allowing the needle to enter into the orifice and cause a mass flow rate reduction. In this way, an automatic control is achieved allowing for a maximum mass flow rate during cool-down and an adjusted mass flow rate at nominal operating condition to compensate the heat load strictly.

Open-cycle systems do not require any power input, and generally the low-pressure gas is directly vented to the atmosphere. They are well adapted to man-handleable and restricted space applications. Typical miniature J–T systems are shown in Fig. 7-10.

For some applications such as electronics cooling, continuous operation is required. In this case, a closed-cycle-type operation may be achieved by connecting a compressor to the J–T expansion unit. These compressors are sophisticated devices because the compression ratios involved are large (200 to 400:1). To minimize the work of compression and achieve a quasi-isothermal operation, multistaged reciprocating compressors with intercooling are generally used. A major problem is gas cleaning to remove any contaminant after compression. Such a compressor is shown in Fig. 7-11.

Microminiature J–T cryocoolers of small cooling capacity (less than 100 mW at 80 K) using photolithographic processes to etch the counterflow heat exchanger on a flat glass plate and a fine capillary for gas expansion, have also been developed by Little [5]. Capable of rapid cool-down because of their small mass, they are well adapted for laboratory study on superconductors or semiconductors.

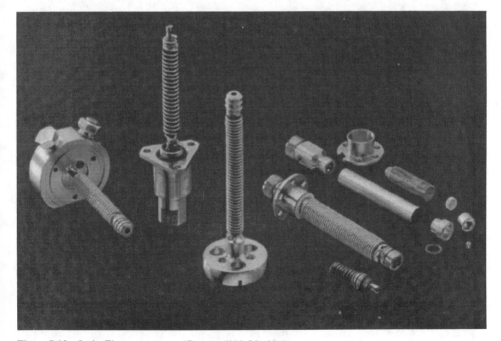

Figure 7-10   Joule–Thomson system. (Courtesy l'Air Liquide.)

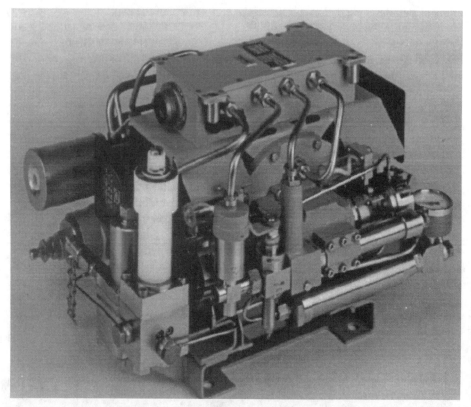

Figure 7-11 Multistaged compressor for Joule–Thomson cooler. (Courtesy Cryotechnologies S.A.)

7-4-2 Gifford–McMahon Cryocoolers

Cryocoolers intended to follow an Ericsson cycle (isobaric–isothermal) were invented and patented at the end of the nineteenth century by Solvay (with a fixed regenerator and expansion piston for work extraction) and Postle (displacer with integrated moving regenerator). Gifford and McMahon of A.D. Little, Inc., industrialized and commercialized this type of cryocooler in the late 1950s, which is nowadays widely produced by several companies in a large range of cooling capacities. Its success comes from a proven high reliability, minimal maintenance due to a low operating frequency (1–2 Hz), and a robust technology. Gifford–McMahon cryocoolers are mainly used integrated into mechanical cryopumps for applications requiring a clean and high vacuum. They are also widely used now by physicists for sample cooling in cryostats and have replaced cryogenic fluids (LN_2 or LH_2).

The high- and low-pressure levels required in the Ericsson cycle are provided by helium compressing units. These units incorporate compressors developed for domestic refrigerators, thus taking advantage of a large-scale production with resulting cost reductions. They include piston, rolling, or scroll-type compressors. The cycle gas used in these cryocoolers is helium. As a monoatomic gas, its isobaric to isochoric specific heat ratio ($\gamma = c_p/c_v = 1.67$) is larger than the one of polyatomic fluids (CFC or hydrocarbons with γ ranging between 1 and 1.3) commonly used in domestic refrigerators. Helium results in a larger temperature rise during compression. To avoid any damage to the compressor valves or any cracking of the lubricant, oil is injected in the helium at the level of the compressor suction line, then acting as a thermal moderator during compression. Most of this oil is later removed from the compressed helium by centrifugation and coalescence. The remaining traces (a few parts per million) are trapped in an activated charcoal adsorber. The compression unit is connected to the cold finger by two (high and low) pressure lines, allowing for a separation of both subsystems without any noticeable efficiency loss.

A schematic of a two-stage cryocooler cold finger with two expansion volumes providing cooling at different temperature levels is shown in Fig. 7-12. This is a common feature that does not increase the mechanical complexity of the cooler too much and improves the efficiency by reducing the temperature difference between cold and hot heat sinks for each stage. Such a cryocooler provides a first level of temperature for cryopumping applications at about 80 K useful for the cooling of baffles for water vapor condensation and thermal shielding of the second stage, which is operated at about 15 K for the cooling of activated charcoal to allow for air, hydrogen, and helium cryotrapping. Such an arrangement of a mechanical cryopump is shown in Fig. 7-13.

To operate and synchronize the valves and displacer motions properly two types of drive mechanisms are commonly used. A first mode of operation uses a mechanical drive with a crankshaft or eccentric cams, or both, kept in rotation by a motor and governing the movement of the displacer and the opening and closing of the valves.

In an alternate mode, the inlet and exhaust of the cycle gas are controlled through a rotary valve driven by a motor, as shown in Fig. 7-12. Then the mechanically driven displacer is replaced by a free displacer moved by differential pressure forces acting on a small-section extension of the displacer. The high- and low-cycle pressures alternately act on one extremity of this small section cylinder, the other extremity remaining at the mean cycle pressure, resulting in a reciprocating force on the displacer.

The forces required to move the displacer are quite small because the resistant forces acting on it are only due to the pressure drop through the regenerator and the sliding piston seal friction. The sealing is not a severe problem, for the pressure is almost the same on both sides of the displacer and the frequency of operation is low. This is a reason why maintenance is only required after about 15,000 hours of operation for the G–M cryocoolers.

The first stage regenerators (300–50 K) are commonly made of metallic wire mesh (stainless steel or bronze) with wire diameters and apertures of about 50 to 100 μm. Because the heat capacity of common materials decreases at low temperature (below 50 K), whereas the heat capacity of the cycle fluid helium increases, the efficiency of the regenerator is strongly affected. To minimize this effect, lead shots (diameter about 200 μm) are used in the second stage regenerator because lead exhibits the largest volumetric specific heat at low temperature among the common materials used. In practice,

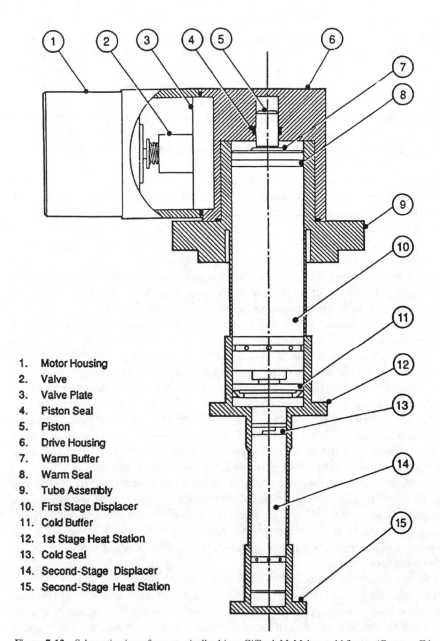

1. Motor Housing
2. Valve
3. Valve Plate
4. Piston Seal
5. Piston
6. Drive Housing
7. Warm Buffer
8. Warm Seal
9. Tube Assembly
10. First Stage Displacer
11. Cold Buffer
12. 1st Stage Heat Station
13. Cold Seal
14. Second-Stage Displacer
15. Second-Stage Heat Station

Figure 7-12 Schematic view of pneumatically driven Gifford–McMahon cold finger. (Courtesy Edwards.)

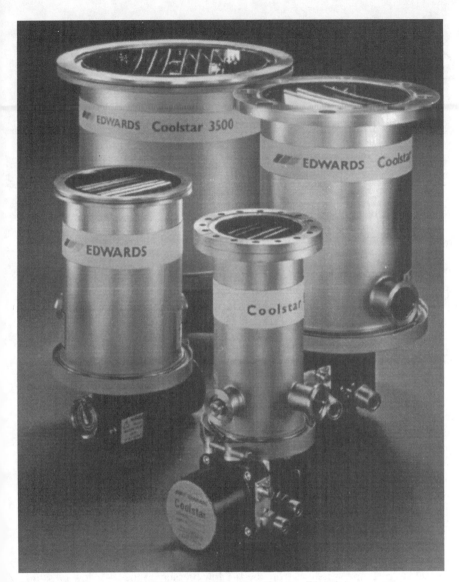

Figure 7-13 Cryopump with Gifford–McMahon cooler. (Courtesy Edwards.)

the regenerator void volumes and the material specific heat decrease result in a limitation of the useful operating temperature of G–M cryocoolers to about 10 K.

The ideal cooling power of a cryocooler is given by the integral $\int v \, dF$ calculated in the expansion volume of the cold finger. For an ideal G–M cooler we get

$$Q_F = \Delta P \times V_c \times N \tag{7-9}$$

where ΔP is the difference between the high and low pressures delivered by the compressor, V_c is the displacer swept volume, and N is the operational frequency.

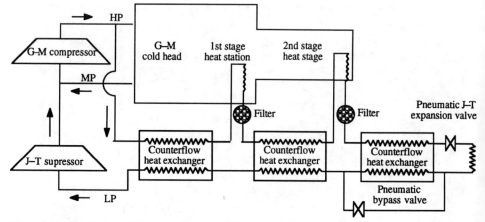

Figure 7-14 Schematic diagram of a compound Gifford–McMahon and Joule–Thomson cycle.

The principal drawback of the G–M cryocooler is its poor efficiency, for no work is actually extracted during expansion. Nevertheless, its high reliability largely outweighs this point for the practical applications for which size and efficiency are not the main points.

7-4-3 Compound Gifford–McMahon and Joule–Thomson Cryocoolers

Gifford–McMahon cryocoolers are reliable but are limited to ultimate temperatures of about 10 K. Various applications or systems such as niobium–titanium superconducting magnets or bolometers and Josephson junctions for detectors still require cooling at liquid helium temperatures. The use of pool-boiling cryostats for such applications may be constraining and expensive for long-term operation. To provide mechanical cooling and avoid any cryogenic fluid refilling and consumption at 4 K, it has been suggested to combine a G–M cooler and a J–T expander.

A schematic diagram of such a compound cycle is given in Fig. 7-14.

The two-staged G–M cryocooler is used for the precooling of the high-pressure helium gas in the J–T loop. The J–T counterflow heat exchangers are inserted between the G–M precooling stations. Part of the high-pressure helium mass flow rate from the G–M cooler compressor is diverted to the J–T loop. An additional compressor is then incorporated to recompress helium from the J–T low pressure to the G–M low pressure.

Several systems based on this technology have been developed at CEA/SBT [6,7] with cooling powers ranging from 100 mW at 2.8 K up to 5 W at 4.5 K. Specific pneumatic valves have been incorporated in the process for automatic cool-down (bypass of the low-temperature counterflow heat exchanger during initial cooling down to 15 K) and automatic temperature control (see Fig. 7-15). The J–T low pressure is used to control the opening of the J–T expansion valve, resulting in a temperature stability of a few millikelvin. An appropriate control of gas purity to prevent plugging at the J–T expansion nozzle allows for long-time, trouble-free operation. A typical system is shown in Fig. 7-15.

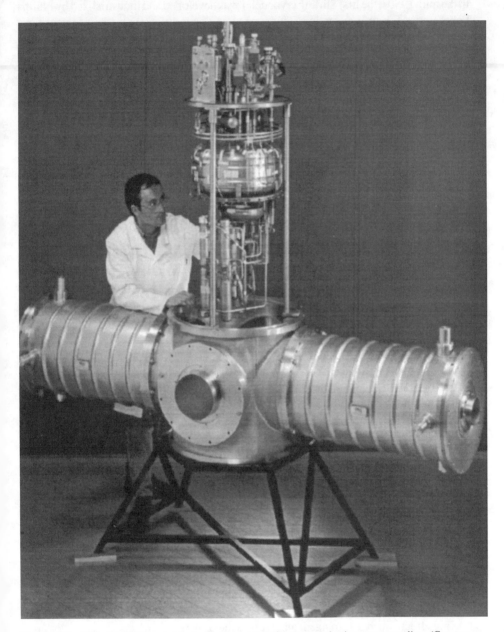

Figure 7-15   Gifford–McMahon and Joule–Thomson cooler for superconducting magnet cooling. (Courtesy CEA/SBT.)

7-4-4 Stirling Cryocoolers

In the mid-1950s, the first Stirling cryocooler was developed and industrialized by Philips Laboratories for air liquefaction. This type of engine is still commercialized nowadays as well as derived products such as two-stage versions for hydrogen liquefaction and multicylinder engines for cooling power of up to a few kilowatts

However, main developments and applications of Stirling cryocoolers are related today to the cooling of infrared detectors and associated cold electronics for night vision and missile guidance and may in the near future lead to the development of applications including high-temperature superconducting materials. For these applications, compactness and efficiency are often the more important criteria; thus the high-frequency-operated miniature Stirling coolers have emerged as the best possible compromise. The typical cooling power requirement for Stirling refrigerators is from about a quarter of a watt up to a few watts in the temperature range 50–80 K, depending on the type and size of the detector to be cooled. For this level of temperature, a single-staged cold finger is sufficient. Main development efforts are aimed to increase the lifetime and the efficiency of these coolers and to lower their size, their electromagnetic noise, and their exported vibrations. A large number of mechanical arrangements have been explored. We shall summarize in this section the main basic configurations.

A Stirling cryocooler is made of two specific elements:

- A pressure oscillator operating at ambient temperature in which a reciprocating piston transmits mechanical work to the cycle gas and generates a pressure oscillation in the refrigerator cold finger.
- A cold finger cylinder in which a displacer containing the regenerator matrix separates two volumes at ambient and cold temperature. When reciprocating in the cylinder, ideally without any work, the displacer forces the gas from one volume to the other. An appropriate phasing of the displacer motion versus the pressure oscillations generated by the oscillator provides the cooling effect.

The cooling capacity of a Stirling cooler operating with a real gas is given by $Q_c = N \int \alpha V_c \, dP$, where α is the expansivity [$\alpha = T/V(\partial V/\partial T)_P$], P the pressure in the cooler, V_c the variable expansion space, and N the frequency of operation. The development of this expression, taking into account the motion and phase shift of both the compression piston and the displacer as well as other parameters such as the cycle mean pressure and the cold tip temperature, has been discussed by Schmidt, and the main results of this analysis are reported by Walker [1].

In an *integral* cooler the pressure oscillator and the cold finger are integrated in the same casing and mechanically driven by the same crankshaft. The two cylinders are often arranged on orthogonal axes, which simplifies the achievement of the 90° phase angle between compression pistons and expansion displacer required for a maximum cooling effect. Such an arrangement is represented in Fig. 7-16.

The main advantages of the integral arrangement are the mechanical control of both piston and expander stroke and phase and the minimization of the connecting dead volume between the pressure oscillator and the cold finger. A disadvantage is that it is

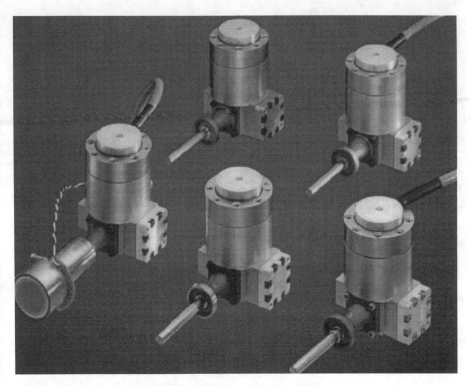

Figure 7-16   An integral-type Stirling cooler. (Courtesy l'Air Liquide.)

very difficult to cancel or at least damp the mechanical vibrations generated by the piston motion and directly transmitted to the tip of the cold finger.

In a *split* arrangement the pressure oscillator and the cold finger are completely independent and connected by a small internal diameter tube. A *split* Stirling cooler is shown in Fig. 7-17. What results from this arrangement is a larger flexibility in the integration of the cooler to the system. It should not be forgotten that the connecting line acts like a dead volume and may reduce the efficiency of the cooler.

Conventional *split* Stirling pressure oscillators are of *rotary* design: the rotor of a brushless motor is directly coupled to a crankshaft coupling mechanism connected to the compression piston. To avoid cycle gas contamination by oil lubrication, sealed ball bearings or dry-rubbing materials are used for the shaft mounting. A component of the force acting on the piston pushes the piston against the cylinder wall, resulting in a friction and wear that limits the life of the oscillator (typically a few thousand hours).

Linear drive systems are widely developed today. In this new arrangement, piston side forces are eliminated, and consequently, rubbing seals have been replaced by clearance seals, resulting in a significant increase of the mean time before failure. Moreover, the use of twin pistons operated in opposition leads to a very significant reduction of induced vibrations. The moving piston is submitted on one side to the cycle pressure oscillations and on its opposite side to the mean cycle pressure, resulting in a gas

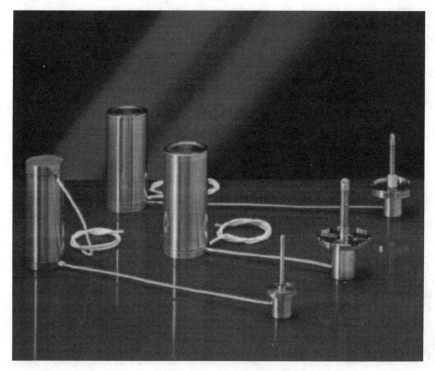

Figure 7-17 A linear split-type Stirling cooler. (Courtesy Cryotechnologies S.A.)

spring-like force acting on it. To minimize the axial force to be delivered by the linear motor, the pressure oscillators are thus operated at the resonance frequency resulting from the inertia and gas-spring mutual compensation (this frequency is typically a few tens of hertz).

In the *split* arrangement there is no more mechanical mechanism to control the stroke of the cold finger displacer and its phase relationship with the oscillator piston. It is obvious for cost reasons (excepted for space applications) that a specific motorization of the displacer with phase control cannot be considered. The motion of the displacer is then obtained by pneumatic means, as shown by the schematic diagram of a cold finger in Fig. 7-18.

Owing to the pressure oscillations generated by the pressure oscillator, a periodic force acts on the displacer (mean pressure in the buffer volume and oscillating pressure in the expansion volume) and drives its reciprocating motion. The frictional damping (rubbing or clearance seal) generates the appropriate phase shift for effective cooling. The main problem associated with pneumatically driven displacers is the variation in time of the damping force, resulting in long-term performance degradation.

For space applications (Earth observation) specific technologies for long-life Stirling coolers have been developed. To avoid any wear, frictionless operation is achieved by clearance sealing and contactless bearings. Prototypes using active magnetic bearings, hydrodynamic gas bearings [8], or flexure bearings have been designed and developed.

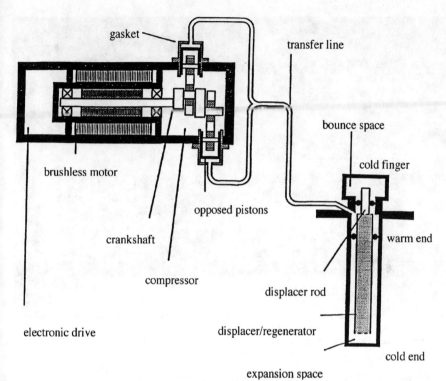

gasket

transfer line

bounce space

cold finger

brushless motor

opposed pistons

warm end

crankshaft

compressor

displacer rod

electronic drive

displacer/regenerator

cold end

expansion space

Figure 7-18   Schematic view of a pneumatically driven Stirling cold finger.

A photo of the linear Stirling cryocooler developed by Jewell et al. at RAL [9] and industrialized and space-qualified by Matra Marconi Space (previously BAe) is given in Fig. 7-19. Both the pressure oscillator and the expansion displacer are driven by a loudspeaker-type linear motor. The phase between both piston and displacer motions is measured by position transducers and electronically controlled. In its latest version, this cooler is capable of about 2 W of cooling power at 80 K with about 60 W of electrical input power to the pressure oscillator. Double-staged versions of this cooler as well as a compound two-stage Stirling and J–T expansion loop system are under development [10].

A summary of different cryocooler types and their relative merits is given in Table 7.3.

7-5 FUTURE TRENDS IN CRYOCOOLER DEVELOPMENT

Cryocoolers are nowadays used in appreciable numbers for various applications. To promote a larger diffusion, strong development efforts are being undertaken mainly to improve their reliability, efficiency, and capability for significant cooling power at low temperature (i.e., liquid helium temperature). The recent results obtained in these developments, which probably prefigure the future trends in cryocooler technology, are reported hereafter.

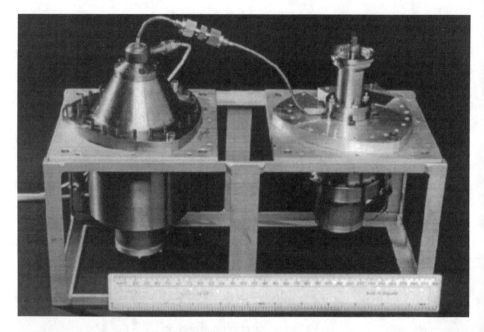

Figure 7-19 Flexure bearing Stirling cooler for space application. (Courtesy RAL.)

7-5-1 Magnetic Materials for Regenerators

The ultimate temperature achievable by G–M or Stirling cryocoolers is limited to about 10 K by the large inefficiency of the regeneration process when temperature decreases. The main reasons for this efficiency drop are the increasing mass of gas kept and cyclically pressurized and expanded in the void volume of the regenerator porous matrix and the volumetric specific heat diminution of most of the commonly used metallic materials for regeneration while the volumetric specific heat of the helium cycle gas increases. The volumetric specific heat of some usual materials for regenerators is reported in Fig. 7-20.

New geometries of regenerators based on perforated thermally conductive plates stacking with thermally insulating spacers are under validation. They will allow for low void volume fractions, moderate pressure drops, and large heat transfers at low temperature.

A way to cope with the helium gas specific heat enhancement is to use materials exhibiting a comparable specific heat anomaly. This is the case in the temperature range of interest (4 to 15 K) of several rare-earth-based materials that undergo a magnetic ordering. Several compounds have been suggested, and their volumetric specific heats have been experimentally determined. Among them, Er_3Ni appears as a good compromise with well-adapted specific heat (see Fig. 7-20), chemical stability, insensitivity to oxidation, and the capability to be prepared in the form of spheres.

Results on two-staged G–M coolers using Er_3Ni spheres in the second regenerator instead of (or in association with) lead shots and achieving ultimate temperatures as

Table 7-3 Summary of cryocooler types

Cooler type	Temperature range	Cooling power range	Advantages	Disadvantages
Joule–Thomson expansion (open cycle)	300 → 80 K	100 mW/1W	Simple, compact, no moving parts	Poor efficiency, limited autonomy (one shot), susceptibility to gas purity
Gifford–McMahon	300 → 30 K 300 → 6 K	5 W/200 W 1 W/20 W	Simple, robust, reliable	Poor efficiency, induced vibrations
Single stage/two stages				
Gifford–McMahon and Joule–Thomson	300 → 2.5 K	100 mW/5 W	Extend the temperature range of the G–M cooler	Poor efficiency, induced vibrations, susceptibility to gas purity
Stirling	300 → 50 K	100 mW/5 W	Compact, good efficiency	Sensitivity to mechanical load on the cold finger, induced vibrations
Pulse-tube	May replace G–M and Stirling	Coolers in the near future	Compact, robust, no moving parts, reliable	Efficiency may be slightly lower than Stirling
Adsorption cooler	≈100 → 0.1 K	μW/few W	Compact, no moving parts, "unlimited" lifetime, fully passive	Limited autonomy, poor efficiency

low as 3 K with cooling power at 4.2 K of a few hundreds milliwatt have recently been published [11]. The long-term mechanical integrity of this brittle material nevertheless remains to be proven. Gifford–McMahon coolers including magnetic material in the regenerator will probably compete in the near future with compound G–M and J–T coolers for 4-K cooling.

Additional information on magnetic materials for cryocoolers may be found in chapter 2 of this handbook.

7-5-2 Gas Mixtures for Joule–Thomson Expansion Coolers

The technological simplicity, reliability, capability for miniaturization, and temperature stability are some qualities of the J–T coolers operated in open-cycle mode that explain their wide use for infrared detectors (night vision, missile guidance) and electronics

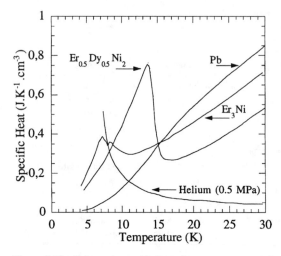

Figure 7-20 Volumetric specific heat of regenerator materials.

cooling. On the other hand, the efficiency of closed-cycle J–T systems in the 80-K temperature range is poor owing to their low specific cooling power and the high pressure required for optimal operation (several hundreds of atmospheres) with a single gas (nitrogen, air, or argon). However, large improvements in specific cooling power and efficiency can be achieved by the use of mixtures of gases as proposed by Alfeev [12]. More recently, at MMR Technologies, Inc., and at CEA/SBT, these results have been confirmed, and analysis of the thermodynamic properties of these mixtures has been performed for performance optimization. Suitable mixtures containing nitrogen and hydrocarbons provide at 80 K, with pressures of the order of 30 bars, the same specific cooling power as pure nitrogen under 150 bars. This reduction in operating pressure allows for large improvements in efficiency and for the use of less sophisticated compressors. Recently, a prototype of a J–T cooler, operated with a Gifford–McMahon-like helium compressor using a gas mixture and capable of 10 W of cooling at 95 K, has been developed by Air Products. Future developments will probably give rise to a new generation of closed-cycle J–T coolers using gas mixtures in the 80-K temperature range.

7-5-3 Pulse-Tube Refrigerators

Miniature Stirling coolers are widely used for fractional watt cooling when miniature size, weight, and high efficiency are required. Nevertheless, the technological complexity of the cold finger, including a moving displacer–regenerator with clearance seal and pneumatic drive, is a limitation to the reliability and ease of integration of these coolers. A new concept of cooler is emerging that allows for the design of a cold finger with no moving part: the pulse tube cooler.

In 1963 Gifford and Longsworth [13] published results concerning a pulse-tube cooler (generally referred to as the basic pulse tube) with no moving part in which a cooling effect was achieved by surface heat pumping. This heat transfer mode is

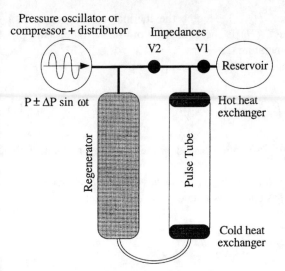

Pressure oscillator or
compressor + distributor

Impedances
V2   V1

Reservoir

$P \pm \Delta P \sin \omega t$

Regenerator

Pulse Tube

Hot heat
exchanger

Cold heat
exchanger

Figure 7-21   Schematic of a pulse-tube cooler.

restricted to low-frequency operation by the gas thermal diffusivity and results in a poor efficiency, only allowing attainment of ultimate temperatures of about 150 K. Owing to this performance limitation, the basic pulse tube has not been further developed. Later on, Mikulin et al. [14] and Zhu et al. [15] proposed new concepts respectively known as orifice and double inlet pulse tubes.

Ultimate temperatures of about 80 and 40 K, respectively, have been achieved by these authors. A schematic of the various arrangements for pulse tubes (basic, orifice, double inlet) is presented in Fig. 7-21. The pulse tube refrigerator consists of two components :

- A subsystem for pressure wave generation. It can be either a pressure oscillator (as in a Stirling cooler) or a compressor associated with a rotating valve distributor (as in a G–M cooler).
- A set of two tubes. The first one is a traditional regenerator connected at its cold end to a second tube: a simple hollow tube. At its ambient temperature end this tube is connected through a flow impedance (needle valve, calibrated orifice, or capillary) to a buffer volume.

The analysis of the heat transfer (enthalpy flow) in the orifice pulse tube arrangement has been proposed by Radebaugh and Storch [16].

The pulse tube refrigerator can be compared with a Stirling cooler. The pressure oscillator generates adiabatic oscillations of the gas in the tube.

If no disturbance (i.e., turbulence) occurs in the hollow tube, a piston-like motion of the gas is achieved. The enthalpy flow in the tube is described in the following paragraphs.

From the energy conservation equation in the adiabatic tube we get

$$\langle \dot{Q}_c \rangle + \langle \dot{Q}_{loss} \rangle = \langle \dot{H} \rangle = \langle \dot{Q}_a \rangle \qquad (7\text{-}10)$$

where $\langle \dot{Q}_c \rangle$ is the cooling power, $\langle \dot{Q}_{loss} \rangle$ denotes the thermal losses (regenerator inefficiency and conduction losses), $\langle \dot{H} \rangle$ is the enthalpy flow in the tube, and $\langle \dot{Q}_a \rangle$ is the heat rejected at ambient temperature.

At any point in the tube we can calculate the enthalpy flow by

$$\langle \dot{H} \rangle = \frac{c_p}{\tau} \int_0^\tau \dot{m} T \, dt \tag{7-11}$$

where τ is the duration of a pressure oscillation period, $\dot{m}$ the mass flow rate, and T the temperature.

From the conservation of mass ($\dot{m} = \rho S u$, with ρ = gas density, S = tube section, u = gas velocity) and the perfect gas equation of state ($\rho = \frac{P}{RT}$) we get

$$\langle \dot{H} \rangle = \frac{c_p S}{RT} \int_0^\tau u P \, dt \tag{7-12}$$

If we assume sinusoidal variations of the pressure ($P = \bar{P} + \Delta T \sin \omega t$) and of the gas velocity ($u = u_0 \sin(\omega t - \phi)$) in the tube, we get

$$\langle \dot{H} \rangle = \frac{1}{2} \frac{c_p S}{R} u_0 \Delta P \cos \phi \tag{7-13}$$

If the proper phasing ($\phi = 0$) is achieved between the pressure wave generated by the oscillator and the gas velocity in the tube, a maximal cooling effect is obtained. In the basic pulse tube configuration the pressure and the velocity are in quadrature and consequently no enthalpy flow (i.e., cooling power) is obtained. By means of the impedance V_1 and of the buffer volume, as represented in Fig. 7-21, the phase ϕ can be properly adjusted, and a cooling effect is obtained.

Extensive work is performed on the pulse tube concept in several laboratories in the world. At CEA/SBT, for example [17], an ultimate temperature of 28 K has been obtained in a single-stage cooler. Developments for low-frequency (using a helium compressor and a rotary valve as in G–M coolers) and high-frequency (using a pressure oscillator as in Stirling coolers) systems are in progress. Performances and efficiencies comparable to Stirling (1–10 W at 80 K) or G–M (100 W at 80 K) coolers have been demonstrated. Multistage systems with magnetic material regenerators are under development for low-temperature cooling ($T < 4$ K).

The technological simplicity of the pulse tube cold finger results in a large reliability and ease of integration. Moreover, the absence of any moving piston and motorization strongly reduces the vibrations and electromagnetic noise exported to the cold tip. Some pulse-tube cold finger laboratory prototypes are shown in Fig. 7-22.

It is obvious that in the near future pulse coolers will strongly compete with traditional G–M, Stirling, and J–T coolers in a large range of temperatures and cooling powers.

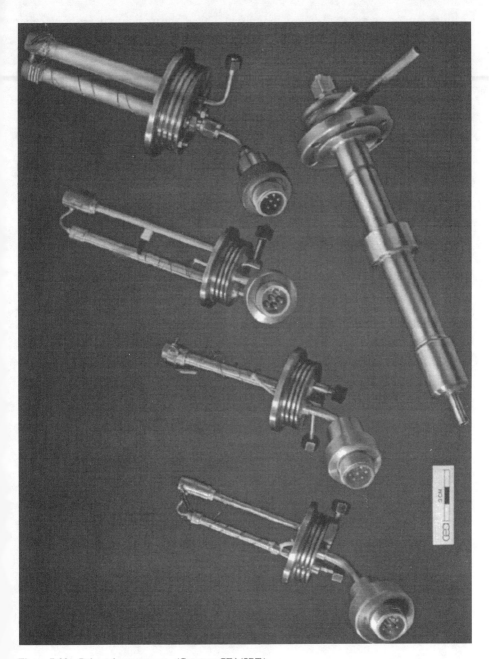

Figure 7-22   Pulse-tube prototypes. (Courtesy CEA/SBT.)

7-5-4 Adsorption Coolers

Adsorption coolers are at the edge of the present subject, and we briefly describe hereafter the basic principle along with an example of application. These systems rely on the capability of porous materials, when cyclically cooled or heated, to adsorb or release a gas. With a few exceptions their range of interest remains below 10 K. This is due in part to the fact that to alternately heat up or cool down the element containing the porous material requires an amount of power or energy that becomes prohibitively large as the temperature increases (owing to the increase of the associated heat capacities).

One can either design a sorption compressor to drive, for example, a J–T loop or a sorption pump to pump on a liquid bath to decrease its temperature. Various prototypes have been developed for both uses. Bard et al. and Wade and Levy [18,19], who have done extensive work on the sorption compressor, have, for instance, developed a 10-K sorption cooler. This concept is based on sequentially heating beds containing metal hydride powders to circulate hydrogen as the refrigerant fluid in a closed-cycle J–T refrigeration system.

Duband et al. [20] have developed various self-contained helium sorption coolers for laboratory uses and space applications. In these sealed systems, initially described by Torre and Chanin [21], a sorption pump holding activated charcoal is heated to release the adsorbed gas until the pressure is sufficient to condense liquid; then the sorption pump is cooled down to readsorb gas and pump on the liquid helium bath to decrease its temperature. For example, Fig. 7-23 shows the ^{3}He adsorption cooler designed to cool

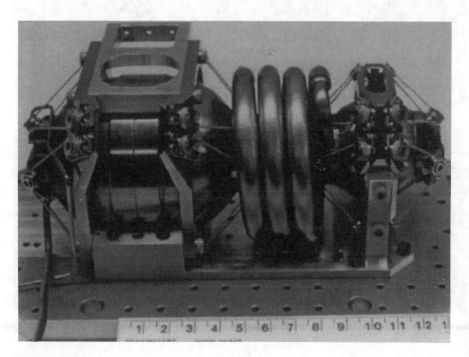

Figure 7-23 Infrared telescope ^{3}He adsorption cooler.

Table 7-4 Questionnaire for the selection of a cryocooler

Question
• Temperature range
• Cooling power range
• Electrical input power availble
• Thermal environment
• Cooldown time
• Continuous cooling
• If above is no, autonomy
• Temperature stability
• Other cryogenic source available for precooling
• Various levels of temperature (one-, two-stage machine, etc.)
• Orientation
• Sensitivity to exported vibrations of operating cooler
• Sensitivity to EMC
• Any requirements on materials (nonmagnetic, etc.)
• Any specific mechanical aspects (axial, transverse, torsional load, etc.)

down the bolometric detectors of the infrared telescope in space, which successfully flew in 1995 and provided the first subkelvin temperature on orbit, to 0.3 K.

7-6 CHOOSING A CRYOCOOLER

There is no straightforward answer to the question of how to choose a cryocooler. However, to help the potential user in his choice, we suggest filling out Table 7-4 as a guide. The answers should give a clear indication to any cryocooler manufacturer on what system best suits the user's needs.

NOMENCLATURE

C_P Constant-pressure specific heat (J/kg · K)
C_v Constant-volume specific heat (J/kg · K)
H Enthalpy (J/kg)
$\dot{m}$ Mass flow rate (kg/s)
N Frequency (Hz)
P Pressure (Pa)
Q Heat (W)
S Entropy (J/kg · K)
T Temperature (K)
V Volume (m^3)
W Work (W)
μ Joule–Thomson coefficient (K/Pa)
ρ Density (kg/m^3)

Subscripts

c   cold
a   ambient

REFERENCES

1. Walker, G., *Cryocoolers (Part 1: Fundamentals and Part 2: Applications)*, (New York: Plenum Publishing Corporation, 1983).
2. Walker, G., *Miniature Refrigerators for Cryogenic Sensors and Cold Electronics*, Monographs in Cryogenics, no. 6 (Oxford: Clarendon Press, 1989).
3. Geist, J. M., and Lashmet, P. K., "Miniature Joule Thomson Refrigeration Systems," *Adv. Cryog. Eng.* 5 (1959):324–333.
4. Strobridge, T. R., *Cryogenic Refrigerators: An Updated Survey*, U.S. Department of Commerce, NBS Technical Note no. 655 (Washington, D.C.: U.S. Government Printing Office, 1974).
5. Little, W. A., "Microminiature Refrigeration," *Rev. Sci. Instrum.* 55 (1984):661–680.
6. Poncet, J. M., Claudet, G., Lagnier, R., and Ravex, A., "Large Cooling Power Hybrid Gifford–McMahon/Joule Thomson Refrigerator and Liquefier," *Cryog.* 34 ICEC Supplement (1992):175–178.
7. Claudet, G., Lagnier, R., and Ravex, A., "Closed Cycle Liquid Helium Refrigerators," *Cryog.* 32, ICEC Supplement (1992):52–55.
8. Duband, L., Ravex, A., and Rolland, P., *Development of a Stirling Cryocooler Using Hydrodynamic Gas Bearings*, Society of Automotive Engineers, SAE Technical Paper Series 941528 (Warrendale, Pennsylvania: Society of Automotive Engineers, 1994).
9. Jewell, C., Bradshaw, T., Orlowska, A., and Jones, B., "Present Life Testing Status of 'Oxford type' Cryocoolers for Space Applications," in *Proc. 7th Int. Cryocooler Conf.*, AFB, NM 87117-5776 (Phillips Laboratory, Kirtland, 1993).
10. Orlowska, A., Bradshaw, T., and Hieatt, J., *Development Status of a 2.5–4 K Closed Cycle Cooler Suitable for Space Use*, Society of Automotive Engineers, SAE Technical Paper Series 941280 (Warrendale, Pennsylvania: Society of Automotive Engineers, 1994).
11. Hashimoto, T., Eda, T., Yabuki, M., Kuriyama, T., and Nakagome, H., "Recent Progress on Application of High Entropy Magnetic Material to the Regenerator in Helium Temperature Range," in *Proc. 7th Int. Cryocooler Conf.* (1993).
12. Alfeev, V. N., Brodyansky, V. M., Yagodin, V. M., Nicholsky, V. A., and Ivantsov, A. V., Br. Patent 1336892 (1973).
13. Gifford, W. E., and Longsworth, R. C., "Pulse Tube Refrigeration," *Trans. ASME J. Eng. Ind.* 63 (1964):264.
14. Mikulin, E. I., Tarasov, A. A., and Shkrebyonock, M. P., "Low Temperature Expansion Pulse Tubes," *Adv. Cryog. Eng.* 12 (1984):629.
15. Zhu, S., Wu, P., and Chen, Z., "A Single Stage Double Inlet Pulse Tube Refrigerator Capable of Reaching 42 K," *Cryog.* 30, ICEC Supplement (1990):257–261.
16. Radebaugh, R., and Storch, P. J., "Development and Experimental Test of an Analytical Model of the Orifice Pulse Tube Refrigerator," *Adv. Cryog. Eng.* 35 (1988):1191.
17. Ravex, A., and Rolland, P., *Status of Pulse Tube Development at CEA/SBT*, Society of Automotive Engineers, SAE Technical Paper Series 941525 (Warrendale, Pennsylvania: Society of Automotive Engineers, 1994).
18. Bard, S. et al., "Development of a Periodic 10 K Sorption Cryocooler," in *Proc. 7th Int. Cryocooler Conf.* (1993).
19. Wade, L. A., and Levy, A. R., "Sorption Cooling of Astrophysics Science Instruments," in *Proc. 30th ESLAB Symp.*, ESA SP-388 (Noordwijk, The Netherlands: ESTEC, 1996).
20. Duband, L., Lange, A., and Bock, J., "Helium Adsorption Coolers for Space," in *Proc. 30th ESLAB Symp.*, ESA SP-388 (Noordwijk, The Netherlands: ESTEC, 1996).
21. Torre, J. P., and Chanin, G., "Miniature Liquid ^{3}He Refrigerator," *Rev. Sci. Instrum.* 56 (1985):318–320.

EIGHT

SUPERCONDUCTING MAGNET TECHNOLOGY

A. Devred, H. Desportes, F. Kircher, C. Lesmond, C. Meuris, and J. M. Rey

CEA Saclay, DAPNIA/SCTM, 91191 Gif Sur Yvette Cedex, France

J. L. Duchateau

CEA Cadarache, DRFC/STID, 13108 Saint-Paul-lez-Durance Cedex, France

8-1 INTRODUCTION

The applications of superconductivity can be divided into four categories:

1. High DC or slow ramping magnets for fundamental and medical research.
2. Industrial applications with possible use in large electrical networks such as alternators, transformers, and current limiters.
3. Radio-frequency (RF) cavities (at high frequency, a superconducting material exhibits a surface resistance that is much lower than the resistance of a normal metal. Thus, using superconducting materials for RF cavities, even in continuous operation, consumes much less power than copper cavities in the pulsed mode).
4. Low-current applications for electronics, mainly Josephson junctions used for measuring very low magnetic fields (SQUIDS) and passive circuits (antennas, resonators, filters, delay lines, etc.).

Although all these applications use the general phenomenon of superconductivity, they are based on different properties of the material. Only the DC magnet technology will be covered in the following sections.

For the construction of magnets, superconducting materials have been used mainly for fundamental research (particle accelerators, fusion devices, etc.). A remarkable exception is their large development in the medical field for use in magnetic resonance imaging (MRI) scanners.

Up to now, all superconducting magnets for applications have been refrigerated with helium in liquid, gaseous, or mixed phase at very low temperature. This is because

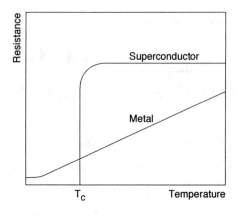

Figure 8-1 Variation of resistance with temperature.

the only materials available for these applications are the so-called low-critical-temperature superconductors in opposition to the more recent high-critical-temperature superconductors.*

After a review of the general properties of superconductors, the main elements that affect the design and construction of superconducting magnets will be considered: conceptual design, conductor and losses, cooling and thermal stability, and insulating materials and protection in case of quench (return to the resistive state). For illustration, some applications will be described at the end of the chapter.

8-2 GENERAL PROPERTIES OF SUPERCONDUCTORS

8-2-1 Critical Parameters

Critical temperature. The first property of a superconducting material, that its electrical resistance falls abruptly to zero under a temperature T_c called the critical temperature, was discovered by Kammerlingh Onnes in 1911. This phenomenon is completely different from the behavior of a normal conductor, even a very pure one, for which the decrease of resistance with temperature is smooth and never reaches a zero value (Fig. 8-1).

Critical magnetic field[†] and critical current density. After the discovery of this property, it was found that a superconducting material also has a critical magnetic field B_c and a critical current density J_c. All these properties are related to each other. In a three-dimensional space (T, B, J), each superconducting material can be characterized by its critical surface (Fig. 8-2). The material is superconducting everywhere below this surface, and resistive above.

Meissner effect. The notion of critical-flux density is related to the Meissner effect, discovered in 1933, which is the absence inside a superconducting material of flux

---

*Additional information on high T_c superconductors may be found in chapter 2 of this handbook.

[†]The magnet builders often improperly use the term "magnetic field" instead of "magnetic flux density" for B.

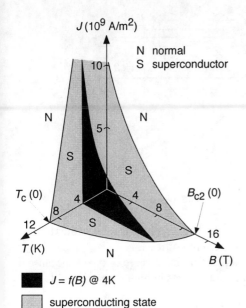

J (10^9 A/m^2)

N normal
S superconductor

Figure 8-2 Critical surface of niobium–titanium.

density, B_i, as expressed by

$$B_i = \mu_0(H_a + M) = 0 \qquad (8\text{-}1)$$

where H_a is the strength of the applied field and M is the magnetization of the material.

This exclusion is produced by superconducting currents flowing at the surface of the superconductor within a very thin depth called the penetration depth. For a superconducting material at some temperature below T_c, the critical flux density is the upper limit of the flux that can be excluded by the material.

8-2-2 Different Types of Superconductors

Type I superconductors. The full exclusion of magnetic flux is typical of so-called type I superconductors (Fig. 8-3(a)). Most of the pure metals belong to this category (Table 8-1). These have almost no practical applications for magnets owing to the very low value of their critical flux density.

Type II superconductors. A more complicated phenomenon happens in so-called type II superconductors. Two critical magnetic fields H_{c1} and H_{c2} can be defined (Fig. 8-3(b)) with the following characteristics:

- For $0 < H < H_{c1}$, there is no flux density in the superconductor; the behavior is the same as for type I superconductors.
- For $H_{c1} < H < H_{c2}$, there is a partial penetration of the flux density in the superconductor. This is called the "mixed state."
- For $H > H_{c2}$, the superconductivity disappears.

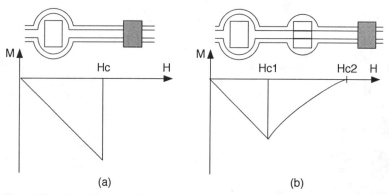

Figure 8-3 Magnetization and flux penetration for (a) type I and (b) type II superconductors.

In the "mixed state," magnetic flux penetrates the superconductor and creates normal cores in the form of tubes surrounded by supercurrent vortices.

All the superconducting materials for magnet applications are of type II because it is the only type that enables the transport of large currents in high magnetic fields.

Pinning centers. The possibility of having large transport currents in type II superconductors is due to the presence of pinning centers created by defects in the crystalline structure that are generated by sophisticated metallurgic processes. They prevent the normal tubes from moving under Lorentz forces and creating a resistance due to flux flow, which would generate power dissipation. The transport current in the superconductor can be increased up to its critical value, which is the one for which the Lorentz force equals the pinning force.

Practical superconducting materials. Among all the superconducting materials, two categories will be considered: alloys and A15 compounds.

The main critical characteristics of the most common materials are given in Table 8-2:

- Niobium titanium alloy (NbTi) and niobium tin (Nb_3Sn) have been used nearly exclusively for all existing applications, and their properties have been continuously improved over the years.
- Tantalum-doped niobium titanium (NbTiTa) and niobium aluminum (Nb_3Al) are more recent materials with enhanced properties, making them promising, but they are still under industrial development.

Table 8-1 Type I superconductors

Material	T_c (K)	$\mu_0 H_c = B_c$ @ 4.2 K (T)
Al	1.2	0.01
Sn	3.7	0.03
Pb	7.2	0.08
Hg	4.1	0.04

Table 8-2 Type II superconductors

Material	T_c(K)	$\mu_0 H_{c2} = B_{c2}$ @ 4.2 K(T)	J_c (A/mm^2) @ 4.2 K (Industrial production)
Alloys			
NbTi	9.5	11	3000 @ 5 T
NbTiTa	9	11.3	1400 @ 8 T
A15 phases			
Nb$_3$Sn	18	23	2000 @ 10 T
Nb$_3$Al	19	30	760 @ 12 T
Nb$_3$Ge	23	35	Not available

8-3 PRACTICAL SUPERCONDUCTING MATERIALS

8-3-1 Niobium Titanium

Metallurgy and superconducting properties. Niobium titanium (NbTi) is by far the most widely used superconducting material in present magnet technology. Its superconducting properties, up to 8- to 10-T magnetic field, cover most of the existing applications with high-current performances and convenient operating temperatures. Furthermore, NbTi is a ductile alloy that can be drawn fairly easily into multifilamentary composites, and its high mechanical properties enable the fabrication of solid coils resisting large magnetic forces without degradation.

The alloy composition can vary according to different optimization criteria. A maximum critical temperature of 10.1 K is reached with 25 wt % Ti, whereas the critical field is maximum at around 44 % Ti. However, the dependence of these parameters on the composition is rather weak and, for practical feasibility, the range of composition is usually chosen between 40 to 50 wt % Ti. A particular effort for enhancing the critical current performances of fine filament composites has been concentrated for many years on the Nb–46.5 wt % Ti alloy under the strong impulse of the SSC Research and Development program in the United States [1]. This special composition has therefore become the most commonly used.

An efficient way of enhancing the upper critical field is alloying the NbTi with a ternary element, mainly tantalum [2]. A tantalum content between 15 and 25% is found to increase B_{c2} by ≈ 0.3 T at 4.2 K, but more significantly by 1.3 T at 1.8 K. However, the optimization of the critical-current density appears more difficult to achieve with ternary alloys, and industrial manufacturing problems have not yet been properly solved.

Continuous progress has been made over the last three decades towards higher critical current and low AC loss performances together with cost-effective industrial production. The critical current is related to the number and to the distribution of flux pinning centers, which result, in the classical method of fabrication of multifilamentary composites, from a combination of cold work and heat treatments to produce α-Ti precipitates in defects of the lattice structure. A more recent method of manufacturing NbTi is by creating artificial pinning centers (APC) [3]. These can be obtained in different ways, such as by incorporating fine fibers of normal material in the superconductor lattice or by a "jelly-roll" technique.

Alternating current losses are decreased by reducing the size of filaments and, if necessary, by using a high resistivity matrix material, resistive barriers, or both, around the filaments. Very fine filaments, in the micrometer or submicron range, must be protected from size effects such as "sausaging" by using high-homogeneous NbTi alloy in the process and by coating the filaments with an antidiffusion barrier, usually niobium.

Practical formulas for critical parameters. Simple scaling rules can be used to predict, with reasonable accuracy over a wide range of field and temperature, the operating characteristics of a given NbTi conductor from a single-point measurement of the critical current density at a reference field and reference temperature [4]. The reference point is generally taken at the field B_{ref} of 5 T and at a temperature T_{ref} of 4.2 K.

First, a general relationship between the upper critical field B_{c2} and temperature, with no transport current, can be expressed by the following formulas, verified experimentally on a large variety of NbTi samples:

$$B_{c2}(T) = 14.5(1 - T/9.2)^{1.7} \tag{8-2}$$

or

$$T_c(B) = 9.2(1 - B/14.5)^{0.588} \tag{8-3}$$

Assuming linear relationships of J_c versus B and T around the reference point, which is also well verified over a wide range, the following expressions can be derived:

$$J_c(B, T) = J_c(B_{ref}, T)^*[B_{c2}(T) - B]/[B_{c2}(T) - B_{ref}] \tag{8-4}$$

with

$$J_c(B_{ref}, T) = J_c(B_{ref}, T_{ref})^*[T_c(B_{ref}) - T]/[T_c(B_{ref}) - T_{ref}] \tag{8-5}$$

For $B_{ref} = 5$ T and $T_{ref} = 4.2$ K, $T_c(B_{ref}) = 7.2$ K, and so

$$J_c(5, T) = J_{ref}^*[(7.2 - T)/3)] \tag{8-6}$$

Another useful quantity is the temperature margin ΔT between the operating temperature T_{op} and the current-sharing temperature T_{cs} corresponding to an operating current chosen below the critical characteristics:

$$\Delta T = T_{cs}(B) - T_{op} = [T_c(B) - T_{op}]^*[1 - J_{op}/J_c(B, T_{op})] \tag{8-7}$$

This ΔT, translated in enthalpy margin, gives a measure of the operating stability margin against thermal disturbances.

8-3-2 Niobium Tin and Niobium Aluminum

Metallurgy and superconducting properties. Niobium tin (Nb_3Sn) belongs to the family of the A15 compound superconductors characterized by the formula A_3B, where A is a transition metal and B can be either a transition or a nontransition metal. The tin atoms form a body-centered cubic sublattice with two atoms of niobium on each face of the cube. The short distance between the niobium atoms in such an arrangement, in comparison with the niobium cell element, is certainly the reason for the good superconducting properties.

The pure stoichiometric Nb_3Sn has a theoretical critical temperature of 18 K and an upper critical flux density at zero temperature of 28 T. This stoichiometric composition is giving the best superconducting properties and is stable at room temperature, which is not always the case for A15 compounds. These ideal properties are generally affected by a small deviation from the stoichiometric composition and by some kind of compression introduced inevitably during the fabrication and reaction process due to the other elements such as the copper matrix.

The critical-current density J_c is governed by grain boundaries. An increase of the pinning strength has been pointed out in relation with a decrease of the grain size.

Unlike NbTi, owing to the flux pinning mechanism, the behavior of Nb_3Sn is mainly isotropic (at least for field angles with respect to the strand axis greater than 45°).

The most effective method to enhance J_c consists of alloying with small quantities of tantalum or titanium leading to the so-called ternary Nb_3Sn. Typically, an Nb–7.5 wt % tantalum alloy is used in the bronze process. This increase is related to the increase of the normal state resistivity, which is well known to increase B_{c2}.

The application of stress in compression and in tension leads to a modification of the A15 structure with associated decrease of B_c and T_c and of course of J_c. Irreversible degradation occurs after tensile strain application greater than 0.5% on practical wires [5].

Practical data to be used for critical properties of Nb_3Sn. The formulas given below are valid for binary as well as for ternary alloys.

The critical non-copper current density J_c can be very well represented by the following laws [6]. The non-copper part of the material to be considered includes the unreacted niobium, niobium tin, the bronze, and the antidiffusion barrier generally existing to prevent the pollution of the pure copper part of the strand:

$$J_c = 1/(1/J_{c1} + 1/J_{c0}) \tag{8-8}$$

$$J_{c0} = J_0[1 - (T/T_{c0})^2] \tag{8-9}$$

$$J_{c1} = C_0[(1 - (T/T_{c0})^2]^2 B^{-0.5}(1 - B/B_{c2})^2 \tag{8-10}$$

$$B_{c2} = B_{c20}[1 - (T/T_{c0})^2][1 - T/(3T_{c0})] \tag{8-11}$$

$$B_{c20} = B_{c20m}(1 - a\varepsilon^{1.7}) \qquad T_{c0} = T_{c0m}(1 - a\varepsilon^{1.7})^{0.333} \tag{8-12}$$

The following values can be assumed for modern ternary Nb_3Sn strands:

$$J_0 = 3.354 \times 10^{10} \text{ A/m}^2 \qquad T_{c0m} = 18 \text{ K} \qquad B_{c20m} = 28 \text{ T}$$
$$a = 1250 \text{ for } \varepsilon > 0 \text{ (tensile)} \qquad a = 900 \text{ for } \varepsilon < 0 \text{ (compressive)}$$

The calibration coefficient C_0 is in the range of 10^{10} AT$^{0.5}$/m^2, typically 1.15×10^{10} for strands manufactured according to the internal tin process, leading to $J_c = 700$ A/mm^2 ($B = 12$ T, $T = 4.2$ K), and 0.9×10^{10} for the bronze process, leading to $J_c = 550$ A/mm^2 ($B = 12$ T, $T = 4.2$ K).

A typical value of -0.25% can be taken for ε for the strand due to the compressive strain induced after heat treatment by the strand matrix (copper and bronze). The critical temperature T_c in operating conditions, which is different from T_{c0}, can be numerically calculated as the one for which the critical current density under strain is equal to zero:

$$J_c(B, T_c, \varepsilon) = 0 \qquad (8\text{-}13)$$

Nb₃Sn strand. These last five years have seen considerable progress in the production of industrial Nb₃Sn wires. Fields of 13 T are needed for fusion applications, in particular for tokamaks, which necessitate large quantities of Nb₃Sn. In the frame of ITER (International Thermonuclear Experimental Reactor), a large program has been built with several Japanese, Russian, European, and American companies.

A typical Nb₃Sn strand of 0.8 mm, such as developed for ITER, consists of several thousand filaments (3–5 μm) embedded in a bronze matrix. This assembly can be constituted by single or by double stacking. The bronze matrix is separated from a pure copper shell by an antidiffusion barrier generally made of tantalum and sometimes associated with a second antidiffusion barrier made of niobium. This antidiffusion barrier is needed to prevent tin pollution of the pure stabilizing copper shell. In certain cases, islands of Nb₃Sn filaments are distributed inside the composites, each of them surrounded by the antidiffusion barrier. In most of the industrial wires, the A15 phase is produced via a solid-state reaction through a bronze matrix. There are several variants of this process. The bronze route is the oldest process. The tin is provided from a bronze matrix manufactured separately. Owing to the maximum concentration of tin (15.7 wt %) in the ductile phase of bronze, an intrinsic limitation of the current density exists. The effective filament diameters can reach low values in the range of 5 μm.

In the internal tin process, the tin diffuses from several tin cores spread out in the copper matrix, including a niobium mesh. During the first stage of the heat treatment at a temperature less than 180 °C to avoid tin melting, the bronze is formed. The main advantages of the process are an easier drawing of the wire (no bronze during this phase) and a higher concentration of tin in bronze during the heat treatment. The effective filament diameters are typically around 25 μm.

The modified jelly-roll process can be considered as a less encountered variant of the preceding one. In this process, a niobium mesh and a copper sheet are cowound around the central tin cores. The niobium mesh is torn out during the drawing process, leading to filaments that can be considered nonconnected.

Another A15 material under industrial development: Nb₃Al. In connection with the ITER program, another A15 compound is in progress. The research concerning the development of this material has been mainly concentrated at JAERI [7] and ENEA. Results given hereafter have to be taken with caution because the state of industrial development of this material is much less advanced than for Nb₃Sn.

The stoichiometric composition is metastable at room temperature and stable only at 1940 °C. The off-stoichiometric compounds generally obtained have critical properties below the theoretical values ($T_c = 18.9$ K, $B_{c2} = 32$ T).

Interest has converged on Nb₃Al owing to its better mechanical properties in comparison with Nb₃Sn. Its lower sensitivity to strain is illustrated in Fig. 8-4. The process used for the production of these strands is a jelly-roll process already mentioned for Nb₃Sn.

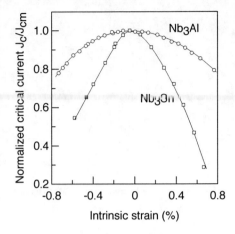

Figure 8-4 Strain effect on the critical current density of Nb_3Sn and Nb_3Al.

Modified Summers formulas of practical use have recently been given in [7] after an extensive study at different fields and temperatures. Detailed influence of strain, which has not been determined yet, has still to be introduced in the equations.

8-3-3 Conductor Assembly

Whether NbTi or Nb_3Sn is used as the basic superconductor, the elementary composite is first produced as a single wire with a number of fine filaments twisted inside a matrix of normal metal, generally pure copper. This wire, or strand, is characterized by its size, number and size of filaments, normal-to-superconductor ratio, RRR of the normal metal, and twist pitch. Its size is typically between a fraction of a millimeter and 1 or 2 mm, rarely bigger, so that its current capacity is limited to a few hundred amperes.

Such a strand can be used directly to wind coils of small size without particular constraints, but in large-scale applications and complex magnet configurations, additional requirements have to be included in the complete conductor design.

For a higher nominal current, an adequate number of strands are assembled in parallel in a fully transposed arrangement. For stability and quench protection, a specified amount of normal metal, or stabilizer, must be added to the composite. Mechanical reinforcement may also be needed. According to the type of cooling adopted in the magnet design, cooling paths, channels, or conduits must be provided in the conductor structure.

The combination of these features gives rise to a large variety of conductor configurations. Typical examples are shown in Fig. 8-5:

- Rutherford flat cables are extensively used in accelerator magnets. To reduce AC losses or coupling currents, the strands can be coated with a high-resistance metal such as Staybrite, or an insulating thin core can be inserted in the cable.
- Copper- or aluminum-clad cables are tightly assembled by a soft-soldering, rolling, or coextrusion process. High-purity aluminum is used for light weight but also offers benefits from its high electrical and thermal conductivity at low temperature.

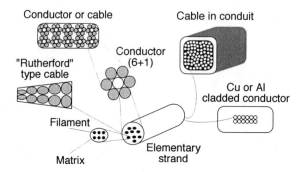

Figure 8-5 Different types of conductors. (Adapted from Tixador, P., *Les Supraconducteurs*, Paris: Hermes, 1995.)

• Cable-in-conduits are specially developed for fusion devices in which forced-flow cooling is strongly advocated in view of their severe operating constraints. The conduit can be made of high-strength material for structural reinforcement.

8-4 CONCEPTUAL DESIGN OF SUPERCONDUCTING MAGNETS

A large variety of technologies can be applied to the design of superconducting magnets to fulfill the different requirements imposed by particular applications. In each case, basic choices have to be made among various techniques according to the specifications and to relevant criteria. The general guidelines followed in a particular design are briefly reviewed.

8-4-1 User's Specifications

Magnets are generally incorporated in special and often complex experimental devices and must conform to the physical needs of the experiment. The specifications cover different aspects.

Magnetic field configuration. A large number of field shapes can be produced by different types of magnets such as solenoids, toroids, helicoids, dipoles, multipoles, Helmholtz coils, mirror coils, or any other type of field-shaped configuration.

The field extends over a specified volume or aperture at a given strength and within particular tolerances with regard to field quality such as uniformity or harmonic content.

Operating mode. Because time-varying fields are the main sources of heat generation in superconductors, the operating mode, whether purely DC or AC or pulsed, is of utmost importance for the determination of the coil characteristics. Ramp rate or cycling duty must be specified precisely, as well as field stability and low-noise requirements.

Long-term stability, as required in NMR devices, is currently achieved by persistent mode operation with the use of superconducting switches.

Environmental constraints. The experimental setup in which the magnet is integrated may impose geometrical constraints. Access to the useful field volume must be kept open in the specified aperture. The available space for the magnet is often restricted, and the boundaries and interfaces have to be well defined. Material thickness and weight may impose another limitation, for example, for radiation transparency in particle detectors or for airborne experiments.

Limitation of stray fields by magnetic shielding may be necessary, and possible interactions with other parts of the system must be identified.

8-4-2 First Design Approach

From the specifications above, a preliminary design of the magnet can be drawn based on existing experience. The first item to be determined is the winding configuration and its rough dimensions to ensure that the required field performances can be reached. At this stage, the main parameters that will guide the next design steps are estimated, such as

- The ampere-turns needed to produce the field
- The stored energy
- The peak field in the conductor region
- An estimate of the magnetic forces and of the needed mechanical structure
- The dependence of these parameters on the average current density in the winding

8-4-3 Conceptual Choices

In order to proceed with a more complete design, a number of conceptual and technical choices have to be made. These are based on the characteristics found in the preliminary design and on constraints laid in the specifications. These choices concern several areas that can be separated for the analysis but are in reality closely connected and need to be defined as a whole.

Cooling mode. The cooling mode is a major area, for it has a direct impact on other essential items such as the type of conductor, the winding structure, and the cryogenic layout.

The cooling mode can be chosen among three main techniques, depending on the coil geometry, on the operating temperature, and on the needed cooling efficiency as follows:

- Pool boiling using liquid helium storage or closed-cycle refrigeration. Helium can be pressurized or subcooled between 5 and 1.8 K (superfluid).
- Forced-flow internal cooling in a hollow or cable-in-conduit type of conductor. Helium can be two-phase or supercritical.
- Indirect cooling based on heat conduction through a compact winding from restricted cooling loops.

The three options must be compared with regard to their applicability from a structural and cryogenic point of view, depending on the configuration and constraints of the considered magnet. A major issue concerns their respective cooling efficiencies in accordance with the estimated heat generation in the winding under the specified operating conditions.

Pool boiling is probably the most efficient cooling mode, provided that cooling channels are widely distributed through the winding with part of the conductor bare and in direct contact with helium. However, this requires a solid and leak-tight helium vessel surrounding the coils, which, for large or complex systems, raises technical difficulties. Also, electrical insulation and mechanical strength of such a porous structure are rather weak and in many cases unacceptable.

Forced-flow internal cooling is also very efficient, and it permits the fabrication of solid and well-insulated coils without the need for a helium vessel. However, other difficulties appear in the fabrication of the conductor and of internal joints, and the cryogenic system becomes much more sophisticated.

Indirect cooling with restricted cooling loops separate from the conductor is the simplest scheme because it avoids the difficulties of both previous systems. However, its efficiency, in terms of stability margin, is sensibly lower, and it can only be used for reasonably low-loss magnets, which is often the case for magnets operating in a pure steady-state regime.

Stability criteria. The concept of stability refers to the ability of a superconducting magnet to operate without accidental transition to the normal state under thermal disturbances. Stability conditions are determined by a balance between the heat removal capacity of the winding and the predictable size of losses and of other possible disturbances and can be evaluated by a number of stability criteria, as explained in section 8-6. The magnet design must incorporate an adequate stability margin, which results from a combination of the cooling method and of the conductor characteristics.

Quench protection. Whatever the degree of stability provided in the design, superconducting magnets must be fully protected against an accidental quench. In such a case, the current must be discharged in a time short enough to prevent an excessive temperature rise due to Joule heating in the resistive conductor without inducing dangerous overvoltages and eventual insulation breakdowns.

Protection methods can vary considerably according to the amount of stored energy to be dumped and to the conductor rating in terms of nominal current and current density. The different methods are described in section 8-8.

Conductor characteristics. The conductor specifications combine all the conditions stated in the preceding paragraphs.

The superconducting material and the operating temperature are chosen according to the field level (peak field on the conductor). The fine structure (filament size, matrix composition, and subdivision) depends on the operating mode and particular field requirements. The nominal current and the overall current density, which are related to the content of stabilizing material, are chosen in connection with the quench protection and stability criteria. The need for structural reinforcement is related to the force containment and stress distribution. The shape and assembly of the finished conductor, integrating all the above features as well as electrical insulation and cooling provision, are determined according to the type of winding and its anticipated method of fabrication.

8-4-4 Complete Design

After the main technical features have been established, the complete design is carried out along practical engineering techniques. The design studies cover all the aspects already mentioned but in a more complete and coordinated way.

Magnetic field computations. The winding geometry has to be defined precisely to achieve the specified field performances. According to the system complexity and to the required tolerances, more or less elaborate methods of calculation are needed, from simple analytical formulas to powerful computer codes. A large number of such codes, in two and three dimensions, are available and enable the most difficult problems to be solved.

In addition to the field map in the useful volume, the field distribution through the whole winding has to be calculated, for it directly affects the operating characteristics of the superconductor to be chosen. It also provides the Lorentz force distribution in the winding, which is needed for stress analysis.

Mechanical design. Three types of forces participate in the mechanical loading of the winding structure: the weight, the thermal stresses induced by differential thermal contraction between inhomogeneous materials, and the magnetic forces. All these forces can be calculated fairly accurately and are combined for complete stress analysis and for the design of the mechanical structure.

Again, according to the system complexity, this analysis can be straightforward or may require elaborate computer codes, that exist from many other areas of science and industry. Some codes are even adapted for coupled treatment of field and forces.

Especially important for superconducting magnets is the knowledge of the fine stress distribution in the winding and in particular at the bonds between components such as conductor, insulation, and structural elements. These stresses, especially shear stresses, have to be kept below conservative ratings to prevent the occurrence of mechanical disturbances that could endanger the conductor stability, in the case of indirectly cooled impregnated windings.

Stability and quench protection. As already discussed for the choice of basic concepts, the stability behavior and the quench process have to be fully evaluated and documented in the final design. The relevant methods of analysis are presented in sections 8-6 and 8-8.

Cryostat and cryogenics. After the cold mass, which was the concern of the previous paragraphs, the design is completed with the overall cryogenic structure, including helium vessels or containers, thermal shields, vacuum vessels, supports, cold box, current leads, cryogenic lines, and instrumentation. These items make use of available technologies, as described in other chapters of this handbook.

8-5 AC LOSSES

The zero-resistance property of superconductors is only valid under DC conditions. As soon as the magnetic field is changed and penetrates the superconductor, an electrical field appears and losses are created.

We will examine here the more common situation of composites and cables submitted to transverse-varying uniform fields.

When the field is varied very slowly, only the hysteresis component of losses has to be considered. It is generated inside the superconducting filaments themselves and depends on the size and the form of these filaments.

The need simply to increase the field of DC magnets within a reasonable time and the interest in pulsed magnets have resulted in consideration of another kind of loss: the coupling current losses generated in the conducting material surrounding the filaments.

Modern composites and cables are twisted and transposed to ensure, as far as possible, an equal balance of current between the strands and to minimize these losses. Schematically, on half a twist pitch, the field variation is capable of driving a so-called coupling current between two filaments or two strands or even two bundles of strands, depending on the arrangement considered.

The tightness of the different twist pitches is one of the major parameters to keep these coupling currents at an acceptable value by decreasing the area of the loops. The smallest value is established on the basis of manufacturing considerations not to damage the assembly at a value around ten times its size.

Another way of controlling the coupling current is to choose very resistive matrixes and even to insulate the strands. On the other hand, the necessity of important quantities of pure copper to stabilize and protect the wires gives another limitation, and a kind of balance has to be found. Studies in that field are progressing to adjust and precisely control the contact resistance between the strands of a given cable to calculate the best balance.

8-5-1 Superconducting Magnetization

Introduction. Bulk type-II superconductors tend to shield their inner core from any change of amplitude or orientation of applied field by creation of magnetization currents at their periphery. The distribution of magnetization currents is such that they produce within the superconductor a magnetic flux density B_i exactly opposite to the applied magnetic flux density change ΔB_a

$$B_i + \Delta B_a = 0 \tag{8-14}$$

In the critical state model developed by Bean [8], the magnetization current density is assumed to be the superconductor critical-current density at the given field and temperature. Unlike eddy currents, magnetization currents are proportional to the amplitude of applied field change (and not to the rate of variation), and they do not decay. They are also called persistent magnetization currents.

Behavior of a superconducting filament. Let us consider a rectilinear and infinite superconducting filament carrying no transport current and initially in a virgin state, and let us vary the applied field from 0 to B_0, where B_0 is perpendicular to the filament axis.

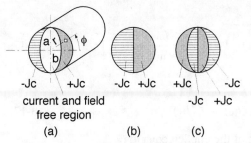

-Jc   +Jc   -Jc +Jc   +Jc   -Jc

                                              -Jc +Jc

current and field
free region

(a)   (b)   (c)

Figure 8-6   Model of persistent magnetization current shells with elliptical inner boundaries [10]: (a) up-ramp from a virgin state, (b) full penetration, and (c) down-ramp after full penetration.

Several models have been developed to determine the persistent magnetization current distribution. In the simplest ones [9,10], the magnetization currents flow in a shell at the filament periphery with an elliptical inner boundary (see Fig. 8-6(a)). As the applied field is increased, the ellipse eccentricity decreases until the magnetization currents fill up the whole filament (see Fig. 8-6(b)). The field at which this occurs is called the penetration field $B_{p,0}$ and is determined by the implicit equation

$$B_{p,0} = \frac{[2\mu_0 J_c(B_{p,0})r_f]}{\pi} \tag{8-15}$$

where μ_0 is the permeability of vacuum, J_c is the superconductor critical-current density at the given temperature, and r_f is the filament radius. If the external field is increased beyond $B_{p,0}$, the distribution of magnetization currents remains the same.

Reference [11] proposes to represent the effects of persistent magnetization currents by a magnetic moment per filament unit length, M_0, given by

$$\boldsymbol{M}_0 = -\frac{4}{3}J_c(B_0)\left[1-\left(1-\frac{B_0}{B_{p,0}}\right)^3\right]r_f^3 \boldsymbol{u} \tag{8-16a}$$

for $\boldsymbol{B}_0$, $B_0 < B_{p,0}$ and

$$\boldsymbol{M}_0 = -\frac{4}{3}J_c(B_0)r_f^3 \boldsymbol{u} \quad \text{for } \boldsymbol{B}_0, B_0 \geq B_{p,0} \tag{8-16b}$$

where B_0 is the absolute value of $\boldsymbol{B}_0$ and $\boldsymbol{u}$ is a unit vector parallel to $\boldsymbol{B}_0$. Let us now assume that, after reaching the maximum value B_0, the field is decreased from B_0 to B_1. Then, the simpler models indicate that a new shell is created at the filament periphery where the magnetization currents flow in opposite directions to the magnetization currents in the initial shell (see Fig. 8-6(c)). Hence, the distribution is constituted by the overlay of two shells: a first one created during the up-ramp from 0 to B_0 with $[-J_c(B_0)]$ magnetization currents on one side and $[+J_c(B_0)]$ magnetization currents on the other side, and a second shell created during the down-ramp from B_0 to B_1 with $[+J_c(B_0) + J_c(B_1)]$ magnetization currents on one side and $[-J_c(B_0) - J_c(B_1)]$ magnetization currents on the other side. In the more sophisticated model, the contribution to the magnetic moment per unit filament unit length of the outermost shell, $\boldsymbol{M}_1$, is estimated as

$$M_1 = \frac{4}{3}[J_c(B_0) + J_c(B_1)]\left[1 - \left(1 - \frac{B_0 - B_1}{B_0 - B_{p.1}}\right)^3\right]r_f^3 u \qquad (8\text{-}17a)$$

for $B_{p1} < B_1 < B_0$ and

$$M_1 = \frac{4}{3}[J_c(B_0) + J_c(B_1)]r_f^3 u \qquad (8\text{-}17b)$$

for $B_1 \leq B_{p.1}$ where $B_{p.1}$ is the solution of the implicit equation

$$B_0 - B_{p.1} = \frac{2\,\mu_0[J_c(B_0) + J_c(B_{p.1})]r_f}{\pi} \qquad (8\text{-}18)$$

Furthermore, the total magnetic moment per filament unit length, M_{tot}, is simply

$$M_{tot} = M_0 + M_1 \qquad (8\text{-}19)$$

If, after reaching B_1, the field is increased once again from B_1 to B_2, a third shell is created at the filament periphery with magnetization currents flowing in opposite directions to the magnetization currents of the second shell. The contribution of the third shell to the magnetic moment per filament unit length can be computed by changing the sign of Eqs. (8-17) and (8-18) and by replacing B_0 by B_1 and B_1 by B_2 in Eqs. (8-17) and (8-18), and so on.

In practice, to determine the magnetization state of a superconducting filament, it is necessary to know the history of applied field variations. Then, for each field variation, one determines the parameters of the persistent magnetization current shell that is created and sums the contributions from the various shells.

Effects of superconductor magnetization. As we have seen, magnetized filaments act as magnetic moments. In the case of superconducting magnets with stringent field-quality requirements, such as particle accelerator magnets, these magnetic moments result in undesirable field distortions that have to be corrected.

Let z_f designate the filament position in the complex plane, and let us introduce the complex magnetic moment M_{tot} defined as

$$M_{tot} = M_{tot.y} + i M_{tot.x} \qquad (8\text{-}20)$$

where $M_{tot.x}$ and $M_{tot.y}$ designate the x- and y-components of the magnetic moment vector M_{tot}.

The magnetic flux density B_{tot} produced far from a magnetized filament can be computed by representing it by a current-line doublet, which consists of a current line of intensity $(-I)$ located at z_f and a current line of intensity $(+I)$ located at $(z_f + d)$, where d is such that

$$Id = -M_{tot}^* \qquad (8\text{-}21a)$$

and

$$|d| \ll |z_f| \qquad (8\text{-}21b)$$

In Eq. (8-21), the symbol (*) indicates the complex conjugate.

Let B_{tot} designate the complex magnetic flux density defined as

$$B_{tot} = B_{tot.y} + i\,B_{tot.x} \qquad (8\text{-}22)$$

where $B_{tot.x}$ and $B_{tot.y}$ are the x- and y-components of B_{tot}.

The expression of B_{tot} at a point z in the disk of radius $|z_f|$ can be shown to be

$$B_{tot} \cong \frac{-\mu_0}{2\pi} \sum_{n=0}^{\infty} (n+1)\frac{M_{tot}^* z^n}{z_f^{n+2}} \qquad (8\text{-}23)$$

for z, $|z| < |z_f|$

Let us introduce the complex magnetic flux density applied to the filament, B_a, defined as

$$B_a = B_{a.y} + i\,B_{a.x} \qquad (8\text{-}24)$$

where $B_{a.x}$ and $B_{a.y}$ are the x- and y-components of the applied magnetic flux density vector B_a.

For a given cycle, the magnetization losses per unit length of filament W can be estimated as [12]

$$W = \mathrm{Re}\left(\int_{cycle} M_{tot}^* \, dB_a \right) \qquad (8\text{-}25)$$

where Re designates the real part of the expression in brackets.

To illustrate the use of Eq. (8-25), let us consider the case of a filament subject to a transverse applied field oscillating between $-B_a$ and $+B_a$, where B_a is large compared with the effective penetration field $B_{p.a}$ given by

$$B_{p.a} = \frac{4\mu_0 J_c(B_{p.a})r_f}{\pi} \qquad (8\text{-}26)$$

Then it can be shown that the magnetization losses per cycle and unit length of filament can be approximated by

$$W \cong \frac{16 J_c(B_a)r_f^3 B_a}{3} \qquad (8\text{-}27)$$

The result above has to be divided by πr_f^2 to derive the losses per unit volume of superconductor.

8-5-2 Coupling Current Losses in Composites and Cables

The conductor time constant. Schematically, when a composite is subjected to a transverse uniform changing magnetic field B_a, coupling currents take place that generate a uniform reaction field ΔB_i in the opposite direction. The resulting internal field B_i is the algebraic addition of these two components. It can be demonstrated that [13]:

$$B_i = B_a + \Delta B_i \qquad (8\text{-}28)$$

$$B_i = B_a - \theta_{10}\dot{B_i} \qquad (8\text{-}29)$$

where θ_{10} is the time constant of the decay of the coupling currents.

It can be demonstrated that the power losses per unit of volume of filamentary zone due to these coupling current can be written as

$$P = 2\frac{\dot{B}_i^2 \theta_{10}}{\mu_0} \qquad (8\text{-}30)$$

where θ_{10} is the time constant of the coupling current of the composite alone in space. If the composite is no longer alone but inserted in an assembly of given shape, the time constant is θ_{20} as follows:

$$\theta_{20} = 2(1 - N)\theta_{10} \qquad (8\text{-}31)$$

where N is the demagnetization factor associated with the sample geometry. If the sample considered is a round cylinder, which is the case for a single multifilamentary composite, $N = 0.5$.

For practical reasons, in certain cases, the energy and power given are related to the composite volume. In this case a new time constant can be defined, θ_1, which is no longer related to the current decay but is such that

$$P = 2\frac{\dot{B}_i^2 \theta_1}{\mu_0} \qquad (8\text{-}32)$$

Another time constant also has to be considered, θ_2, which is related to the more classical eddy currents appearing in the copper shells of the composites. This component can be added to the first one such as

$$\theta = \theta_1 + \theta_2 \qquad (8\text{-}33)$$

In the following formulas θ will be used, and the power and energy are given per unit volume of composite.

Losses in a conductor subjected to an exponential external field variation

$$B_a = \Delta B(1 - e^{-t/\tau}) \qquad (8\text{-}34)$$

If there is no current saturation of the external filament layers,

$$W = \frac{\Delta B^2}{\mu_0}\left\{\frac{\theta}{\theta + \tau}\left(\frac{R_f}{R_2}\right)^2 + \frac{\theta_2}{\theta_2 + \tau}\left[1 - \left(\frac{R_f}{R_2}\right)^2\right]\right\} \qquad (8\text{-}35)$$

where R_f is the radius of the filamentary zone and R_2 the radius of the composite.

Losses in a conductor subjected to a slow ramp rate

$$B_a = \Delta B\frac{t}{\tau} \qquad (8\text{-}36)$$

$$P = \frac{2\Delta B^2 \theta}{\mu_0 \tau^2} \qquad W = \frac{2\Delta B^2 \theta}{\mu_0 \tau} \qquad \text{if } \tau \gg \theta \qquad (8\text{-}37)$$

Time constant calculations. A difficulty is to evaluate the time constant of the multi-filamentary composites or of the conductors that are considered. The measurement of this time constant by magnetization or calorimetric method is not an easy task. A few examples are given hereafter. More details are given in Ref. [14].

Time constant of a composite. The formula given hereafter is valid only for a composite made of a filamentary zone surrounded by a pure copper shell with p as the twist pitch of the composite, ρ_t the transverse resistivity of the filamentary zone, and ρ_{cu} the resistivity of the copper shell:

$$\theta_1 = \frac{\mu_0}{2} \frac{R_f^2}{R_2^2} \left(\frac{p}{2\pi}\right)^2 \left(\frac{1}{\rho_t} + \frac{1}{\rho_{cu}} \frac{R_2^2 - R_f^2}{R_2^2 + R_f^2}\right) \tag{8-38}$$

Particular attention has to be paid to the calculation of ρ_t. If the filaments (radius r_f) are surrounded by a layer of thickness e_b of a material with a resistivity ρ_b and immersed in a matrix of resistivity ρ_m, the following formula can be taken from Ref. [15] if e_b is small compared with r_f:

$$\rho_t = \rho_m \frac{(1-\lambda) + \chi(1+\lambda)}{1+\lambda + \chi(1-\lambda)} \tag{8-39}$$

$$\chi = \frac{\rho_b}{\rho_m}\left(\frac{e_b}{r_f}\right) \tag{8-40}$$

where λ is the superconductor proportion in the filamentary zone.

The case of a pure copper matrix can be covered by this formula, taking into account that a resistive interface exists anyway between the filaments and the matrix, which can be estimated as [15]

$$\rho_b e_b = 6 \times 10^{-15} \ \Omega \ \mathrm{m}^2$$

Time constant of a twisted cable. An example of a twisted cable is presented in Fig. 8-7. It is usually considered for fusion applications.

Even if several stages are included in such a cable, in a simplified approach it is possible to consider only one dominating stage (see Ref. [16] for detailed calculations).

$$\theta_n = \frac{\mu_0}{2\rho_n}\left(\frac{p_n^*}{2\pi}\right)^2 \frac{1}{1 - \nu_{n-1}} \tag{8-41}$$

where p_n^*, ρ_n, and ν_n are, respectively, the effective twist pitch length, the effective resistivity, and the average void fraction of cabling stage n.

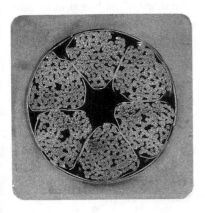

Figure 8-7   Twisted cable in conduit.

Then we have

$$p_n^* = p_n - \frac{r_{n-1}}{R_{n-1}} p_{n-1} \qquad \text{and} \qquad \rho_n = \frac{\rho_b e_b}{\varepsilon_n R_{n-1}} \tag{8-42}$$

where p_n, R_n, r_n, and ε_n are, respectively, the apparent twist pitch length, the outer radius, the twist radius, the contact area ratio of cabling stage n, and $\rho_b e_b$ is the product of the resistivity and of the thickness of the contact resistive barrier. When $n = 2$, r_1 is the strand filamentary area radius and R_1 is the strand radius.

Time constant of a flat cable. A flat cable is usually considered for particle accelerator magnets.

A model for calculation is presented in Ref. [17]. In addition to the interstrand losses, intrastrand coupling losses have to be considered. Two cases can be envisaged.

Time constant dominated by crossing strands

$$\theta = \frac{\mu_0}{\rho} \frac{l_p^2 b^2}{240 c^2} \tag{8-43}$$

where ρ is the equivalent resistivity of the material situated between the two strand axes belonging to the two different layers (strand matrix, coating, and eventual metallic strap between the two layers), c is the thickness of this layer, b the width of the cable, and l_p the twist pitch of the cable.

Time constant dominated by adjacent strands It is the case if there is an insulating strap between the two layers

$$\theta = \frac{\mu_0}{98} \frac{l_p^2}{\rho} \tag{8-44}$$

8-6 THERMAL STABILITY

In superconducting magnets, the conductor is subjected to different types of losses, either internal or external, which need to be evaluated efficiently so that the temperature remains below its critical characteristics. The heat transfer mechanism between the conductor and its cooling environment must be adapted to the size and shape of the heat disturbances and depends on the cooling mode adopted for the magnet. The three types of cooling techniques generally used lead to different heat transfer processes, and their stability conditions need to be analyzed separately. These cooling modes concern

- Indirectly cooled or compact impregnated coils in which the conductors are not in contact with the helium refrigerant. The heat is removed by pure solid conduction from the heated zone to the cold source either by bath or restricted cooling loops.
- Coils with cooling channels distributed through the winding in a transverse flow arrangement where liquid helium is in direct contact with the conductors. The thermal behavior of the conductor is essentially governed by the convective heat transfer characteristics between conductor and liquid helium in the case of He I or by the heat transport mechanism along helium channels characteristic of He II.

• Internally cooled conductors with confined helium paths in a parallel-flow arrangement, such as hollow or cable-in-conduit conductors. These are generally cooled by forced flow of either two-phase or supercritical helium, and their thermal behavior is mainly governed by the specific heat of the helium volume close to the heated area.

8-6-1 General Stability Concepts

Disturbances. Different types of internal losses, such as hysteresis and AC losses, are evaluated in section 8-5 with their analytical expressions. Other disturbances can arise from external heat or beam radiation or from mechanical instabilities created by thermal or electromagnetic stresses in the windings. This last source, though generally weak and fugitive, becomes significant in systems with low cooling efficiency such as indirect cooling.

A magnet is stable if, after a given disturbance has deposited a certain amount of energy in the conductor, with possible excursion into the normal state, the cooling medium is able to absorb the energy produced and to recover the conductor to its initial superconducting state and initial temperature. The aim of stability studies is to evaluate the balance between a disturbance spectrum (in terms of space distribution, duration, and amplitude) and the dynamic response of the conductor.

Thermal behavior of the conductor. The temperature distribution of a superconducting system is given by the heat diffusion equation and appropriate boundary conditions:

$$C \frac{\partial T}{\partial t} = \text{div}(\lambda \cdot \boldsymbol{grad} \cdot T) + W \tag{8-45}$$

with C as the volumetric specific heat of the solid, λ as the thermal conductivity tensor, and W as the power dissipated per unit volume of material, including the power produced by the initial disturbance $P(x, y, z, t)$ and the Joule heating in the conductor $G(T)$. The latter can be expressed as

$$G = 0 \qquad\qquad T_b \leq T \leq T_{cs} \tag{8-46a}$$

$$G = \rho J^2 \frac{T - T_{cs}}{T_c - T_{cs}} \qquad\qquad T_{cs} \leq T \leq T_c \tag{8-46b}$$

$$G = \rho J^2 \qquad\qquad T \geq T_c \tag{8-46c}$$

where T_b is the bath temperature, T_c the critical temperature at the operating field B, T_{cs} the transition current sharing temperature, J the overall current density in the conductor of cross section A, and ρ the equivalent electrical resistivity ($\rho = \rho_{cu} A / A_{cu}$ in the case of a copper stabilizer).

Depending on the cooling mode, the winding will be modeled as

• A nonisotropic homogeneous three-dimensional medium ($\lambda_x \neq \lambda_y \neq \lambda_z$) for impregnated coils; the boundary conditions are set at the borderline of the winding (either bath or cooling loop).

• An isotropic one-dimensional homogeneous medium, with uniform temperature over a cross section, for coils in which the heat transfer to helium is dominant compared with the heat transfer between neighboring conductors (coils with cooling channels wetting the conductors or internally cooled cables). As a consequence of neglecting the transverse temperature gradients and of reducing the model to one dimension, the boundary conditions at the conductor surface are integrated in the heat diffusion equation as follows:

$$C(T)\frac{\partial T}{\partial t} = \frac{\partial}{\partial z}\left[\lambda(T)\frac{\partial T}{\partial z}\right] + P(z,t) + G(T) - Q(T) \qquad (8\text{-}47)$$

where $Q(T)$ represents the power evacuated by helium per unit volume of conductor.

8-6-2 Stability Criteria of Windings Cooled by Helium Channels

Stekly criterion: full-recovery current [18]. By assuming a heat transfer to helium proportional to the temperature difference between the conductor and helium and neglecting the heat flux by conduction along the conductor (which is the same as considering disturbances extending uniformly along the length), a dimensionless stability parameter can be expressed as

$$\alpha = \frac{\rho I_c^2}{Ahp(T_c - T_b)} \qquad (8\text{-}48)$$

where p is the wetted perimeter of the conductor and h the heat transfer coefficient per unit surface.

The stability criterion is stated as follows:

• If $\alpha \leq 1$, the conductor is fully stable, which means that recovery is achieved at all currents up to the critical current.
• If $\alpha > 1$, the conductor is globally stable, which means that it will recover, whatever the size of the disturbance, for all currents $I \leq I_c/\sqrt{\alpha}$.

This criterion can be extended to the case of nonlinear heat transfer. In this case the conductor is globally stable for currents below a "full-recovery current" I_r such that

$$G(I_r, T) \leq Q(T) \,\forall T \qquad (8\text{-}49)$$

Equal-area Maddock criterion: cold-end recovery current. Maddock et al. [19] define a stability criteria by a graphical model that takes into account the longitudinal conduction. The conductor is assumed to be of infinite length, with the end at the bath temperature T_b, and both powers dissipated in the conductor and transferred to helium are single functions of the conductor temperature.

The conductor is globally stable, which means that it will recover after a disturbance has transited its entire length into the normal state, if the two surface areas a and b shown in Fig. 8-8(a) fulfill the condition $a > b$ also expressed by the condition

$$\int_{T_b}^{T_2} [Q(T) - G(T)]\lambda(T)\,dT \geq 0 \qquad (8\text{-}50)$$

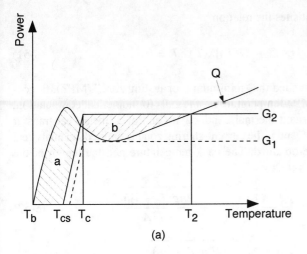

(a)

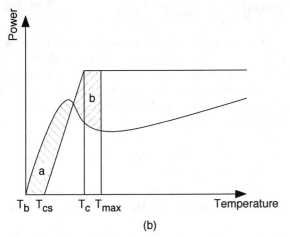

(b)

Figure 8-8 Stability criteria for bath-cooled windings: (a) Stekly and Maddock criteria, and (b) Minimum Propagating Zone.

The cold-end recovery current, or minimum propagating current, is the current for which the two areas are equal. This cold-end recovery current is higher than the previous full-recovery current.

Concepts of MPZ and MQE. Superconducting magnets can in some cases operate reliably at currents higher than the recovery current. The previous criteria were based on disturbances creating an infinite normal zone (global stability). For currents above the recovery current, the conductor can still recover if the disturbance has not exceeded a characteristic size (limited stability).

Wilson and Iwasa [20] have extended the equal-area theorem to the case of limited normal zones. For a given current above the recovery current, there is a steady temperature profile with a peak temperature T_{max} such that the two areas a and b shown in

Fig. 8-8(b) are equal, which satisfies the relation

$$\int_{T_b}^{T_{max}} [Q(T) - G(T)]\lambda(T)\, dT = 0 \qquad (8\text{-}51)$$

This stationary solution is called the "minimum propagating zone" (MPZ). In general, the determination of the MPZ temperature profile calls for numerical computation. In the particular case of a constant thermal conductivity and of a linear heat transfer coefficient, $Q = h(T - T_b)p/A$, and if the current-sharing zone is omitted, an analytical expression of the MPZ can be obtained. The peak temperature and the length of the normal zone are given, respectively, by

$$T_{max} = T_b + \frac{\rho J^2 A}{hp}\left[1 - \sqrt{1 - \frac{2hp(T_c - T_b)}{\rho J^2 A}}\right] \qquad (8\text{-}52)$$

$$l_n = -2\sqrt{\frac{\lambda A}{hp}} \ln\sqrt{1 - \frac{2hp(T_c - T_b)}{\rho J^2 A}} \qquad (8\text{-}53)$$

The MPZ, unstable stationary temperature distribution, provides useful indications about the domain of stability of the superconducting state: any energy deposition that develops a temperature profile above that of the MPZ leads to a growth of the normal zone over the entire conductor, whereas, for a disturbance generating a profile below that of the MPZ, the recovery to the superconducting state is practically ensured.

The energy contained in the MPZ profile is given by

$$E_{max} = A\int_{z\to-\infty}^{z\to+\infty}\int_{T_b}^{T_{MPZ}(z)} C(T)\, dT\, dz \qquad (8\text{-}54)$$

This energy is often used as an approximate measure of the "minimum quench energy" (MQE), which is the minimum heat input, delivered instantaneously to a spot, necessary to induce a quench.

The critical energy depends on the duration and on the space distribution of the disturbance. For a very short disturbance, the critical energy may be smaller than the MQE if the initial temperature profile is particularly sharp.

The concept of MPZ is also applicable to the scheme of impregnated windings. Similar equations can be written using the heat transfer mechanism by both longitudinal and transverse conduction through the winding in a three-dimensional geometry. An unstable stationary solution is derived for the MPZ.

8-6-3 Stability of Internally Cooled Conductors

The stability concept of cables cooled internally by forced-flow supercritical helium or by pressurized superfluid helium differs from that of windings cooled by transverse helium channels communicating with a bath. In this case, the available helium enthalpy is restricted and is not replaced (within the concerned time scale). The stability is very sensitive to the operating temperature T_{op} and to the temperature margin, $T_{cs} - T_{op}$, which

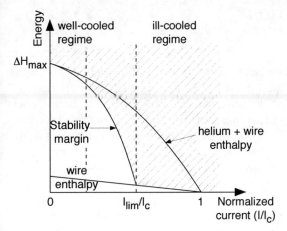

Figure 8-9 Stability margin of a cable-in-conduit conductor.

determines the total energy removable by the helium content (also called the "enthalpy margin" [J/m^3]) expressed by

$$\Delta H_{max} = \frac{A_{He}}{A} \int_{T_{op}}^{T_{cs}} C_{He}\, dT \qquad (8\text{-}55)$$

where A_{He} is the cross section of helium contained in the cable, A is the cross section of metal, and C_{He} is the constant-pressure volumetric heat of helium per unit volume (the metal enthalpy is negligible).

The stability of such a system is difficult to evaluate because the heat exchange between conductor and helium is strongly time-dependent. The transient heat transfer coefficient can be very high during a short time (a few ms), but the helium temperature increases rapidly during the heat pulse. The heat diffusion equation of the conductor is coupled, through the heat exchange, to that of helium and is usually solved by numerical computation.

The concept of stability margin proposed by Hoenig and Montgomery [21] as the "uniform heat density instantaneously deposited in a long length of conductor that just causes a quench," can be used as a figure of merit for the comparison of different cable-in-conduit conductors. The critical energy density is strongly dependent on the current, as shown in Fig. 8-9 [22,23]. Above a certain current, the stability margin is very small (ill-cooled conditions). In this region, only a small fraction of the available enthalpy, ΔH_{max}, is used. In order to remain in the well-cooled regime, the operating current must be well below this limit. If the heat transfer coefficient h is assumed to be constant, the limit is given by

$$\rho J^2 = \frac{p}{A} h (T_c - T_{op}) \qquad (8\text{-}56)$$

The current limit depends on the copper cross section ($I_{lim} \propto \sqrt{A_{cu}}$) and on the strand diameter d ($I_{lim} \propto 1/\sqrt{d}$ for a given overall metal cross section).

8-7 ELECTRICAL INSULATION

8-7-1 Specification

The electrical insulation of superconducting magnets must fulfill special requirements related to electrical, thermal, and mechanical properties. Although in steady-state DC operation there is no voltage across the coils, during transient periods, such as when ramping up and down or more particularly in case of emergency fast dump of the current, high voltages can be created in parts of the circuit and can endanger the magnet safety. Voltage breakdowns must be totally prevented because, in view of the large stored magnetic energy, they would generally lead to the destruction of the magnet.

The materials commonly used in superconducting magnets have intrinsically high electric properties, but, because they are also submitted to high mechanical stresses under thermal and magnetic constraints, great care must be taken to avoid any damage, either during coil construction or under operation.

8-7-2 The Different Insulation Materials

Typical breakdown voltages for materials used as electrical insulation in superconducting magnets are given in Table 8-3.

Phenolic resins used as varnish insulation for superconducting wires are often used on small SC magnets. A common commercial varnish is known as Formvar.

Because of their very high breakdown voltage and radiation resistance, thermoplastic films such as polyimide [24] are widely used in SC magnets, especially in particle accelerators.

Fiber-reinforced epoxy* compounds are very common insulating materials because of their relatively high mechanical properties. Furthermore, they can be used in different ways in manufacturing such as prepreg [25], fully cured parts, G10 and G11, and the vacuum impregnation technique [26–28]. There is some scatter in the available values of thermal properties of epoxy resins and epoxy-based composites. This is due to the difference in the cross-link density of the polymers and to the fiber volumetric fraction and orientation in the composites. At large radiative fluxes, the strength of epoxy composites decreases [29]. Irradiation effects do not change breakdown voltage significantly [24] but only the mechanical properties.

Liquid helium sometimes has a part in the insulation of bath coils.

The case of Nb_3Sn magnets has to be considered separately. Because the thermal cycle required to synthesize the superconducting Nb_3Sn phase is done at high temperature (660–700 °C), polymer insulation cannot be used before the thermal cycle. Usually glass fiber is used as a spacer during the thermal cycle and is followed by a vacuum impregnation. Both Nb_3Sn phase and glass fiber are very brittle after the cycle, and so the process needs special care.

---

*Additional information on composite materials can be found in chapter 2 of this handbook.

Table 8-3 Electrical and thermal properties for insulating materials used in superconducting magnets compared with copper

Insulating materials	Thermal conductivity at 4.2 K (W/m · K)	C_p at 4.2 K (J/kg · K)	Integrated thermal contraction from 293 to 4.2 K (%)	Breakdown voltage DC condition (kV/mm)
Liquid helium	0.028	4500	–	30 at 4.2 K
Gas helium	0.008	7300	–	15 at 4.4 K
				0.5 at 77 K
				0.2 to 0.3 at RT
Glass–epoxy composite	0.07 ± 0.02	0.4 to 2	0.16 to 0.38 depending on fiber orientation	
• Unidirectional				
parallel to fiber	0.13 ± 0.05		0.1 to 0.55	
transverse to fiber			0.26 to 0.8	
• Woven 48% fiber				
longitudinal	0.07 ± 0.02		depending on fiber	
through thickness	0.06 to 0.075		volumic fraction	
Glass fiber	0.12 ± 0.02			
Glass	0.1			
Phenolic resin (varnish)	0.6	3.2	0.9	118 at 300 K
Polyimide film	0.045	17	0.4 ± 0.1	301 at 4.2 K
Epoxy resin	0.04 to 1.1	1.4 ± 0.6	1.15 ± 0.06 rigid 1.1 flexible 1.5	
Polyethyleneterephtalate	0.008	0.96	0.42	543 at 4.2 K
Polytetrafluoroethylene	0.043 ± 0.003	2.96	2.1 ± 0.6	33 at 4.2 K
Polyethylene	0.012	0.8 crystalline 2 amorphous	1.5	360 at 4.2 K
Nylon	0.012		1.5	
Copper used in superconductor		0.09	0.29	

8-7-3 Temperature Dependence of the Insulation Material Properties

The problem for organic insulation materials is to match the thermal contraction difference that exists between metallic parts and insulation. Typical values of integrated thermal contraction from 293 to 4.2 K are presented in Table 8-3.

Thermoplastic polymer films, such as polyimide, lead to some problems in prestressed magnets due to the creep of the thermoplastic at room temperature. Preliminary tests to measure the creep are often needed for the design of prestressed coils.

Organic polymers used as matrix for composite insulation are usually brittle at room temperature because of their high cross-link density, but the rupture strain of the fibers is lower than the one of the matrix. At cryogenic temperature the contrary is observed [30], the first failure occurring in the matrix. Therefore, the rupture strain of the polymer is the limiting criterion for its use at cryogenic temperature. Because, as in a composite, the strain is the same for both matrix and fiber, only the strain limitation should be taken into consideration in the mechanical analysis. Failure mechanisms of brittle matrix composites have been extensively studied. At liquid helium temperature, the failure strain of the polymer occurs between 0.8 and 1.15%. This failure strain is on the same order as the differential thermal contraction between the polymeric and metallic materials, which means that the remaining strain margin of a superconducting coil in the operating conditions is small. The energy released by the failure or cracks of the polymer matrix is a type of disturbance that can affect the conductor stability, as mentioned in section 8-6.

The difference between the integrated thermal contraction of metals and composite materials often leads to high calculated shear stresses at the insulation–conductor interface. This is due to the fact that the calculation considers an equivalent elastic modulus for the composite insulation, which is dominated by the high fiber modulus. Actually, the bonding occurs between the polymer matrix of low modulus and the metal. Therefore, the actual shear stresses at the metal interface are much lower.

The breakdown voltages of helium [31] decrease approximately by a factor of 2 when it changes from the liquid to the gaseous state, as shown in Table 8-3. Further decrease is observed as the temperature of the gas increases, the breakdown voltage varying with the temperature reciprocal. Therefore, the part played by helium in the insulation must be limited and carefully controlled.

8-7-4 Influence of the Cooling Technique on the Insulation

The cooling mode of the magnet plays an important role in the design of the insulation.

Magnets receiving large radiative fluxes, or which have to remove important losses, often require a direct contact between the cryogenic fluid and the conductor. This can be realized in bath coils with bare conductors or more commonly nowadays with porous insulation using polyimide films and glass fiber ribbons that allow helium flow through the porosity of the fiber cloth. Magnets using internally cooled conductors do not lead to specific problems. The radiation resistance of the polymer is the limiting criterion for the use of organic material in magnets receiving large particle fluxes.

For magnets using indirect cooling systems, the thermal conductivity of the insulation must be high, and the bonding between the conductor and the insulation must be strong. In particular, shear stresses between conductors and between the coil and its cooling structure must be kept at a low level.

Extrapolation of thermal properties from 4.2 to 1.8 K should be avoided because of the increase of thermal resistivity due to the Kapitza effect.*

8-7-5 Impregnated Superconducting Coils

Because vacuum impregnation using epoxy resin is a very common technique for insulation, some remarks have to be written on it. The vacuum impregnation technique

---

*See chapter 10 of this handbook.

requires the use of a very low viscosity resin [32,33]. The impregnation process is possible if the viscosity is lower than 200 mPa · s. Because vacuum is used to ease the resin flow through the glass fiber cloth, the following requirements have to be taken into account:

- The use of solvent to reduce the viscosity of the resin–hardener mixture has to be avoided.
- The vacuum has to be controlled to avoid the evaporation of the hardener during the impregnation process.

There is always a risk of bubble formation using this technique. Most of the studies [28] done on vacuum impregnation for superconducting magnets are based on Darcy's law that relates the flow of the liquid in the porous insulation to the pressure gradient appearing in the liquid. Although this represents the liquid flow well, it neglects the wetting phenomenon at the liquid–solid–vacuum interface. Because epoxy resin has excellent wetting properties on metallic surfaces and glass fibers, the metallic surfaces and glass fibers have to be well outgassed; otherwise, the epoxy will first dissolve the gas molecules absorbed on the surfaces. The dissolved gases in the liquid resin will form bubbles, creating regions of reduced thermal conductivity after curing. Outgassing conditions prior to the resin impregnation are therefore of major importance. If vacuum impregnation is well executed, the monolithic structure that is finally realized does not allow any movement of the conductor inside the coil.

8-8 QUENCH PROTECTION

In the event of a quench, and if no appropriate measures were taken, a magnet could be endangered by overheating owing to the high level of current density in the superconductor. Although the superconducting magnets are designed with an adequate level of stability with respect to disturbances affecting the windings, the probability of undergoing quenches cannot be altogether precluded. An accidental quench may originate, for instance, from the loss of liquid helium as a result of cryogenic failure or of vacuum failure. Therefore, the design of the magnets and the conception of their protection systems must allow the magnets to quench safely.

Because the basic process of a quench is the conversion of the magnetic energy into heat inside the volume of winding transited into the resistive state, all protection techniques consist in decreasing the current as fast as possible (i.e., without the appearance of overvoltages across or through the windings). The most common technique entails discharging the energy into an external resistor.

8-8-1 Quench Mechanism

The quench is characterized by the irreversible transition of a zone of the conductor from the superconducting state to the normal (resistive) state. The heat dissipated in the initial zone by the Joule effect due to the magnet current entails warming up to the critical temperature of the surrounding volumes, which quench in turn, resulting in a continuous expansion of the normal zone. The propagation of the quench is governed by heat diffusion determined by the thermal conductivities of the materials.

Longitudinal propagation velocity of the normal zone. In an isolated superconducting wire, the normal zone expands along the conductor, under the combined actions of heat conduction and ohmic effect, at a constant velocity

$$v_l = \frac{J}{C} \sqrt{\frac{\rho \lambda_l}{T_c - T_0}}$$ (8-57)

where J is the conductor current density and C and ρ, respectively, are the averaged specific heat and resistivity of the whole conductor at the critical temperature T_c.

Transverse propagation velocity of the normal zone. In a winding, the normal zone also expands in the directions perpendicular to the conductor resulting from the heat diffusion across the insulation. The transverse velocities are much slower because they are also proportional to the square root of the thermal conductivities in those directions, which are principally determined by the thermal conductivity and the thicknesses of the insulation. The equivalent conductivity in the transverse direction is

$$\lambda_t = \frac{e}{e_i} \lambda_i$$ (8-58)

where λ_i is the insulation thermal conductivity and e and e_i the conductor and insulation thickness in the transverse direction, respectively.

The velocity in the transverse direction is then

$$v_t = v_l \sqrt{\frac{\lambda_t}{\lambda_l}}$$ (8-59)

Current diffusion: Effect on velocity. When the conductor quenches, the current is expelled from the superconducting material and is diffused into the surrounding stabilizer where, after a transient phase, its density becomes uniform. A characteristic time of the diffusion phase can be defined as

$$t_m = e_t^2 / \pi^2 D_m$$ (8-60)

where e_t is the transverse dimension of the stabilizer and D_m the magnetic diffusivity ($D_m = \rho / \mu_0$). During that period, the current in the stabilizer, being restricted to a smaller area, dissipates more power than with a uniform density. As a result, the propagation velocity of the normal zone can be much faster than that given by Eq. (8-57), which is benificial for protection, as seen in section 8-8-3.

8-8-2 Maximum Temperature and Voltage

Maximum temperature. Though there is no strict limit for the temperature rise, the usual designed value is of the order of 100 K. The reason is that because all the materials

Table 8-4 Linear expansions as function of temperature for usual materials

Material	$\int_4^{100} dl/l$	$\int_{100}^{293} dl/l$
Stainless steel	35×10^{-5}	296×10^{-5}
Copper	44×10^{-5}	326×10^{-5}
Aluminum	47×10^{-5}	415×10^{-5}
Iron	18×10^{-5}	198×10^{-5}
Epoxy fiberglass	47×10^{-5}	279×10^{-5}

entering the coil structure have almost no thermal expansion when warmed up from liquid helium temperature to 100 K, no significant thermal stresses appear in the windings. For the same reason, it is also advantageous to keep a low thermal gradient throughout the windings. Table 8-4 compares the thermal expansions from 4 to 100 K and from 100 to 293 K for usual coil materials.

Maximum voltage. In superconducting magnets, the thickness of the insulation may have to be limited because of different constraints such as cooling efficiency or thermal stability.

In some cases, parts of the conductor or of the current leads are exposed to liquid or gaseous helium, which have rather weak dielectric properties (the breakdown voltage of helium at 300 K is only about 300 V/mm). For these reasons, voltages created during the quench process have to be kept as low as possible. A practical limit is often taken on the order of 500 to 1000 V. The peak voltage does not appear necessarily at the magnet terminals but can be across part of the winding that has not yet transited to the normal state. This has to be determined in each particular case.

Hot spot criterion. The hot spot temperature is easily estimated from the knowledge of the current decay with time if we assume local adiabaticity. This assumption is a fair approximation because the quench time is short, but in all cases it is conservative. The balance between the Joule heat and the enthalpy growth of the length Δl of the conductor at the hot point gives

$$\rho \frac{\Delta l}{A} I^2 \, dt = C A \, \Delta l \, dT \qquad (8\text{-}61)$$

where A is the conductor cross section and C the volumic specific heat. Rearranging the equation and integrating give

$$\int_0^\infty J^2 \, dt = \int_{T_o}^{T_m} \frac{C}{\rho} \, dT = U(T_m) \qquad (8\text{-}62)$$

The function U contains only the properties of the materials used in the winding and therefore has a universal validity allowing the determination of the final temperature T_m of the hot point. Figure 8-10 shows the function U for copper, aluminum, and a typical winding made of a copper–NbTi monolithic conductor impregnated with epoxy resin. The conspicuous effectiveness of the residual resistivity of the materials should be noted.

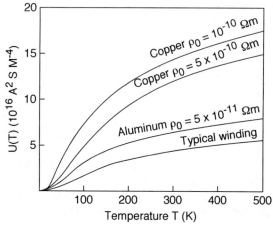

Figure 8-10 The function $U(\theta)$ for various conductors and for a typical small magnet winding. (From Wilson, M. N., *Superconducting Magnets*, Oxford: Clarendon Press, 1989.)

An upper limit of the hot spot temperature is readily obtained with the two following assumptions:

- There is no propagation of the quench (internal resistance is negligible).
- The magnet energy is dumped through a constant external resistor R.

In this case the decay of the current is exponential with the time constant $t = L/R$ (L being the magnet inductance). Thus

$$\int_0^\infty J^2\,dt = J_0^2 \frac{\tau}{2} = U(T_m) \tag{8-63}$$

where J_0 is the initial current density at $t = 0$.

For a magnet whose stored energy is E, if the rated current I_0 and the dump voltage V across the magnet terminals are chosen, the current density J_0 is determined by the maximum T_m allowed for the peak temperature according to the following equation:

$$U(T_m) = J_0^2 \frac{\tau}{2} = J_0^2 \frac{L}{2R}\frac{I_0^2}{I_0^2} = \frac{J_0^2}{I_0}\frac{E}{V} \tag{8-64}$$

During a quench and the following discharge, the internal resistance of the magnet increases by the normal zone propagation and the Joule heating. Therefore, the decrease of the current is faster than that without propagation, and the value of the integral of Eq. (8-63) is lower. Consequently, the final hot spot temperature is lower than that calculated with Eq. (8-63), particularly when the current density is high. Equation (8-62) is still valid if the actual current decay is known by calculation or measurement.

To predict the peak temperature, calculations with the help of elaborate computer codes are needed. There are a large number of such codes generally developed for specific applications such as the following:

- The program QUENCH [35] includes the normal zone expansion with the velocities entered as input parameters. The resistance and the heat capacity of the windings are calculated from the individual constituent characteristics versus temperature introduced as data in the computer code. The temperature of the successive quenching volumes is calculated at each step of time, yielding the final hot spot temperature.
- Codes of thermal diffusion in three dimensions using the finite element method are available. The geometry of the conductor, of the coils, of the coil structure, and the properties of all the materials are given in input. The programs can describe the evolution of the quench with time and compute the characteristics of the process such as propagation velocities in the three directions, temperature distribution through the windings and the structures, resistances, voltages, energies, and so forth.

Quench back. The decay of the magnet current during its discharge into the dump resistor produces a magnetic flux variation throughout the coils and their structures. In the conductor, as described in section 8-5, coupling currents and eddy currents generate losses. In the coil mechanical structures made of low resistive material, such as aluminum alloy, the eddy currents may reach large intensities and generate enough heat to cause the quench of other coil parts still in the superconducting state. These quench-back processes can result in very fast growth of the coil resistance; a significant fraction of the stored energy is dissipated rather evenly inside the windings with smooth temperature gradients and reduced peak temperatures.

8-8-3 Protection Techniques

Quench detector. When a quench occurs, a resistive voltage appears that has to be detected in any phase of the magnet operation (ramping up, steady-state current, ramping down). The quench signal, whose detection threshold is usually of the order of 1 V, must be extracted from the coil inductive voltage, which is one or two orders of magnitude greater. To eliminate the inductive voltage, mainly two types of quench detectors are utilized.

The first type, shown in Fig. 8-11(a), uses a resistor bridge circuit. It needs an electrical tap in the magnet winding. The bridge has to be balanced under the sole inductive voltages of the two magnet parts (at the first ramping up). Therefore, the unbalanced current i_q is proportional to the resistive voltage appearing in one part of the magnet.

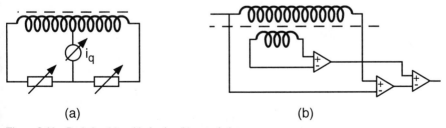

| (a) | (b) |

Figure 8-11   Resistive (a) and inductive (b) quench detectors.

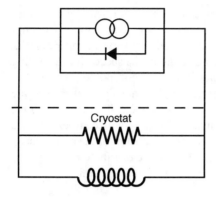

Figure 8-12 Self-protected magnet.

The second type, shown in Fig. 8-11(b) consists of an electronic device subtracting the inductive voltage part from the total magnet voltage. The inductive voltage is measured by means of a secondary coil coupled to the magnet.

Protection circuit schemes. The systems of protection depend on the magnet designs. Several schemes of protection circuits are shown in Figs. 8-12 to 8-15 according to the magnet features.

Protection of small compact magnets. For small impregnated magnets of low energies (hundreds of kilojoules) and high current densities (hundreds of amperes per square millimeter), there is no need of a quench detector because the internal resistance rapidly reaches a high value. Figure 8-12 shows the protective circuit: there is no breaker, and the power source has its proper protective system against output overvoltage. In the event of a quench, the power source is switched off, and the current is discharged through the free-wheel diode of the source. Nevertheless, a protective resistor must be mounted in parallel across the magnet to prevent the destructive damage caused by a line rupture.

External resistor. As soon as a quench originates, the stored energy is extracted outside the magnet windings into an external resistor by the opening of breaker(s) triggered by the quench detector. From the point of view of magnet protection, the two circuits shown in the following figures are equivalent. In Fig. 8-13(a), the resistor is connected in parallel

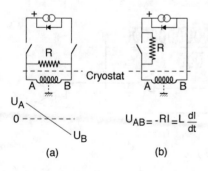

$$U_{AB} = -RI = L\frac{dI}{dt}$$

(a)   (b)

Figure 8-13 Protection by (a) external parallel and (b) series resistor.

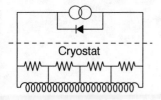

Figure 8-14 Protection by subdivided internal resistor.

across the magnet directly between the current lead terminals. Such an arrangement ensures the full safety of the magnet against any external failure. In Fig. 8-13(b) the resistor is in series with the magnet with a breaker connected in parallel. This arrangement does not protect the magnet from severe damage in the event of a rupture of the electrical line or of the power supply. It has the advantage that the currents of the magnet and of the source are always equal with no current derived in parallel.

Internal subdivided resistor. The resistor is subdivided into elements located inside the cryostat and connected in parallel across the magnet sections, as shown in Fig. 8-14. If a magnet section quenches, the resistor element in parallel provides a shunting path for the current, thus tempering the thermal effects in this section. However, such a scheme can entail an imbalance of forces between sections, which in some cases is not acceptable.

Segmented external resistor. For the magnets with large stored energies, when the discharge voltage RI_0 is too high (e.g., several thousand volts), the external resistor is segmented into elements that are connected between the magnet coils, as in Fig. 8-15. Breakers are mounted in parallel with each resistor. With n segments, the elements have a resistance $r = R/n$, and the voltage is limited to $\pm RI_0/n$ all along the magnet during the discharge. The main disadvantage is to multiply the number of current leads.

Quench propagators. Quench propagators such as heaters or thermally conductive strips can be placed in the windings to initiate quenches in all parts of the magnet as soon as a quench is detected. The aim of such devices is to propagate the quench artificially in order that the heat released be distributed evenly throughout the magnet at a uniform temperature without creating a high peak temperature. Because the complete magnet reverts to the normal state, its resistance reaches a high value, so that most of the stored energy is dissipated in the magnet. The role of the external dump resistor as energy extractor becomes negligible, and therefore it can even be lowered to zero (e.g., by

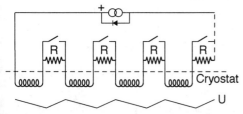

Figure 8-15 Protection by segmented external resistor.

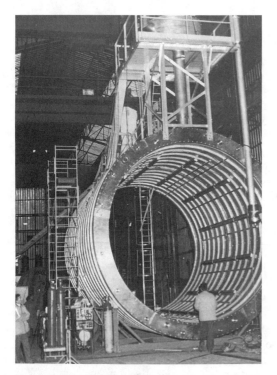

Figure 8-16 The Aleph solenoid.

means of diodes). This technique, also named the internal dump technique, seems to be the sole method suitable for very big magnets whose stored energies are huge — several tens of gigajoules — because it solves the high voltage problem and avoids the need for bulky and expensive dump resistors of so large a thermal capacity.

8-9 SOME APPLICATIONS

Several applications using superconducting magnets have been widely developed, mainly in the field of fundamental research:

1. High-magnetic field generators that can use superconducting coils only (up to 24 T) or a hybrid set of superconducting and copper coils.
2. High-energy particle accelerators such as the Tevatron at Fermi Lab (USA) in service since 1983 [36], HERA at DESY (Germany) put in operation in 1991 [37], and LHC (the Large Hadron Collider) at CERN (Switzerland–France), the start up of which is scheduled during the year 2005 [38].
3. Particle detectors associated with very large accelerators. Among many are solenoids Cello [39] and H1 at DESY, solenoids Aleph (Fig. 8-16 and [40]) and Delphi at CERN, and the future projects of ATLAS toroid [41] and Compact Muon Solenoid (CMS) [42] to be installed on the LHC.

Table 8-5 Main specifications

Characteristics	High field	Accelerator	Detector	Fusion	MRI
Type of magnet					
Configuration	Solenoid, Split coil	Dipole, quadrupole, higher multipole	Solenoid, toroid	Toroid poloidal, solenoid, helicoidal, mirror	Lumped solenoids
Maximum magnetic induction	3 to 24 T	5 to 9 T	1.5 to 5 T	9 to 13 T	1 to 4 T
Operating mode	DC	DC plus slow ramp rate	DC	DC, fast cycling, high external B	Persistent
Main concerns	Field as high as possible, access, homogeneity	Compactness, field homogeneity series production	Transparency, reliability	Compactness, cooling, reliability, mechanical structure, high AC losses	Field homogeneity, helium consumption, access

4. Plasma fusion devices, mainly using tokamak machines. The Tore Supra tokamak (CEA—EURATOM) has been in operation since 1989 [43]. The ITER tokamak, result of a worldwide collaboration, is under engineering design [44].

The most developed industrial application of superconducting magnets is their use in magnetic resonance imaging (MRI) devices for medical scanners. The specific characteristics of the superconducting magnets used in these applications are summed up in Tables 8-5 (main specifications) and 8-6 (conceptual choices).

Following the completion of very successful projects, the most ambitious projects in each field by the beginning of 1997 are listed below.

1. For high magnetic field generation, the 45-T project of the National High Magnetic Field Laboratory (NHMFL) at Florida State University (USA). The 45-T field in a 32-mm bore diameter is produced using a hybrid magnet system [45] with field contributions by the resistive insert and the superconducting outset of 31 and 14 T, respectively.

The superconducting outsert magnet contains three separate subcoils, two using Nb_3Sn cable-in-conduit conductor and one using NbTi cable-in-conduit conductor. The cryostat has a 2.4-m outer diameter and a 2.5-m height. This system is expected to be tested by the end of 1998.

2. For high energy accelerator, the LHC project will use a 27-km circumference with 1200 twin-aperture dipoles, 14.2-m long, with a central field of 8.35 T, and 380 twin-aperture quadrupoles, 3.1-m long, with a field gradient of 220 T/m (Fig. 8-17). All magnets will work at 1.8 K to accelerate two proton beams up to an energy of 7000 Gev,

Table 8-6 Conceptual choices

Characteristics \ Type of magnet	High field	Accelerator	Detector	Fusion	MRI
SC material	Nb₃Sn, NbTi, HT$_c$	NbTi	NbTi	NbTi, Nb₃Sn	NbTi
Conductor type	Strand, monolith, cable	Cable	Cable plus aluminum stabilizer plus eventual mechanical reinforcement	Bare conductor or cable in conduit with mechanical reinforcement	Monolith
Cooling mode	Pool boiling, internal cooling	Two-phase flow	Indirect cooling by conduction	Bath or circulation assuming large wet perimeter of the conductor	Large helium tank or cryocoolers, very low consumption needed
Temperature	4.2 or 1.8 K	4.5 or 1.8 K	4.5 K	4.5 or 1.8 K	4.2 K
Stability	Low margin to critical conditions	Low margin to critical conditions	Margin to critical conditions ≥ 2 K	Margin to critical conditions ≥ 2 K	Medium margin to critical conditions
Protection	Dump resistor	External, dump resistors plus heaters, internal diodes	External dump resistor plus quench-back tube or heaters	Segmented dump resistor	Self-protected, internal dump

which will later collide at four points. This project has very new features compared with previous superconducting particle accelerators in operation:

(a) High magnetic field and forces in the magnets.
(b) Twin-aperture structure (two magnetic elements of the same structure are put in the same cryostat).
(c) Use of superfluid helium on very large distances.
(d) High-beam losses due to the luminosity of the machine.

3. For particle detectors, the size of the detector follows the accelerator's size. The next two most important projects for LHC will be the following:
   (a) The ATLAS magnet system, which consists of three parts:
      (1) An inner thin solenoid producing a magnetic induction of 2 T in a cylinder 5-m long and 2.5-m in diameter,
      (2) The barrel toroid, composed of eight coils inside their own cryostats (Fig. 8-18). The main characteristics of the toroid are an inner bore of 9.4 m, an outer bore

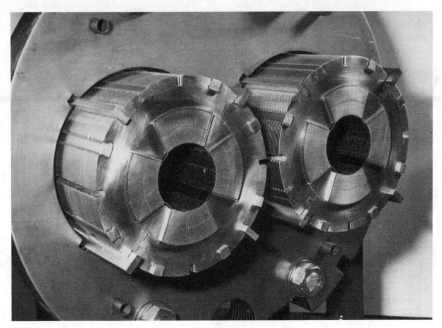

Figure 8-17 Large Hadron Collider quadrupole cross section.

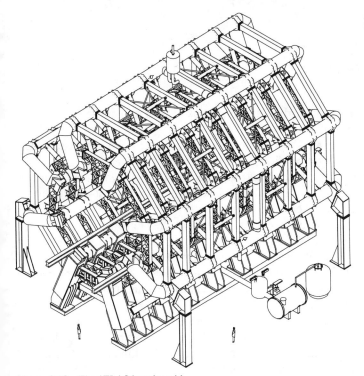

Figure 8-18 The ATLAS barrel toroid.

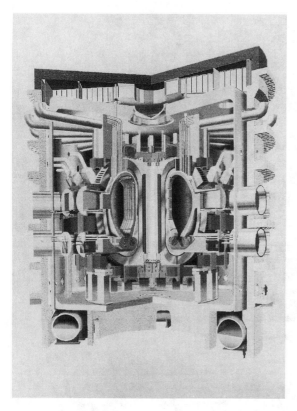

Figure 8-19   The ITER magnet system.

  of 20.1 m, an axial length of 25.3 m, a peak field on the conductor of 4 T, and
  a stored energy of 1.1 GJ.
 (3) The two end cap toroids with an outer diameter of 11 m and an axial length
  of 5.6 m providing a bending power in the range 4–8 T · m.
(b) The CMS solenoid, for which a magnetic field of 4 T in a 5.9-m free warm bore
 and a 12.4-m length is requested. This solenoid will be the biggest with the largest
 stored energy (2.5 GJ) ever built.
 Both projects are under detail design and are expected to be put in operation on
 the LHC during the year 2005.
4. For plasma fusion, the ITER project has the objective of achieving a controlled ignited burn time of 1000 s with a nominal fusion power of 1500 MW. The machine is
 a tokamak with a toroidal geometry and a plasma major radius of 8.15 m (Fig. 8-19).
 The superconducting magnetic system consists of
 (a) 20 toroidal D-shaped coils that produce the main confining field. The maximum
  field of 12.5 T on the conductor imposes the use of Nb_3Sn. The conductor is
  a 60-kA cable-in-conduit one cooled by supercritical helium at 4.5 K. The total
  stored energy for the toroidal system is 100 GJ.

(b) A central solenoid, that induces and maintains the plasma current. This winding is 12-m high with a mean radius of 2.3 m. The maximum field of 13 T on the conductor also imposes the use of a 45-kA Nb_3Sn cable.

(c) The poloidal coils, which control the plasma position and shape. Two coils, operating at a field up to 8 T, use a Nb_3Sn conductor. Three others, operating at a lower field, use a NbTi conductor. The coil diameter ranges from 13 to 32 m.

Presently in an engineering design phase, the project is expected to be followed by a construction phase, which will last for about 10 years.

5. For magnetic resonance imaging, superconducting magnets using NMR phenomena for medical imaging have been the first large-scale commercial application of superconductivity. Practically all the systems with a magnetic field larger than 0.35 T use a superconducting magnet, and about 10,000 such systems are now in operation worldwide.

Being operated in persistent mode (the magnet is short-circuited on itself), these magnets can have a very high long-term field homogeneity and stability. Such a development has enabled an evolution of the conceptual design of these magnets, now smaller, lighter, and less helium-consuming than ten years ago. The evolution is still going on with the development of open magnetic systems permitting access to the patient during examination and the use of more and more performing cryocoolers.

NOMENCLATURE

a	Coefficient for strain effect	%
A	Cross section	m^2
b	Cable width	m
B	Magnetic flux density (field)	T
B_a, B_a, x, B_a, y	Applied magnetic field	T
B_c	Critical magnetic field	T
B_{c20}	Upper critical magnetic field at 0 K and under strain	T
B_{c20m}	Upper critical magnetic field at 0 K and no strain	T
B_i, B_i	Internal magnetic field	T
$B_{p,0}, B_{p,1}$	Penetration field	T
B_{ref}	Reference magnetic field	T
$B_{tot}, B_{tot,x}, B_{tot}$	Field produced by a doublet	T
B_0, B_0	Applied magnetic field,	T
c	Insulating space between two strands	m
C	Specific heat per unit volume	$J \cdot m^{-3} \cdot K^{-1}$
C_0	Calibration coefficient for Nb_3Sn	$A \cdot T^{0.5} \cdot m^{-2}$
d	Characteristic doublet distance	m
e	Transverse thickness	m
E	Stored energy	J
G	Joule effect power per unit volume	$W \cdot m^{-3}$

h	Heat transfer coefficient	$W \cdot m^{-2} \cdot K^{-1}$
H_a	Applied magnetic field	$A \cdot m^{-1}$
H_{c1}	Lower critical magnetic field	$A \cdot m^{-1}$
H_{c2}	Upper critical magnetic field	$A \cdot m^{-1}$
I, I_0	Current	A
I_c	Critical current	A
J	Current density	$A \cdot m^{-2}$
J_c	Critical-current density	$A \cdot m^{-2}$
J_{c0}, J_{c1}	Contributions to J_c	$A \cdot m^{-2}$
J_{ref}	Critical current density at B_{ref} and T_{ref}	$A \cdot m^{-2}$
J_0	Critical current density at 0 K and 0 T	$A \cdot m^{-2}$
l_p	Cable twist pitch	m
L	Inductance coefficient	H
M	Magnetization	$A \cdot m^{-1}$
$M_{tot}, M_{totx}, M_{toty}$	Total magnetic moment per unit length	$A \cdot m$
M_0, M_1	Magnetic moment per unit length	$A \cdot m$
N	Demagnetization factor	
p	Cooled perimeter	m
p_n	Apparent twist pitch of stage n cable	m
p_n^*	Effective twist pitch of stage n cable	m
P	Loss or perturbation power per unit volume	$W \cdot m^{-3}$
Q	Power exchanged with helium per unit volume of conductor	$W \cdot m^{-3}$
r_f	Filament radius	m
r_n	Twist radius of stage n cable	m
R	Dump resistance	Ω
R_f	Filamentary zone radius	m
R_n	Outer radius of stage n cable	m
R_2	Composite radius	m
t	Time	s
T	Temperature	K
T_b	Bath temperature	K
T_c	Critical temperature	K
T_{c0}	Critical temperature at 0 T under strain	K
T_{c0m}	Critical temperature at 0 T and no strain	K
T_{cs}	Current-sharing temperature	K
T_m	Maximum temperature	K
T_{op}	Operating temperature	K
T_{ref}	Reference temperature	K
T_0	Initial temperature	K
U	Protection function	
v_l	Longitudinal propagation velocity	$m \cdot s^{-1}$
v_t	Transverse propagation velocity	$m \cdot s^{-1}$
V	Voltage	V
W	Loss energy per unit length or volume	$J \cdot m^{-1}$ or $J \cdot m^{-3}$

z	Complex coordinate	
z_f	Filament position in the complex plane	
α	Stability parameter	
ΔB, $\Delta \mathbf{B}_a$	Change of applied magnetic field,	T
ΔB_i	Change of internal magnetic field,	T
ϵ	Strain	%
ϵ_n	Contact ratio of stage n cable	%
θ	Flat cable time constant	s
θ_n	Time constant of stage n twisted cable	s
θ_1	Losses time constant	s
θ_{10}	Coupling current time constant	s
θ_2	Eddy current time constant	s
θ_{20}	Assembly coupling current time constant	s
λ	Superconductor fraction	
λ, λ_x, λ_y, λ_z	Thermal conductivity tensor and components	$W \cdot m^{-1} \cdot K^{-1}$
λ_l	Longitudinal thermal conductivity	$W \cdot m^{-1} \cdot K^{-1}$
λ_t	Transverse thermal conductivity	$W \cdot m^{-1} \cdot K^{-1}$
λ_0	Matrix or stabilizer thermal conductivity	$W \cdot m^{-1} \cdot K^{-1}$
μ_0	Permeability of free space	$4\pi 10^{-7} H \cdot m^{-1}$
v_n	Average void fraction of stage n cable	
ρ	Equivalent resistivity	$\Omega \cdot m^{-1}$
ρ_b	Barrier resistivity	$\Omega \cdot m^{-1}$
ρ_{cu}	Copper resistivity	$\Omega \cdot m^{-1}$
ρ_m	Matrix resistivity	$\Omega \cdot m^{-1}$
ρ_n	Effective resistivity of stage n cable	$\Omega \cdot m^{-1}$
ρ_t	Transverse resistivity	$\Omega \cdot m^{-1}$
τ	External field variation time constant	s
τ	Current decay time constant	s

REFERENCES

1. Lee, P. J., and Larbalestier, D. C., *IEEE Trans. Appl. Supercond.* 3, no. 1 (1993):833–841.
2. Lee, P. J. et al., *IEEE Trans. Appl. Supercond.* 3, no. 1 (1993):1354–1357.
3. Scanlan, R. M. et al., *IEEE Trans. Appl. Supercond.* 3, no. 1 (1993):1351–1358.
4. Lubell, M. S., *IEEE Trans. Magn.* MAG-19, no. 3 (1983):754–757.
5. ten Haken, B., Godecke, A., ten Kate, H., and Specking, W., *IEEE Trans. Magn.* 32, no. 4 (1996):2739–2742.
6. Summers, L. T. et al., *IEEE Trans. Magn.* 27, no. 2 (1991):1763–1766.
7. Ando, T., et al., *IEEE Trans. Magn.* 32, no. 4 (1996):2324–2327.
8. Bean, C. P., *Phys. Rev. Lett.* 8, no. 6 (1962):250–253.
9. Wilson, M. N., *Superconducting Magnets* (Oxford: Clarendon Press, 1983), 162 ff.
10. Schmüser, P., *AIP Conf. Proc.* 249, no. 2 (1992):1099–1158.
11. Rem, P. C., "Numerical Models for AC Superconductors," Ph.D. diss., Twente University, 1986.
12. Ogitsu, T., "Influence of Cable Eddy Currents on the Magnetic Field of Superconducting Particle Accelerator Magnets," Ph.D. diss., Tsukuba University, 1994.
13. Ries, G., *IEEE Trans. Magn.* MAG-13, no. 1 (1977):524.

14. Duchateau, J. L., Ciazinski, D., and Turck, B., "Coupling Current Losses in Composites and Cables (Analytical calculations)," in *Encyclopaedia of Applied Superconductivity*, COMETT, to be published.
15. Turck, B., ICMC (Kobe, Japan: Butterworths, 1982), 179–182.
16. Schild, Th., and Ciazynski, D., *Cryog.* 36 (1996):1039.
17. Turck, B., "Energy Losses in a Flat Transposed Cable," Los Alamos Internal Report LA -7635-MS (February 1979).
18. Stekly, Z. J. J., and Zar, J. L., *IEEE Trans. Nucl. Sci.* NS-12 (1965):367.
19. Maddock, B. J. et al., *Cryog.* 9 (1969):261.
20. Wilson, M. N., and Iwasa, Y., *Cryog.* 18 (1978):17
21. Hoenig, M. O., and Montgomery, D. B., *IEEE Trans. Magn.* MAG-11 (1975):569.
22. Ciazynski, D., and Turck, B., *Cryog.* 33 (1993):1066.
23. Bottura, L., *Cryog.* 34 (1994):787.
24. Kernohan, R. H. et al., *J. Nucl. Mat.* 85 and 86 (1979):379.
25. Evans, D., and Morgan, J. T., *Nonmetallic Materials and Composites at Low Temperatures* 3 (New York: Plenum Press, 1985), 195–200.
26. Green, M. et al., *Nonmetallic Materials and Composites at Low Temperatures* 1 (New York: Plenum Press, 1979), 409–420.
27. Hacker, H. et al., *Adv. Cryog. Eng.* 30 (1984):51–60.
28. Evans, D., and Morgan, J.T., *Adv. Cryog. Eng.* 38 (1992):413–420.
29. Klabunde, C. E. et al., *J. Nucl. Mat.* 117 (1983):345–350.
30. Rey, J.M. et al., *Composite Polym.* 5, no. 3 (1992).
31. Fallou, B. et al., *Cryog.* 10 (1970):142.
32. Evans, D., and Morgan, J. T., *Nonmetallic Materials and Composites at Low Temperatures* 2 (New York: Plenum Press, 1982), 73–87
33. Rey, J. M. et al., *Nonmetallic Materials and Composites at Low Temperatures* 8, 1996, to be published.
34. Devred, A., *J. Appl. Phys.* 66, no. 6 (1989).
35. Wilson, M., Rutherford Laboratory Report RHEL/M151 (1968).
36. Koepke, K. et al., *IEEE Trans. Magn.* MAG-15, no. 1 (1979):658–661.
37. Wolf, S., *IEEE Trans. Magn.* 24, no. 2 (1988):719–722.
38. "The Large Hadron Collider Conceptual Design," CERN/AC/95-05 (1995).
39. Desportes, H., Le Bars, J., and Mayaux, G., *Adv. Cryog. Eng.* 25 (1980):175–184.
40. Baze, J. M. et al., *IEEE Trans. Magn.* Mag-24, no. 2 (1988):1260–1263.
41. "ATLAS Technical Proposal," CERN/LHC 94-43 (December 1994).
42. "The Compact Muon Solenoid Technical Proposal," CERN/LHCC94-38 (December 1994).
43. Tore Supra team, *IEEE Trans. Magn.* 25, no. 2 (1989):1473–1480.
44. Green, B. J., and Huguet, M., *IEEE Trans. Magn.* 32, no. 4 (1996):2224–2229.
45. Miller, J. R. et al., *IEEE Trans. Magn.* 30, no. 4 (1994):1563–1571.

BIBLIOGRAPHY

Rose-Innes, A. C., and Rhoderick, E. H., *Introduction to Superconductivity* (Oxford: Pergamon Press, 1994).
Wilson, M. N., *Superconducting Magnets* (Oxford: Clarendon Press, 1989).
Iwasa, Y., *Case Studies in Superconducting Magnets* (New York: Plenum Press, 1994).
Tixador, P., *Les Supraconducteurs* (Paris: Hermes, 1995).
CERN Accelerator School. "Superconductivity in Particle Accelerators," Geneva: CERN Reports 89-04 (1989) and 96-03 (1996).
Dresner, L., *Stability of Superconductors* (New York: Plenum Press, 1995).
Westbrook, J. H., and Fleischer, R. L., eds., *Intermetallic Compounds, Principles and Practice* (New York: John Wiley & Sons, 1995).
Hartwig, G., *Polymer Properties at Room and Cryogenic Temperatures* (New York: Plenum Press, 1994).

NINE

CRYOGENIC EQUIPMENT

D. E. Daney

MS-J580, LANL, Los Alamos, NM 87545

J. E. Dillard and M. D. Forsha

Barber-Nichols Inc., 6325 W 55th Avenue, Arvada, CO 80002

9-1 CRYOGENIC TRANSFER SYSTEMS

9-1-1 Introduction

Many concerns in the design of ambient and higher-temperature systems are also common to cryogenic fluid transfer systems. For example, correlations developed for ambient temperature fluids for pressure drop through valves, fittings, and pipes apply to cryogenic fluids as well. The contribution that valves and fittings make to the total system pressure drop, however, is sometimes not well recognized.* Because in many cases this contribution dominates, it is important to consider all sources of pressure loss. Some specific cryogenic design considerations are

1. *Optimization of the heat leak to the transfer line.* The quality of transfer line insulation is primarily an economic problem of minimizing the sum of the capital cost (of the insulation system) and the operations cost (incurred by the heat leak, taking into account the duty cycle). Large-diameter or low-duty-cycle LNG and LN2 lines are often insulated with glass or plastic foam, whereas liquid helium and liquid or slush hydrogen are vacuum insulated with MLI[†] — sometimes with a vapor-cooled or liquid-nitrogen-cooled shield. In general, the lower the temperature, the better the insulation required, because the refrigeration is more expensive.

---

*For example, reports in the 1970s from two different sources indicated that the friction factor for liquid and supercritical helium was anomalously high—by a factor of 1-1/2 to 2. These reports were based on measurements of the overall pressure drop—with some correction for bends and fittings—of large, complex helium flow loops. Subsequent, more controlled measurements with simpler configurations by other investigators [1,2], however, demonstrated no anomalous effect for helium.

[†]Multilayer insulation (see chapter 3 of this handbook).

2. *Cavitation and two-phase flow.* When cryogens are transferred with little subcooling, two-phase flow may occur at positions where the pressure falls below saturation owing to the combined effects of pressure drop and heat transfer. Cavitation may occur locally in the low-pressure regions of flowmeters and valves with the vapor bubbles collapsing in the pressure recovery regions of these devices [3].
3. *Thermal–acoustic oscillations.* Helium and slush hydrogen systems are susceptible to thermal–acoustic oscillations in pressure taps, valve stems, and other conduits with large length-to-diameter ratios that traverse between these cryogens and ambient temperature. The oscillations can have heat pumping rates on the order of watts; their frequency is typically tens of hertz.
4. *Pressure collapse and low-frequency pressure oscillations.* Slush hydrogen and sub-cooled liquid croygen flow systems are susceptible to pressure collapse in relief valve standpipes, valve stems, and so forth, in which a temperature-stratified layer of liquid maintains the subcooling pressure on the flow system. If flow turbulence disturbs the stratification, the pressure collapses as vapor condenses on the slush or subcooled cryogen. The cryogen then surges into the warmer regions of the pipe, where it flashes, causing a pressure pulse. The resulting low-frequency oscillations can pump large quantities of heat into the cryogen.
5. *Negative gauge pressures.* Systems at negative gauge pressure, such as slush hydrogen and pumped helium, are susceptible to contamination by air and water vapor that enter through leaky valve stems, relief valves, and pipe joints. These leaks may plug relief valve lines with ice and solid air. Air, if it reaches the cryogen, frequently condenses in submicron-size particles, giving hydrogen and helium a milky appearance. Because these crystals have settling times of hours or longer, they are easily transported throughout a system. They tend to collect in stagnant zones, such as downstream of valve seats, where they may block the flow. In hydrogen systems, accumulated oxygen crystals represent a potential safety hazard. Special precautions such as the use of welded-bellows valve packing and avoidance of compression fittings (welded or soldered joints are preferred) can reduce these problems.
6. *Thermal contraction.* Contraction of stainless steel from ambient to cryogenic temperatures is about 0.003 in./in., which, on a 100-ft length of pipe, is 3.6 in. Bellows placed periodically along straight pipe runs, are used to eliminate thermal cool-down stresses. On lengths up to several feet, thermal contraction can be accommodated with bends on smaller-diameter lines.
7. *Trapped line segments.* Segments of cryogenic piping that can be isolated between valves must be provided with relief valves to prevent rupturing the line by trapped cryogens as they warm up. The isometric pressure rise experienced by liquid nitrogen warming to 300 K, for example, is about 2900 bar.

Valves. Figures 9-1 and 9-2 illustrate typical cryogenic valves. Thin-wall stainless steel valve stems and vacuum jackets minimize the heat leak to the cryogen. Enclosing the valve stem in a stainless steel sheath allows an all-welded construction, which assures integrity of the vacuum insulation and makes replacement of the valve plug easy. The annular space between the valve stem and its sheath is typically 0.1 mm or less to prevent convection and its associated heat leak. Valve plugs are typically fabricated

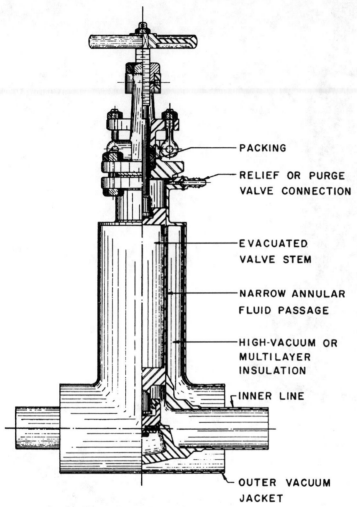

Figure 9-1 Typical vacuum-jacketed liquid helium valve showing thin-walled evacuated stem design with warm-end connection on helium gas space (from Ref. [3]).

from fluorocarbons such as Kel-F. Either an O-ring or packing seals the cryogen gas space.

For small diameters (10 mm or less) the author has had good success using all-welded construction Nupro valves with a welded bellows valve stem seal and either Kel-F or copper valve plugs. These valves are fitted with extended stems and placed in the cryostat vacuum space. The low-temperature bellows valve stem seal eliminates both the possibility of thermoacoustic oscillations and leaks into subatmospheric systems.

Couplings. Vacuum-jacketed bayonet fittings, illustrated in Figs. 9-3 and 9-4, are used to make low-heat-leak joints in cryogenic lines. The reentrant configuration of the bayonet isolates the cryogenic region from ambient temperature with thin-wall stainless-steel (or

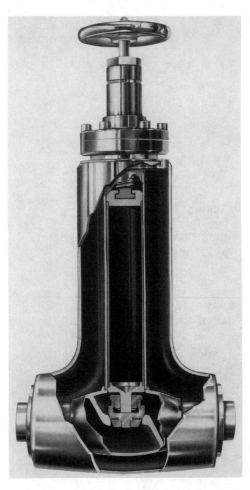

Figure 9-2 Typical vacuum-jacketed cryogenic valve (Courtesy CVI, Inc.).

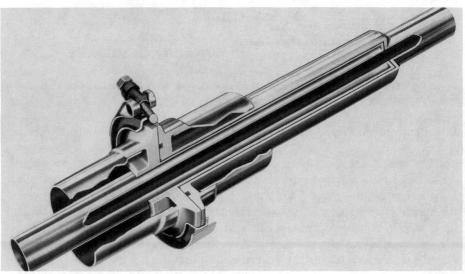

Figure 9-3 Liquid helium bayonet assembly; a warm-end O-ring seal is shown. A narrow mating annulus eliminates the need for a liquid end seal. (Courtesy CVI, Inc.)

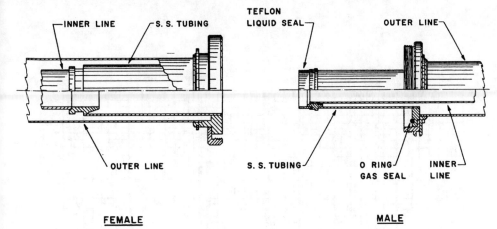

Figure 9-4 Air Force-type hydrogen bayonet, 2-in. diameter and 7-in. length (from Ref. [3]).

other low-thermal-conductivity material) mating sheaths on the two components. An O-ring at the warm-end joint seals the cryogen gas space. A close fit between the mating components, and frequently a Teflon nose seal, reduces convection in the annular gas space. The preferred orientation is with the cold end down, or at least horizontal, to reduce convection in the annulus and ensure that the warm-end seal does not become cold and leak.

9-1-2 Pressure Drop

Single-phase flow. The pressure drop in tubes of uniform cross section with single-phase, steady flow and modest property changes along the flow path is

$$p_2 - p_1 = \underbrace{\frac{G^2}{\alpha}\left(\frac{1}{\rho_2} - \frac{1}{\rho_1}\right)}_{\text{flow acceleration}} + \underbrace{f\left(\frac{L_e'}{D_e}\right)\frac{G^2}{2\rho_m}}_{\text{friction}} + \underbrace{g\rho_m(z_1 - z_2)}_{\text{elevation}} \qquad (9\text{-}1)$$

where the equivalent diameter D_e is defined by

$$D_e = \frac{4A}{\mathcal{P}} \qquad (9\text{-}2)$$

and the total equivalent length is given by

$$L_e' = L + L_e, \qquad (9\text{-}3)$$

the sum of the pipe length L, and the equivalent length of the valves and fittings L_e. Figure 9-5 gives the friction factor f for commercial pipe, and Table 9-1 gives the equivalent length for various valves and fittings. Figures 9-6 and 9-7 give the equivalent length of smooth bends and miter bends.

Sudden enlargements and contractions are another source of pressure change in transfer systems. The pressure change due to a sudden contraction in a pipe or at a pipe

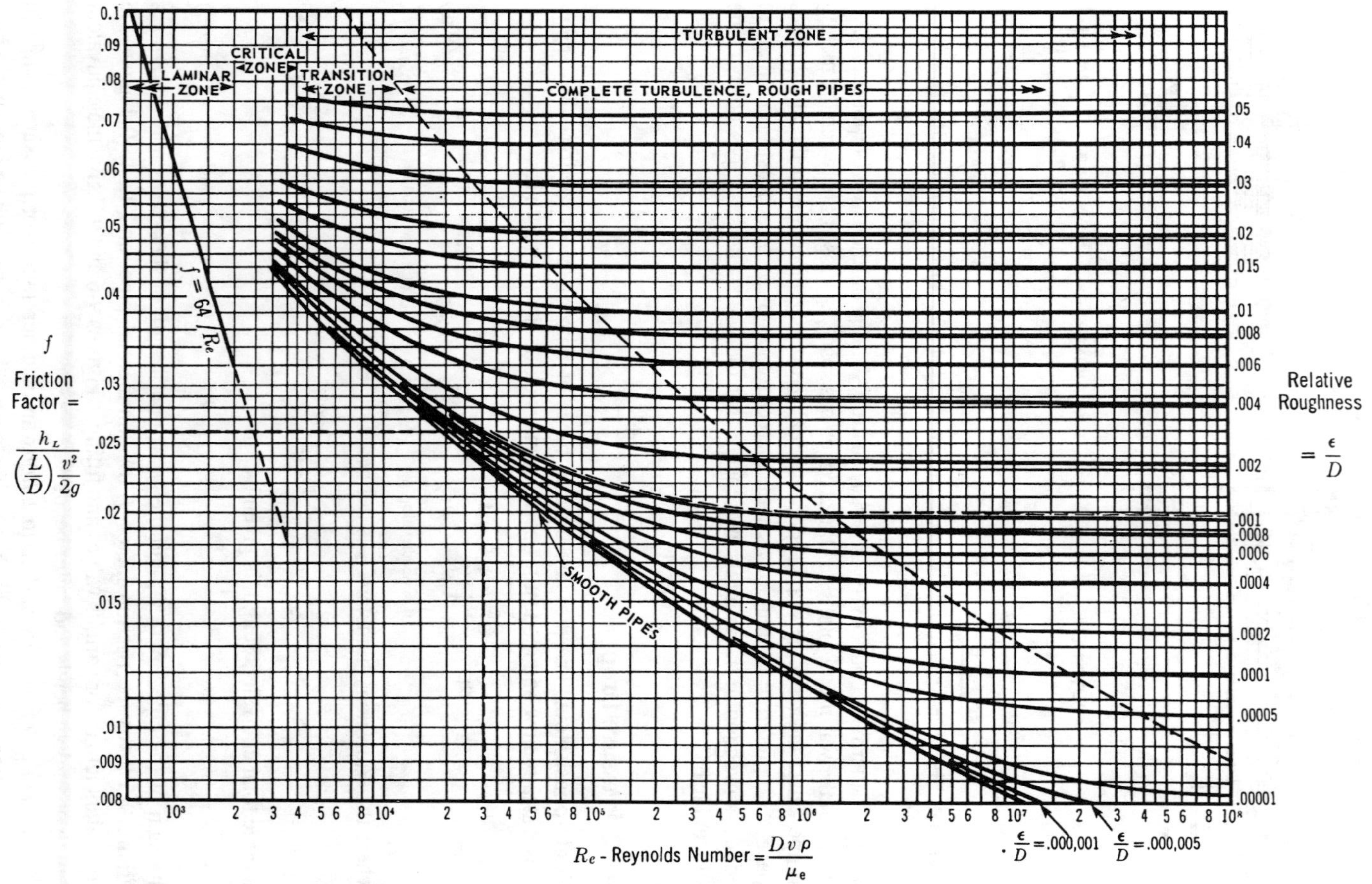

Figure 9-5 Friction factor for commercial pipe. (Courtesy Crane Valve.)

Table 9-1 Equivalent length of various valves and fittings (Courtesy Crane Valve)

		Description of product		Equivalent length in pipe diameters (L/D)
Globe valves	Stem perpendicular to run	With no obstruction in flat,- bevel , or plug-type seat	Fully open	340
		With wing or pin guided disc	Fully open	450
	Y-pattern	(No obstruction in flat-, bevel-, or plug-type seat)		
		With stem 60° from run of pipe line	Fully open	175
		With stem 45° from run of pipe line	Fully open	145
Angle valves		With no obstruction in flat-, bevel-, or plug-type seat	Fully open	145
		With wing or pin guided disc	Fully open	200
Gate valves	Wedge, disc, double disc, or plug disc		Fully open	13
			Three-quarters open	35
			One-half open	160
			One-quarter open	900
	Pulp stock		Fully open	17
			Three-quarters open	50
			One-half open	260
			One-quarter open	1200
Conduit pipe line gate, ball, and plug valves			Fully open	3[a]
Check valves	Conventional swing		0.5^{b} ... Fully open	135
	Clearway swing		0.5^{b} ... Fully open	50
	Globe lift or stop; stem perpendicular to run or Y-pattern		2.0^{b} ... Fully open	Same as globe
	Angle lift or stop		2.0^{b} ... Fully open	Same as angle
	In-line ball	2.5 vertical and 0.25 horizontal^{b} ... Fully open		150
Foot valves with strainer	With poppet lift-type disc		0.3^{b} ... Fully open	420
	With leather-hinged disc		0.4^{b} ... Fully open	75
Butterfly valves (8-in. and larger)			Fully open	40
Cocks	Straight-through	Rectangular plug port area equal to 100% of pipe area	Fully open	18
	Three-way	Rectangular plug port area equal to 80% of pipe area (fully open)	Flow straight through	44
			Flow through branch	140
Fittings	90° standard elbow			30
	45° standard elbow			16
	90° long radius elbow			20
	90° street elbow			50
	45° street elbow			26
	Square corner elbow			57
	Standard tee	With flow through run		20
		With flow through branch		60
	Close pattern return bend			50

[a] Exact equivalent length is equal to the length between flange faces or welding ends.

[b] Minimum calculated pressure drop (psi) across valve to provide sufficient flow to lift disc fully.

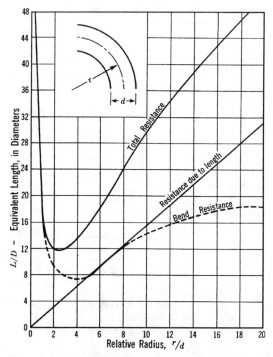

Figure 9-6 Resistance of 90° bends (Courtesy Crane Valve.).

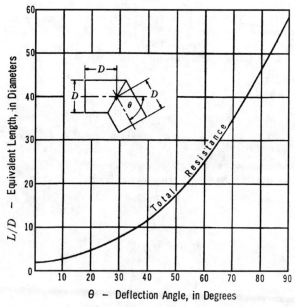

Figure 9-7 Resistance of miter bends (Courtesy Crane Valve.).

entrance is

$$P_0 - P_1 = \rho_m \frac{V_1^2 - V_0^2}{2} + \rho_m K \frac{V_1^2}{2}. \tag{9-4}$$

For a sudden enlargement or discharge at the pipe exit, the pressure change is

$$P_2 - P_3 = \rho_m \frac{V_3^2 - V_2^2}{2} + \rho_m K \frac{V_2^2}{2}. \tag{9-5}$$

Figures 9-8 and 9-9 give the resistance coefficient K for various situations.

Bellows and *corrugated lines* are common in cryogenic piping systems—both for accommodating thermal contraction and for making flexible sections. Measured values for the pressure drop of gaseous nitrogen, liquid nitrogen, and He II flowing through corrugated bellows are about four times higher than through tubing of the same internal diameter [7]. One manufacturer of flexible transfer lines gives pressure drops a factor of three higher based on nominal pipe sizes. Data specific to a particular configuration should be used when they are available.

Coiled tubing in components such as heat exchangers gives rise to secondary flows and enhanced flow losses. An expression developed by Ito [8]

$$\frac{f}{4} = 0.076(R_e)^{-0.25} + 0.00725 \left(\frac{d}{D_h} \right)^{0.5} \tag{9-6}$$

gives good agreement with experimental results for liquid and supercritical helium [1].

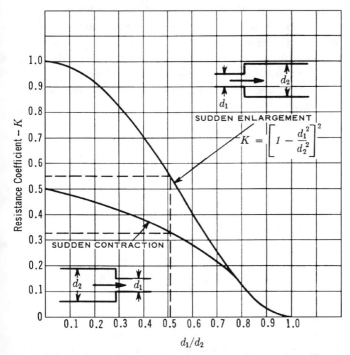

Figure 9-8 Resistance due to sudden enlargements and contractions. (Courtesy Crane Valve.)

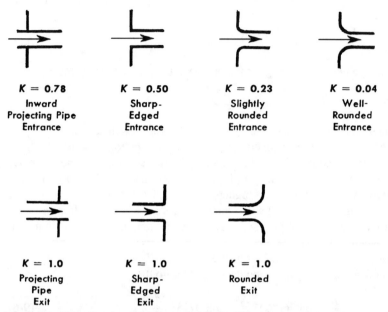

| $K = 0.78$ | $K = 0.50$ | $K = 0.23$ | $K = 0.04$ |
| Inward Projecting Pipe Entrance | Sharp-Edged Entrance | Slightly Rounded Entrance | Well-Rounded Entrance |

| $K = 1.0$ | $K = 1.0$ | $K = 1.0$ |
| Projecting Pipe Exit | Sharp-Edged Exit | Rounded Exit |

Figure 9-9 Resistance due to pipe entrance and exit. (Courtesy Crane Valve.)

Near-critical-flow conditions frequently occur in helium systems because of the low critical pressure of helium ($p_c = 2.2 \times 10^5$ Pa, $T_c = 5.2$ K). Forced-flow helium cooling systems, particularly, may operate in the near-critical region. If the thermodynamic path of a fluid operating in this regime crosses the transposed critical line,* the fluid may experience large changes in density that render Eq. (9-1) inaccurate. Arp [9] derived generalized flow equations for one-dimensional, single-phase flow. These equations are independent of the equation of state and use thermodynamic parameters that are only weakly divergent across the transposed critical line. Arp's generalized pressure drop equation is

$$(1 - M^2)K_s\frac{1}{p}\frac{dp}{dx} = -(1 + \phi M^2)\frac{1}{2}\left(\frac{\mathcal{P}}{4A}\right)M|M|f - \phi M^2\frac{\Lambda}{\dot{m}c^2} + \frac{M^2}{A}\frac{dA}{dx} - \frac{1}{c^2}\frac{d\Phi}{dx}$$

$$\underbrace{}_{\text{friction}} \qquad \underbrace{}_{\substack{\text{heat}\\\text{transfer}}} \quad \underbrace{}_{\substack{\text{area}\\\text{change}}} \quad \underbrace{}_{\substack{\text{potential}\\\text{energy}}}$$

$$(9\text{-}7)$$

For integration of other properties along the flow path, the reader is referred to Arp's original text [9].

Slush hydrogen. Slush hydrogen is a slurry of liquid and solid hydrogen at or near its triple point (para-hydrogen triple-point temperature = 13.803 K, triple-point pressure =

---

*The continuation of the liquid–vapor equilibrium line beyond the critical point is referred to as the transposed critical line. Its locus is commonly taken along the maxima of the specific heat. See chapter 1 of this handbook for further information.

7.04 kPa) and has been considered as an advanced aerospace propellant because of the advantages it offers in storability and cooling capacity [10–14]. Slush hydrogen with a 60% solid fraction is 16.5% more dense than normal-boiling-point (NBP) liquid, and its enthalpy is 86.2 J/g less (compared to a latent heat of vaporization of 445.5 J/g at the NBP). Although somewhat difficult to generate continuously in large quantities, slush hydrogen is readily transferred through well-insulated cryogenic transfer lines and can be pumped with a centrifugal pump so long as the minimum pump passages exceed about 7 mm [10,14]. Considered on a volume basis, the latent heat of fusion of solid hydrogen is approximately the same as the latent heat of vaporization of liquid helium, and thus "helium quality" thermal insulation is recommended. Figure 9-10 summarizes the results of measurements of the friction factor of slush hydrogen made in a 16.6-mm-diameter by 15-m-long straight test section [10,11]. At low flow velocities and high solid fractions, the friction factor of slush is nearly twice that of the liquid; at higher velocities and lower solid fractions, the slush friction factor is *lower* than that of the liquid. Similar reductions in friction factor have been observed in other slurry flows [15].

Thermal acoustic oscillations (TAOs). Thermal acoustic oscillations are common to helium [16–22] and slush hydrogen systems [23–25] but can also occur in nitrogen, oxygen, and argon systems [26] if the cold end of the tube in which the oscillations occur is immersed below the liquid level. These spontaneous oscillations, which pump large quantities of heat into a cryogenic environment, occur when a large temperature gradient exists in a slender tube connecting ambient and cryogenic temperatures. Rott's original analysis of the problem [27,28], which assumed a step change in temperature along the tube, has been modified by Gu [29,30] using a steep but continuous temperature profile based on experiment. Gu's stability map for a 1-m-long helium-filled tube, Fig. 9-11, was verified by experiment. For lengths other than 1 m, use a corrected tube radius $r' = r/\sqrt{L}$. If additional volume is present at the warm end, correct the warm-to-cold length ratio using $\xi' = (L_h + L_{hs})/L_c$, where L_h and L_c are the actual lengths of the warm and cold sections, respectively, and L_{hs} is the equivalent length of the additional volume. It is calculated using $L_{hs} = V_s/\pi r^2$, where V_s is the additional volume and r is the tube radius. At the left stability boundary in Fig. 9-11, the viscous boundary layer fills the tube, damping the oscillation. At the right stability boundary, the thermal boundary layer area is insufficient to pump enough heat to sustain the oscillation against frictional losses.

If a tube geometry that lies in the unstable region of Fig. 9-11 cannot be avoided, several methods for damping the oscillations are available, as summarized by Gu [30]:

1. Helmholtz Resonator
   The Helmoltz resonator is an extra volume connected to the closed end of an oscillating tube that increases the volume of the warm end. The stability curve of Rott shows that the most susceptible configuration occurs when $\xi = 1$. Therefore, if the volume and length of the warm end are increased to make $\xi \gg 1$, the stability curve will move up and to the right in Fig. 9-11 and increase the area of the stability region. For example, a Helmholtz resonator was used to eliminate oscillations in a pressure tap of a slush hydrogen system [31]. Figure 9-12 shows this scheme.

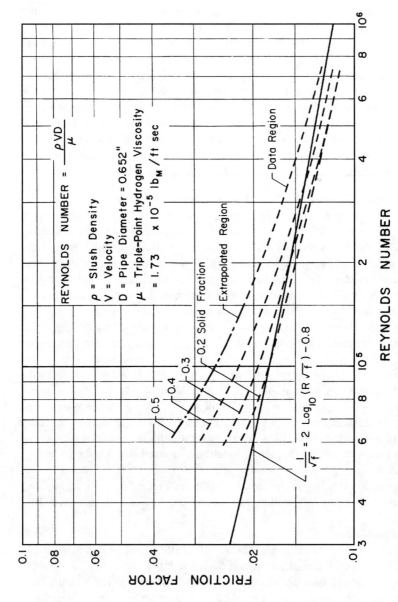

Figure 9-10 Friction factor for slush hydrogen (from Ref. [10]).

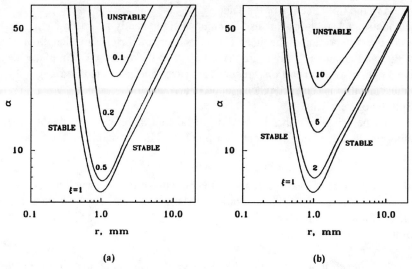

Figure 9-11 Critical radius for TAOs in a helium system with $T_h = 295$ K. (a) $\xi \leq 1$; (b) $\xi \geq 1$ (from Ref. [30]).

2. Wire in Tube
   Figure 9-11 also shows that the volume of a resonator can be greatly reduced if a copper wire is inserted inside the warm end of the tube. Nylon fish line is also effective in damping oscillations [31].

3. Low-Pressure Check Valve
   A low-pressure check valve effectively dampens TAOs in a vent line [31]. With the check valve closed, the vent line acts as a closed cold-end tube in which no oscillations will occur. This approach is usually used when the oscillation pressure is as high as 1 to 2 psi.

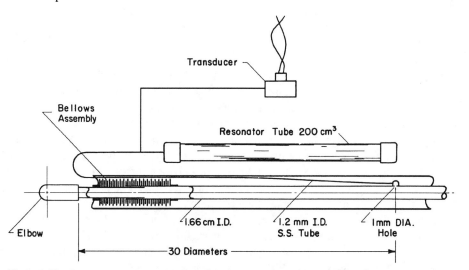

Figure 9-12 Pressure tap arrangement on slush hydrogen system used to eliminate thermoacoustic oscillations (from Ref. [31]).

4. Perforation in the Cold Section of the Tube

Thermal acoustic oscillations can also be damped significantly by drilling a number of holes in the cold portion of the tube. The holes decrease the effective length of the tube in the cold chamber. If holes are drilled close to the warm–cold interface, the effective length of the cold portion is reduced to nearly zero. As noted from Fig. 9-11, the greatest stability is achieved when ξ approaches zero.

5. Heat-Sinking of Vent Tube

Stability can be achieved either by cooling or heating the closed end of the tube, depending on the location of the operation point (i.e., by changing the temperature T_h/T_c).

6. Connection of the Vent and Fill Lines

From the observations of Clement [17] it is apparent that oscillations will not occur if both ends of the tube are open. This condition can be approximated by interconnecting the vent and fill lines, which is an effective technique if both the fill and vent lines are maintained at atmospheric pressure.

Thermally induced flow oscillations (density-wave oscillations) may occur in supercritical and two-phase flow systems if the system is operating in a regime where the fluid undergoes large density changes on heating (e.g., a thermodynamic path that crosses the transposed critical line). Chugging-type flow that one hears on cool-down of an open-ended transfer line is an example. The oscillations can also occur, however, in quasisteady flow of supercritical helium, with temperature oscillations of several K, as illustrated in Fig. 9-13 [32].

The phase (or space lag) between the inlet and outlet flows that is required for oscillatory instability in a heated conduit can be understood by referring to Fig. 9-14, assuming a simple incompressible flow model (which considers thermal expansion, but no pressure effects) with a large exit flow impedance. Focusing attention on the exit restriction, we note that the velocity at this point is given by

$$V_d \approx \sqrt{\frac{\Delta p_{d\text{-}f}}{\rho_d}} \tag{9-8}$$

When warmer than average fluid (lower density) arrives at the exit restriction, the velocity increases and the fluid in the line accelerates to satisfy continuity. The residence time of the fluid in the heated section decreases, resulting in less heating per unit mass and hence in cooler fluid being delivered to the exit restriction after some time lag. As the cooler fluid flows through the exit restriction, the fluid in the heated section decelerates, giving it an increased residence time and greater-than-average heating. Thus, a positive perturbation in the exit temperature induces a negative perturbation or reflection that arrives at the exit after the transit time of the fluid in the line. The period of oscillation is twice the transit time, and the mass flow rate at the inlet and exit is 180° out of phase. This phase difference results because, in the absence of pressure effects, the inlet and exit velocities are in phase, making the inlet mass flow $\dot{m}_b$ proportional to $1\sqrt{\rho_d}$ (i.e., $\dot{m}_b \approx V_b \approx V_d \approx \sqrt{1/\rho_d}$). According to Eq. (9-8), however, the exit mass flow, $\dot{m}_d$, is proportional to $\sqrt{\rho_d}$, giving the 180° phase shift between inlet and exit mass flow rates.

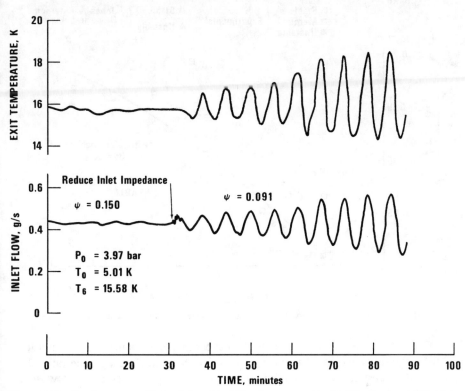

Figure 9-13 Density wave oscillation induced in 185-m-long supercritical helium line by reducing inlet impedance; $Q = 37.2$ W (from Ref. [32]).

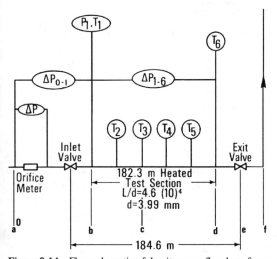

Figure 9-14 Flow schematic of density-wave flow loop for supercritical helium (from Ref. [32]).

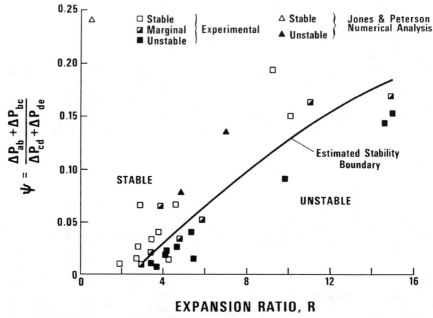

Figure 9-15 Stability map for density-wave oscillations in supercritical helium (from Ref. [32]).

Figure 9-15 is a stability map (based on experiments by Daney, Ludtke, and Jones [32]) for density wave oscillations in supercritical helium. Here ψ is the ratio of the pressure drop upstream of the transposed critical line to the pressure drop downstream of the transposed critical,

$$\psi = \frac{\Delta p_{ab} + \Delta p_{bc}}{\Delta p_{cd} + \Delta p_{de}} \tag{9-9}$$

and $R = \Delta v_{bd}/v_b$ is the fluid expansion ratio. Downstream impedance is destabilizing, and upstream impedance is stabilizing.

9-2 PUMPS

9-2-1 Introduction

Cryogenic pumps, which are now commonplace, commercially available products, are used both for transferring liquid and slush cryogens between vessels and for circulating liquid and supercritical cryogens around coolant loops. When feasible, pressure transfer is the easiest, most cost-effective method of transfer. Pumps are often preferred for larger systems but are required for systems with a receiver pressure greater than the supply pressure.

Positive displacement pumps are best suited for high pressure rises and low flow rates. Available piston pumps give pressure rises of over 700 bar. *Centrifugal pumps* are favored for lower head rises and higher flow rates, although pumps with capacities as low as 0.1 L/s are feasible [33]. *Axial flow pumps* have been used to circulate cryogens, but their use is restricted to situations that require only the very low head these pumps produce. *Fountain effect pumps* (discussed in chapter 10) are used to transfer superfluid helium in the zero-*g* environment of space [34]. They can operate with a zero net positive suction head and have no moving parts.

The overall *efficiency* η of a pump is the ratio of its hydraulic power to the input power,

$$\eta = \frac{\rho g Q H}{\text{input power}} = \frac{Q \, \Delta p}{\text{input power}} = \frac{\dot{m} \, \Delta h_s}{\text{input power}} \tag{9-10}$$

where Q is the volumetric flow rate, H is the head rise across the pump,

$$H = \frac{p_2 - p_1}{\rho g} + \frac{V_2^2 - V_1^2}{2g} + z_2 - z_1 \tag{9-11}$$

and Δh_s is the isentropic enthalpy rise.

The term *transfer efficiency* is sometimes used to describe pump transfer systems. It is the ratio of the fluid delivered to the fluid consumed (the difference being the boil-off due to pump and transfer line losses). Although somewhat useful in defining total system performance, the transfer efficiency is not a good indicator of pump performance because it depends as much on the thermodynamic state at the pump inlet (i.e., the degree of subcooling) as it does on the pump efficiency.

Cavitation, the formation of vapor in the flow stream when the local pressure in a pump falls below the local saturation pressure by some necessary amount owing to flow acceleration, causes a reduction in the developed head of a pump and may erode pump components, such as impellers and inducers. The magnitude of the depression in the pressure below saturation pressure that induces cavitation depends on the thermodynamic and transport properties of a particular fluid [35,36]. The difference between the pump inlet pressure and the inlet saturation pressure (expressed in terms of head) is the *net positive suction head* (NPSH). The NPSH required to prevent cavitation in a pump depends on the pump type, construction, operating conditions, and fluid.

9-2-2 Centrifugal Pumps

Centrifugal pumps, as illustrated by the small experimental liquid helium pump [37] in Fig. 9-16, are simple devices with one moving assembly (motor shaft, ball bearings, and impeller in this case). This pump consists of (1) a stationary, two-piece *pump housing*, which includes a *vaneless diffuser* for efficient recovery of fluid kinetic energy; (2) a rotating, radial flow *impeller*, which imparts pressure and kinetic energy to the fluid; (3) an *inducer*, which is an axial flow, low-head preimpeller that suppresses cavitation in the impeller by boosting the pressure at the impeller inlet; and (4) a *drive motor* and *drive shaft* and bearings that power the impeller. The motor in this submersible pump is immersed in the liquid cryogen, so motor losses are transferred to the cryogen, which cools the motor and bearings. Bleed ports in the pump housing control the coolant flow. The submersible design offers the possibility of higher rotational speeds because the drive shaft is a short, cantilevered extension of the motor shaft. The overall pump

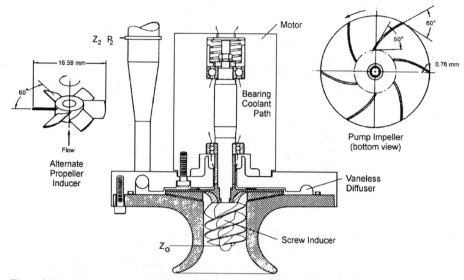

Figure 9-16 Small centrifugal pump for liquid helium with submersible motor (from Ref. [37]).

efficiency of the submersible design tends to be lower because all the motor losses are adsorbed at the operating temperature.

Warm drive pumps, illustrated in Figs. 9-17 through 9-19, remove the motor losses to ambient temperature but have conduction heat leak down the drive shaft and shaft housing. The drive shaft must be designed so that it does not operate near its critical speed yet has a relatively small heat leak. The pumps illustrated are designed with hermetic housings, and thus there are no dynamic seals in the assembly. This arrangement (1) eliminates the small but inevitable leakage that escapes through a dynamic seal during normal operation, (2) eliminates the possibility of massive leaks that can occur with seal failure, and (3) eliminates air leaking into the system during vacuum purging for charging of the system with pure gas because it will hold a hard vacuum (which a dynamic seal typically will not). This characteristic is especially important with flammable gases or liquids.

In contrast to the *open impeller* design illustrated in Fig. 9-19, Fig. 9-20 illustrates a *shrouded impeller*. Open impellers are easier to fabricate but have slightly lower efficiencies due to windage losses. The shrouded impeller requires close-fitting seals to minimize recirculation losses around the outside of the shroud. Smaller impellers have less advantage shrouded because the clearances on axial seals do not scale.

Conventional centrifugal pumps use a *full emission* design, but an unconventional *partial emission* design offers advantages in high-head, low-flow applications. Figure 9-21 compares impeller and diffuser flow passages for the two designs. The conventional full-emission design uses backward-curved blades on the impeller and a collector scroll that allows flow from all impeller channels to pass continually to the pump discharge. The partial emission design uses straight radial blades on the impeller and a diffuser that only allows flow from a small sector of the impeller channels to pass to the pump discharge. In some applications where the performance of a conventional full

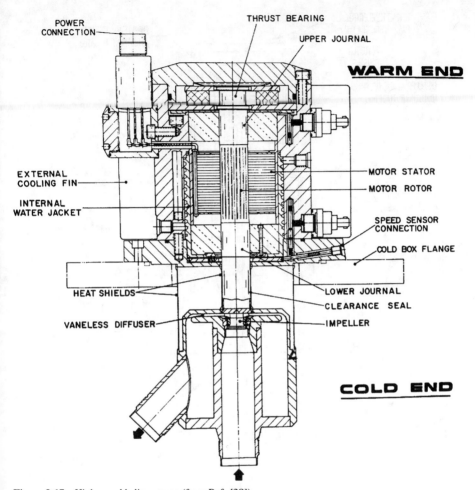

Figure 9-17 High-speed helium pump (from Ref. [38]).

emission pump would be unacceptably poor, a partial emission pump can be used in lieu of a fixed displacement pump.

Selecting a particular pump design (impeller type, diameter, and rotational speed) involves a trade-off between efficiency, reliability, and long life because pump efficiency tends to increase with rotational speed, whereas reliability and long life are more difficult to achieve with increased impeller speed. The relationship between impeller speed and efficiency is correlated using the concepts of specific speed and specific diameter:

$$\text{specific speed} \quad N_s = \frac{N Q^{0.5}}{H^{0.75}} \tag{9-12}$$

$$\text{specific diameter} \quad D_s = \frac{D H^{0.25}}{Q^{0.5}} \tag{9-13}$$

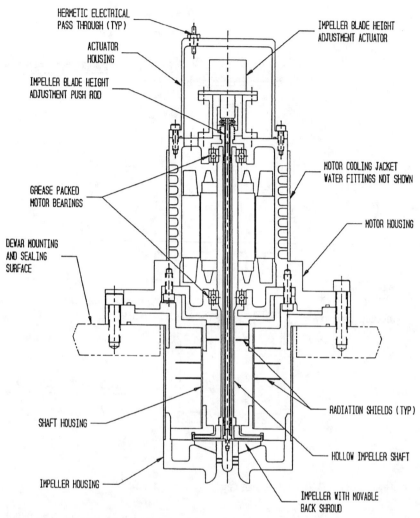

Figure 9-18   Liquid helium circulating pump.

where N = impeller speed (rpm)
D = impeller diameter (ft)
Q = volume flow rate (ft³/s)
H = isentropic head rise (ft)

Dynamic similarity of the flow occurs at like values of N_s and D_s because Reynolds number has only a secondary effect. With gravitational acceleration included in the head term (replacing H by gH), specific speed and diameter are dimensionless, but U.S. engineering practice uses dimensional quantities as above.

A universal performance map, Fig. 9-22, correlates the pump efficiency. The efficiency contours show that high-specific-speed, conventional full-emission pumps give

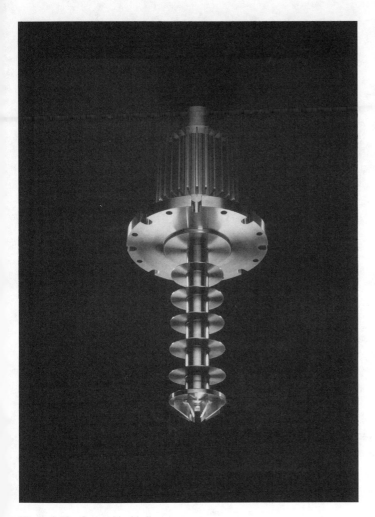

Figure 9-19 Supercritical helium pump.

the best performance; however, at specific speeds below about 30, a partial emission pump is more efficient. Thus, at lower specific speeds, partial emission pumps are favored and can be used in some applications ($N_s < 20$) where positive displacement pumps might normally be used. Use of partial emission pumps brings the advantages of centrifugal pumps (i.e., generous clearances, no rubbing parts, and low bearing loads).

Until recently pump speeds have usually been limited to 3600 rpm (synchronous speed of 60 Hz, 2-pole motors) because of the high cost of high-frequency drives or gear boxes. Recent advances in solid-state electronics have made variable frequency drives (VFDs) an economic option for pumps, and higher-speed drives are becoming common. The advantages of higher rotational speeds are illustrated by Table 9-2, which compares the designs of two pumps for the same application—same head and flow rate but different operating speeds.

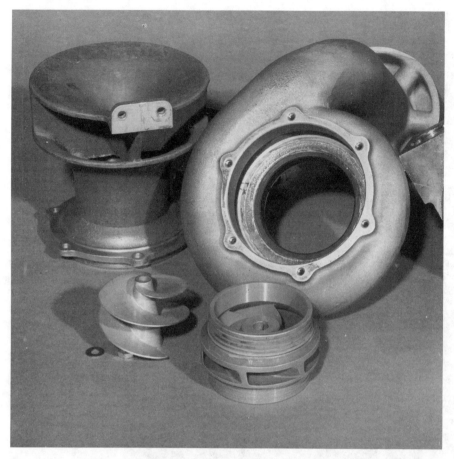

Figure 9-20 Disassembled Saturn SIV-B pump used in slush hydrogen pump tests. Clockwise from upper left are inlet housing, discharge volute, shrouded impeller, and inducer.

Typical pump performance curves, known as *characteristic curves*, are illustrated in Fig. 9-23 and 9-24. The variation in the performance of a particular pump with rotational speed N is

$$\frac{Q_1}{Q_2} = \frac{N_1}{N_2} \qquad \frac{H_1}{H_2} = \left(\frac{N_1}{N_2}\right)^2 \qquad \frac{P_1}{P_2} = \left(\frac{N_1}{N_2}\right)^3 \qquad (9\text{-}14)$$

where P is the pump power.

The effect of cavitation on centrifugal pump performance is illustrated in Fig. 9-25, which shows the deterioration in the developed head as the NPSH is reduced [37]. A comparison of the lower two curves shows the effect of inducer design. Replacing a simple propeller inducer with a variable pitch screw inducer reduced by a factor of nearly three the NPSH required to prevent cavitation. For a particular impeller and

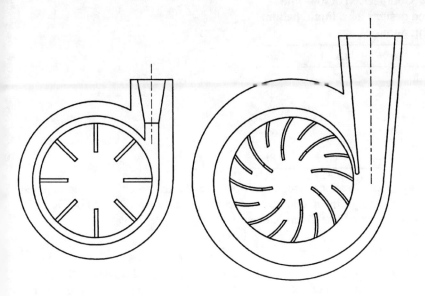

Partial Emission   **Full Emission**

Figure 9-21   Comparison of full emission and partial emission flow paths.

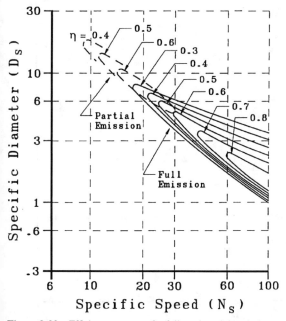

Figure 9-22   Efficiency contours for full- and partial-emission centrifugal pumps.

**Table 9-2 Comparison of low- and
high-speed designs for a liquid helium
circulating pump**

	Case 1	Case 2
Pump head (ft)	130	130
Flow rate (gpm)	48	48
Pump speed (rpm)	3600	7600
Impeller diameter (in.)	5.25	2.65
Specific speed	30.6	64.6
Specific diameter	4.54	2.27
Best possible efficiency	60	81

inducer design, both rotational speed and flow rate at fixed speed affect the required
NPSH. A comparison of the middle two curves (680 L/h versus 500 L/h) of Fig. 9-25
shows the effect of flow. The Thoma cavitation coefficient, defined as

$$\sigma = \frac{NPSH}{H} \tag{9-15}$$

is frequently used to correlate pump cavitation performance as illustrated by Fig. 9-26,
which gives σ as a function of specific speed for the liquid and slush hydrogen pump

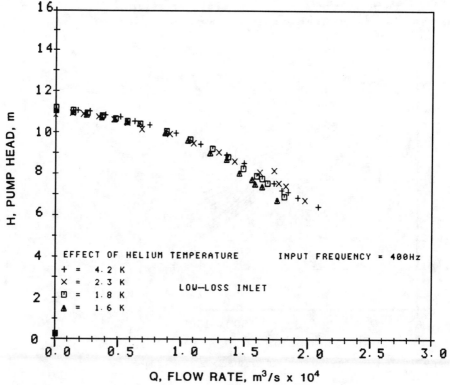

Figure 9-23 Performance of liquid helium pump illustrated in Fig. 9-16 in He I and He II (from Ref. [33]).

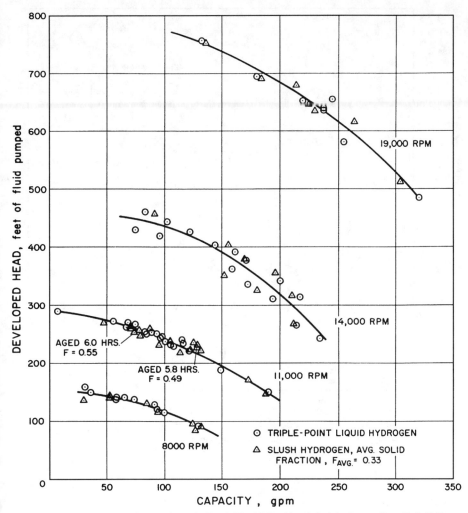

Figure 9-24 Performance of pump shown in Fig. 9-20 with liquid and slush hydrogen (from Ref. [14]).

shown in Fig. 9-20. Note that for this figure the specific speed N_s is defined with Q measured in gallons per minute, not cubic feet per second as used elsewhere.

A comparison of the top two curves (4.2 K, 500 L/h versus 1.8 K, 500 L/h) of Fig. 9-25 illustrates the effect of the thermodynamic and transport properties of the fluid being pumped. The unusual negative NPSH for He I in these tests is attributed both to the properties of He I and a sophisticated inducer design. The abrupt decrease in head of the 4.2 K curve occurred when the liquid level fell below the pump inlet and the pump started ingesting vapor. The actual NPSH for cavitation may be well below the -100 mm shown. Cavitation theory and tests under static conditions are not particularly useful in predicting the minimum NPSH for pumps because the pressure reductions from theory and static tests (e.g., ultrasonic techniques) may be orders of magnitude greater than those observed in flowing cryogens [35,39].

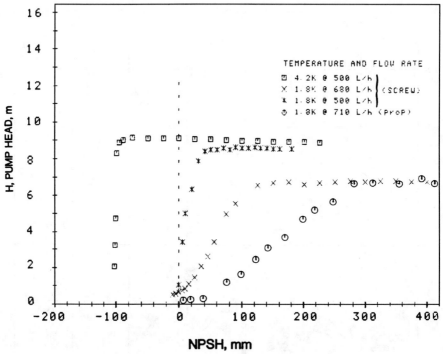

Figure 9-25 Cavitation characteristics of pump in Fig. 9-16 (from Ref. [33]).

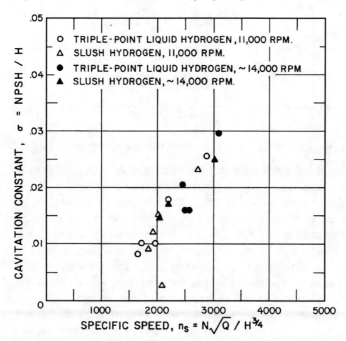

Figure 9-26 Cavitation constant for S-IVB pump (Fig. 9-20) with liquid and slush hydrogen (from Ref. [14]).

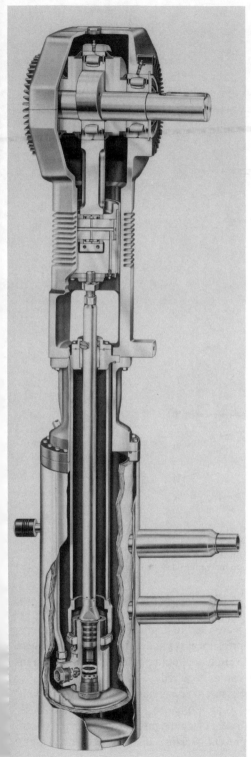

Figure 9-27 Small-bore commercial high-pressure pump. (Courtesy CVI Inc.)

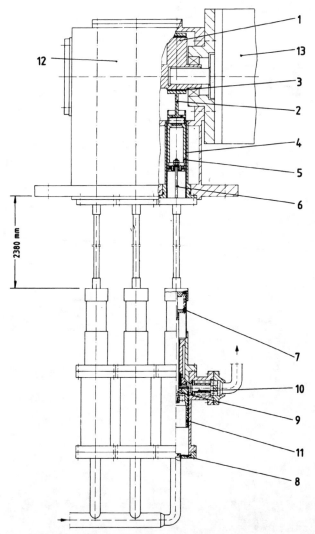

Figure 9-28   Three-cylinder piston pump for circulation supercritical helium (from Ref. [40]).

9-2-3 Positive Displacement Pumps

Positive displacement (reciprocating) pumps are used in applications requiring a very high pressure (head) rise such as filling high-pressure gas cylinders from a liquid cryogen supply. These pumps have also been used to circulate liquid or supercritical helium in cooling loops where pressure rises of a few bar are required.

Figure 9-27 is an example of a high-pressure commercial pump that, depending on the bore and stroke, delivers from 0.04 L/s at 700 bar to 1.9 L/s at 70 bar. These single-action pumps used for filling gas cylinders place the piston rod in compression. Consequently, the rod diameter is large to prevent buckling, and the heat leak is high, which is unimportant in this application.

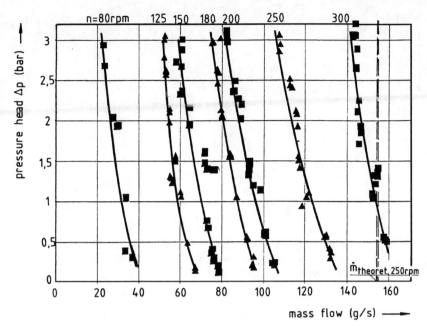

Figure 9-29 Pump characteristics for three-cylinder piston pump. Inlet conditions are 4 bar and 4.5 K (from Ref. [40]).

Figure 9-28 shows a three-cylinder piston pump used to circulate supercritical helium [40]. As illustrated in Fig. 9-28, the pistons (11) are driven by the upper crank mechanism with eccentric disks (1), connecting rods (2) rolling on needle bearings (3), and crossheads (5) guided in dry bushings (6). The piston rods (6) lift the pistons so that the rods are in tension, thus minimizing their cross section and heat leak. Return springs (7) maintain the piston rods in tension and prevent their buckling on the return stroke. The fluid is sucked into the space below the piston through a gravity valve (8) on the up stroke, and through the inlet valve (9) on the down stroke. The fluid leaves the pump through the exit valve (10). The piston has two guide rings and five sealing rings, all made with wear resistant Teflon compound.

Figure 9-29 shows the performance of this pump; its characteristic curves are nearly vertical. This behavior is in sharp contrast to that of centrifugal pumps, which have more horizontal characteristic curves over much of their flow range. The isentropic efficiency of the pump varies from 67% at the highest flow rate and head rise, to 22% at the lowest flow rate and head rise.

9-3 COLD COMPRESSORS

9-3-1 Introduction

Cold compressors are frequently used to boost the pressure of the low-pressure return stream in helium refrigerators operating at temperatures below about 4.4 K. Cold compressors offer the following advantages [41]: (1) reducing the volume of the low-pressure

Refrigeration [W]

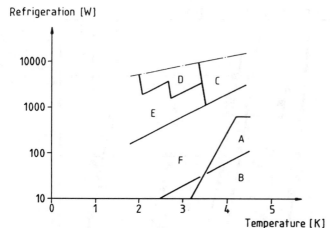

Figure 9-30 Range of application of different types of cold compressors; (a) ejector, (b) piston compressor, (c) turbocompressor, one stage to 1.2 bar, (d) turbocompressor, multistage to 1.2 bar, (e) turbocompressor, last stage below 1.2 bar (f) no cold compressor (from Ref. [41]).

side of the heat exchangers by reducing the volumetric flow rate; (2) eliminating subatmospheric piping outside the refrigerator cold box, thus reducing the possibility of air leaking into the helium refrigerant; and (3) improving the thermodynamic efficiency of the refrigeration cycle in some cases.

The effect of cold compressors on refrigerator efficiency is complex, but in general they can reduce losses associated with nonideal gas properties at the coldest temperatures. Because the specific heat of the low-pressure return stream is greater than that of the high-pressure stream at the lowest temperature part of a helium refrigerator, there is excess refrigeration in the low-pressure stream that cannot normally be used [41]. A cold compressor takes advantage of this surplus refrigeration. Ejectors use some of the available work (exergy) normally lost in a J–T expansion to compress the low-pressure stream.

Types of cold compressors include *ejectors* (jet pumps), *piston compressors*, and *turbocompressors* (both single and multistage). Figure 9-30 shows the approximate range of applicability of each type of compressor, as given by Quack [41]. With reference to the ranges of application delineated in the figure, the following comments are noteworthy:

A. The ejector is a simple device without moving parts. Its poor thermodynamic efficiency limits its use to lower capacities.
B. Piston compressors can be used for small volumetric throughputs. The lower the dead volume, the lower the attainable temperature.

Ranges C, D, and E are for cold turbocompressors.

C. Here the exhaust pressure of 1.2 bar can be reached in one stage of compression.
D. Here the final exhaust pressure of 1.2 bar requires several stages of compression.

E. Some pressure increase can be obtained from one or several stages of turbo compression, but it is not practical to try to reach 1.2 bar by cold compression.
F. There remains quite a large field where no technical solution for cold compression is now feasible. The volumetric flow rate is too large for a piston compressor and too small for a turbo compressor. The only technical solution available today is warming the gas up to room temperature and compressing it with room-temperature vacuum pumps.

9-3-2 Turbo Compressors

Several combinations of drive type (gas turbine, oil turbine, and electric motor) and bearing type (gas, oil, and magnetic) are used in cold turbo compressors, as illustrated in Figs. 9-31 through 9-34.

A matrix of bearing and drive combinations feasible for cold compressors appears in Table 9-3. Leakage of oil or warm bearing gas into the process stream is a major consideration in the matrix. For exhaust pressures greater than 1.2 bar, a number of drive and bearing combinations are feasible. For exhaust pressures below 1.2 bar, electric motor drive with magnetic bearings or ball bearings are in operation along with gas turbine drive with gas bearings.

The low density of low-pressure helium requires relatively high-tip-speed compressors to achieve adequate compression ratios. Figure 9-35 shows the effect of compressor

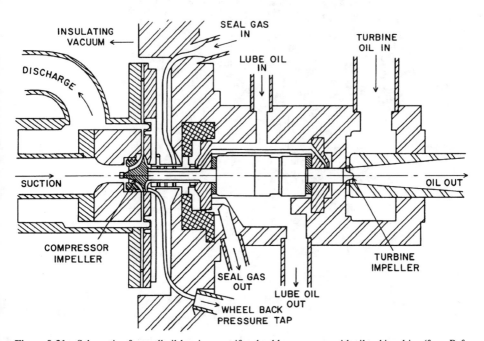

Figure 9-31 Schematic of a small oil-bearing centrifugal cold compressor with oil turbine drive (from Ref. [42]).

Table 9-3 Bearings and drives for cold compressor (from Ref. [44])

	Gas Turbine	Oil Turbine	Electric motor with gear	Electric motor direct	Exhaust pressure
Gas	++	−	−−	++	> 1 bar
bearings	++	−	−−	+	< 1 bar
Oil	+	++	+	++	> 1 bar
bearings	−	−	−	−	< 1 bar
Magnetic	+	−	+	++	> 1 bar
bearings	+	−	−	++	< 1 bar
Ball	+	+	−	++	> 1 bar
bearings	+	−	−	++	< 1 bar

Note: −− = not feasible,
  − = feasible, but problematic,
  + = feasible,
  ++ = machines in operation.

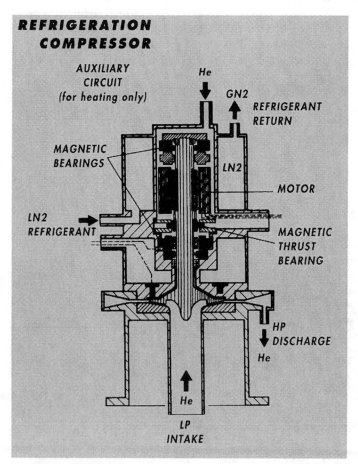

Figure 9-32 Cross section of cryogenic centrifugal compressor with active magnetic bearings and LN₂ cooled electric motor drive (from Ref. [43]).

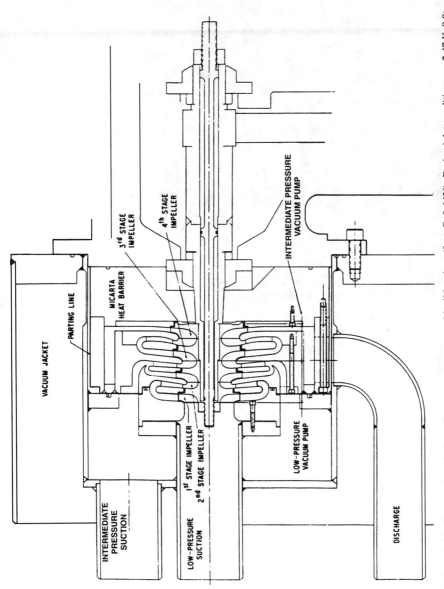

Figure 9-33 Cross section of a large four-stage compressor with oil bearings (from Ref. [42]). Design inlet conditions are 2.47 K 0.0t bar, and discharge conditions are 10.53 K, 1.36 bar.

VACUUM JACKET

PARTING LINE

MICARTA HEAT BARRIER

3rd STAGE IMPELLER

4th STAGE IMPELLER

INTERMEDIATE PRESSURE VACUUM PUMP

INTERMEDIATE PRESSURE SUCTION

1st STAGE IMPELLER

2nd STAGE IMPELLER

LOW-PRESSURE SUCTION

LOW-PRESSURE VACUUM PUMP

DISCHARGE

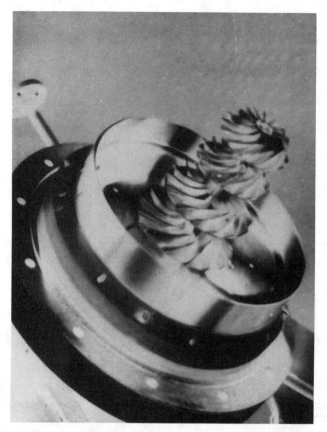

Figure 9-34 Photograph of turbine wheel assembly of compressor illustrated in Fig. 9-33 (from Ref. [42]).

speed on the performance of the last two stages of the compressor illustrated in Fig. 9-33.

9-3-3 Ejectors

Cold ejectors, introduced in helium refrigerators by Lacaze [45] and Rietdijk [46], are jet pumps that use available work (exergy) in the high pressure cold stream of a refrigerator to reduce the pressure of a subcooler bath, as illustrated in Fig. 9-36. Ejectors may be used alone or with a cold compressor.

In an ejector, Fig. 9-37, high-pressure supercritical helium at point 1 expands through a nozzle to form a high-velocity, low-pressure jet, which entrains the secondary (suction) flow that enters the ejector at point 2. The two streams combine in the mixing chamber and emerge from the diffuser as a two-phase flow at intermediate pressure, point 3. The flow in these simple devices is rather complex. Fluid enters the primary nozzle as supercritical, low-velocity flow and exits as supersonic and probably metastable liquid.

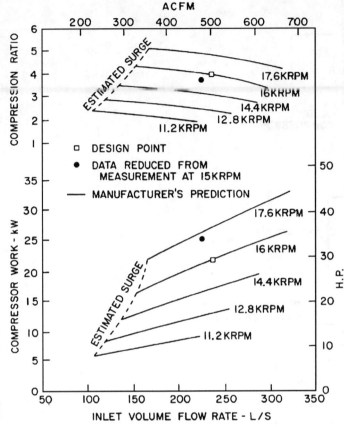

Figure 9-35 Compressor performance map for stages 3 and 4 of pump illustrated in Fig. 9-34 (from Ref. [42]).

In the mixing zone the primary jet becomes two-phase and decelerates to subsonic flow in a shock wave as it mixes with and accelerates the secondary flow. For these reasons, optimum ejector design is somewhat empirical. The performance of a helium ejector is illustrated by Fig. 9-38. Although the efficiency of ejectors, typically on the order of 20%, is lower than that of cold compressors, their simplicity of construction offers advantages for small-to-medium-capacity refrigerators.

9-4 CURRENT LEADS

9-4-1 Introduction

Current leads, which conduct electrical current into cryogenic equipment, vary in capacity from milliamperes or less for instrument leads to kiloamperes for large, superconducting magnets. *Conduction-cooled current leads*, which are simply wires or rods that

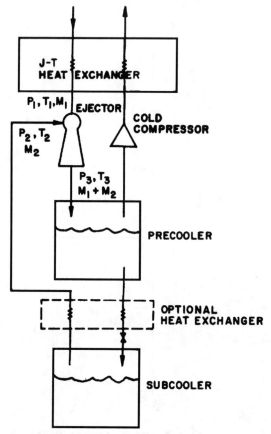

Figure 9-36 Flow diagram of an ejector in series with a cold compressor (from Ref. [47]).

span ambient and cryogenic temperatures, are favored for low-capacity leads because they are simple to build. *Gas-cooled current leads*, which are cooled by the counter-flow of cryogenic gas (usually boil-off gas), are preferred for high-capacity leads below liquid nitrogen temperature because they are more efficient. *Hybrid leads*, which use a metallic conductor for their upper stage (300 to about 77 K) and a high-temperature superconductor for their lower stage, are under investigation because they offer the promise of a several-fold improvement of efficiency compared with gas-cooled leads. The goal in the design of current leads is to minimize the heat leak per unit current, Q/I, while maintaining thermal stability.

Figure 9-39 shows how current affects the temperature profile of both conduction and gas-cooled metallic leads. At the optimum current for a particular lead, $(Q/I)_{min}$, the temperature gradient is zero at the ambient temperature end [49–51]. Thus, all the electrical losses in an optimized current lead are conducted to the low-temperature end. At greater than optimum currents, a maximum temperature occurs somewhere in the

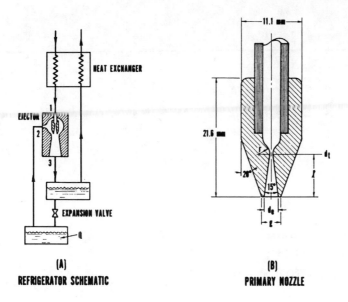

(A)
REFRIGERATOR SCHEMATIC

(B)
PRIMARY NOZZLE

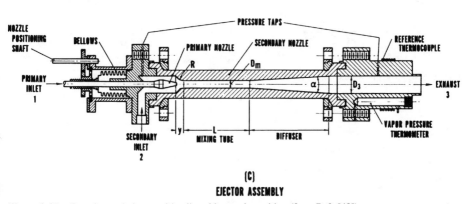

(C)
EJECTOR ASSEMBLY

Figure 9-37 Experimental ejector with adjustable nozzle position (from Ref. [48]).

central portion of the lead. If the maximum temperature exceeds the metallurgical limit (melting point) of the conductor, *burnout* occurs.

Intuition might suggest that purer metals with low electrical resistivities would be preferred for current leads because they can support higher current densities. This is not the case, however, because the thermal conductivity of purer metals is also higher, with the result that the optimum (minimum) value of the cold-end heat input $(Q/I)_{\min}$ is nearly independent of the material for a variety of pure metals and alloys. The relationship between the electrical resistivity ρ and the thermal conductivity k is given by the Wiedemann–Franz law

$$kρ = L_0 T \qquad (9\text{-}16)$$

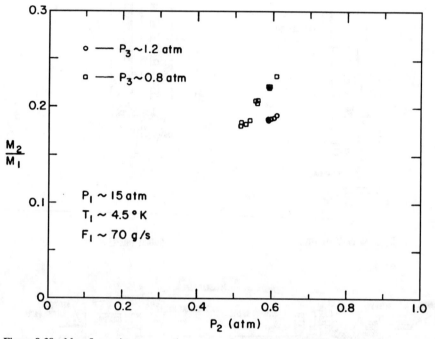

Figure 9-38 Mass flow ratio versus suction pressure for an ejector in a 3.7 K refrigerator (from Ref. [47]).

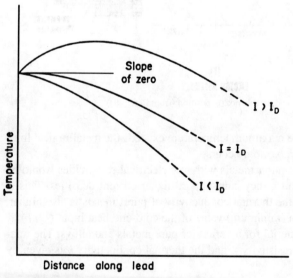

Figure 9-39 Dependence of current lead temperature profile with current (from Ref. [50]).

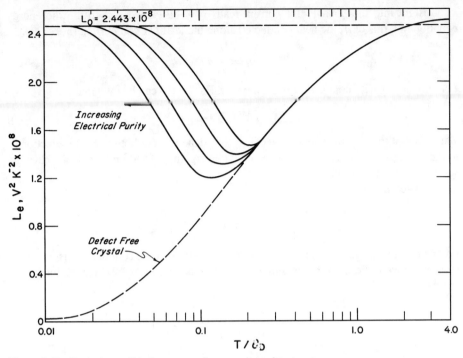

Figure 9-40 Dependence of the Lorentz number on purity and temperature.

where L_0, the Lorentz number, is nearly constant for pure metals. For the ideal case of elastically scattered electrons, $L_0 = 2.45(10)^{-8} A^2\Omega^2/K^2$. Analytical solutions to the current lead equations give

$$(Q/I)_{\text{minimum}} \approx \sqrt{L_0} \qquad (9\text{-}17)$$

Thus, $(Q/I)_{\text{minimum}}$ is fixed for fixed L_0. Experiment shows some variation of L_0 with material and temperature, as illustrated in Fig. 9-40. Although purer metals have a slightly lower average L_0, they should generally be avoided because they have higher temperature peaks for a given overload current and a lower heat capacity per unit current that leads to faster thermal runaway [52]. Thus, less pure metals offer superior stability and near-optimum efficiency. Analytical solutions to the current lead equations also show that tapering a lead will not improve its efficiency [50,53].

9-4-2 Conduction-Cooled Current Leads

The steady-state energy conservation equation for a conduction-cooled lead is

$$\frac{d^2T}{dx^2} = -\frac{I^2/A^2}{\sigma k} \qquad (9\text{-}18)$$

Both the electrical conductivity σ and the thermal conductivity k are generally functions of temperature, and thus Eq. (9-18) must be numerically integrated to predict the exact performance of a particular lead material.

Insight into the behavior of current leads may be gained by writing the energy equation in terms of q, the heat conducted along the lead per unit current ($q = Q/I$)

$$q\,dq = \frac{k}{\sigma}\,dT \tag{9-19}$$

For conductors with constant Lorentz number, Eq. (9-19) can be integrated to give

$$q_{L_{opt}} = \bar{L}_0^{1/2}\left(T_H^2 - T_L^2\right)^{1/2} \tag{9-20}$$

Thus, the optimum (minimum) value of $q_{L_{opt}}$ is independent of both material selection—to the first order—and cross-section profile; that is, tapered and uniform leads have the same optimum performance.

The geometry is given by

$$I\int_0^x \frac{dx}{A(x)} = \int_T^{T_L} \frac{k(T)\,dT}{q(T)} \tag{9-21}$$

For many commercial conductors, including copper, the thermal conductivity is relatively constant down to liquid nitrogen temperature. In that case Eq. (9-21) can be integrated to give

$$(LI/A)_{opt} = \frac{\pi}{2}\frac{\bar{k}}{\bar{L}_0^{1/2}}C_{os}^{-1}\left(\frac{T_L}{T_H}\right) \tag{9-22}$$

for constant cross section.

The heat conducted to the low temperature region by an optimum copper lead and the optimum lead geometry are given in Figs. 9-41 and 9-42 for ETP (electrolytic tough pitch) copper. McFee [50], assuming constant properties, calculated the off-optimum lead performance to be

$$\frac{Q_L}{(Q_L)_{min}} = \frac{1}{2}\left(\frac{I}{I_{opt}} + \frac{I_{opt}}{I}\right) \tag{9-23}$$

which is plotted in Fig. 9-43. Equation (9-23) shows that a current twice the design value results in only a 25% increase in heat flow over that of a lead optimized for twice the current. Note that Eq. (9-23) applies only to conduction-cooled leads. Gas-cooled leads have a different response to overcurrent and, depending on conductor purity, might burn out at twice the design current.

9-4-3 Gas-Cooled Current Leads

The unsteady-state, energy conservation equations for gas-cooled current leads are

$$\frac{\partial}{\partial x}\left(kA\frac{\partial T}{\partial x}\right) + \frac{I^2\rho}{A} = \frac{C}{v}A\frac{\partial T}{\partial t} + hA_s(T - T_g) \tag{9-24}$$

for the conductor, and

$$\frac{dT_g}{dx} = \frac{hA_s}{\dot{m}c_p}(T - T_g) \tag{9-25}$$

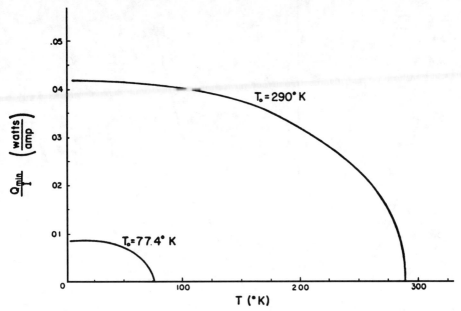

Figure 9-41   Heat conducted to low-temperature region by optimum, conduction-cooled copper lead connecting temperature T_0 to lower temperature T (from Ref. [50]).

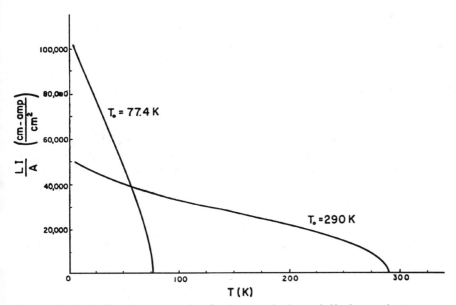

Figure 9-42   Ratio of length to cross section of optimum conduction-cooled lead connecting temperature T_0 to lower temperature T (from Ref. [50]).

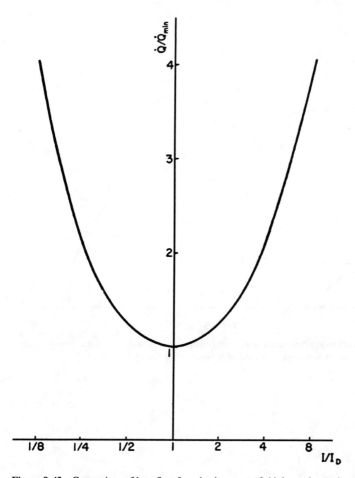

Figure 9-43 Comparison of heat flow from lead a current I, higher or lower than design value I_D, with heat flow that would occur if the lead were optimized for a new current I (from Ref. [50]).

for the coolant gas. As with Eq. (9-18), numerical integration of Eqs. (9-24) and (9-25) is required for a particular lead geometry and material. Odenov [53] recast the problem in terms of q' ($q' = Q/I\bar{L}_0^{1/2}$) and the gas-to-conductor heat transfer efficiency β ($\beta = 1$ for perfect heat transfer, and $\beta = 0$ for zero heat transfer—conduction cooling case). His governing equation is

$$\frac{dq'}{dT} + \frac{T}{q'} - Aq' = 0 \tag{9-26}$$

Here

$$A \equiv \frac{\beta c_p}{r} \tag{9-27}$$

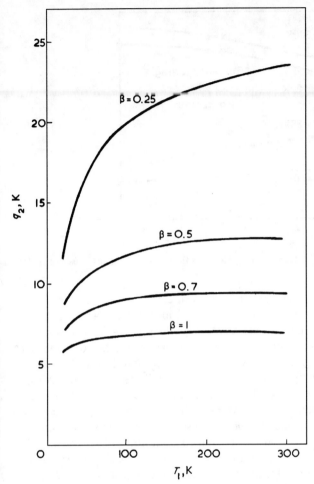

Figure 9-44 Heat conducted to 4.2 K in a gas-cooled lead as a function of lead warm-end temperature (from Ref. [53]).

where r is the latent heat of vaporization of the liquid evaporated by the heat conducted down the lead. Odenov's* analytical solution to Eq. (9-26) for an optimum lead is

$$T_1 = \left(q_2'^2 - A q_2'^2 T_2 + T_2^2\right)^{1/2} \times \exp\left[\frac{A q_2'^2}{B} \operatorname{arccot}\left(\frac{2T_2 - A q_2'^2}{q_2' B}\right)\right] \qquad (9\text{-}28)$$

where $B^2 = 4 - (A q_2')^2$.

Note that for a particular fluid (defined by A and T_2), the heat flow per unit current into the bath depends only on the warm-end temperature and the average Lorentz number. For $\beta = 0$ (conduction cooling), Eq. (9-28) reduces to Eq. (9-20). Figure 9-44 shows

---

*Odenov solved the more general problem of additional heat input to the bath and the lower end of the lead superconducting. Equations (9-26) and (9-28) are for the simpler case discussed above.

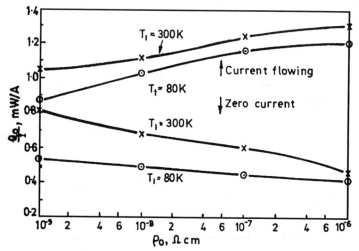

Figure 9-45 Heat dissipation at 4.2 K for an optimized lead as a function of the residual resistance ρ_0 (from Ref. [55]).

the solution of Eq. (9-28) for liquid helium. The heat conducted into the bath is only a weak function of the warm-end temperature. For an ideal Wiedemann–Franz metal $(L_0 = 2.45 \times 10^{-8}\ A^2\Omega^2/K^2)$, Eq. (9-28) gives $Q_0/I = 1.08$ mW/A for an autonomous helium-cooled lead. This value compares well with a numerical solution of 1.13 mW/A [54]. For nonideal metals, such as copper, the low-temperature heat leak is a weak function of the residual resistivity, as illustrated by Fig. 9-45. The slight reduction in heat leak associated with high-purity copper (low ρ_0) is at the expense, however, of a tendency towards thermal instability (burnout) [52]. At nondesign currents, high-purity copper is less efficient than lower purity materials, such as brass, as illustrated by Fig. 9-46.

The geometry of gas-cooled leads is determined from Eq. (9-21), which applies to both types of leads. Because of their lower values of $q(T)$, gas-cooled leads have a more slender aspect ratio than conduction-cooled leads. Figure 9-47 shows $(LI/A)_{opt}$ as a function of the residual resistance for helium-cooled copper leads. Table 9-4 gives the optimum lead geometry for a variety of materials; an empirical expression for the optimum geometry is [57]

$$\left(\frac{LI}{A}\right)_{opt} = 286(\rho_{4.2})^{-0.5} \tag{9-29}$$

Because current leads made from lower resistivity materials have a larger cross section and hence greater heat capacity, they can frequently be designed to operate at their rms current rather than at their peak current.

9-4-4 Hybrid Current Leads

The advent of high-temperature superconductors (HTSs)[†] provides a means for escaping the minimum low-temperature heat conduction value of 1.1 mW/A imposed by the

---

[†]Additional Information on high-temperature superconductors may be found in chapter 2 of this handbook.

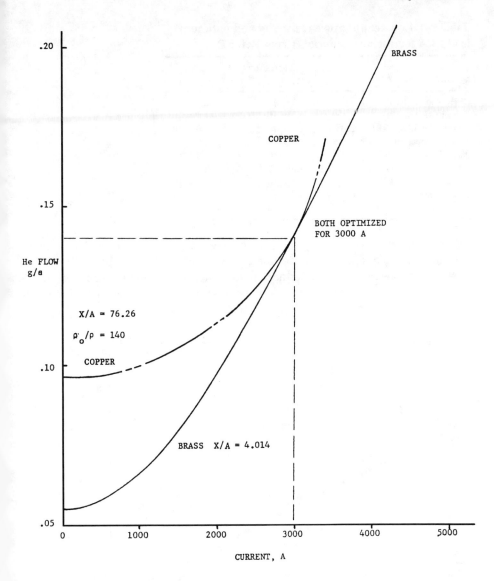

Figure 9-46 Comparison of helium boil-off for brass and copper vapor-cooled current leads (from Ref. [56]).

Wiedemann–Franz law. Because their thermal conductivity is low and their electrical resistivity vanishes, HTSs can be used as the lower stage of hybrid HTS-metal current leads, which have significantly lower low temperature losses. Mumford proposed this arrangement in 1988 [58]. Figure 9-48 illustrates such a lead. The upper metallic stage may be either conduction-cooled or vapor-cooled by helium boil-off gas, nitrogen boil-off gas, or gas taken from an intermediate stage of a refrigerator.

In contrast to helium temperature leads for which the low-temperature heat load is 43 times lower for gas-cooled leads than for conduction-cooled leads [53], gas cooling offers only a slight advantage for nitrogen temperature leads, as illustrated by Table 9-5.

Table 9-4 Low-temperature resistivity and optimum lead LI/A for various materials (from Ref. 57)

Material	4.2 K resistivity (Ω m)	IL/A value (A per m)
OFHC copper (RRR = 180)	8.7×10^{-11}	2.7×10^{7}
Copper (RRR = 30)	5.3×10^{-10}	1.1×10^{7}
1100-O aluminum (RRR = 25)	1.0×10^{-9}	9.0×10^{6}
Type-M copper pipe (RRR = 6.5)	3.1×10^{-9}	5.6×10^{6}
Phos. deox. copper (RRR = 3)	6.7×10^{-9}	3.5×10^{6}
6061-T6 aluminum (RRR = 2)	1.4×10^{-8}	2.4×10^{6}
70 Cu 30 Zn brass (RRR = 2)	2.8×10^{-8}	1.7×10^{6}
5456 Aluminum (RRR = 1.4)	3.3×10^{-8}	1.6×10^{6}
304 Stainless steel (RRR 1.1)	3.7×10^{-7}	4.7×10^{5}

The elimination of gas cooling in the upper stage of a hybrid lead results in greater flexibility in lead design. The conduction-cooled upper segment can be flexible so that lead penetrations into the cryostat need not be aligned with the terminals of the device being supplied current. Furthermore, because conduction-cooled hybrid leads are efficient, cryogen-free systems using cryocoolers are feasible.

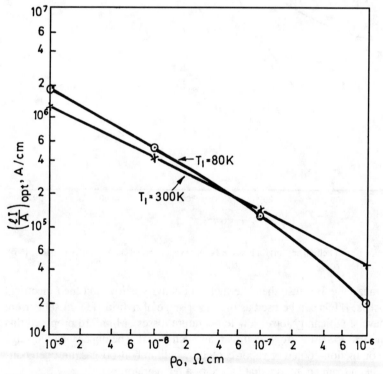

Figure 9-47 Optimum geometry as a function of the residual resistance for a gas-cooled current lead connecting temperature T_1 to 4.2 K (from Ref. [55]).

Table 9-5 Cryogenic loads for different liquefaction modes (from Ref. [59])

	$\dot{Q}_L$ per kA[a]	P_e per kA[b]
Optimized all-metal CL, 300–4.2 K	1.14 W, vapor cooled	1.7–3.4 kW, vapor cooled[c]
Optimized metal CL, 300–77 K	≈30 W, vapor cooled ≈41 W, conduction cooled	380–580 W, vapor cooled[c] 400–600 W, conduction cooled[d]
HTCL conduction cooled, 77–4.2 K	0.12 W, Bi-2212 tube 0.32 W, Y-123 tube	40–80 W, Bi-2212 tube[d] 180–350 W, Y-123 tube[d]

[a] Heat loads $\dot{Q}_L$ at refrigeration temperature
[b] Electric power consumption P_e of refrigerator
[c] Liquefaction of 300 K vapors
[d] Liquefaction of cold vapors

The gain in efficiency achieved by HTS hybrid leads depends on the type of HTS conductor as well as its configuration. Table 9-5 illustrates, however, that the total electric power consumption of hybrid leads tends to be dominated by the losses in the upper normal conducting stage. In the best case the overall power consumption is reduced by a factor of nearly four. Melt-cast BSCCO leads have superior thermal performance but are brittle. For this reason silver-sheathed BSSCO tapes are also under investigation because

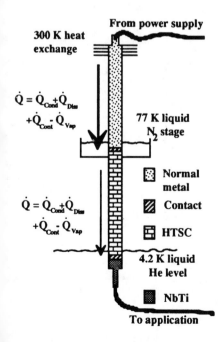

Figure 9-48 Hybrid current lead and its heat loads (from Ref. [59]).

they are more robust. For magnet leads, a parallel path of normal conductor—a safety lead—can dump energy from the magnet in case the HTS lead breaks or is driven normal.

Unlike metal leads, tapered HTS leads are more efficient but difficult to fabricate from silver-sheathed tapes. Because the electrical loss of an HTS lead is essentially zero when it operates below its critical current, it may be possible to exceed the critical current and operate in the flux-flow loss regime. However, leads operating in this regime may be unstable.

In cryogen-free systems the heat intercept at the junction of the normal conductor and the HTS presents a problem because the intercept should have a high thermal conductance and yet be electrically insulated from the cryostat. Several solutions to this problem are available:

1. Move the electrical isolation point outside the cryostat. The cryocooler is grounded to the lead with a high-conductance metallic connection (copper braid or leaves), and the cooler is electrically isolated.
2. Use a thin layer of plastic film, epoxy, or G-10 glass–epoxy, which has low thermal conductivity and make the surface area large enough to give an acceptable thermal conductance. The thickness must be great enough to give an adequate breakdown voltage.
3. Clamp a sheet crystalline dielectric, such as sapphire or aluminum nitride, between the lead and the cooled surface. At low temperature these crystalline dielectrics have thermal conductivities comparable with copper.
4. Use an annular heat pipe in which the central conductor is electrically insulated from the outer cooled shell by epoxy dielectric joints, as illustrated in Fig. 9-49. The heat

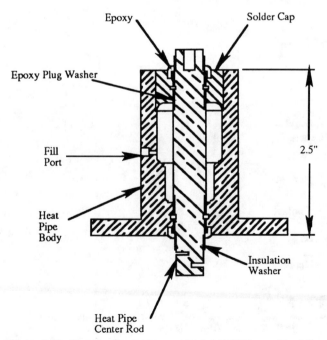

Figure 9-49   Heat pipe thermal intercept for hybrid HTS current lead (from Ref. [60]).

pipe is filled at ambient temperature with nitrogen gas at about 135 bar so that when cooled to operating temperature the annular space is partially filled with liquid nitrogen, which evaporates from the inner conductor (removing heat from the lead) and condenses on the outer shell that is thermally coupled to the cryocooler.

The development of hybrid leads follows the development of high current capacity, robust HTS conductors. Because of the potential improvement in efficiency offered by these leads, they are under consideration for a number of applications.

9-5 HEAT EXCHANGERS

9-5-1 Introduction

Heat exchangers for cryogenic equipment range in size from 25,000 m^2 surface area for natural gas liquefiers to less than 1 cm^2 for microminiature J–T coolers for electronics. Regardless of size, the purpose of cryogenic heat exchangers is to conserve refrigeration,* subject to constraints of size or cost. The effort justified in a heat exchanger design varies with the application, of course. In heat exchangers for large LNG or air separation plants, small reductions in the heat exchanger irreversibilities may result in substantial savings of input power costs over the life of the plant, and thus a detailed, sophisticated analysis may be called for. In helium-temperature refrigerators and small coolers, an optimum design may be required for the device to work at all. On the other hand, all that may be required in a small laboratory heat exchanger may be a back-of-the-envelope calculation and a few coils of copper tubing.

The goal of conserving refrigeration may be expressed more precisely as one of optimizing the performance of a heat exchanger by minimizing its losses, subject to a constraint such as holding the surface area, N_{tu}, or volume constant. These losses are measured in terms of the loss in the availability function Λ (exergy) and are given by

$$\Delta \Lambda_{\text{loss}} = T_0 \Delta S_{\text{loss}} \tag{9-30}$$

where T_0 is the ambient temperature and ΔS_{loss} is the net entropy generation in the heat exchanger. The two major sources of loss in heat exchangers are those due to the temperature difference between the process streams exchanging heat and those due to friction (pressure drop). The entropy generation in a heat exchanger section of length dx is [61,62]

$$\Delta S_{\text{loss}} = \frac{q' \Delta T}{T^2 (1 + \Delta T/T)} + \frac{\dot{m}}{\rho T} \left(-\frac{dp}{dx} \right) \cong \frac{q' \Delta T}{T^2} + \frac{\dot{m}}{\rho T} \left(-\frac{dp}{dx} \right) \geq 0 \tag{9-31}$$

The $1/T^2$ dependence of the heat exchanger loss illustrates the importance that efficient heat exchangers play in cryogenic processes. The losses for transferring a fixed quantity of heat at a fixed ΔT are 5100 times greater at 4.2 than at 300 K! For a series of counterflow heat exchangers of fixed size that span some temperature range, Grassman and Kopp [61] show that the losses are minimized by making $\Delta T \approx T$. They also show that the heat transfer coefficient should increase as the temperature is lowered.

---

*Vaporizers, of course, are an exception.

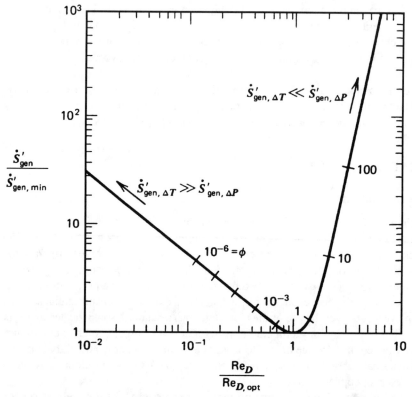

Figure 9-50 Relative entropy-generation rate for forced-convection heat transfer through a smooth tube (from Ref. [62]).

An essential feature of Eq. (9-31) is that a proposed design change (e.g., making the passage longer or more narrow) induces changes in the opposite direction in the two terms of the expression. Thus, there exists an optimum design for which the overall irreversibilities are a minimum, as illustrated by Fig. 9-50, in which the irreversibility distribution ϕ is defined as

$$\phi = \frac{\text{fluid-flow irreversibility}}{\text{heat transfer irreversibility}}. \qquad (9\text{-}32)$$

For this example, $\phi_{opt} = 0.17$, so the optimum does not occur when the two irreversibility mechanisms are perfectly balanced, although setting $\phi = 1$ is a fair (back-of-the-envelope) way of guessing the optimum. In heat exchanger design it should be recognized that there is a limit to the advantage gained by increasing the heat exchanger size.

Some characteristics common to many cryogenic heat exchangers are

1. Compact size (high heat transfer area to volume ratio) so as to reduce their outside surface area and hence the heat leak.
2. High surface area per unit mass flow and a high heat transfer coefficient so as to achieve high effectiveness and low losses.

3. Low pressure drop so as to keep frictional irreversibilities in balance.
4. High pressure in some cases (for some processes such as J–T refrigerators, the high-pressure channels may see pressures of 200 bar or more).
5. Operation in regions with nonideal fluid properties in some cases.
6. Operation in a high-vacuum insulation space in some cases (in which case the outer shell must typically be leaktight to better than 10^{-8} or 10^{-9} std cm^3/s helium leak rate).

9-5-2 Types of Heat Exchangers

Heat exchangers may be classified according to designation as recuperative or regenerative, flow arrangement, or according to type of construction.

Recuperative heat exchangers. Flow arrangements typical of recuperative heat exchangers and their accompanying temperature profiles are illustrated in Fig. 9-51. The counterflow arrangement is the workhorse of cryogenic heat exchangers because it has

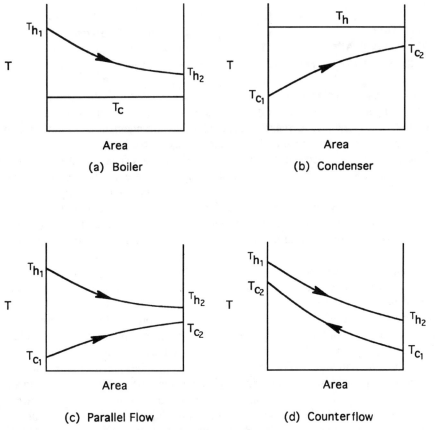

Figure 9-51 Axial temperature distribution in heat exchangers.

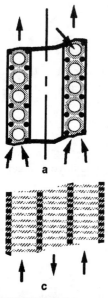

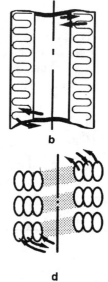

a) **FINNED TUBE**
c) **PERFORATED PLATE**

b) **CORRUGATED HOSE**
d) **FLATTENED TUBE**

Figure 9-52   Some J–T heat exchangers used in small cryocoolers (from Ref. [63]).

the lowest losses. For balanced flow, $(\dot{m}c_p)_h = (\dot{m}c_p)_c$, the temperature difference, and hence the temperature difference portion of the loss, approaches zero as the area of a counterflow heat exchanger increases (the parallel-flow arrangement is seldom used in cryogenic heat exchangers because of its inherently high losses).

Construction types of simple cryogenic counterflow heat exchangers are illustrated in Figs. 9-52 and 9-53. Two of the simplest arrangements are a pair of copper tubes soldered together and wound in a coil for compactness and a coil of copper tubing in an annular space—typically with boil-off gas in the annulus in counterflow with a pressurized stream in the tube. Commercial internally finned tubing can be incorporated in some of these simple configurations to improve the surface area and heat transfer coefficient.

Some more complex configurations used when size, economics, or process require large size or a low-loss heat exchanger are coiled tubular (Hampson), plate-fin, and perforated plate. Figure 9-54 illustrates a large tubular-type heat exchanger. It has several tube-side streams. The tubes are coiled around the core in a number of layers and collected at both ends of the exchanger in headers. The core cylinder gives mechanical stability, and its minimum diameter is determined by the maximum curvature of the tube for which no flattening occurs. Successive layers of tubes are wound in opposite directions and separated by spacing strips to give uniform crossflow on the shell side.

Figure 9-55 illustrates a brazed aluminum plate-fin heat exchanger. This type heat exchanger is quite flexible in its flow configuration with up to 11 streams and 4 refrigeration temperature levels designed into a single shell. It is compact (up to 450 ft^2

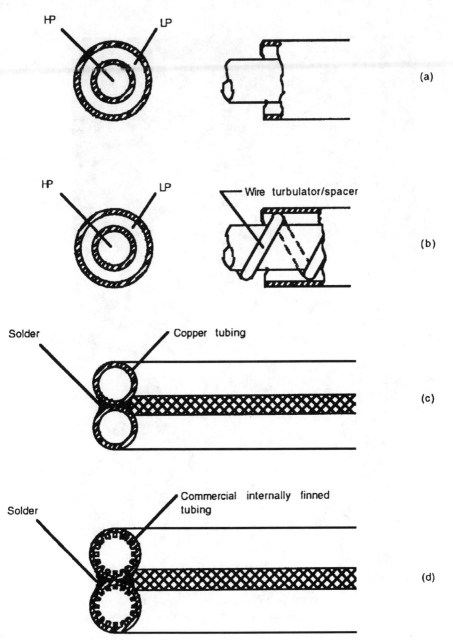

Figure 9-53 Some simple tubular heat exchanger configurations: (a) concentric tubes, (b) concentric tubes with spacer–turbulator, (c) soldered refrigeration tubing pairs, (d) soldered, internally finned tube pairs.

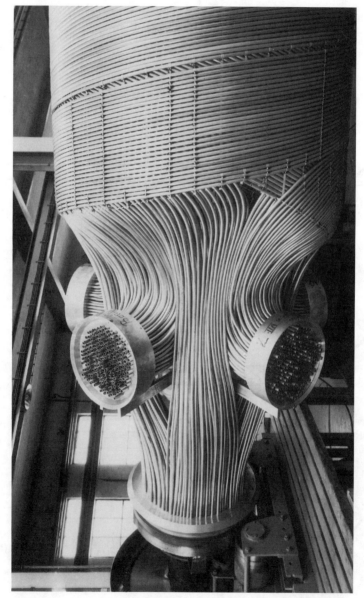

Figure 9-54 Typical large-coiled tubular heat exchanger (from Ref. [64]).

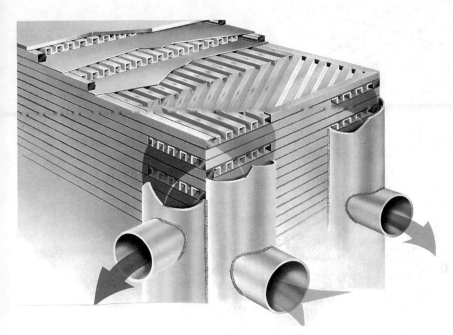

Figure 9-55   Brazed aluminum plate-fin heat exchanger. (Courtesy Altec International Inc.)

surface area per cubic foot of heat exchanger volume), and lightweight because of its aluminum construction. Design pressures up to 60 bar are possible.

Figure 9-56 illustrates the core of a perforated-plate heat exchanger [65–67] used in small cryogenic refrigerators. These are very compact as indicated by Table 9-6. Although plastic separators between flow passages appear in the figure, more recent practice uses stainless steel spacers with diffusion bonding [68], or vacuum brazing [69] to prevent leaks between channels and through the outer shell. The leakage problem previously hindered the development of this class of heat exchanger. Sixsmith et al. [70] developed a similar heat exchanger with slots, that gives about a 40% higher heat transfer coefficient than circular holes.

The reversing heat exchanger scheme of Fig. 9-57 [71] is frequently used to remove carbon dioxide and water from the feed stream of cryogenic air separation plants. The flow in channels A and B periodically reverses so that impurities frozen out in A (while the raw airstream flows into A) are swept out by clean gas after the flow is reversed. Proper operation of reversing heat exchangers requires careful attention both to the phase equilibria of the frozen contaminants and to the temperature distribution in the heat exchanger. Reversing heat exchangers are usually oriented with the cold end up so that flow of melted contaminants is towards the warm end.

Regenerators are quite simple devices that exhibit very complex behavior. A regenerator with counterflow—the arrangement used in cryogenic applications—is illustrated in Fig. 9-58. As with the reversing heat exchangers described above, the regenerator is a periodic flow device. In the first part of the cycle, flow at some temperature T_0 enters the regenerator matrix from the left. As the gas (or fluid) flows through the regenerator,

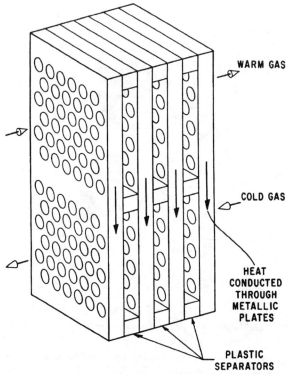

Figure 9-56 Perforated-plate heat exchanger principle (from Ref. [65]).

it exchanges heat with the matrix and is warmed (assuming $T_0 < T_L$) while the matrix cools some. In the second part of the cycle, gas flows into the regenerator from the right at some temperature T_L and is cooled as it progresses towards the low-temperature end of the regenerator. The matrix warms back to its original condition.

In the limit of infinite regenerator heat capacity (no temperature swing of the matrix), the counterflow regenerator behaves just like a counterflow heat exchanger. Real

Table 9-6 Comparison of heat transfer capacity of some compact cryogenic heat exchangers (from Ref. [68])

Type	Schematic	Heat transfer capacity per unit volume UA/V [W/m³ K]
Perforated plate	See Fig. 9-56	39,000
Fin tube		28,000
Aluminum-plate fin		8,800

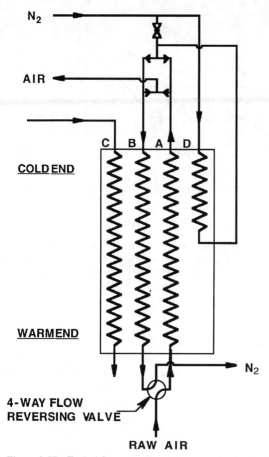

N₂

AIR

C B A D

COLD END

WARM END

N₂

**4-WAY FLOW
REVERSING VALVE**

RAW AIR

Figure 9-57   Typical flow arrangement in a reversing heat exchanger for an air separation plant.

regenerators, however, and particularly cryogenic regenerators operating below about 15 K (where the volumetric heat capacity of the matrix is reduced to the same order of magnitude as that of the gas) see significant swings in the matrix temperature, as illustrated by Fig. 9-59.

A regenerator's effectiveness is based on the mass average of the gas exit temperature, which varies with time, as illustrated by Fig. 9-60. Not only is the effectiveness a function of regenerator size (N_{tu}) and the ratio of fluid heat capacities (C_{min}/C_{max}), it also depends on the ratio of the heat capacity of the regenerator matrix to the heat

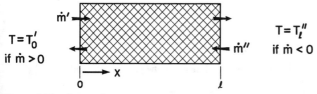

$T = T_0'$
if $\dot{m} > 0$

$\dot{m}'$

$T = T_l''$
if $\dot{m} < 0$

$\dot{m}''$

x

0   l

Figure 9-58   Counterflow regenerator schematic.

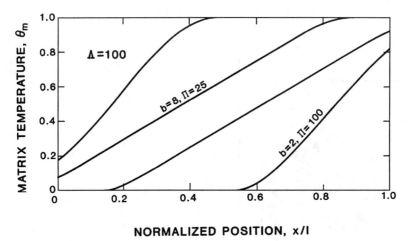

NORMALIZED POSITION, x/l

Figure 9-59 Swing in the matrix temperature of a cryogenic regenerator. The matrix temperature is shown at the end of each half cycle for two regenerators, each with an effectiveness of 0.98. The inner pair of curves are for one regenerator, and the outer pair of curves are for the other. The temperature swings are larger than normally encountered (from Ref. [72]).

capacity of the fluid (C_r/C_f) and the ratio of the fluid void volume heat capacity to the heat capacity of the fluid that passes through the regenerator (C_{void}/C_f).

Cryogenic regenerators range in size from large pebble-filled regenerators used in liquid air plants (in a manner analogous to reversing heat exchangers) to small wire screen or lead-shot-filled regenerators used in Stirling, G–M, and pulse-tube cryocoolers. Typical matrix packing materials are pebbles, ceramic balls, and corrugated metal ribbon in larger regenerators; and bronze screen and lead spheres in cryocoolers. Regenerators

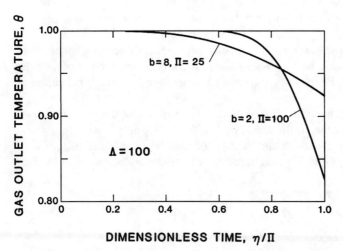

DIMENSIONLESS TIME, η/Π

Figure 9-60 Variation of the gas outlet temperature with time for the two regenerators in Fig. 9-59 (from Ref. [72]).

operating below 10 K use materials such as Er_3 (erubium 3 nickel), which has a high heat capacity at low temperatures owing to a magnetic transition [73].

9-5-3 Heat Exchanger Design*

The first law of thermodynamics applied to a steady-flow heat exchanger with two channels gives

$$dH_h = (A_s U/\dot{m}_h)(T_h - T_c)\, d\Psi \qquad (9\text{-}33)$$

for the enthalpy change of the warm stream, and

$$dH_c = \pm(\dot{m}_h/\dot{m}_c)\, dH_h \qquad (9\text{-}34)$$

for the enthalpy change of the cold stream, where the plus sign refers to counterflow and the minus sign to parallel flow. In Eq. (9-33)

$$d\Psi = d A_s/A_s \qquad (9\text{-}35)$$

and U is a function of temperature and pressure.

Depending on the thermodynamic region of the gases (or fluids) in the heat exchanger, T_h and T_c may be simple or complex functions of H_h and H_c, and further simplification of the preceding equations may or may not be appropriate. If the heat exchanger operates in the near-critical region, where the specific heat is a strong function of both temperature and pressure (see Fig. 1-9), numerical integration of Eqs. (9-33) and (9-34) using a thermodynamic property code gives the most accurate and informative result. The integration may be obtained with finite difference or element techniques, or the problem may be treated as an initial value or propagation problem with initial values at one end of the heat exchanger (e.g., T_{h1} and T_{c2}) used to march through the heat exchanger to obtain values at the other end (T_{h2} and T_{c1}). Because the inlet stream conditions at opposite ends of the heat exchanger (T_{h1} and T_{c1}) are usually the knowns, iteration of the solution is required until the assumed value of T_{c2} gives the correct inlet condition T_{c1}. In regions where there is a particularly strong dependence of pressure, it is necessary to solve the pressure drop equations simultaneously with Eqs. (9-33) and (9-34). Figure 9-61, which gives the temperature distribution of a helium counterflow heat exchanger operating in the near-critical region, shows the effect that nonuniform heat capacity may have on the stream-to-stream temperature difference. In such cases the temperature difference in the middle of the heat exchanger is considerably larger than that at either end. In some cases the opposite situation may arise with a temperature pinch occurring in the middle of the exchanger. In these cases a heat exchanger design would be faulty if based on the log mean temperature difference at the ends.

If a heat exchanger design requires only modest accuracy, using average properties, even in the near-critical region, gives results with accuracies on order of 15% or better in the ineffectiveness [74]. In the noncritical region, harmonic averaging of the specific heat gives values of effective N_{tu} within a few percent for balanced flow, with larger errors for unbalanced flow [75].

---

* Design of He II heat exchangers is covered in chapter 10 of this handbook.

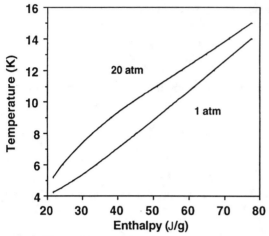

Figure 9-61   Temperature distribution of a counterflow heat exchanger operating in the near-critical region.

If the specific heat of each stream is constant, then Eqs. (9-33) and (9-34) may be combined to give

$$\frac{d(T_h - T_c)}{T_h - T_c} = \left(\pm \frac{1}{C_h} - \frac{1}{C_c} \right) U A_s \, d\Psi \tag{9-36}$$

with

$$C_h = (\dot{m}c_p)_h \quad \text{and} \quad C_c = (\dot{m}c_p)_c \tag{9-37}$$

Introducing the concept of heat exchanger effectiveness

$$\varepsilon = \frac{C_h(T_{h1} - T_{h2})}{C_{min}(T_{h1} - T_{c1})} = \frac{C_c(T_{c2} - T_{c1})}{C_{min}(T_{h1} - T_{c1})} \tag{9-38}$$

which is the ratio of the actual heat transferred to the thermodynamically maximum possible gives for counterflow [76,77]

$$\varepsilon = \frac{1 - e^{-N_{tu}(1 - C_{min}/C_{max})}}{1 - (C_{min}/C_{max})e^{-N_{tu}(1 - C_{min}/C_{max})}}. \tag{9-39}$$

For balanced counterflow ($C_{min} = C_{max}$), Eq. (9-38) becomes

$$\varepsilon = \frac{N_{tu}}{1 + N_{tu}} \tag{9-40}$$

The number of transfer units (N_{tu}) is the dimensionless size of the heat exchanger and is given by $N_{tu} = A_s U / \dot{m}c_p$.

Because most cryogenic heat exchangers have an effectiveness close to 1, it is usually more instructive to consider the ineffectiveness $1 - \varepsilon$, which is proportional to the heat exchanger loss and is more indicative of heat exchanger performance. For balanced counterflow the ineffectiveness is

$$1 - \varepsilon = \frac{1}{1 + N_{tu}} = \frac{\Delta T}{T_{h1} - T_{c1}} \tag{9-41}$$

The overall heat transfer coefficient U is given by [76]

$$\frac{1}{U_r} = \frac{1}{\varepsilon f f_c h_c} \frac{d A_r}{d A_c} + R_w \frac{d A_r}{d A_w} + \frac{1}{\varepsilon f f_h h_h} \frac{d A_r}{d A_h} \qquad (9\text{-}42)$$

where A_r is the reference surface area (usually A_c or A_h); for a flat plate $R_w = x_w/k_w$, and for a cylinder

$$R_w = \left[\frac{\ln(r_0/r_i)}{2\pi k_w} \right] \frac{d A_r}{dL} \qquad (9\text{-}43)$$

The overall surface efficiency εff is defined as

$$\varepsilon ff = \eta \frac{A_f}{A} + \frac{A_u}{A} \qquad (9\text{-}44)$$

where $A \equiv A_u + A_f$, the unfinned plus finned surface area. The fin effectiveness for a rectangular fin on a flat wall is

$$\eta = \frac{\tanh mL}{mL} \qquad (9\text{-}45)$$

where

$$m = \sqrt{\frac{2h}{k\delta}} \qquad (9\text{-}46)$$

Figure 9-62 presents the fin effectiveness for straight and circular fins. The effectiveness for other configurations is presented graphically in Ref. [78].

The ineffectiveness as a function of N_{tu} is shown in Fig. 9-63 for balanced flow and Fig. 9-64 for unbalanced flow ($C_{min}/C_{max} = 0.95$). For heat exchangers with high effectiveness such as those used in cryogenic applications, axial heat conduction can lead

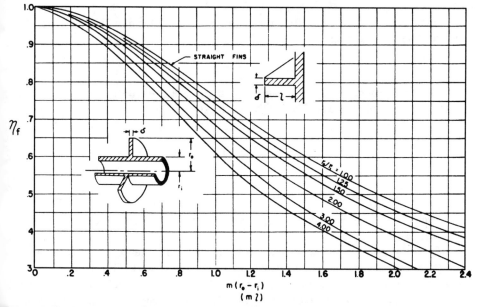

Figure 9-62 Fin effectiveness for straight and circular fins (from Ref. [77]).

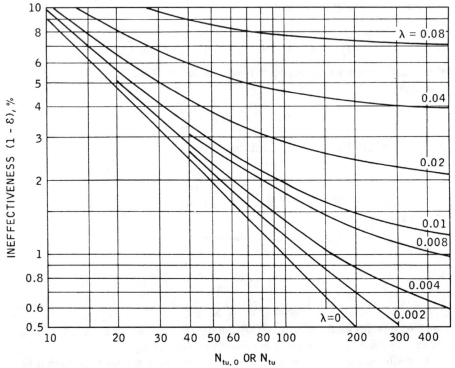

Figure 9-63 Heat exchanger ineffectiveness for balanced flow ($C_{min}/C_{max} = 1$) heat exchangers and balanced flow regenerators with $C_m/C_{min} > 5$. The effect of axial conduction is given by the parameter λ (from Ref. [77]).

to significant reductions in the effectiveness, as illustrated in the figures, which show the dimensionless conduction

$$\lambda = \frac{k A_c}{L C_{min}} \qquad (9\text{-}47)$$

as a parameter. For ranges of parameters other than those given, the ineffectiveness with axial conduction may be calculated with an expression developed by Kroeger [79]

$$1 - \varepsilon = \frac{1 - C_{min}/C_{max}}{\Psi e^{r_1} - C_{min}/C_{max}} \qquad (9\text{-}48)$$

with

$$r_1 = (1 - C_{min}/C_{max})\frac{N_{tu}}{1 + \lambda N_{tu} C_{min}/C_{max}} \qquad (9\text{-}49)$$

and with Ψ taken from Fig. 9-65. Kroeger also gives ineffectiveness curves for a number of values of $\dot{C}_{min}/C_{max}$.

Two other sources of irreversibility that limit the performance of high-design N_{tu} cryogenic heat exchangers are heat leak from the environment and flow maldistribution. Precise evaluation of these effects requires detailed computer models of the particular heat exchanger. Chowdhury and Sarangi [80] derived an analytical solution for the effects of heat leak on a simple, coaxial, counterflow heat exchanger. For the case of a

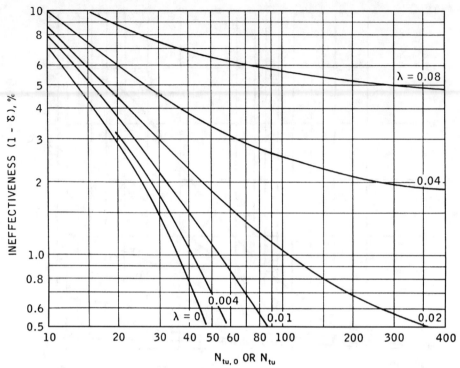

Figure 9-64 Heat exchanger ineffectiveness for unbalanced flow $(C_{min}/C_{max} = 0.95)$ heat exchangers and balanced flow regenerators with $C_m/C_{min} > 5$. The effect of axial conduction is given by the parameter λ (from Ref. [77]).

counterflow heat exchanger operating between ambient and liquid air temperatures, they developed a chart, Fig. 9-66, which relates the effective N_{tu} to the design N_{tu} as a function of $v = C_{min}/C_{max}$, and a heat leak parameter $\alpha = U_0 A_0/U_i A$ (the ratio of the shell-to-ambient thermal conductance to the thermal conductance between streams). For a typical value of $\alpha = 10^{-4}$ for cryogenic air plant heat exchangers, Fig. 9-66 shows that the effective N_{tu} has a limiting value of 100—regardless of the design N_{tu} of the heat exchanger. Increasing this heat exchanger size much above N_{tu} design causes little reduction in the heat transfer irreversibility, while increasing the pressure drop irreversibility.

Flow maldistribution in multiparallel-passage heat exchangers degrades their performance because the gain in effectiveness in the low-flow channels is less than the loss of effectiveness in the high-flow channels. This phenomenon arises from the $1/(1 + N_{tu})$ dependence of the ineffectiveness. Because the effects of flow maldistribution become more severe as the design N_{tu} increases, they are a major concern in the design of cryogenic heat exchangers. The lower susceptibility of coiled-tubular heat exchangers to flow maldistribution effects has been a factor encouraging their use in base-load LNG plants. Fleming [81] analyzed flow maldistribution effects for several flow passage arrangements, and Weimer and Hertzog [82] used detailed computer models to analyze effects in plate-fin and coiled tubular heat exchangers. Some conclusions from their studies are

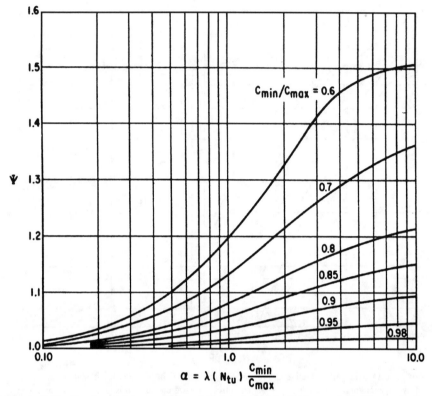

Figure 9-65 Function Ψ for computation of heat exchanger ineffectiveness including conduction effects (from Ref. [79]).

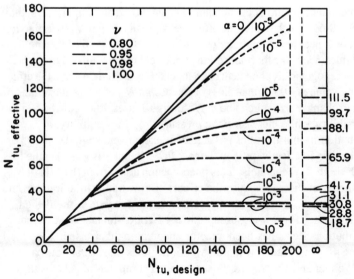

Figure 9-66 Relation of effective N_{tu} to the design N_{tu}, heat capacity ratio ν and heat leak parameter α (from Ref. [80]).

1. If the flow distribution is nonuniform, little is gained by increasing the design N_{tu}; rather, the distribution should be improved by careful attention to header design and channel uniformity.
2. The effect of flow maldistribution can be reduced either by mixing the uniform side flow throughout the exchanger or by adding headers to the exchanger and mixing the flow from both streams at intervals along its length.
3. Because of the complexity of exchangers in cryogenic service, it is difficult quantitatively to generalize the effects of maldistribution with simple models. Detailed computer simulation is recommended.

9-5-4 Regenerator Design

The time-dependent, one-dimensional equations of a regenerator, neglecting transverse temperature gradients in the matrix packing, and assuming incompressible flow, are

$$\frac{\partial T}{\partial t}(\rho A c_p) = -\dot{m} c_p \frac{\partial T}{\partial x} - h A_s (T - T_m) \tag{9-50}$$

for the fluid and

$$\frac{\partial T_m}{\partial t}(\rho A C)_m = h A_s (T - T_m) \tag{9-51}$$

for the matrix. Introducing a dimensionless position ξ and dimensionless time η, flow direction M, a matrix to void volume heat capacity ratio b, and a normalized temperature θ, Eqs. (9-50) and (9-51) are transformed to dimensionless equations

$$\frac{\partial \theta}{\partial \eta} = -Mb\frac{\partial \theta}{\partial \xi} - b(\theta - \theta_m) \tag{9-52}$$

for the fluid and

$$\frac{\partial \theta_m}{\partial \eta} = (\theta - \theta_m) \tag{9-53}$$

for the matrix.

For a regenerator with periodic flow reversal and equal flow periods, the boundary and flow conditions are

$$\begin{array}{ll} \text{at } \xi = 0 \\ \theta = 1 & \text{when } n\Pi < \eta < (n+1)\Pi, \quad \text{and} \quad M = +1 \\ \text{at } \xi = 1 \\ \theta = 0 & \text{when } (n+1)\Pi < \eta < (n+2)\Pi, \quad \text{and} \quad M = -1 \end{array} \tag{9-54}$$

The term on the left-hand side of Eqs. (9-50) and (9-52) is usually small, and thus usually neglected. For regenerators operating at temperatures below about 15 K, however, this term becomes significant and should be included in an accurate analysis. Hausen [83] first solved the regenerator equations with periodic flow. A review of techniques for solving these equations is given in Ref. [84].

Figures 9-67 and 9-68 give the regenerator ineffectiveness as a function of $N_{tu,0}$, which is given by

$$\frac{1}{N_{tu,0}} = \frac{1}{(C_h/C_{min})\Lambda_h} + \frac{1}{(C_c/C_{min})\Lambda_c} \tag{9-55}$$

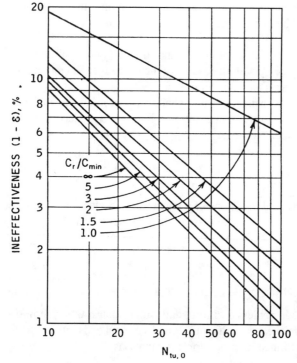

Figure 9-67 Regenerator ineffectiveness as a function of N_{tu} and matrix capacity-rate ratio for $C_{min}/C_{max} = 1$ (from Ref. [77]).

and the reciprocal of the heat load on the regenerator $C_r/C_{min} = \Lambda/\Pi$. For balanced flow $(C_h = C_c)$, Eq. (9-55) becomes

$$N_{tu,0} = \frac{1}{2}\Lambda \qquad (9\text{-}56)$$

As previously noted, when the heat load on the regenerator matrix is zero $(C_r/C_{min} = \infty)$, the effectiveness of both the counterflow regenerator and counterflow heat exchanger is identical. The effect of void volume heat capacity on regenerator performance is illustrated in Fig. 9-69 for a regenerator with $N_{tu,0} = 50$ $(\Lambda = 100)$ [73]. The lower curve $(b = \infty)$ is for the case of negligible void volume heat capacity. The behavior of regenerators with significant void volume heat capacity can be counterintuitive. In some regenerators with low matrix heat capacity, increases in matrix heat capacity may reduce the effectiveness rather than increase it.

9-5-5 Heat Transfer Coefficients and Pressure Drop

The multitude of heat transfer surfaces available is testament to the ingenuity of heat exchanger designers. We give heat transfer correlations for a few of the simpler configurations and refer the reader to the references—especially *Compact Heat Exchangers* by Kays and London [77]—for a more comprehensive treatment. The uncertainty in the correlations is typically on the order of 10 to 20%.

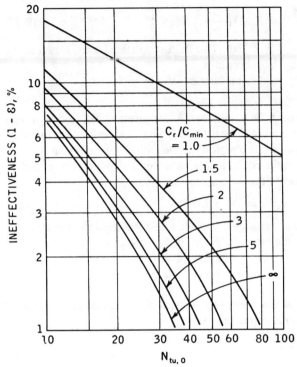

Figure 9-68 Regenerator ineffectiveness as a function of N_{tu} and matrix capacity-rate ratio for $C_{min}/C_{max} = 0.95$ (from Ref. [77]).

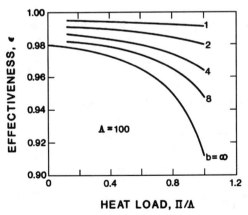

Figure 9-69 Regenerator effectiveness versus the thermal load Π/Λ for various ratios of matrix-to-void-volume heat capacity b (from Ref. [73]).

Heat transfer inside tubes. For *circular tubes*, the heat transfer is correlated by the expression

$$\left(\frac{hd}{k_b}\right) = 0.023 \left(\frac{Gd}{\mu_b}\right)^{0.8} (Pr)_b^{0.4} \tag{9-57}$$

for $2300 < Re < 10^7$ and $0.5 < Pr < 120$. The fluid properties are evaluated at the bulk temperature, as indicated by the subscript b.

For *short tubes* ($L/d < 60$), modify the heat transfer by

$$h_m/h_\infty = 1 + (d/L)^{0.7} \tag{9-58}$$

where h_m is the mean transfer over the length, and h_∞ is given by Eq. (9-57). Equation (9-58) illustrates the improvement in heat transfer given by perforated plate heat exchangers, which operate in the entrance region regime with d/L values near one.

In *helical coils* the heat transfer coefficient is enhanced by an induced secondary flow. For fully developed turbulent flow the enhancement is

$$h_c/h = 1 + 3.5d/D_h \tag{9-59}$$

For *annular or rectangular passages*, replace the tube inside diameter d in Eq. (9-57) with the equivalent diameter D_e given by Eq. (9-2). For an annulus, D_e is $D_o - D_i$, the difference between the outside and inside diameter.

To evaluate pressure drop inside tubes, refer to section 9-1-2.

Heat transfer outside tubes. For flow normal to banks of tubes, such as in coiled tubular heat exchangers, the heat transfer is correlated by

$$\left(\frac{h_m d_o}{k}\right) = C \left(\frac{G_{max} d_o}{\mu_b}\right)^{0.6} (Pr)_b^{1/3} \tag{9-60}$$

where $C = 0.33$ for staggered tubes and 0.26 for in-line tubes. The heat-transfer coefficient h_m is the mean for 10 or more tubes, and G_{max} is based on the minimum flow area between tubes.

Evaluate the pressure drop for turbulent flow ($2000 < G_{max} d_0/\mu_b < 40{,}000$) across tube banks using

$$\Delta p = 4f'N \frac{G_{max}^2}{2\rho} \left(\frac{\mu_w}{\mu_b}\right)^{0.14} \tag{9-61}$$

where N is the number of tube rows normal to the flow. 2 For *in-line tubes*

$$f' = \left[0.044 + \frac{0.08x_L}{(x_T - 1)^n}\right] \left(\frac{d_o G_{max}}{\mu}\right)^{-0.15} \tag{9-62}$$

and for *staggered tubes*

$$f' = \left[0.23 + \frac{0.11}{(x_T - 1)^{1.08}}\right] \left(\frac{d_o G_{max}}{\mu}\right)^{-0.15} \tag{9-63}$$

where $n = 0.43 + 1.13/x_L$. Here x_L is the ratio of longitudinal pitch to tube diameter, and x_T is the ratio of transverse pitch to tube diameter.

Plate-fin surfaces. An example of the heat transfer and friction correlations for a plate-fin heat exchanger is illustrated in Fig. 9-70, which uses the hydraulic radius ($r_h = D_h/4$).

Regenerator surfaces. For a *randomly packed bed of spheres* the heat transfer is correlated by

$$\left(\frac{hD_p}{k}\right) = 0.80\left(\frac{G_0 D_p}{\mu}\right)^{0.7}(Pr)^{1/3} \qquad (9\text{-}64)$$

with the mass flux G_0 based on the cross-sectional area of the empty bed. Obtain the bed pressure drop from

$$\left(\frac{\rho\,\Delta p}{G_0^2}\right)\left(\frac{D_p}{L}\right)\left(\frac{\varepsilon^3}{1-\varepsilon}\right) = 150\frac{1-\varepsilon}{D_p G_0/\mu} + 1.75 \qquad (9\text{-}65)$$

The packing density ε for randomly packed spheres is 0.59.

For *woven screen* regenerators the heat transfer is correlated by Fig. 9-71 and the pressure drop by Fig. 9-72.

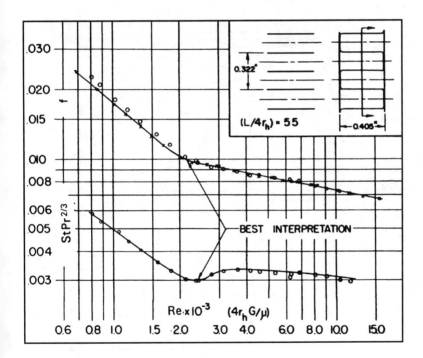

Fin pitch = 6.2 per in.= 244.1 per m
Plate spacing, b = 0.405 in.= 10.29×10^{-3} m
Flow passage hydraulic diameter, $4r_h$ = 0.0182 ft = 5.54×10^{-3} m
Fin metal thickness = 0.010 in. aluminum = 0.254×10^{-3} m
Total transfer area/volume between plates, β = 204 ft²/ft³ = 669.3 m²/m³
Fin area/total area = 0.728

Figure 9-70 Heat transfer and friction factor correlations for a typical plate-fin heat exchanger (from Ref. [77]).

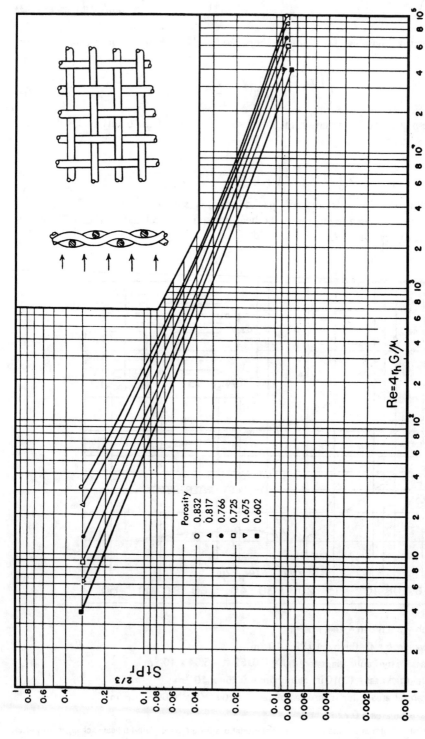

Figure 9-71 Heat transfer characteristics for gas flow through an infinite randomly stacked woven-screen matrix. The mass flux is given by $G = \dot{m}/\dot{\rho}A_{\mathrm{fr}}$, and the hydraulic radius is given by $r_{\mathrm{h}} = p/\alpha$ (from Ref. [77]).

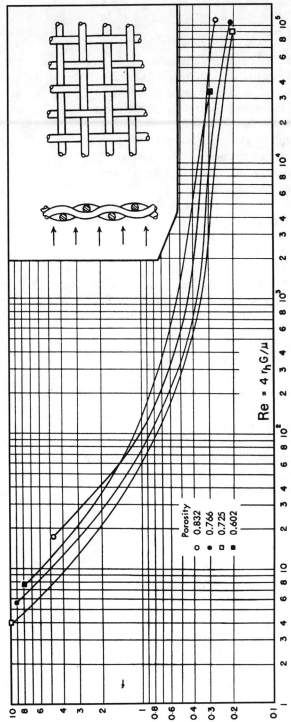

Figure 9-72 Flow friction characteristics for gas flow through an infinite randomly stacked woven-screen matrix. The mass flux is given by $G = \dot{m}/\rho A_{\mathrm{fr}}$, and the hydraulic radius is given by $r_{\mathrm{h}} = p/\alpha$ (from Ref. [77]).

Porosity	
○	0.832
●	0.766
□	0.725
■	0.602

$$Re = 4 r_h G/\mu$$

NOMENCLATURE

SI units are used throughout in the equations except for pump specific speed and specific diameter, as noted in the text. Some figures taken from original publications use centimeter-gram-second (cgs) or other units. In most equations, any set of consistent units may be used. Parameters listed without units are dimensionless.

A	Parameter defined by Eq. (9-27)	
A	Fluid flow cross section, current lead cross section	m^2
A_c	Heat exchanger conduction path cross section	m^2
A_{fr}	Heat exchanger or regenerator total frontal area	m^2
A_s	Heat exchanger surface area	m^2/m
b	Regenerator matrix to fluid heat capacity ratio, $(\rho AC)_m / \rho A c_p$	
c	Velocity of sound	m/s
c_p	Specific heat at constant pressure	J/kg
C	Heat capacity	J/kg
C_{max}	Maximum of C_c or C_h	W/K
C_{min}	Minimum of C_c or C_h	W/K
C_c	Heat capacity of heat exchanger cold stream, Eq. (9-37)	W/K
C_h	Heat capacity of heat exchanger warm stream, Eq. (9-37)	W/K
d_i	Pipe inside diameter	m
d_o	Pipe outside diameter	m
D	Impeller diameter	ft
D_e	Equivalent diameter defined by Eq. (9-2)	m
D_i	Annulus inside diameter	m
D_0	Annulus outside diameter	m
D_h	Helix diameter	m
D_s	Specific diameter, Eq. (9-13)	$s^{1/2}/ft^{1/4}$
f	Fanning friction factor (Other definitions of friction factor differ by a numerical value of 1/4 or 1/2.)	
g	Local acceleration of gravity	m/s^2
G	Mass flux	$kg/s \cdot m^2$
h	Enthalpy	J/kg
h	Heat transfer coefficient	$W/m^2 \cdot K$
H	Pump head rise	m
H_c	Enthalpy of heat exchanger cold stream	J/kg
H_h	Enthalpy of heat exchanger warm stream	J/kg
I	Current	A
k	Thermal conductivity	$W/m \cdot K$
K	Resistance coefficient	
K_s	Isentropic compressibility, $(\frac{\rho}{T} \frac{\partial T}{\partial \rho})_s$	
L	Pipe length	m
L_e	Equivalent length of valves and fittings	m
L_e'	$L + L_e$	m
L_0	Lorentz number, kg/T	$A^2 \Omega^2/K^2$
$\dot{m}$	Mass flow rate	kg/s

M	Mach number	
N	Impeller speed	rpm
N_s	Pump specific speed	rpm ft$^{3/4}$/s$^{1/2}$
N_{tu}	Number of heat exchanger transfer units, $A_s U/\dot{m}c_p$	
$NPSH$	Net positive suction head	m
p	Pressure	Pa
p	Matrix porosity	
P	Pump power	W
$\mathcal{P}$	Wetted perimeter	m
q	Q/I	W/A
q'	$Q/(I\bar{L}_0^{1/2})$	K
Q	Heat transfer rate	W
Q	Pump volumetric flow rate	ft^3/s
r	Latent heat of vaporization	J/kg
r	Tube diameter	mm
R_e	Reynolds number, Gd/μ	
S	Entropy	J/kg · K
t	Time	s
T	Temperature	K
T_0	Ambient temperature	K
U	Overall heat transfer coefficient, Eq. (9-42)	W/m^2 · K
v	Specific volume	m^3/kg
V	Velocity	m/s
x	Axial position	m
z	Elevation	m
α	Flow uniformity factor. For highly turbulent, slug-like flow $\alpha = 1$, and for laminar flow (parabolic velocity distribution) $\alpha = 0.75$.	
α	$A/A_{fr} \cdot L$	1/m
Λ	Heat transfer per unit length	W/m
Λ	Availability function, $H - T_0 S$	J/kg
Λ	Dimensionless regenerator length, $\frac{hA_sL}{\dot{m}c_p}$	
β	Current lead transfer efficiency	
ε	Heat exchanger effectiveness, Eq. (9-38)	
εff	Overall surface efficiency, Eq. (9-44)	
η	Pump efficiency	
η	Fin effectiveness	
η	Dimensionless regenerator time, $\frac{hA_st}{(\rho AC)_m}$	
λ	Heat exchanger conduction parameter, Eq. (9-47)	
ξ	Ratio of warm to cold tube length	
ξ	Dimensionless regenerator position, $\frac{hA_sx}{\dot{m}c_p}$	
μ	Viscosity	Pa · s
Π	Dimensionless regenerator period, $\frac{hA_sP}{(\rho AC)_m}$	
ρ	Electrical resistivity	Ωm

ρ	Density	Kg/m^3
ρ_m	Mean fluid density	Kg/m^3
ρ_1	Fluid density at position 1	Kg/m^3
ρ_2	Fluid density at position 2	Kg/m^3
σ	Thoma cavitation constant	
σ	Electrical conductivity	1/Ωm
ϕ	Grüneisen parameter, $(\frac{\rho}{T}\frac{\partial T}{\partial \rho})_s$	
ϕ	Irreversibility distribution, Eq. (9-32)	
Φ	Potential energy function (gz for gravity)	m^2/s^2
Ψ	Pressure drop ratio defined by Eq. (9-9)	
Ψ	Dimensionless heat exchanger length	

Subscripts

c1	Cold stream inlet
c2	Cold stream exit
g	Gas
h1	Warm stream inlet
h2	Warm stream exit
H	High-temperature end
L	Low-temperature end
m	Regenerator matrix
opt	Optimum
min	Minimum
s	Constant entropy

REFERENCES

1. Daney, D. E., and Ludtke, P. R., "Friction Factors for Flow of Near Critical Helium in Curved Tubes," *Cryog.* 18 (1978):345.
2. Junghans, D., Friction Factor of Supercritical Helium in a Straight Tube, *Cryog.* 20 (1980):633.
3. Kropschot, R. H., Birmingham, B. W., and Mann, D. B., eds., *Technology of Liquid Helium*, U.S. Department of Commerce, National Bureau of Standards Monograph 111 (Washington, D.C.: U.S. Government Printing Office, 1968).
4. Figure courtesy of CVI Incorporated, P.O. Box 3138, Columbus, Ohio 43216, USA.
5. Crane Technical Paper No. 410 (Joliet, Illinois: Crane Valve, 1969).
6. Daney, D. E., "Behavior of Turbine and Venturi Flowmeters in Superfluid Helium," *Adv. Cryog. Eng.* 33 (1988):1071.
7. Weisend, J. G., II, and Van Sciver, S. W., "Pressure Drop from Flow of Cryogens in Corrugated Bellows," *Cryog.* 30 (1990):935–941.
8. Ito, H. J., "Friction Factors for Turbolent Flow in Curved Pipes," *J. Basic Engr.* D81 (1959):123.
9. Arp, V. D., "Thermodynamics of Single-Phase One-Dimensional Fluid Flow," *Cryog.* 15 (1975):285.
10. Sindt, C. F., "A Summary of the Characterization Study of Slush Hydrogen," *Cryog.* 10 (1970):372.
11. Sindt, C. F. Ludtke, P. R., and Daney D. E., *Slush Hydrogen Fluid Characterization and Instrumentation*, U.S. Department of Commerce, National Bureau of Standards Technical Note 377 (Washington D.C.: U.S. Government Printing Office, 1969).
12. Daney, D. E., Arp, V. D. and Voth, R. O., "Hydrogen Slush Production with a Large Auger," *Adv. Cryog. Eng.* 35 (1990):1767.

13. Voth, R. O., Ludtke, P. R., Daney, D. E., and Brennan, J. A., *Production, Characterization, and Flow of Slush Hydrogen*, National Aerospace Plane. Tech. Memo. 1165 (1992).

14. Daney, D. E., Ludtke, P. R., and Sindt, C. F., *Slush Hydrogen Pumping Characteristics Using a Centrifugal-Type Pump*, in Adv. Cryog. Eng. (1969):438.

15. Stepanoff, A. J., "Pumping Liquid-Solid Mixtures," *Mech. Eng.* 86 (Sept. 1964):29.

16. Taconis, K. W., Beenakker, J. J. M., Nier, A. O. C., and Aldrich, L. T., "Measurements Concerning the Vapor-Liquid Equilibrium of Solutions of ^{3}He in ^{4}He below 2.19 K," *Physica* 15 (1949):733.

17. Clement, J. R., and Gaffney, J., "Thermal Oscillations in Low Temperature Apparatus," *Adv. Cryog. Eng.* 1 (1954):302.

18. Bannister, J. D., "Spontaneous Pressure Oscillating in Tubes Connecting Liquid Helium Reservoirs to 300 K Environments," in *Liquid Helium Technology* (*Proc. Comm I.* Boulder, Annexe 1966–5, IIR) Pergamon Press, London (1967):127.

19. Yazaki, T., Tominaga, A., and Narahara, Y., "Experiments on Thermally Driven Acoustic Oscillations of Gaseous Helium," *J. Low Temp. Phys.* 41 (1980):45.

20. Liburdy, J. A., and Wofford, J. L., "Acoustic Oscillation Phenomena in Low Velocity Steady Flow with Heating," *Advanc. Cryog. Eng.* 25 (1980):528.

21. von Hoffman, T., Lienert, U., and Quack, H., "Experiments on Thermally Driven Gas Oscillations," *Cryog.* 13 (1973):490–492.

22. Daney, D. E., Ludtke, P. R. and Jones, M. C., "Thermal Acoustic Oscillations in Current Leads Cooled with Supercritical Helium," *IEEE Trans. Magn.*, MAG-13 (1977):412.

23. Daney, D. E., Ludtke, P. R., Sindt, C. F., and Chelton, D. B., "Slush Hydrogen Fluid Characterization and Instrumentation Analysis," U.S. Department of Commerce, Natinoal Bureau of Standards, Report No. 9701 (Washington, D.C.: U.S. Government Printing Office, 1967).

24. Mann, D. B., Sindt, C. F., Ludtke, P. R., and Chelton, D. B., "Slush Hydrogen Fluid Characterization and Instrumentation Analysis," U.S. Department of Commerce, National Bureau of Standards, Report 9265 (Washington, D.C.: U.S. Government Printing Office, 1966).

25. Ludtke, P. R., *Slush Hydrogen Flow Facility*, U.S. Department of Commerce, National Bureau of Standards Report 9752 (Washington, D.C.: U.S. Government Printing Office, 1969).

26. Dmitreviskiy, Yu. P., and Melnik, Yu. M., "Observation of Thermal-Acoustic Oscillations in Hydrogen, Nitrogen, Oxygen and Argon," *Cryog.* 16 (1976):25.

27. Rott, N., "Damped, and Thermally Driven Acoustic Oscillations in Wide and Narrow Tubes," *ZAMP* 20 (1969):230.

28. Rott, N., "Thermally Driven Acoustic Oscillations, Part 2: Stability Limit for Helium," *ZAMP* 24 (1973):24.

29. Gu, Y., and Timmerhaus, K. D., "Experimental Verification of Stability Characteristics for Thermal Acoustic Oscillations in a Liquid Helium System," *Adv. Cryog. Eng.* 39B (1994):1733.

30. Gu, Y., "Thermal Acoustic Oscillations in Cryogenic systems," Ph.D. thesis, University of Colorado, Boulder, Department of Chemical Engineering (1993).

31. Ludtke, P. R., *Slush Hydrogen Flow Facility*, U.S. Department of Commerce, National Bureau of Standards, Report 9752 (Washington, D.C.: U.S. Government Printing Office, 1969).

32. Daney, D. E., Ludtke, P. R., and Jones, M. C., "An Experimental Study of Thermally-Induced Flow Oscillations in Supercritical Helium," *ASME J. Heat Transfer* 101 (1979):9.

33. Ludtke, P. R., Daney, D. E., and Steward, W. G., "Performance of a Small Centrifugal Pump in HeI and HeII," *Adv. Cryog. Eng.* 33, (1988):515.

34. DiPirro, M. J., and Kittel, P., "The Superfluid On-Orbit Transfer (SHOOT) Flight," *Adv. Cryog. Eng.* 33 (1988):893.

35. Daney, D. E., "Cavitation in Flowing Superfluid Helium," in *Proc. Space Cryog.* Workshop (Plemum, Massachusetts: Butterworth & Co., Ltd., 1988):132.

36. Edmonds, D. K., and Hord, J., "Cavitation in Liquid Cryogenics," *Adv. Cryog. Eng.* 14 (1969):274.

37. Ludtke, P. R., and Daney, D. E., "Cavitation Characteristics of a Small Centrifugal Pump," *Cryog.* 28 (1988):96.

38. Jasinski, T., Stacy, W. D., Honkonen, S.C., and Sixsmith, H., "A Generic Pump/Compressor Design for Circulation of Cryogenic Fluids," *Adv. Cryog. Eng.* 31 (1986):991.

39. Nissen, J. A., Budegom, E., Brodie, L. C., and Semura, J. S., "New Measurements of the Tensile Strength of Liquid ^{4}He," *Adv. Cryog. Eng.* 33 (1988):999.

40. Lehmann, W., and Minges, J., "Operating Experience with a High Capacity Helium Pump Under Super-critical Conditions," *Adv. Cryog. Eng.* 29 (1984):813.

41. Quack, H., "Cold Compression of Helium for a Refrigerator Below 4K," *Adv. Cryog. Eng.* 33 (1988):647.

42. Brown, D. P., Gibbs, R. J., Schlafke, A. P., Sondericker, J. H., and Wu, K. C., "Operating Experiences and Test Results of Six Cold Helium Compressions," *Adv. Cryog. Eng.* 33 (1988):663.

43. Gistan, G. M., Villard, J. C., and Turcat, F., "Application Range of Cryogenic Centrifugal Compressors," *Adv. Cryog. Eng.* 356, (1990):1031.

44. Quack, H., Technische Universitat Dresden personal communication, update of table from Ref. 41 (1997).

45. Lacaze, A., *60e Exposition Société Francaise de Physique* (Paris: 1964), 68.

46. Rietdijk, J. A., "The Expansion-Ejector—A New Device for Liquefaction and Refrigeration at 4K and Lower," in *Liquid Helium Technology (Proc. Comm. I. Boulder, Annexe 1966-5, IIR)* (London: Pergamon Press, 1967):241.

47. Schlafke, A. P., Brown, D. P., and Wu, K. C., "Combined Cold Compressor/Ejector Helium Refrigerator Cycle," *Adv. Cryog. Eng.* 29 (1984):487.

48. Daney, D. E., McConnell, P. M., and Strobridge, T. R., "Low Temperature Nitrogen Ejector Performance," *Adv. Cryog. Eng.* 18 (1973):476.

49. Meissner, W., *Annalen der Physik IV* 47 (1915):1001.

50. McFee, R., "Optimum Input Leads for Cryogenic Apparatus," *Rev. Sci. Instr.* 30 (1959):98.

51. Grassman, P., and von Hoffman, T., "Optimization of Current Leads for Superconducting Systems," *Cryog.* 14 (1974):349.

52. Jones, M. C., Yeroshenko, V. M., Starostin, A., and Yaskin, L. A., "Transient Behavior of Helium-Cooled Current Leads for Superconducting Power Transmission," *Cryog.* 18 (1978):337.

53. Odenov, S. V., "Heat Transfer and Thermal Exchange Processes in Low Temperature Current Leads," *Cryog.* 13 (1973):543.

54. Agsten, R., "Thermodynamic Optimization of Current Leads into Low Temperature Regions," *Cryog.* 13 (1973):141.

55. Lock, J. M., "Optimization of Current Leads into a Cryostat," *Cryog.* 9 (1969):438.

56. Morgan, G. H., *Design of AC Cryogenic Power Leads*, Brookhaven National Laboratory, Power Transmission Project, Technical Note No. 48 (1975). Accelerator Depart. Brookhaven National Laboratory, Upton, N.Y., 11973.

57. Green, M. A., A Design Method for Multiple Tube Gas-Cooled Electrical Leads for the g-2 Superconducting Magnets, *Adv. Cryog. Eng.* 41a (1996):573

58. Mumford, F. J., "Superconducting Current Leads Made from High T_c Superconductor and Normal Metal Conductor," *Cryog.* 29 (1989):206.

59. Herrman, P. F., Cottevieille, C., Duperray, G., Leriche, A., Verhaege, T., Albrecht, C., and Bock, J., "Cryogenic Load Calculation of a High T_c Current Lead," *Cryog.* 33 (1993):555.

60. Daugherty, M. A., Daney, D. E., Prenger, F. C., Hill, D. D., Williams, P. M., and Boenig, H.J., "Assembly and Testing of a Composite Heat Pipe Thermal Intercept for HTS Current Leads," *Adv. Cryog. Eng.* 41a, (1996):579.

61. Von Grassman, P., and Kopp, J., "Zur günstigsten Wahl der Temperatur Differenz und der Wärme-ubergangzahl in Wärmeaustauschern (on the Choice of Temperature Difference and Heat Transfer Coefficient in Heat Exchangers)," *Kältetechnik* 9 (1957):306.

62. Bejan, A., *Advanced Engineering Thermodynamics*, (New York: John Wiley and Sons, 1988).

63. Longsworth, R. C., "4K Gifford–McMahon/Joule Thomson Cycle Refrigerators," *Adv. Cryog. Eng.* 33 (1988):693.

64. Courtesy of LINDE AG, *see also*: Abadzic, E. E., and Scholz, H. W., "Coiled Tubular Heat Exchangers," *Adv. Cryog. Eng.* 18 (1973):42.

65. Fleming, R. B., "A Compact Perforated-Plate Heat Exchanger," *Adv. Cryog. Eng.* 14 (1969):197.

66. McMahon, H. Q., Bowen, R. J., and Bleyle, Jr., G. A., *Trans. ASME* 72 (1950):623.

67. Vonk, G., "A New Type of Compact Heat Exchanger with a High Thermal Efficiency," *Adv. Cryog. Eng.* 13 (1968):582.

68. Izumi, H., Harada, S., and Matsubara, K., "Development of Small Size Claude Cycle Helium Refrigerator with Micro Turbo-Expander," *Adv. Cryog. Eng.* 31 (1986):811.

69. Hendrichs, J. B., "A New Method for Producing Perforated Plate Recuperators," *Adv. Cryog. Eng.* 41b (1996):1329.
70. Sixsmith, H., Valenzuela, J., and Swift, W. L., "Small Turbo-Brayton Cryocoolers," *Adv. Cryog. Eng.* 33 (1988):827.
71. Timmerhaus, K. D., and Schoenhals, R. J., "Design and Selection of Cryogenic Heat Exchangers," *Adv. Cryog. Eng.* 19 (1974):445.
72. Daney, D. E., and Radebaugh, R., "Non-Ideal Regenerator Performance—The Effect of Void Volume Fluid Heat Capacity," *Cryog.* 24 (1984):499.
73. Sahashi, M., Tokai, Y., Kuriyama, T., Nakagome, H., Li, R., Ogawa, M., and Hashimoto, T., "New Magnetic Material R3T System with Extremely Large Heat Capacities Used as Heat Regenerators," *Adv. Cryog. Eng.* 35b (1990):1175.
74. Oonk, R. L., and Hustvedt, D. C., "The Effect of Fluid Property Variations on the Performance of Cryogenic Helium Heat Exchangers," *Adv. Cryog. Eng.* 31 (1986):415.
75. Chowdhury, K., and Sarangi, S., "The Effect of Variable Specific Heat of the Working Fluids on the Performance of Counterflow Heat Exchanges," *Cryog.* 24 (1984):679.
76. Rohsenow, W. M., and Choi, H. Y., Heat, Mass and Momentum Transfer (Englewood Cliffs, New Jersey: Prentice–Hall, 1961).
77. Kays, W. M., and London, A. L., *Compact Heat Exchangers*, 3rd ed. (New York: McGraw–Hill, 1984).
78. Gardner, K. A., "Efficiency of Extended Surfaces," *Trans. ASME* 67 (1945):621–631.
79. Kroeger, P. G., "Performance Deterioration in High Effectiveness Heat Exchangers due to Axial Heat Conduction Effects," *Adv. Cryog. Eng.* 12 (1967):363.
80. Chowdhury, K., and Sarangi, S., "Performance of Cryogenic Heat Exchangers with Heat Leak from the Surroundings," *Adv. Cryog. Eng.* 29 (1984):273.
81. Fleming, R. B., "The Effect of Flow Distribution in Parallel Channels of Counterflow Heat Exchangers," *Adv. Cryog. Eng.* 12 (1967):352.
82. Weimer, R. F., and Hartzog, D. G., "Effects of Maldistribution on the Performance of Multistream, Multipassage Heat Exchangers," *Adv. Cryog. Eng.* 18 (1973):52.
83. Hausen, H., *Wärmeübertragung im Gegenstrom, Gleichstrom und Kreuzstrom* (Berlin: Springer–Verlag, 1950).
84. Schmidt, F. W., and Willmott, A. J., *Thermal Energy Storage and Regeneration* (New York: Hemisphere Publishing Co., 1981).

TEN

He II (SUPERFLUID HELIUM)

S. W. Van Sciver

NHMFL/FSU, 1800 E. Paul Dirac Drive, Tallahassee, FL 32310

10-1 INTRODUCTION

Superfluid helium (or He II) has special properties that are generally different from those of all other common cryogenic fluids. For this reason, this handbook devotes a complete chapter to the subject. The purpose of this chapter is to survey the subject of He II properties and applications so that engineers and scientists can use the information for analysis of data and system design. Emphasis is on the engineering aspects of the fluid with occasional, where necessary, reference to fundamentals. Much of this chapter has been abstracted and updated from *Helium Cryogenics* [1], which was written by the author about 15 years ago. Readers may find that reference particularly useful for understanding the origin of the physical principles behind the equations. For more in-depth development of the physical properties, the reader is referred to one of several reference texts on liquid helium [2–4].

The interest in applications of He II has grown in recent years so that now there exist a considerable number of large-scale systems that utilize this unique fluid as a coolant. Included among these are cryogenic systems for large-scale superconducting magnets, electron accelerators, and a range of space-based applications. Over the years, these applications have encouraged a database development for He II that can be used for design. This chapter on He II represents an attempt to bring the He II database into one location to simplify its use by scientists and engineers. To this end, the chapter is organized as follows. We begin with a survey of the unique properties of He II, including the transport equations. The next section describes the heat and mass transfer issues unique to He II. Finally, we discuss, by example, the application of He II in technical devices.

The data and correlations given in this chapter all use SI units unless otherwise specified. Graphical representations of He II properties are given in the text, and more detailed tabular values are listed in the appendix. Most of the data presented were obtained from the property database software, HEPAK [5]. Other values are available in tabular form in the literature [6].

10-2 PROPERTIES OF He II

10-2-1 Phase Diagram

The phase diagram of liquid helium clearly shows the unique characteristics of this fluid (see Fig. 10-1). In addition to the standard features such as the critical point and liquid–vapor coexistance line, one can see that the liquid can exist in either of two very different states. He I is the normal liquid with characteristics that are typical of classical fluids, whereas the superfluid state, which is more correctly referred to as He II, has physical features that are truly exceptional. Most notable of these features are the transport properties, with a vanishingly small viscosity and an apparent thermal conductivity many orders of magnitude larger than liquids or even high-conductivity solids. The λ line separates these two liquid states. This designation was adopted because the specific heat near the transition has the shape of the Greek letter λ. The λ transition temperature

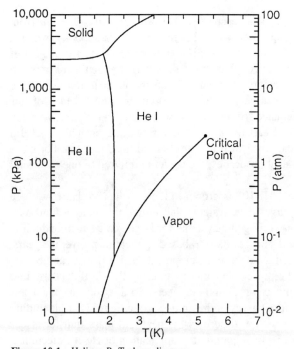

Figure 10-1 Helium *P–T* phase diagram.

**Table 10-1 Lambda transition as a function
of temperature, pressure, and density**

Temperature (K)	Pressure (bar)	Density (kg/m^3)
1.780	29.420	179.3
1.800	28.270	178.4
1.820	27.100	177.5
1.840	25.890	176.6
1.850	25.280	176.1
1.860	24.660	175.6
1.880	23.400	174.6
1.900	22.110	173.5
1.920	20.790	172.3
1.940	19.440	171.1
1.960	18.060	169.9
1.980	16.650	168.5
2.000	15.200	167.1
2.020	13.710	165.6
2.040	12.190	163.9
2.060	10.620	162.1
2.080	9.000	160.2
2.100	7.328	158.0
2.110	6.470	156.9
2.120	5.593	155.6
2.130	4.696	154.3
2.140	3.775	152.9
2.150	2.824	151.3
2.160	1.835	149.6
2.170	0.795	147.7
2.175	0.251	146.6
2.176	0.050	146.2

is 2.176 K at saturated vapor pressure and decreases gradually with increasing pressure until it intersects the solid coexistence boundary at 1.763 K, $p = 2.974$ MPa.

The phase diagram of helium is also unique in that it lacks a triple point of coexistence between liquid, vapor, and solid because the solid state can exist only under an external pressure. The intersection of the λ line with the two phase coexistence regions of liquid and vapor or solid and liquid is not a triple point, although it occasionally is identified incorrectly as such. The λ transition represents a second-order phase transition, and there is no latent heat of formation of the He II state. The coexistence of He II and He I in equilibrium conditions is not possible. The actual values of the pressure, temperature, and density of liquid helium at the λ transition are listed in Table 10-1.

10-2-2 State Properties

The properties of He II at saturated vapor pressure are given in Table 10-2. The saturation density ρ is one of the most important thermodynamic properties of liquid helium because it is needed to derive the equation of state. Plotted in Fig. 10-2 is the saturated density

Table 10-2 Properties of He II on the saturated vapor–pressure line

T (K)	P (Pa)	ρ_l (kg/m³)	ρ_v (kg/m³)	C_p (J/kg · K)	S (J/kg · K)	h_{fg} (kJ/kg)	κ (Pa⁻¹)	β (K⁻¹)
1.000	15.57	145.157	0.0075	100.2	16.34	20.08	1.214×10^{-7}	0.00018
1.030	20.67	145.156	0.0097	121.5	19.61	20.23	1.214×10^{-7}	0.00010
1.060	27.07	145.156	0.0123	146.3	23.44	20.37	1.215×10^{-7}	0.00000
1.090	34.98	145.156	0.0155	174.8	27.91	20.52	1.215×10^{-7}	-0.00010
1.120	44.68	145.157	0.0193	207.5	33.09	20.66	1.216×10^{-7}	-0.00022
1.150	56.45	145.159	0.0238	244.7	39.05	20.8	1.217×10^{-7}	-0.00035
1.180	70.58	145.161	0.0290	286.7	45.88	20.93	1.218×10^{-7}	-0.00048
1.210	87.42	145.163	0.0350	334	53.66	21.07	1.220×10^{-7}	-0.00063
1.240	107.3	145.167	0.0420	386.9	62.48	21.2	1.221×10^{-7}	-0.00078
1.270	130.7	145.171	0.0500	445.8	72.41	21.33	1.223×10^{-7}	-0.00095
1.300	157.9	145.176	0.0591	511.1	83.57	21.46	1.225×10^{-7}	-0.00112
1.330	189.3	145.182	0.0693	583.1	96.03	21.58	1.228×10^{-7}	-0.00129
1.360	225.5	145.188	0.0809	662.3	109.9	21.70	1.230×10^{-7}	-0.00148
1.390	267	145.196	0.0937	749.1	125.3	21.82	1.233×10^{-7}	-0.00167
1.420	314.1	145.205	0.1081	843.8	142.3	21.94	1.235×10^{-7}	-0.00187
1.450	367.4	145.214	0.1240	946.9	161	22.05	1.238×10^{-7}	-0.00208
1.480	427.5	145.225	0.1416	1059	181.5	22.15	1.241×10^{-7}	-0.00229
1.510	494.8	145.236	0.1608	1180	203.9	22.25	1.244×10^{-7}	-0.00251
1.540	570.1	145.249	0.1820	1310	228.4	22.35	1.247×10^{-7}	-0.00273
1.570	653.7	145.263	0.2050	1451	255	22.45	1.251×10^{-7}	-0.00297
1.600	746.4	145.278	0.2301	1603	283.9	22.53	1.254×10^{-7}	-0.00321
1.630	848.6	145.295	0.2572	1766	315.2	22.62	1.258×10^{-7}	-0.00347
1.660	961.1	145.312	0.2866	1940	349	22.69	1.262×10^{-7}	-0.00373
1.690	1084	145.332	0.3182	2127	385.4	22.77	1.266×10^{-7}	-0.00402
1.720	1219	145.352	0.3521	2328	424.5	22.83	1.270×10^{-7}	-0.00433
1.750	1366	145.375	0.3885	2543	466.6	22.89	1.275×10^{-7}	-0.00466
1.780	1525	145.399	0.4274	2774	511.8	22.95	1.280×10^{-7}	-0.00502
1.810	1697	145.425	0.4688	3023	560.2	22.99	1.286×10^{-7}	-0.00542
1.840	1884	145.453	0.5128	3290	612.1	23.03	1.292×10^{-7}	-0.00588
1.870	2084	145.483	0.5595	3579	667.6	23.06	1.299×10^{-7}	-0.00640
1.900	2299	145.516	0.6090	3893	727	23.07	1.307×10^{-7}	-0.00699
1.930	2530	145.553	0.6611	4236	790.7	23.08	1.316×10^{-7}	-0.00770
1.960	2776	145.593	0.7161	4614	858.9	23.08	1.326×10^{-7}	-0.00855
1.990	3038	145.638	0.7738	5036	932.1	23.06	1.337×10^{-7}	-0.00957
2.000	3129	145.654	0.7936	5187	957.8	23.05	1.341×10^{-7}	-0.00996
2.030	3413	145.706	0.8550	5686	1039	23	1.354×10^{-7}	-0.01133
2.060	3714	145.765	0.9190	6267	1126	22.94	1.369×10^{-7}	-0.01309
2.090	4031	145.833	0.9857	6970	1222	22.86	1.385×10^{-7}	-0.01546
2.120	4365	145.915	1.0549	7881	1327	22.75	1.404×10^{-7}	-0.01888
2.150	4715	146.016	1.1265	9269	1447	22.62	1.426×10^{-7}	-0.02487
2.170	4958	146.106	1.1755	11330	1540	22.51	1.447×10^{-7}	-0.03530
2.180	5082	146.158	1.2004	6708	1592	22.47	1.433×10^{-7}	-0.00630

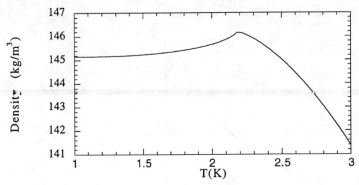

Figure 10-2 Density of liquid helium under saturated vapor pressure.

of liquid helium below 3 K. A maximum density occurs at 2.182 K or 6 mK above T_λ in saturated liquid helium. Below T_λ the density is only weakly temperature-dependent and becomes essentially constant for $T < 2.0$ K. He II has a negative thermal expansion coefficient.

The slope of the density profile is a direct measure of the volume expansivity at saturated vapor pressure. This quantity is plotted in Fig. 10-3. By definition the volume expansivity at saturated vapor pressure is given by

$$\beta = -\frac{1}{\rho}\left(\frac{\partial \rho}{\partial T}\right) \tag{10-1}$$

Note that β has a discontinuity at T_λ.

To obtain the expansion coefficient at constant pressure, one should use the relationship

$$\beta_{\mathrm{p}} = \beta_{\mathrm{sat}} + \kappa \left(\frac{\partial p}{\partial T}\right)_{\mathrm{sat}} \tag{10-2}$$

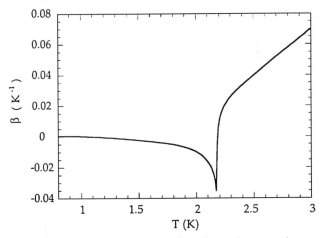

Figure 10-3 Volume expansivity of liquid helium under saturated vapor pressure.

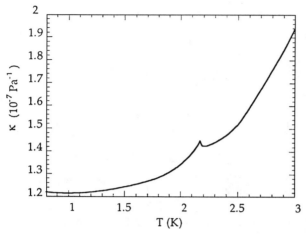

Figure 10-4 Bulk compressibility of liquid helium.

where bulk isothermal compressibility is defined by

$$\kappa = -\frac{1}{V}\left(\frac{\partial V}{\partial p}\right)_T \tag{10-3}$$

The bulk isothermal compressibility is plotted in Fig. 10-4. Typical values for κ are about $1.2 \times 10^{-7}\,\mathrm{Pa^{-1}}$ below 1 K, increasing to $2 \times 10^{-7}\,\mathrm{Pa^{-1}}$ at 3 K. Note that the compressibility has a discontinuity at the λ point, which is consistent with the signature of a second-order phase transition.

The specific heat of saturated liquid helium is shown in Fig. 10-5. At very low temperatures, $T < 0.6\,\mathrm{K}$, the specific heat appears to obey a cubic dependence,

$$C = 20.4T^3 \tag{10-4}$$

in SI units (J/kg · K). Although in this case C refers to the specific heat at saturated vapor pressure, at low temperatures the differences between C, C_p and C_v are small. The

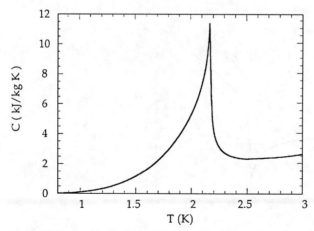

Figure 10-5 Specific heat of liquid helium under saturated vapor pressure.

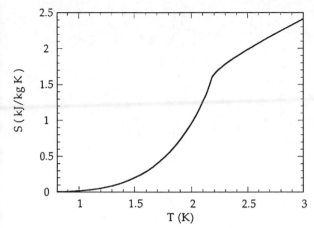

Figure 10-6 Entropy of liquid helium under saturated vapor pressure.

cubic dependence comes from the primary excitations in this regime being longitudinal phonons.

At higher temperatures, the temperature exponent of the specific heat increases by about a factor of 2. Historically, the region has been divided into two segments where the temperature dependence goes as

$$C = 108T^{6.7} \qquad \text{for} \quad 0.6 < T < 1.1 \text{ K} \tag{10-5}$$

and

$$C = 117T^{5.6} \qquad \text{for} \quad 1.1 < T < T_\lambda \tag{10-6}$$

in SI units (J/kg · K). In this regime, the higher exponent to the temperature dependence comes from roton excitations that begin to dominate the spectrum as T_λ is approached.

The entropy in this regime displays the same temperature dependence as the specific heat because S is related to C through the integral $S = \int \frac{C}{T} \, dT$. Figure 10-6 displays the entropy at saturated vapor pressure.

The latent heat of vaporization λ of a liquid helium is displayed in Fig.10-7. This quantity is only defined along the saturated vapor pressure curve by the Clausius–Clapeyron equation

$$\left(\frac{dp}{dT} \right)_{\text{sat}} = \frac{h_{\text{fg}}}{T(v_g - v_l)} \tag{10-7}$$

where v_g and v_l are the specific volumes of the gas and liquid, respectively. The heat of vaporization represents the energy required to take a unit of helium from the liquid to the vapor state. It is, therefore, an indirect measure of the strength of the intermolecular bonds associated with the formation of the liquid state.

The surface tension σ has units of J/m^2 and is associated with the energy increase due to the free-liquid surface. A polynomial fit to σ in the He II regime follows the form

$$\sigma(T) \cong \sigma_0 - \sigma_1 T + \sigma_2 T^2 \tag{10-8}$$

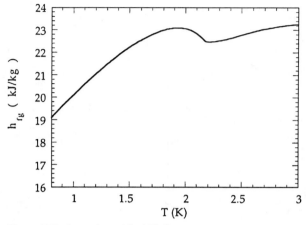

Figure 10-7 Latent heat of liquid helium.

where $\sigma_0 = 0.3534$ mJ/m^2, $\sigma_1 = 1.737 \times 10^{-2}$ mJ/m$^2 \cdot$ K, and $\sigma_2 = 2.154 \times 10^{-2}$ mJ/m$^2 \cdot$ K^2. Plotted in Fig. 10-8 is the fit to experimental values for σ.

10-2-3 Transport Properties

The behavior of He II when subjected to a mass or heat flow clearly demonstrates the unique character of this fluid. The observed effects cannot, in general, be treated by classical fluid mechanics models. The most accepted approach to understanding the transport properties is by means of the two-fluid model. This model treats He II as a mixture of two interpenetrating fluids: the normal fluid component and the superfluid component. The normal fluid component contains the excitations and therefore carries entropy and heat. It has a density ρ_n, velocity v_n, and viscosity, η_n. The superfluid component is in the condensed state and carries no entropy. The superfluid density is

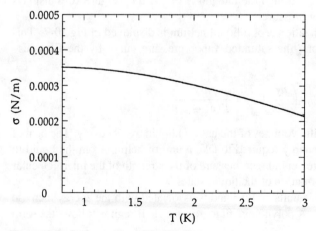

Figure 10-8 Surface tension of liquid helium.

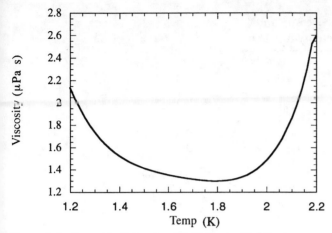

Figure 10-9 Normal fluid viscosity of He II ($1\ \mu_p = 10^{-7}$ Pa · s).

designated by ρ_s and velocity by v_s and it has zero viscosity. The two-fluid model explains many of the unique transport properties of the He II phase. In the following sections, the results of the two-fluid model are stated in the form of correlations for He II properties. The important thing to keep in mind is that these results are based on a phenomenological theory combined with experimental data.

The normal fluid density obeys the relationship

$$\frac{\rho_n}{\rho} = \left(\frac{T}{T_\lambda}\right)^{5.6} \tag{10-9}$$

and $\rho_n + \rho_s = \rho$. This relationship is consistant with the temperature dependence of the specific heat and entropy. The normal fluid viscosity is a quantity determined through heat transport or flow measurements. Figure 10-9 displays the temperature dependence of η_n numerical values are listed in Table 10-3.

Sound propagation. Ordinarily first sound is associated with pressure and density variations in the fluid. The differential equation used to describe sound propagation has the standard solution with a characteristic velocity c_1 given by

$$c_1^2 = \left(\frac{\partial p}{\partial \rho}\right)_s = \frac{\gamma}{\rho\kappa} \tag{10-10}$$

where the partial differentiation is taken at constant entropy and γ is the ratio of the specific heats C_p/C_v. In this case, ρ is the total density. The two-fluid model predicts the existence of second sound, which is entropy fluctuations rather than the density fluctuations of ordinary sound. The wave equation for second sound relates entropy and temperature through

$$\frac{\partial^2 s}{\partial t^2} = \frac{s^2 \rho_s}{\rho_n}\frac{d^2 T}{dx^2} \tag{10-11}$$

**Table 10-3 Normal fluid viscosity and
laminer heat flow conductivity function**

T(K)	Viscosity (μPa·s)	$g(T)$ (W/m^{3}K)× 10^{-13}
1.20	2.135	3.08
1.22	2.035	4.03
1.26	1.867	6.77
1.28	1.797	8.67
1.30	1.735	11.03
1.32	1.680	13.94
1.34	1.633	17.47
1.36	1.591	21.77
1.38	1.554	26.96
1.40	1.522	33.18
1.44	1.470	49.30
1.46	1.448	59.71
1.48	1.430	71.88
1.50	1.413	86.16
1.52	1.399	102.85
1.54	1.386	122.20
1.56	1.374	144.94
1.60	1.354	201.08
1.62	1.345	235.78
1.64	1.337	275.56
1.66	1.329	321.19
1.68	1.322	373.07
1.70	1.316	432.22
1.72	1.311	499.82
1.74	1.306	576.22
1.76	1.303	661.50
1.78	1.300	758.24
1.80	1.300	865.32
1.82	1.302	984.22
1.84	1.305	1118.40
1.86	1.312	1263.00
1.88	1.322	1420.90
1.90	1.336	1591.30
1.92	1.354	1775.30
1.94	1.378	1972.20
1.96	1.407	2178.60
1.98	1.444	2391.80
2.00	1.488	2617.60
2.02	1.540	2846.10
2.04	1.603	3075.70
2.06	1.677	3310.70
2.10	1.867	3777.20
2.12	1.987	3999.40
2.14	2.129	4229.60
2.16	2.303	4456.50
2.18	2.525	4677.10

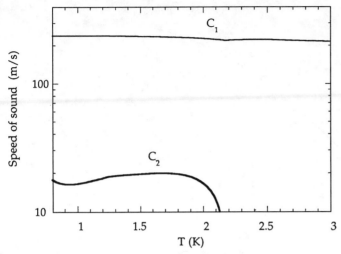

Figure 10-10   Velocities of first and second sound in liquid helium.

and second sound propagates with a characteristic speed c_2 as expressed by

$$c_2 \cong \frac{\rho_s}{\rho_n} \frac{T_s^2}{C_v} \tag{10-12}$$

Second sound has been measured extensively from T_λ to near absolute zero and as a function of pressure [7]. Values for c_2 are compared to c_1 in Fig. 10-10. Note that c_2 is approximately constant over the range 1–2 K. At lower temperatures the second sound velocity increases rapidly as the temperature approaches absolute zero.

Laminar flow and the critical velocity. Laminar flow conditions occur in He II whenever the fluid velocity is below the critical velocity. These conditions can occur even in static He II because heat transport causes a relative velocity of the two fluid components. In He II there are two relevant critical velocities: u_{sc}, which is associated with the onset of turbulence in the superfluid component, and u_{nc} for the normal fluid component. The velocity u_{sc} depends strongly on the method by which it is measured. Most experimental data are correlated to the empirical relationship

$$u_{sc} \approx d^{-1/4} \quad \text{in cgs units} \tag{10-13}$$

On the other hand, the normal fluid critical velocity is interpreted in terms of classical turbulent onset such that

$$u_{nc} \approx \frac{\eta_n Re_c}{\rho d} \tag{10-14}$$

where the critical Reynolds number is $Re_c \approx 1200$. Note that this relationship involves the normal fluid viscosity but the total density.

Laminar heat flow. Heat flow in He II is carried by the normal fluid component in a process known as internal convection or counterflow. In laminar flow, which occurs for

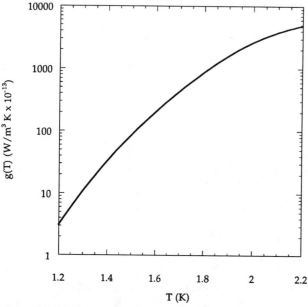

Figure 10-11 Laminar flow heat conductivity function at saturated vapor pressure.

low velocities in narrow channels, the heat conductivity equation may be written in a form similar to Fourier's law as

$$q = -\frac{(\rho s d)^2 T}{\beta \eta_n}\frac{dT}{dx} = -g(T)\frac{d^2}{\beta}\frac{dT}{dx}, \tag{10-15}$$

although the function of proportionality varies as the square of the diameter. The laminar flow heat conductivity function $g(T)$ increases strongly with temperature dominated by the dependence of $(\rho s)^2 T \approx T^{12}$. Figure 10-11 displays $g(T)$ between 1.2 K and T_λ. Table 10-3 gives numerical values for this coefficient at saturated vapor pressure.

Laminar mass flow. In the laminar flow regime, owing to the isentropic nature of the system, the pressure drop due to flow is related to the temperature gradient through London's equation as follows:

$$\frac{dp}{dx} = \rho s \frac{dT}{dx} \tag{10-16}$$

The fountain effect, a unique feature of He II, can be understood in terms of this expression. Specifically, in ideal superflow, a temperature gradient induces a pressure gradient, which in practice can lead to net mass flow of the fluid.

In the laminar flow regime, the heat-flow-induced pressure gradient is related to the temperature gradient through London's equation. The result is given by

$$q = -\frac{\rho s d^2 T}{\beta \eta_n}\frac{dp}{dx} = -g(T)\frac{d^2}{\rho s \beta}\frac{dp}{dx} \tag{10-17}$$

where β is the same geometrical factor as in Eq. (10-15). This relationship can easily be integrated over finite lengths and temperature difference to give practical results.

Turbulent flow. Above the critical velocity u_{sc}, other dissipative processes begin to play a significant role. In particular, the turbulent state, consisting of quantized vortex lines intermixed with the normal fluid component, destroys the isentropic nature of the superfluid state. In this regime, additional dissipative processes come into play, and the appropriate heat conductivity equation is modified as follows:

$$q = -g(T)\frac{d^2}{\beta}\frac{dT}{dx} - \left[f^{-1}(T)\frac{dT}{dx} \right]^{1/3} \tag{10-18}$$

where the additional term is approximately proportional to $(dT/dx)^{1/3}$.

The expression $f^{-1}(T)$ the He II heat conductivity function for turbulent flow. This function is fitted to the equation

$$f^{-1}(T, p) = f^{-1}(T_\lambda, p)[t^{5.6}(1 - t^{5.6})]^3 \tag{10-19}$$

At saturated vapor pressure, $f^{-1}(T, p)$ has a maximum at 1.923 K and a peak value of about 13,000 kW^3/m^5 · K. The temperature and pressure dependence of this function is given in Fig. 10-12. Numerical values are given in Table 10-4. In general, these data are accurate to about $\pm 10\%$ at saturated vapor pressure and compare favorably with experiment up to about 7 bars [1].

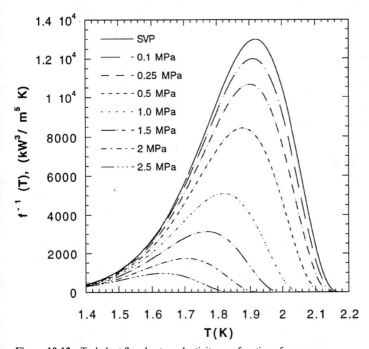

Figure 10-12 Turbulent flow heat conductivity as a function of pressure.

Table 10-4 Turbulent He II heat conductivity function $f^{-1}(T,P)$

T (K)	SVP	0.1 MPa	0.25 MPa	0.5MPa	1 MPa	1.5 MPa	2 MPa	2.5 MPa
1.4	396.88	389.91	374.74	356.23	343.23	322.94	291.98	279.18
1.42	492.09	483.16	464.00	440.23	421.71	394.09	352.60	331.46
1.44	607.04	595.63	571.54	541.13	515.08	477.78	422.59	389.82
1.46	745.02	730.50	700.32	661.55	625.36	575.38	502.50	453.88
1.48	909.64	891.23	853.58	804.33	754.62	688.14	592.62	522.84
1.5	1104.84	1081.57	1034.78	972.45	904.87	817.11	692.86	595.36
1.52	1334.81	1305.52	1247.60	1169.02	1078.03	963.05	802.68	669.54
1.54	1603.96	1567.21	1495.81	1397.13	1275.74	1126.23	920.88	742.74
1.56	1916.77	1870.84	1783.17	1659.73	1499.25	1306.30	1045.52	811.63
1.58	2277.66	2220.49	2113.27	1959.50	1749.17	1502.09	1173.75	872.13
1.6	2690.81	2619.91	2489.35	2298.61	2025.27	1711.38	1301.68	919.55
1.62	3159.86	3072.31	2914.01	2678.47	2326.23	1930.69	1424.35	948.79
1.64	3687.69	3580.03	3388.95	3099.42	2649.33	2155.11	1535.63	954.68
1.66	4275.95	4144.16	3914.56	3560.40	2990.12	2378.07	1628.42	932.58
1.68	4924.68	4764.10	4489.55	4058.54	3342.20	2591.24	1694.78	879.06
1.7	5631.79	5437.10	5110.43	4588.75	3696.87	2784.58	1726.45	792.94
1.72	6392.53	6157.71	5771.08	5143.29	4042.96	2946.41	1715.47	676.33
1.74	7198.86	6917.20	6462.18	5711.32	4366.75	3063.84	1655.15	535.73
1.76	8038.89	7703.03	7170.71	6278.62	4652.08	3123.42	1541.29	382.86
1.78	8896.31	8498.36	7879.58	6827.27	4880.66	3112.10	1373.74	234.57
1.8	9749.90	9281.59	8567.29	7335.65	5032.79	3018.70	1157.98	111.09
1.82	10573.23	10026.21	9207.86	7778.62	5088.44	2835.73	906.67	31.12
1.84	11334.63	10700.85	9771.03	8128.11	5028.94	2561.60	640.58	1.49
1.86	11997.49	11269.75	10222.94	8354.22	4839.10	2203.13	388.07	
1.88	12521.14	11693.80	10527.32	8426.88	4510.05	1777.95	181.76	
1.9	12862.33	11932.24	10647.41	8318.24	4042.50	1316.21	50.37	
1.92	12977.62	11945.21	10548.69	8005.91	3450.25	860.57	2.39	
1.94	12826.67	11697.28	10202.53	7476.91	2763.44	462.82		
1.96	12376.63	11161.98	9590.84	6732.33	2030.59	174.52		
1.98	11607.65	10327.35	8711.42	5792.32	1317.94	27.72		
2	10519.24	9202.22	7583.96	4700.74	703.69	0.00		
2.02	9137.17	7822.67	6255.61	3528.19	263.46			
2.04	7520.03	6257.67	4805.26	2371.58	41.55			
2.06	5763.86	4612.16	3344.14	1347.17	0.00			
2.08	4002.59	3024.66	2009.69	572.35				
2.1	2400.26	1655.30	947.80	129.50				
2.12	1129.61	657.73	276.12	1.99				
2.14	328.41	125.60	18.18					
2.16	21.57	0.35						

In relatively large-scale engineering design calculations (e.g., $d > 1$ mm), the turbulent term in the heat conductivity equation dominates, allowing one to use the following simplified expression for design calculations:

$$q = -\left[f^{-1}(T) \frac{dT}{dx} \right]^{1/3} \qquad (10\text{-}20)$$

This expression may be used much as Fourier's law for determining heat conduction in He II.

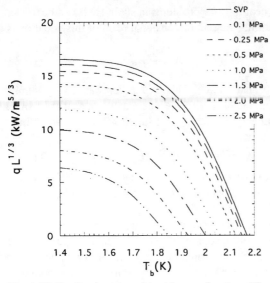

Figure 10-13 Steady-state peak heat flux as a function of T and P in a one-dimensional channel containing turbulent He II for $T_b = 1.8\,\text{K}$. (— = infinite channel; - - - = adiabatic end condition; - - - - = isothermal end condition.)

Steady-state peak heat flux. If the interest is in the heat transport in a finite-length channel with a sizable ΔT, it is possible to determine the heat flux value by integrating Eq. (10-20) over the channel length L and matching boundary conditions. Thus, the maximum heat flux q^* is then established according to the maximum allowable temperature difference $(T_\lambda - T_b)$ as

$$q^* L^{1/3} = \left[\int_{T_b}^{T_\lambda} f^{-1}(T)\, dT \right]^{1/3} \tag{10-21}$$

Figure 10-13 and Table 10-5 display $q^* L^{1/3}$ versus bath temperature and pressure.

Table 10-5 Integrated He II turbulent flow heat conductivity function versus pressure

T_b (K)	$P = SV/P$	0.1 MPa	0.25 MPa	0.5 MPa	1 MPa	1.5 MPa	2 MPa	2.5 MPa
1.4	16.530	16.066	15.422	14.199	11.849	9.942	8.006	6.383
1.5	16.449	15.981	15.333	14.100	11.714	9.765	7.763	6.027
1.6	16.234	15.758	15.102	13.845	11.375	9.331	7.193	5.235
1.7	15.726	15.235	14.562	13.255	10.618	8.395	6.020	3.714
1.8	14.652	14.132	13.431	12.037	9.115	6.615	3.925	1.299
1.9	12.611	12.048	11.307	9.788	6.474	3.676	0.886	
2.0	9.135	8.525	7.749	6.110	2.518			
2.1	3.995	3.391	2.669	1.182				

Transient heat transfer. Transient heat transfer problems in static He II can be treated with a nonlinear heat diffusion equation. The one-dimensional form of this equation is

$$\rho C_p \frac{\partial T}{\partial t} = \frac{\partial}{\partial x} \left[f^{-1}(T) \frac{\partial T}{\partial x} \right]^{1/3} + q_{ext} \tag{10-22}$$

where q_{ext} is any externally applied heat source. This expression has a very similar appearance to the ordinary diffusion equation with the one exception that it involves the cube root of the temperature gradient. On the basis of Eq. (10-22) one can define a characteristic diffusion time τ_d given by

$$\tau_d = a\rho C f^{1/3} \Delta T^{2/3} L^{4/3} = L^{4/3}/D_{eff} \tag{10-23}$$

where the coefficient a is a constant of order unity and D_{eff} is the effective diffusivity of He II. Note that, unlike ordinary diffusion, τ_d varies as the 4/3 power of the characteristic length.

The He II diffusion equation has been successfully compared with experiment for a variety of conditions such as localized pulsed source [8] and step-function clamped flux [9,10]. For example, when one considers step function clamped flux problem, where heat is applied at one end of a channel of length L, there are primarily three boundary conditions at $x = L$:

- Isothermal at $x = L$:$T(L, t) = T_b$
- Adiabatic at $x = L$:$dT/dt(L) = 0$
- Infinite channel: $T(\infty, t) = T_b$

For a given heat flux q there exists a time Δt^* during which heat can be effectively transferred before boiling sets in. This condition is the transient equivalent of Eq. (10-21), which eventually will produce the steady-state solution for isothermal boundary conditions. Figure 10-14 displays the Δt^* versus q for different length channels and boundary conditions assuming constant properties at 1.8 K. Note that for an infinite channel, $\Delta t^* \approx q^{-4}$, which is consistent with experiment [11].

Forced-flow heat transfer. Forced-flow heat transfer to He II may similarly be analyzed using the appropriate nonlinear heat equation

$$\rho C_p \frac{\partial T}{\partial t} = \frac{\partial}{\partial x} \left[f^{-1}(T) \frac{\partial T}{\partial x} \right]^{1/3} - \rho C_p u \frac{\partial T}{\partial x} + q_{ext} \tag{10-24}$$

where the additional term is introduced to account for ordinary convection processes. Because of the nonlinear and temperature dependent properties, Eq. (10-24) can only be solved using numerical techniques. Solutions require fixed boundary conditions and have been successfully compared with experiments involving local or distributed heat sources [12,13].

In steady state, the simplified one-dimensional heat equation can be solved either by approximate analytic methods for constant properties or more accurately through numerical methods. This problem has been solved for numerous cases including local [14,15] and distributed heat sources [16] as well as heat transfer boundary conditions as occur in heat exchangers [17–19].

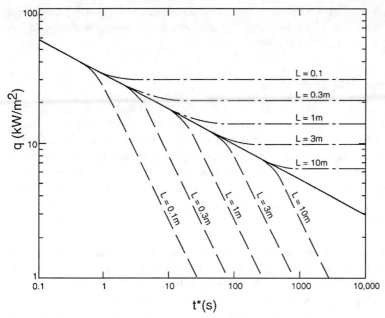

Figure 10-14 Time to film-boiling for transient heat transfer to an He II channel for different boundary conditions.

Pressure drop in turbulent flow. The pressure drop associated with flow of turbulent He II has been analyzed for a variety of channel geometries [20–22]. The most notable feature of these measurements is the similarity of friction factor to that for classical fluids. In other words, the pressure drop may be correlated with the expression

$$\Delta p = 2 f_d \rho u^2 \left(\frac{L}{D}\right) \qquad (10\text{-}25)$$

where the friction factor f_d is similar to that observed for classical fluids. For example, smooth-tube friction factors for He II in the Reynolds number regime $Re_d > 2 \times 10^4$ appear to follow the von Kármán–Nikuradse correlation

$$\frac{1}{f_d^{1/2}} = 1.737 \ln \left(Re_d f_d^{1/2}\right) - 0.396 \qquad (10\text{-}26)$$

where the Reynolds number is defined by $Re_d = \rho u d / \eta_n$. Similarly for $1500 < Re_d < 2 \times 10^4$, the Blausius correlation

$$f_d = \frac{0.0791}{Re_d^{1/4}} \qquad (10\text{-}27)$$

is preferred.

For noncircular cross-section channels, present evidence suggests that the friction factor may also be correlated by classical models.

The preceding discussion for the most part assumes that the helium flow is fully developed and turbulent. This allows both the use of the turbulent pressure drop correlations and the turbulent heat transport relation. More complex phenomena can occur, particularly in flow systems consisting of narrow channels in laminar flow, which can lead to fountain-effect-driven flows. For such complex behavior, a more complete modeling approach is necessary (see, for example, Ref. [23]).

10-2-4 Surface Heat Transfer

A unique characteristic of heat transfer in He II is the process that occurs at an interface between a solid and the liquid. In contrast to ordinary convection heat transfer, surface heat transfer in He II is more controlled by the nature of the interface, including the properties of the solid material, rather than the condition of the bulk liquid. At relatively low heat flux, there is no boiling at the surface, and the heat transfer is dominated by a phenomenon known as Kapitza conductance. For heat fluxes greater than the peak value q^* the surface is blanketed by a film of He I or vapor or both. In this region the heat transfer is controlled primarily by the character of this film.

Kapitza conductance. Thermal boundary conductance occurring at the interface between a solid and liquid He II is of great technical interest because it often results in the largest temperature differences in a He II heat transfer problem. Although there have been many theories [24] on the subject, Kapitza conductance is usually defined in terms of empirical data. Ideally, the Kapitza conductance is defined in the limit where q and ΔT_s are vanishingly small as

$$h_{K_0} = \lim_{\Delta T_s \to 0} \left(\frac{q}{\Delta T_s} \right) \tag{10-28}$$

where ΔT_s is $(T_s - T_b)$ and the subscript 0 refers to the limit as $\Delta T_s \to 0$. In the limit of small ΔT, h_{K_0} may be described by a fairly simple relationship

$$h_K = \alpha T^n \tag{10-29}$$

where n is between 2 and 4 and α is an empirically determined quantity. Listed in Table 10-6 are the highest values obtained experimentally for a variety of metals and nonmetals [25]. These values appear to correlate with the Debye temperature Θ_D, which is characteristic of the material. However, it is important to note that these experimental values vary considerably—in some cases by as much as an order of magnitude.

Experimental measurements have shown that the magnitude of h_K at a given temperature varies by as much as an order of magnitude among samples. Part of this variation can be attributed to surface condition: oxidation, impurities, or condensates. Generally, the high values in Table 10-6 are for surfaces that are cleaned carefully either chemically or mechanically and perhaps recrystallized at room temperature to reduce surface strain. Practical materials will have lower Kapitza conductance coefficients. For copper, approximate empirical forms for the Kapitza conductance in this temperature range have been suggested:

$$h_K \approx 900T^3 \qquad \text{for clean surfaces} \tag{10-30}$$
$$h_K \approx 400T^3 \qquad \text{for dirty surfaces} \tag{10-31}$$

Table 10-6 Highest experimental values for the Kapitza conductance at 1.9 K (from Ref. [25])

Solid	Θ_D (K)	h_K@1.9 K (kW/m² · K)	Value of α ($n = 3$) (kW/m² · K⁴)
Hg	72	30	4.4
Pb	100	32	4.7
In	111	11	1.6
Au	162	8.8	1.3
Ag	226	6	0.9
Sn	195	12.5	1.8
Cu	343	7.5	1.1
Ni	440	4.0	0.6
W	405	2.5	0.4
Nb	275	3.3	0.43
KCl	230	6.9	1.0
SiO₂ (quartz)	290	5.7	0.8
Si	636	4.2	0.6
LiF	750	4.5	0.6
Al₂O₃	1000	1.6	0.23

in W/m² · K. Most observed values fall in this range. In comparing Eqs. (10-30) and (10-31) with the values in Table 10-6, it is fair to assume that technical surfaces will have Kapitza conductances in the range of 30 to 50% of the highest experimental values. However, great care should be exercised when applying these correlations without experimental confirmation.

For large heat fluxes, $q > 1$ kW/m², the Kapitza conductance can no longer be adequately described by the linear coefficient, Eqs. (10-28) and (10-29). Rather, on the basis of experimental data and theory, a more general form for the surface heat flux is usually written as

$$q = a\left(T_s^m - T_b^m\right) \tag{10-32}$$

where a and m are also adjustable parameters. Note that if one equation is able to fit the experimental data for one sample over the whole temperature difference range, then it should be possible to expand Eq. (10-32) to obtain the low-heat-flux temperature dependence. Similar to the behavior of the experimental data for small ΔT, the high-heat-flux Kapitza conductance values also vary considerably with sample preparation. Figure 10-15 shows the measured surface temperatures for different materials in this heat flux regime. Also, listed in Table 10-7 is a summary of the fit coefficients in Eq. (10-32) for the data displayed in Fig. 10-15. Displayed are the surface preparation, surface temperature at a heat flux $q = 1$ W/cm², and the best-fit functional form to these data. Note that most of the fits give values of $m = 3 \pm 0.5$. Also, the best fit to the coefficient in Eq. (10-31) is for $a \approx 0.5$ kW/m² · K^{n+1}, but with substantial variation. It is interesting to note that the variation in Kapitza conductances at large ΔT is not nearly as great as is obtained in the limit ΔTs → 0, where an order-of-magnitude deviation in h_K is seen.

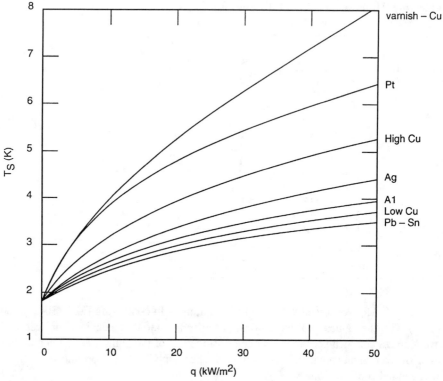

Figure 10-15 Surface temperature increase due to Kapitza conductance at high heat flux and $T_b = 1.8$ K.

Finally, there is considerable experimental evidence to show that the Kapitza conductance is not a function of fluid velocity [26,27]. This feature comes about because of the microscopic nature of the heat exchange in Kapitza conductance. As a result, technical application of published data can be accomplished without concern for the flow conditions of the helium, provided the fluid temperature does not exceed T_λ.

Table 10-7 High-heat-flux Kapitza conductance fitting parameters for different metals at 1.8 K (from Ref. [1])

Metal	Surface	T_s (K) @ 10 kW/m^2	a (kW/m$^2 \cdot$ K^{m+1})	m
Copper	As received	3.1	0.486	2.8
	Polished	2.67	0.455	3.45
	Oxidized	2.46	0.52	3.7
	PbSn solder	2.43	0.76	3.4
	Varnish coat	4.0	0.735	2.05
Platinum	Machined	3.9	0.19	3.0
Silver	Polished	2.8	0.6	3.0
Aluminum	Polished	2.66	0.49	3.4

Table 10-8 Typical film-boiling heat transfer coefficients (from Ref. [1])

Sample	T_b (K)	T_s (K)	Δ_p (kPa)	h (kW/m² · K)
Wire ($d = 76\ \mu$m)	1.8	150	0.42	1.1
Wire ($d = 25\ \mu$m)	1.8	150	0.56	2.2
Flat rectangular plate	1.8	75	0.14	0.22
(39 mm × 11 mm)				
	1.8	75	0.28	0.3
	1.8	75	0.84	0.55
Flat surface ($d = 13.7$ mm)	2.01	40	0.13	0.69
	2.01	25	0.237	0.98
Horizontal cylinder	1.88	40	0.10	0.2
($d = 14.6$ mm)				
Wire ($d = 200\ \mu$m)	2.05	150	0.14	0.66
Cylinder ($d = 1.45$ mm)	1.78	80	0.06	0.22

Film-boiling heat transfer. The film-boiling regime of heat transfer is of significant technical importance, for its occurrence can lead to catastrophic events in cryogenic systems where good heat transfer must be maintained continuously. Unfortunately, boiling heat transfer in He II is the least understood process and is subject to engineering correlation rather than model calculation.

In He II above the peak heat flux, the fluid at the heat transfer surface exists in several different phases. Consequently, the physical interpretation of the heat transfer processes is more difficult than in single-phase He II. For heat fluxes above q^* there occurs a discontinuous jump in the surface temperature. This transition marks the formation of a stable film of helium vapor, liquid He I, or both, blanketing the heat-transfer surface. Theoretical efforts to model this process have met with some success, and the most commonly analyzed problem consists of a stable film boiling in saturated He II [28,29]. For design purposes, the best approach remains that of empirically determining the best values for the film-boiling heat transfer coefficient. Listed in Table 10-8 are published values for this coefficient. Note both the strong geometrical and pressure dependence to this process.

10-3 TECHNOLOGY OF He II APPLICATIONS

This section summarizes the status of He II technology for applications. Emphasis is on major technical areas that have unique characteristics as compared with the classical technology. The principal areas discussed include refrigeration techniques, heat exchangers, pumping methods, and flow metering.

10-3-1 Refrigeration Techniques

J–T refrigeration cycles. The most direct method of obtaining He II is by reducing the vapor pressure over the saturated liquid to a pressure below T_λ ($p < 50$ kPa). This state can be relatively easily obtained by attaching a high-capacity vacuum pump to a closed

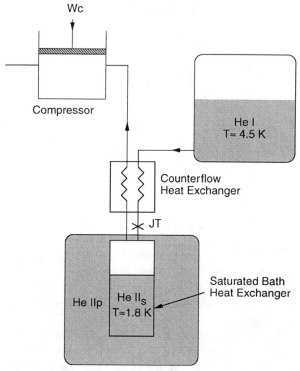

Figure 10-16 Schematic of a simple He II refrigerator.

volume of liquid helium. One disadvantage of such an approach is that it is relatively inefficient and can not provide continuous refrigeration owing to the finite volume of liquid.

Most practical He II refrigeration systems exist as an addendum to a normal helium closed-cycle refrigerator. Thus, the normal starting point for a low-temperature ($T < 4.2$ K) refrigeration circuit is from an isothermal bath of He I. A schematic of an He II refrigeration system that uses this concept is shown in Fig. 10-16. The He II circuit consists primarily of a counterflow heat exchanger, J–T valve, and a pump or compressor to bring the low-pressure helium back to suction pressure of the main compressors. Because the return flow is at low pressure ($p \approx 1$ kPa), the counterflow heat exchanger must be of unconventional design to allow efficient heat transfer at low-pressure drop. An alternative approach allows for the recompression of the helium with a cold compressor, which improves the heat transfer process on the return side.

The importance of the counterflow heat exchanger is made apparant by considering the T–S diagram for helium, Fig. 10-17. Without the counterflow heat exchanger, the helium will enter the J–T valve at essentially He I reservoir temperature, 4.2 K or above. In this case, the isenthalpic expansion is between points (1) and (2) in Fig. 10-17. The corresponding maximum yield for this process is

$$ y = \frac{h_v - h_1}{h_v - h_l} \tag{10-33} $$

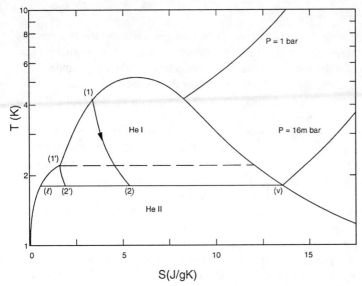

Figure 10-17 The T–S diagram for low-temperature helium showing two different expansion processes to 1.8 K.

where the subscripts apply to the various locations on the T–S diagram. For this set of initial conditions, the maximum yield would be 62%. With the counterflow heat exchanger, it is possible to reduce the temperature of the incoming fluid to just above T_λ. It is difficult to get much lower than 2.2 K because the J–T valve will act as a fountain pump, and its performance will be degraded. With a 2.2-K inlet temperature, the isenthalpic expansion will be between points (1') and (2') with a corresponding maximum yield of 89%.

Once the He II is discharged from the J–T valve, it enters the heat exchanger, which absorbs heat from the surroundings. Design of He II heat exchangers is discussed in the next section. The mass flow through the circuit depends on the heat load and efficiency of the expansion process.

$$\dot{m} = \frac{Q}{y h_{fg}} \tag{10-34}$$

With the latent heat of He II being about 24 kJ/kg, a 20-W heat load corresponds to a minimum mass flow rate of about 1 g/s.

For relatively small He II refrigeration systems, the most common approach to obtaining the low-pressure stage is to use a vacuum pump with roots blower. These units come in various sizes and when combined with an He II heat exchanger can produce refrigeration up to about 100 W at 1.8 K (5 g/s at 1.5 kPa). For large He II refrigeration systems, cold compressors [30,31] are preferred on the return side, for they increase efficiency and reduce the size of the counterflow heat exchanger. These units can provide refrigeration in the kilowatt range at 1.8 K. Chapter 9 of this handbook provides further information on cryogenic machinery.

10-3-2 Heat Exchangers

He II heat exchangers are indispensable components for superconducting magnets and other systems cooled with pressurized He II. However, because of the unusual properties of He II, specifically the high effective heat conductivity and strong temperature-dependent heat capacity, conventional heat-exchanger design methods, such as effectiveness or NTU, are not applicable. In this section, we review the current status of He II heat exchanger design and analysis.

Several different He II heat exchangers have been designed and developed for applications [32–34]. The most common of these is the static-bath-type system shown schematically in Fig. 10-18. The principal component of this system is a saturated He II reservoir in thermal contact through its surface to a surrounding pressurized He II reservoir. Any heat generated in the pressurized He II reservoir must be transferred through the solid wall to the saturated bath, where it is removed by evaporation of the liquid. For this type of system, there are two issues of concern. First, the surface area of the heat exchanger must be large enough to transfer the heat with minimal ΔT between the two reservoirs. Normally, the surface heat transfer process is controlled by the Kapitza conductance of the heat exchanger material. It is important to make the heat exchanger of copper or other high-conductivity material to avoid a significant conduction thermal resistance. The other issue in the design of these systems involves the heat transport in the bulk liquid. In other words, there must be sufficient He II cross section in the saturated bath to transport the heat by counterflow with a small temperature gradient.

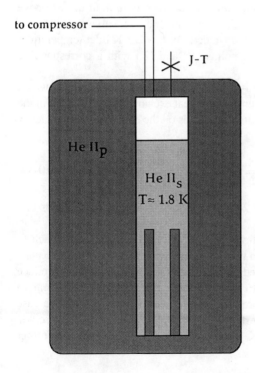

to compressor

J-T

He II$_p$

He II$_s$

$T \approx 1.8$ K

Figure 10-18 Static He II heat exchanger.

Another common type of He II heat exchanger is the tube-in-shell, which is primarily used for systems where the pressurized He II is confined to a cooling loop (Fig. 10-19). An added complexity to the design of this type of heat exchanger occurs when the He II loop has a forced flow. In this case, the design requirements are somewhat different. As in the saturated bath heat exchanger, tube-in-shell type units must meet the surface area requirements for acceptable ΔT between the two bulk He II reservoirs. Also important is that the He II cross section within the tube be large enough to transport the heat flux. This

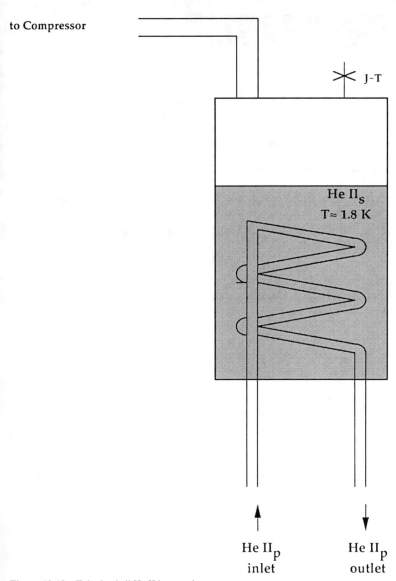

to Compressor

J-T

He II$_s$

$T \approx 1.8$ K

He II$_p$
inlet

He II$_p$
outlet

Figure 10-19   Tube-in-shell He II heat exchanger.

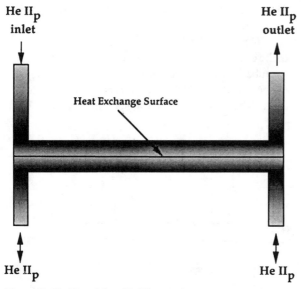

He II$_p$
inlet

He II$_p$
outlet

Heat Exchange Surface

He II$_p$

He II$_p$

Figure 10-20 Forced-flow He II heat exchanger.

part of the design is complicated by the unusual properties of the bulk He II, particularly in forced flow.

Finally, forced-flow He II heat exchangers have also been developed for specialized applications [33]. In this case, the two He II reservoirs are contained in closed loops with one or both being pumped through the system at a velocity u Fig. (10-20). The configuration can be either parallel or counterflow. Design requirements similar to those for the tube-in-shell design apply. The surface area must be sufficient, but also the cross section of the two channels must be large enough to avoid exceeding heat transport limits in the bulk fluid.

He II heat exchanger energy equations. The beginning point for the numerical analysis of an He II heat exchanger is the steady-state He II heat equation with heat transfer

$$\rho u C_p \frac{dT}{dx} - \frac{\partial}{\partial x}\left[f(T)^{-1}\frac{dT}{dx} \right]^{1/3} + \frac{Ph}{A}\Delta T = 0 \qquad (10\text{-}35)$$

where $f(T)^{-1}$ is the He II heat conductivity function appropriate for fully developed turbulent conditions, ΔT is the temperature difference between the two He II reservoirs, and h is the overall heat transfer coefficient between the two reservoirs. Normally, h is dominated by the Kapitza conductance coefficient at the two He II solid interfaces. The total heat transfer coefficient between two reservoirs of He II when separated by a high-conductivity metal wall may be approximated by

$$h = h_0 \left(\frac{T_1 + T_2}{2T_\lambda} \right)^3 \qquad (10\text{-}36)$$

where T_1 and T_2 are fluid temperatures within the hot and cold reservoirs.

For a saturated-bath heat exchanger with $u = 0$, the He II heat equation simplifies to yield

$$\frac{d}{dx}\left[f(T)^{-1}\frac{\partial T}{dx}\right]^{1/3} - \frac{Ph}{A}(T - T_b) = 0 \qquad (10\text{-}37)$$

This equation has an analytic solution for constant properties; however, the fully temperature-dependent equation must be solved by numerical methods.

For He II heat exchangers, the steady-state one-dimensional energy equations for the parallel and counterflow are obtained by applying the steady-state He II energy equation separately to the two fluid streams coupled by the heat transfer process. The appropriate energy equation for each channel may then be written as

$$\rho u_1 C \frac{dT_1}{dx} - \frac{d}{dx}\left[f(T_1)^{-1}\frac{dT_1}{dx}\right]^{1/3} + \frac{Ph}{A}(T_1 - T_2) = 0 \qquad (10\text{-}38)$$

$$\pm\rho u_2 C \frac{dT_2}{dx} - \frac{d}{dx}\left[f(T_2)^{-1}\frac{dT_2}{dx}\right]^{1/3} + \frac{Ph}{A}(T_2 - T_1) = 0 \qquad (10\text{-}39)$$

where T_1 and T_2 are fluid temperatures within the hot and cold channels, respectively. The third term in each case, $\pm\frac{Ph}{A}(T_2 - T_1)$, is the heat transfer flux between channels.

Owing to the high effective thermal conductivity of He II, these heat exchangers have exhibited some unusual temperature distributions not seen for the classical fluids, such as the minimum temperature observed in the tube-in-shell heat exchanger [35] and a crossover of the temperature curves in the parallel-flow heat exchanger [36].

The measured temperatures in both parallel and counterflow He II heat exchangers have been correlated with a finite difference numerical model [36]. The numerical model used to fit the experimental results has one adjustable parameter, the coefficient h_0, which is dominated by the Kapitza conductance between the He II and solid surface. Reasonable values for this coefficient can be obtained by combining Eq. (10-36) with the appropriate coefficients given in Table 10-5.

The heat removal capability of an He II heat exchanger is dependent on the mass flow and bath temperature. With an increase in the mass flow rate, temperature in both channels decreases, and more heat can be taken away from the heat source upstream. This result is consistent with the behavior of classical fluid heat exchangers.

The He II heat transport within the heat exchanger is affected by the mass flow rate. At low fluid velocity, the He II internal convection mechanism dominates the heat transfer process. On the other hand, at high fluid velocity the internal convection contribution becomes small, allowing the heat exchanger to be treated in terms of the forced convection and heat transfer through the wall. This observation suggests the existence of a transition velocity u_t. This velocity can be defined by scaling the terms in the He II energy equation to obtain

$$u_t = (\rho C f^{1/3} \Delta T^{2/3} L^{1/3})^{-1} \qquad (10\text{-}40)$$

where, in this case, ΔT corresponds to the temperature difference within a given stream of He II that is different from the temperature difference between the two separate streams. For fluid velocities well below u_t, the heat exchanger can be designed with simplified forms of Eqs. (10-38) and (10-39) that neglect the forced convection terms. On the other hand, at velocities much greater than u_t, the He II heat exchanger may be designed based on the classical heat exchanger methods. The transition velocity is rather strongly temperature-dependent and thus will vary along the length of the heat exchanger. However, taking advantage of these limits may in some cases simplify the design analysis.

A satisfactory definition of effectiveness in an He II heat exchanger has yet to be developed, and therefore such methods are not recommended for He II heat exchanger design.

10-3-3 Pumping Methods

Circulation of He II through closed systems requires a prime mover or pumping device. In the past, there has been some uncertainty about the suitability of classical circulating equipment (i.e., mechanical pumps) suitable for He II service. This issue has brought about some development and testing efforts. In addition, however, He II can be forced to flow by application of the fountain effect, which can circulate He II without the need for moving parts.

Mechanical Pumps. There are primarily two classes of mechanical circulation pumps that can be used with He II: piston type and centrifugal type. Most of the experience to date is with centrifugal-type units [37–39] of modest size. In general, these pumps perform with He II in much the same way they do with classical fluids. Pump characteristics, such as efficiency and head versus speed performance, show data similar to that expected from pump design models. These results allow designers to model performance for applications using classical scaling laws. Details of this modeling procedure are not presented here, and the reader is referred to the engineering literature [40].

Helium II properties do affect the onset of cavitation in centrifugal pumps, particularly when pumping saturated He II. The high conductivity of the He II normally dissipates the pump heat into the surroundings. As the pump speed increases, the local temperature also increases, eventually reaching the saturation condition, which causes bulk boiling or the He II–He I transition. At this point boiling initiates within the pump. If the pump is circulating pressurized He II, the transition is to the He I state, allowing flow to continue subject to the limitations of the normal fluid cavitation characteristics. In pumping saturated He II, cavitation onset produces large vapor regions in the pump head, which severely degrades pump performance [39].

Fountain pumps and phase separators. Fountain effect pumps (FEPs) are unique to He II. Arp [41] has compared this pumping method to conventional centrifugal pumps for He II service. Essentially, this type of pump uses the fountain effect to force He II to flow through a porous plug. A heater at the outlet of the pump provides the chemical potential difference to drive the fluid. Such a device has been developed and demonstrated for space-based applications [42]. A photograph of the fountain effect pump developed for the SHOOT project is shown in Fig. 10-21 [43]. Such a device consists of a sintered ceramic disk or plug with a heater located on the downstream side. Typical pore size is of the order of 0.1 μm.

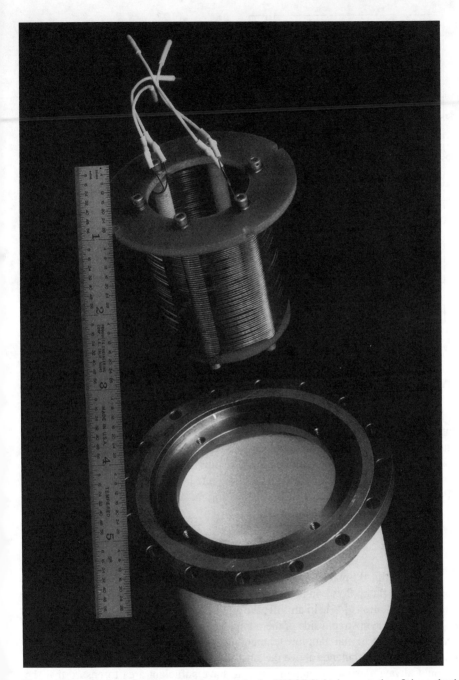

Figure 10-21 The fountain effect pump developed for the SHOOT flight demonstration. It is an alumina–silica composite ceramic with a 0.4-μm effective pore size. This pump demonstrated a flow rate of 30 g/s in flight (from Ref. [43]).

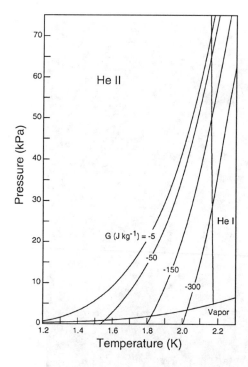

Figure 10-22 Constant chemical potential trajectories on the $P–T$ helium phase diagram. Lines correspond to the ideal fountain pressure.

An ideal fountain pump obeys the London equation and produces a pressure head corresponding to the temperature difference generated by a heater downstream of the flow. If one integrates the London equation, Eq. (10-16), along lines of constant chemical potential, the corresponding static pressure head is given in Fig. 10-22. Thus, for an ideal fountain pump, the maximum pressure head is about 50 kPa for a bath at 1.8 K. Higher pump heads can be realized by running several pumps in series. However, the pump head decreases significantly with increasing mass flow rate [44].

For an ideal fountain pump, the corresponding mass flow rate is given by the relationship

$$Q = \dot{m} S_0 T_0 \qquad (10\text{-}41)$$

where the subscript 0 applies to the conditions at the pump outlet. This relationship suggests that the pump flow can be increased by simply adding more heat downstream, but there are limitations [45]. In an FEP, the addition of heat increases the temperature of the helium on the upstream side of the pump. This heat must be extracted by an He II refrigeration system to maintain low temperature at the pump inlet. Another important limit is the onset of turbulence above the superfluid critical velocity. To avoid this limit one should always design a fountain pump to have sufficient area to ensure that the velocity does not exceed u_c (typically about 10 cm/s for porous media). For a porosity of 30%, this velocity corresponds to an approach velocity of about 3 cm/s, a value that has been achieved in pump tests [46]. Equation (10-41) can be rearranged in terms of the inlet conditions to yield

$$\dot{m} = \frac{\dot{Q}}{6.6\,\Delta p/\rho + s_i T_i} \tag{10-42}$$

where s_i is the entropy at the inlet to the fountain pump and Δp is the hydraulic pressure head.

The design of practical FEPs goes beyond the discussion above. To maintain ideal flow conditions in the pump, the approach velocity must be maintained below a few centimeters per second. Thus, the pump surface area is frequently much larger than the pipe cross section in the attached flow circuit. If these conditions are exceeded, pump performance will degrade; however, the FEP will continue to pump the helium until the inlet temperature exceeds T_λ. The advantage of a fountain pump is in its ease of application. The pump consists of a heater and porous plug. There are no moving parts. On the other hand, the low thermodynamic efficiency of a fountain pump makes it only useful in specialized applications [47–50].

Helium II vapor phase separators (VPS) have been developed for containment of He II in space applications [51–53]. A VPS consists of a porous plug, frequently made from sintered stainless steel powder, that extracts the heat from an He II reservoir by allowing evaporation at the surface of the plug. In this application, the characteristic pore size is larger than for the FEP because it is necessary to have some flow of the normal fluid component to ensure operation. A photograph of a sintered stainless steel VPS developed for the IRAS cryogenic system is shown in Fig. 10-23 [54].

An He II vapor phase separator provides a pressure difference across it given by London's equation, Eq. (10-16). In use, the upstream side of the phase separator is wetted with He II while the downstream side is exposed to low-pressure helium vapor. The phase separator works in the following way: Heat generated in the He II reservoir is carried through the porous plug by counterflow to the liquid–vapor interface, which preferrably occurs within the body of the plug. The heat is then removed by evaporation of the liquid at low pressure. The associated temperature difference across the plug provides the fountain pressure to hold the liquid within the Dewar. The total mass flow is determined by this rate of heat generation. For purely laminar flow that occurs in an ideal phase separator at $u < u_c$, the critical velocity, the mass-flow rate, is given by

$$\dot{m} = \frac{\rho d^2}{\beta \eta_n}\left(\frac{sT}{sT + h_{fg}}\right)\frac{\Delta p}{L} \tag{10-43}$$

where β is a shape factor. This relationship appears to fit experimental data for small mass-flow rates. If the velocity within the plug exceeds u_c, turbulence in the superfluid degrades the performance, and the mass flow increases more slowly with Δp.

The design of a porous plug phase separator is dependent on first knowing the mass flow needed to extract the heat load from the He II reservoir. The pressure drop across the plug is determined by the desired operating temperature of that reservoir. The physical dimensions and pore size of the porous plug follow from analysis of Eq. (10-42). Most phase separators developed for space applications consist of a sintered stainless steel structure [54,55]. The typical pore size is between 1 and 10 μm. Other phase

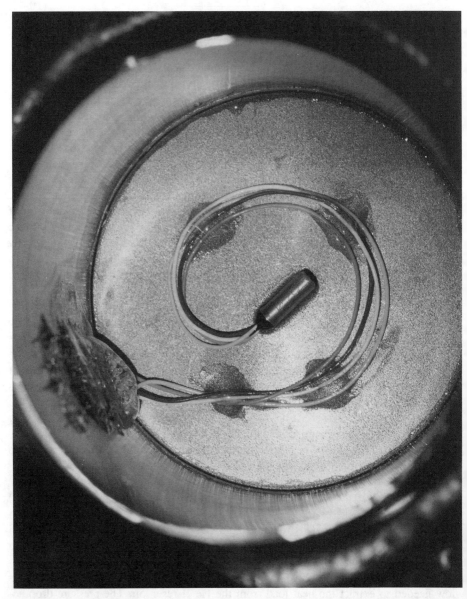

Figure 10-23 Helium II phase separator for the IRAS SFHe tank. The plug is approximately 50 mm in diameter and manufactured by MOTT Metalurgical from sintered nickel. The attached germanium thermometer is for determining the downstream helium temperature (from Ref. [54]).

eparator designs use a columnar structure consisting of many parallel channels of similar dimensions to the pore size in the sintered plugs [55]. Also, a variable-length slit design has been developed for a phase separator when active control is desirable [56].

10-3-4 He II Flowmetering Techniques

A wide variety of classical methods to measure either flow velocity or mass-flow rates have been developed for He II service. In addition, the superfluid properties of He II provide some new opportunities for flowmetering. Experience with different flowmetering techniques is reviewed below.

Turbine flowmeters. A turbine flowmeter contains a bladed wheel that rotates when the liquid moves past it. These devices essentially measure volumetric flow because the bladed wheel interacts with the fluid in a way that is only weakly dependent on fluid density. Thus, a turbine flowmeter is similar to a centrifugal pump. The rotational frequency of the turbine wheel is usually measured with a magnetic pickup and compared against a calibration for the given fluid. Signal conditioning equipment converts the frequency to a voltage output that is nearly linearly related to flow rate.

Turbine flowmeters have had good success in classical fluid, including He I, except at low flow rates, where they tend to show hysteresis [57]. Turbines necessarily contain moving parts, and thus they are more likely to fail or be susceptible to freezeup from any impurity gases in the experimental loop. Turbine flowmeters containing jewel (crystal) bearings with internal stresses or severe defects fracture from the thermal shock. Ceramic or metal ball bearings usually survive many thermal cycles between liquid helium and room temperatures. A turbine flowmeter with a magnetically levitated rotor has recently been developed for liquid helium service [58].

Turbine flowmeters have been successfully applied to He II service by Kashani et al. [59] and Daney [60,61]. As occurs with centrifugal pumps, turbine flowmeters display no unique performance characteristics except a tendency to cavitate in saturated He II at high flow rates. Cavitation can be suppressed by adding a flow constriction to the outlet to increase the local pressure, although this modification will increase the unrecovered pressure drop through the system.

Venturi flowmeters. There are a variety of flowmeters that base their operations on Bernoulli's principle that pressure drop occurs because of fluid acceleration through a narrow construction. Examples of these are venturi flowmeters, orifice plates, and flow nozzles. For an ideal inviscid fluid, a measurable pressure drop can occur without adding to the unrecovered pressure drop in the system. Real fluids experience significant pressure losses in these devices. The venturi flowmeter has the notable advantage of having minimum increased pressure loss and close-to-ideal performance. There have been several attempts to adapt venturi flowmeters for He II service [62–63].

The general expression used to describe mass flow through a venturi flowmeter is

$$\dot{m} = C_D \frac{\pi D^2}{4} \left(\frac{1}{\beta^4} - 1 \right)^{-1/2} (2\rho \, \Delta p)^{1/2} \qquad (10\text{-}44)$$

where D is the inlet diameter, β is the throat to inlet diameter ratio, and C_D is the discharge coefficient and is a measure of the degree of ideality in the flow. Note that because $\dot{m} \approx \Delta p^{1/2}$ the span of pressure drop is large compared with that of the mass-flow rate. Practical limitations on pressure transducer technology usually limit the usable range of a venturi flowmeter to about one order of magnitude in $\dot{m}$.

Daney [60] measured the discharge coefficient of a venturi flowmeter equipped with a low-temperature, differential-pressure transducer of the variable reluctance type. The measured values of the discharge coefficient were observed to be very close to the ideal value of $C_D = 1$. Thus, the indications are that venturi operation is unaffected by the superfluid character of He II up to moderate fluid velocities. Both Daney [61] and Walstrom et al. [20] studied cavitation of He II in venturi flowmeters. Cavitation can be observed as a discontinuous shift to the saturation pressure in the throat of the device.

Fluidic flowmeters. Fluidic flowmeters use hydrodynamic instabilities to generate oscillations in a flow stream. The oscillations are then detected with pressure transducers, thermistors, or thin-film temperature sensors. One type of fluidic flowmeter relies on the Coanda effect for its operation [64]. The Coanda effect refers to the deflection and attachment of a jet toward an adjacent surface. Feedback loops are provided to cause fluidic oscillation. In the turbulent flow regime the oscillation frequency of a fluidic flowmeter is linearly related to the fluid velocity.

The operation of fluidic flowmeters for He II service has been verified [65] when the flow oscillations were detected by measuring the pressure difference between two pressure ports located above the oscillating jet. The amplitude of this oscillating pressure signal is proportional to the volumetric flow rate. Thus, a clear advantage of this device is a wider range of detectable flow rates for a given pressure transducer. On the other hand, a clear disadvantage of a fluidic flowmeter is a rather large unrecoverable pressure drop compared with other devices.

Acoustic flowmeters. Acoustic or ultrasonic flowmeters work by measuring the differences in transit times of sound waves traveling with or against the bulk flow. In liquid helium, the speed of sound is temperature-dependent, and thus to be accurate the flowmeter requires isothermal conditions. This allows the elimination of the sound velocity from the analysis. The expression used to calculate the bulk fluid flow velocity is then written as

$$u = \frac{1}{2}\left(\frac{z_2}{t_2} - \frac{z_1}{t_1}\right) \tag{10-45}$$

where $z_{1,2}$ is the separation distance between the source and transducers 1 or 2 along the flow axis and $t_{1,2}$ is the transit time for a signal to reach transducers 1 or 2. Hofmann and Vogeley [66] developed an ultrasonic flowmeter for He II. In this case, inaccuracies in the dimensional measurements were eliminated by first measuring the difference in arrival times for static He II.

In the application of an acoustic flowmeter, the distance between the transducers must be sufficient to produce a measurable difference in the transit times, given the large velocity of first sound, about 200 m/s in He II. At the same time, the transducers must not be too far from the source to avoid attenuation of the pulses. A reasonable value is

$z \approx 100$ mm. Ultrasonic flowmeters have the advantage that they permit measurement of flow velocity without introducing a major disturbance to the flow. Because of limits to sensor resolution, this type of device is not very suitable for relatively low velocities, $v \ll c_1$.

Temperature-pulse flowmeters. Temperature-pulse flowmeters operate by measuring the time-of-flight of a thermal disturbance within a moving fluid. As a result, the method is a direct measure of fluid velocity. Usually the flowmeter works by the following sequence of events: (1) a quantity of fluid is warmed by a pulsed electrical heater, (2) the region of warmed fluid is carried downstream by the bulk fluid flow and passes over one or two thermometers, and (3) the thermometer output and knowledge of the distances between heater and thermometers are then used to determine the flow velocity.

Several groups have experimented with this type of flowmeter for He II. Kashani and Van Sciver [67] showed that heated regions of He II appear to propagate at the bulk fluid velocity. Walstrom, et al. [20] experimented with time-of-flight fluid velocity measurements. However, this approach has limited usefulness because of the rapid diffusion of the heat pulse in the bulk fluid. An alternative method would be to create a small region of He I and follow its propagation with flow; however, this approach would require the deposition of a large heat pulse with the associated disturbance of the helium [65].

Second sound flowmeters. The propagation of second sound (temperature or entropy waves) has been used to measure bulk flow velocity in He II. In this case, a heat pulse propagates at the second sound velocity, which is about 20 m/s or a factor of 10 lower than c_1, thus allowing for improved resolution at low velocities. Further, the signal is received by sensitive thermometry rather than a pressure transducer. In every other respect, a second sound flowmeter works the same as an acoustic flowmeter. The velocity may be determined by either a time-of-flight method or a phase shift approach; thus, Eq. (10-43) still applies. A prototype second sound flowmeter was developed by Holmes and Van Sciver [68]. This device used thin-film temperature sensors for detecting the signal.

Other flowmetering methods. A flowmetering method that has received considerable interest in recent years is that of Laser Doppler (LD) velocimetry. This method works by tracking neutral density particles suspended in the flow, thus providing a direct measure of fluid velocity. The LD method is particularly useful for making local velocity measurements because the lasers can be focused to a small spot (≈ 1 mm). Laser Doppler velocimetry is also complex in its application and requires very sophisticated and expensive hardware, thus, its use is limited primarily to research studies.

Although laser Doppler flowmetering has not applied to bulk flowing He II, there have been several successful attempts to use the method for studying counterflow in He II. Murakami and coworkers [69,70] have demonstrated the use of LD to study an He II counterflow jet. A critical aspect of this method is the selection of suitable neutral density particles to achieve light scattering. Murakami's group was successful using glass microspheres and small particles of solid hydrogen–deuterium mixtures. With this method they were able to characterize the flow of the normal fluid component in a counterflow jet. The LD method appears to work well in its limited applications to He II, but it remains to be seen whether it can be effectively implemented in flowing He II. See chapter 4 on cryogenic instrumentation for further information.

10-4 SUMMARY

The use of He II as a coolant in large-scale technical devices has expanded to the extent that it now represents a significant branch of cryogenic engineering. Development of such systems requires both a knowledge of conventional cryogenics principles as well as specific understanding of the behavior of He II. The present chapter is designed to provide the tools necessary to assist with future developments of He II cryogenic systems.

NOMENCLATURE

a	Kapitza coefficient (W/m$^2 \cdot$ K^{m+1}), empirical coefficient
A	Cross-sectional area (m^2)
c	Sound speed (m/s)
C	Specific heat (J/kg $\cdot$ K)
d	Diameter (m)
D	Diffusivity (m^2/s)
f_d	Friction factor
$f(T)^{-1}$	Turbulent He II heat conductivity function (W^3/m$^5 \cdot$ K)
$g(T)$	Laminar He II heat conductivity function (W/m$^3 \cdot$ K)
h_{fg}	Latent heat (J/kg)
h	Heat transfer coefficient (W/m$^2 \cdot$ K)
h	Specific enthalpy (J/kg)
L	Length (m)
m	Mass (kg)
p	Pressure (Pa)
P	Perimeter (m)
q	Heat flux density (W/m^2)
Q	Heat flux (W)
S	Entropy (J/kg $\cdot$ K)
t	Time (s), reduced temperature
T	Temperature (K)
u	Velocity (m/s)
V	Volume (m^3)
v	Specific volume (m^3/kg)
y	Yield
z	Distance (m)
α	Kapitza coefficient (W/m$^2 \cdot$ K^4)
β	Bulk expansivity (K^{-1}), empirical parameter
γ	Ratio of specific heat
ρ	Density (kg/m^3)
τ_d	Diffusion time constant (s)

κ	Compressibility (Pa^{-1})
η	Viscosity (N · s/m^2)
σ	Surface tension (N/m)
Θ_D	Debye temperature (K)

Subscripts

b	Bath
c	Critical
eff	Effective
g	Gas phase
K	Kapitza
l	Liquid phase
n	Normal, exponent
p	Constant pressure
s	Superfluid, surface
sat	Saturated vapor pressure
t	Transition
v	Constant volume
λ	At lambda temperature

REFERENCES

1. Van Sciver, S. W., *Helium Cryogenics* (New York: Plenum Press, 1986).
2. Wilks, J., *Liquid and Solid Helium* (Oxford: Clarendon Press, 1967).
3. Keller, W. E., *Helium-3 and Helium-4* (New York: Plenum Press, 1967).
4. Atkins, K. R., *Liquid Helium* (Cambridge: Cambridge University Press, 1959).
5. HEPAK is licensed by Cryodata, Niwot, Colorado.
6. Donnelly, R. J., Riegelmann, R. A., and Barenghi, C. F., *The Observed Properties of Liquid Helium at Saturated Vapor Pressure*, University of Oregon Report, June 1993.
7. Heiserman, J., Hulin, J. P., Maynard, J., and Rudnick, I., *Phys. Rev.* B 15(1976):3862.
8. Dresner, L., *Adv. Cryog. Eng.* 27 (1982):411.
9. Dresner, L., *Adv. Cryog. Eng.* 29 (1984):323.
10. Seyfert, P., Lafferranderie, J., and Claudet, G., *Cryog.* 22 (1982):401.
11. Van Sciver, S. W., *Cryog.* 19 (1979):385.
12. Kashani, A., and Van Sciver, S. W., *Adv. Cryog. Eng.* 31 (1986):489.
13. Kashani, A., Van Sciver, S. W., and Strikwerda, J. C., *J. Num. Heat Transfer A,* 16 (1989):213.
14. Van Sciver, S. W., *Adv. Cryog. Eng.* 29 (1984):315.
15. Kashani A., and Van Sciver, S. W., *Adv. Cryog. Eng.* 31 (1986):315.
16. Walstrom, P. L., *J. Low Temp. Phys.* 73 (1988):391.
17. Shajii, A., Huang, Y., Daugherty, M., Witt, R. J., and Van Sciver, S. W., *Adv. Cryog. Eng.* 35 (1990):165.
18. Huang, Y., Chang, Y., Witt, R., and Van Sciver, S. W., *Cryog.* 32 Supplement (1992):264.
19. Dresner, L., in *Cryogenic Properties, Processes and Applications,* vol. 82 (American Institute of Chemical Engineers, 1986).
20. Walstrom, P. L., Weisend, J. G. II, Maddocks, J. R., and Van Sciver, S. W., *Cryog.* 28 (1988):101.
21. Daughterty, M. A., and Van Sciver, S. W., *IEEE Trans. Magn.* 27 (1991):2108.
22. Hofmann, A., Khalil, A., and Kramer, H. P., *Adv. Cryog. Eng.* 33 (1988):471.
23. Snyder, H. A., Mord, H. J., and Newell, D. A., *Cryog.* 32 (1992):291.
24. Pollack, G. L., *Rev. Mod. Phys.* 41 (1969):48.
25. Snyder, N. S., *Cryog.* 10 (1970):89.

26. Kramer, H. P., in *Proc. 12th Intern. Cryo. Eng. Conf.* (London: Butterworths, 1988), 299–302.
27. Weisend, J. G. II, and Van Sciver, S. W., in *Superfluid Helium Heat Transfer,* vol. 134, (New York: American Society of Mechanical Engineers, 1990), 1–7.
28. Rivers, W. J., and McFadden, P. W., *Trans. ASME, J. Heat Transfer* 88C (1966):343.
29. Labuntzov, D. A., and Ametistov, Ye. V., *Cryog.* 19 (1979):401.
30. Gistau, G.M., Bonneton, M., and Mart, J. W., *Adv. Cryog. Eng.* 33 (1988):591.
31. Rode, C. H., Arenius, D., Chronis, W. C., Kashy, D., and Keesee, M., *Adv. Cryog. Eng.* 35 (1990):275.
32. Gistau, G. M., and Claudet, G., *Adv. Cryog. Eng.* 31 (1986):607.
33. Hofmann, A., in *Proc. 11th Intern. Cryog. Eng. Conf.* (London: Butterworths, 1986), 306–311.
34. Welton, S. et al., *Adv. Cryog. Eng.* 41 (1996):
35. Shajii, A., Huang, Y., Daugherty, M. A., Witt, R. J., and Van Sciver, S. W., *Adv. Cryog. Eng.* 35 (1990):165.
36. Huang, Y., and Van Sciver, S. W., *Cryog.* 36 (1996):535.
37. Steward, W. G., *Cryog.* 26 (1986):97.
38. Ludtke, P. R., Daney, D. E., and Steward, W. G., *Adv. Cryog. Eng.* 33 (1988):515.
39. Weisend, J.G. II, and Van Sciver, S. W., *Adv. Cryog. Eng.* 33 (1988):507.
40. *Marks' Standard Handbook for Mechanical Engineers*, Chapter 8 (New York: McGraw–Hill, 1979).
41. Arp, V., *Cryog.* 26 (1986):103.
42. DiPirro, M. J., and Castles, S. H., *Cryog.* 26 (1986):84.
43. DiPirro, M. J., NASA-Goddard Space Flight Center, Greenbelt, Maryland, Personal communication (1996).
44. Kittel, P., *Adv. Cryog. Eng.* 33 (1988):465.
45. Kittel, P., in *Proc. 11th Intern. Cryog. Eng. Conf.* (London: Butterworths, 1986), 317–322.
46. DiPirro, M. J., Quinn, E. R., and Boyle, R. F., in *Proc. 12th Intern. Cryog. Eng. Conf.* (London: Butterworths, 1988), 646–651.
47. Kittel, P., *Cryog.* 29 (1989):493.
48. Hofmann, A., in *Proc. 11th Intern. Cryog. Eng. Conf.* (London: Butterworths, 1986), 306–311.
49. DiPirro, M. J., and Boyle, R. F., *Adv. Cryog. Eng.* 33 (1987):487.
50. Maytal, B., Nissen, J. A., and Van Sciver, S. W., *Cryog.* 30 (1990):930.
51. Urbach, A. R., Vorreiter, J., and Mason, P., in *Proc. 7th Intern. Cryog. Eng. Conf.* (Surrey, England: IPC Science and Technology Press, 1978), 126–133.
52. Volz, S. M., DiPirro, M. J., Castles, S. H., Ryschewitsch, M. G., and Hopkins, R., *Adv. Cryog. Eng.* 37B (1992):1183.
53. Karr, G. R., and Hendricks, J. B., *Adv. Cryog. Eng.* 29 (1984):669.
54. Urbach, A. R., Ball Aerospace, Boulder, Colorado, Personal communication (1996).
55. Petrac, D., and Mason, P. V., in *Proc. 7th Intern. Cryog. Eng. Conf.* (IPC Science and Technology Press, 1978), 120–125.
56. Denner, H. D., Klipping, G., Klipping, I., and Schmidtchen, U., *Cryog.* 24 (1984):403.
57. Cairnes, D. N. H., and Brassington, D. J., in *Proc. 4th Intern. Cryog. Eng. Conf.* (IPC Science and Technology Press, 1972), 361–363.
58. Rivetti, A., Martini, G., Goria, R., and Lorefice, S., *Cryog.* 27 (1987):8.
59. Kashani, A., and Van Sciver, S. W., *Adv. Cryog. Eng.* 31 (1986):489.
60. Daney, D. E., *Adv. Cryog. Eng.* 33 (1988):1071.
61. Daney, D. E., *Cryog.* 27 (1987):132.
62. Rivetti, A., Martini, G., and Birello, G., *Adv. Cryog. Eng.* 39 (1994):1051.
63. Kashani, A., Wilcox, R. A., Spivak, A.L., Daney, D. E., and Woodhouse, C. E., *Cryog.* 30 (1990):286.
64. Tippetts, J. R., Ng, H. K., and Riyle, J. K., Fluidics Q 5 (1973):28.
65. Van Sciver, S. W., Holmes, D. S., Huang, X., and Weisend, J. G. II, *Cryog.* 31 (1991):75.
66. Hofmann, A., and Vogeley, B., in *Proc. 11th Intern. Cryog. Eng. Conf.* (London: Butterworths, 1984), 448–451.
67. Kashani, A., and Van Sciver, S. W., *Adv. Cryog. Eng.* 33 (1988):417.
68. Holmes, D. S., and Van Sciver, S. W., *Adv. Cryog. Eng.* 35 (1990):247.
69. Murakami, M., Naki, H., Ichikawa, N., Hanada, M., and Yamazaki, T., in *Proc. 11th Intern. Cryog. Eng. Conf.* (London: Butterworths, 1986), 582–586.
70. Murakami, M., and Ichikawa, N., *Cryog.* 29 (1989):438.

ELEVEN

SAFETY

F. J. Edeskuty and M. Daugherty

MS-J576, LANL, Los Alamos, NM 87545

11-1 INTRODUCTION

Safety is primarily important in cryogenic engineering to protect personnel and property. A secondary reason for the importance of safety is that cryogenic equipment can be very expensive. To ensure the safety of a cryogenic project it is necessary that the system be designed and constructed to be as safe as possible and that it be operated safely. Safe operation of a cryogenic system requires that the operation be thoroughly understood and that attention to safety practices is strictly followed. Past experience with operations that do not include the use of cryogenic fluids is not sufficient because the properties of cryogenic fluids and materials can vary considerably over the range of temperature from ambient temperature down to operating temperatures. For the design of the system and its operation, a thorough knowledge is required of all of the physical principles involved. Also, thorough and continuing training of operators is necessary [1].

11-2 SOURCES OF HAZARDS

In working with any cryogenic fluid, hazards that can arise include those that are phys-iological and those that originate from physical (or mechanical) behavior of the fluids themselves or the structural materials in which they are contained. If work involves a com-bustible cryogen or a combustion-enhancing substance like oxygen or oxygen-enriched air, unwanted fires or even explosions can also be a concern [1].

11-3 PHYSIOLOGICAL HAZARDS

Physiological hazards arise because of the very low temperatures of the cryogens, which can cause freezing of human tissue or hypothermia. Also of concern is the very large expansion of cryogenic fluids as they evaporate with the resultant gas warming to ambient temperature (on the order of a thousand-fold multiplication in volume). Toxicity can give rise to an additional hazard, although with the more commonly encountered cryogens (oxygen, nitrogen, hydrogen, and helium) this is not a problem.

11-3-1 Cold Damage to Living Tissue

The very cold temperatures of all cryogens is an obvious hazard if the fluid is allowed to come into contact with human tissue. Such contact can result in almost instantaneous freezing, and the resulting damage to the tissue is in some respects similar to a thermal burn. Thus the term "cryogenic burn" is often encountered. Although it is of obvious importance to prevent contact with either the liquid cryogen or the cold gas accompanying the liquid, an equally important precaution is to preclude the possibility of contact of flesh with any cold metal that is at cryogenic temperatures. A typical place where such cold metal might be encountered is in the vent system through which cold vapors could be passing. Obvious precautions include such measures as locating all ports where cryogenic fluids or cold vapors could be released in places where these fluids could not possibly impinge upon personnel. An equally important precaution is that of thermally insulating any cold part of the system so that cold surfaces are not exposed where they could be inadvertently touched.

In working with systems at cryogenic temperatures, protective clothing should be worn. Because the eyes are especially vulnerable, face shields or goggles should be used. As much of the body as practical should be covered by wearing long-sleeve shirts and long trousers with pant legs not being tucked into boots. Thermally insulating gloves should also be worn.

Contact with cold fluids or cold metal can freeze human tissue extremely fast. Freezing occurs when the tissue is cooled to a temperature of about −3 °C (below 0 °C because of the freezing point lowering as a result of dissolved solutes). If, in spite of the necessary precautions being taken, a freezing of tissue should occur, first aid treatment should consist of making the patient comfortable, gently removing any covering clothing (taking care not to tear any skin), and then gently warming the frozen part, preferably by immersion in warm water (40 to 42 °C, not above 44 °C). Medical attention should promptly be sought [2].

Cold temperatures can harm human beings even if no tissue is frozen. Body heat is maintained by metabolism, muscle action, and shivering. If the body can not generate heat at the rate the heat is being removed, body temperature will continuously decrease, and hypothermia can result. If the body core temperature drops below 35 °C, a general deterioration of the functioning of the body organs can occur as well as that of the nervous, cardiac, and respiratory systems. At temperatures below 28 °C, ventricular fibrillation becomes more likely [3]. In most cases, a person in an environment where hypothermia could be a problem can leave or escape. However, care should be taken to prevent situations in which a person might not be able to escape a rapid flow of exhausting cryogenic fluid, either because of the lack of an available exit or because of being rendered physically incapable of leaving. For this reason it is advisable to provide more than one path of egress from an experimental site and to forbid workers from working alone where a possibility of cold venting fluid could exist.

Table 11-1 Change in volume from liquid at normal boiling point to ambient temperature gas at 1 atmosphere

Substance	Ratio V_{gas}/V_{liquid}
Helium	701
p-Hydrogen	788
Neon	1341
Nitrogen	646
Argon	779
Oxygen	797
CO_2	762

11-3-2 Asphyxiation

Table 11-1 illustrates the large expansion that occurs when a given volume of cryogenic liquid evaporates and is warmed to ambient temperature. The table indicates that a relatively small quantity of a liquid cryogen, other than oxygen, can either displace, or at least dilute, the breathable atmosphere in a location near the spill of the liquid. This becomes even more hazardous in a closed location such as a small room. Table 11-2 gives the consequences of oxygen depletion. However, these results must be taken as only an indication because there are differences in the response from one person to the next. Also, local atmospheric pressure can play a part. The important point is that depletion of the atmosphere to the point where the oxygen concentration is less than 19.5% has been classified as an oxygen deficient atmosphere [4].

Oxygen depletion is a serious hazard. It is even more insidious because one symptom of anoxia is a general feeling of well being, or even euphoria, with the consequence that in this condition a person might not even try to extricate himself or herself from a hazardous location. A particularly dangerous situation for oxygen depletion is in the entry of personnel into tanks. This should never be attempted without a thorough, well-thought-out safety plan, including a method of removing a person, if necessary, without endangering an additional person. Even in the outdoors a hazardously depleted

Table 11-2 Symptoms and effects of oxygen deficiency (from Ref. [4])

Oxygen content (volume %)	At rest symptoms and effects
15–19	Possible impaired coordination; may induce early symptoms in persons with lung, heart, or circulatory problems.
12–15	Deeper respiration, faster pulse, and impaired judgment, coordination, and perception.
10–12	Further increase in respiration depth and rate, lips blue, poor coordination, and judgment.
8–10	Nausea, vomiting, ashen face, mental failure, fainting, unconsciousness.
6–8	4–5 minutes, all recover with treatment; 6 minutes, fatal in 25 to 50% of cases; 8 minutes, fatal in 50 to 100% of cases.
4–6	Coma in 40 seconds and then convulsions, breathing failure, and death.

concentration of oxygen can persist, especially in low areas where the colder, more dense gases may be slow to disperse. Precautions against the hazard of oxygen depletion include limiting the amount of cryogenic fluid within enclosed spaces where personnel can be present, and oxygen monitoring.

11-3-3 Toxicity

Although carbon dioxide is not toxic (and usually not considered a cryogen), it is worth mentioning that an atmosphere with too much carbon dioxide can not allow the body to get rid of the carbon dioxide that is formed by normal respiration. Breathing of an atmosphere with 10% carbon dioxide can result in unconsciousness in less than 1 minute. An upper limit of 5000 ppm has been established for an 8-hour work day [5].

The truly toxic cryogens are carbon monoxide, fluorine, and ozone. Carbon monoxide has an affinity to combine with the hemoglobin in the blood that is 300 times as great as that of oxygen. Thus the body is starved of oxygen by chemical asphyxia. Breathing an atmosphere with 4000 ppm can result in death in less than 1 hour [6]. An upper limit for a 40-hour work week has been established at 25 ppm [7].

Fluorine presents a hazard by inhalation as well as from contact with the skin, where it can cause burns. The exposure limit is 1 ppm for a 40-hour work week. Fluorine's pungent odor allows the human nose to be a good detector, for it can detect concentrations down to about 0.14 ppm [8]. Ozone is also toxic and is presumed to be fatal at concentrations above 50 ppm. The upper limit for human exposure has been placed at 0.1 ppm [9].

11-4 PHYSICAL (OR MECHANICAL) HAZARDS

Physical hazards result from the effect of the low temperatures on structural materials being used to contain the cryogens and from some of the properties of the cryogens themselves.

11-4-1 Embrittlement

Cold temperatures can embrittle some materials at temperatures much warmer than those of cryogens. Recent investigations of the steel from the Titanic have shown that cold embrittlement may have played a part in the massive damage to that vessel in the cold iceberg environment of the North Atlantic Ocean. A cryogenic example of embrittlement is that of the rupture of a tank containing liquefied natural gas (LNG) in Cleveland, Ohio, in 1944. The steel chosen for this structure contained 3.5% nickel. This material has been shown to become brittle at the temperature of LNG (about 110 K). The tank rupture spilled over 4000 m^3 and resulted in over 100 deaths and 200 injuries [10].

An insight into the mechanism for cold embrittlement can be obtained from the behavior of the yield and tensile stresses of a material as a function of temperature. Figure 11-1 shows the behavior of an aluminum alloy that is a good material for cryogenic applications. As the temperature is lowered, the tensile strength increases at a greater rate than does the yield strength. Thus, the difference between these two parameters, which is an indication of ductility, also increases as temperature is lowered. Figure 11-2,

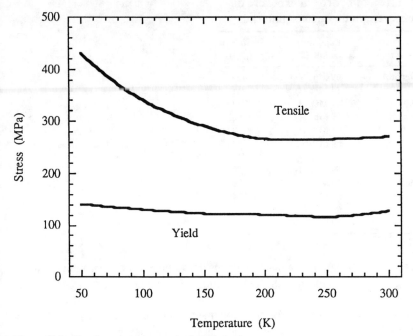

Figure 11-1   Tensile and yield strength of 5086 aluminum.

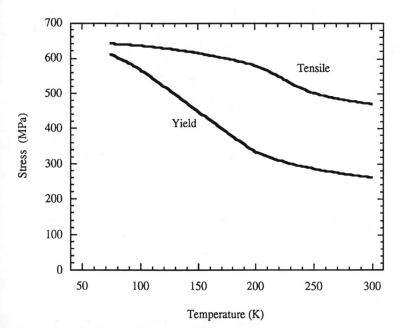

Figure 11-2   Tensile and yield strength of 430 stainless steel.

Table 11-3 Effect of hydrogen exposure on the ultimate strength of various materials

Material (notched samples)	Exposure (at 300 K)	Strength (MPa)
4140 (high strength)	69 Mpa N_2	2496
	14 MPa H_2	931
	41 MPa H_2	834
4140 (low strength)	69 Mpa N_2	1660
	41 MPa H_2	1427
	69 MPa H_2	1407
K Monel PH	69 MPa N_2	1731
	69 MPa H_2	779
K Monel (annealed)	69 MPa N_2	993
	69 MPa H_2	724
C1025	69 MPa N_2	730
	69 MPa H_2	552

in contrast, shows the behavior of a material that is not suitable for cryogenic service. In the case of Fig. 11-2, the yield strength increases more rapidly than the tensile strength as the temperature is lowered with the consequence that eventually these two strengths are almost equal, indicating a brittle material. Good materials for cryogenic service include such metals as aluminum alloys, 300 series (austenitic) stainless steels, and copper [1].

If the structural materials are used to contain hydrogen, another type of embrittlement is possible. Although there are three types of hydrogen embrittlement, the type of concern here is termed "environmental hydrogen embrittlement," which can occur by subjecting the equipment to hydrogen, usually at elevated pressure. Table 11-3 shows the consequences of hydrogen action on three different metals resulting in varying degrees of deterioration in their structural strengths. Several mechanisms have been proposed for the effect of hydrogen on metals, and it has been said that if the conditions are sufficiently stringent, hydrogen will affect almost any material.

Tests comparing strain to failure have shown that the magnitude of the effect of hydrogen is a function of temperature and is maximized at temperatures between 200 and 300 K. Thus, one might think that hydrogen embrittlement is not a problem for cryogenic service. However, most cryogenic equipment that will contain hydrogen will see some service at ambient temperature, and large temperature gradients frequently exist in equipment. Therefore, cryogenic materials for service with hydrogen must be chosen to be as resistant to hydrogen as possible. As with metals for cryogenic service, good materials for hydrogen service include aluminum alloys, copper, and stable austenitic stainless steels. In addition, it is important to avoid plastic strain in metals because straining the material in a hydrogen atmosphere promotes the embrittlement of the material [1].

11-4-2 Buildup of Pressure

One of the most commonly encountered hazards of handling cryogenic fluids comes from the unwanted buildup of pressure. That such large pressures can result does not come

**Table 11-4 Pressure required
to maintain liquid density at
room temperature**

Substance	Pressure
Nitrogen	296 MPa
Hydrogen	172 MPa
Helium	103 MPa

as a surprise when one considers the large thermal expansion coefficient of the liquids and their very large expansion as evaporation and warming of the gases to ambient temperature occurs (see Table 11-1). However, the pressures that can be obtained by confining a volume of cryogenic liquid are much higher than one might compute by merely considering the volume ratios shown in Table 11-1 and using the ideal gas law to compute a pressure.

As the pressure of a gas is increased sufficiently, the value of PV/RT becomes significantly greater than 1 and continues to increase monotonically as the pressure is increased further [11]. Table 11-4 shows the approximate maximum pressures that can be reached by attempting to maintain liquid density as the temperatures of three common cryogens are raised to ambient temperature. One way to attempt to maintain liquid density of a cryogenic liquid while allowing its temperature to rise to ambient levels is to have a pipe filled with liquid and then close two valves in series. Of course, the pressures would usually not be reached because the pipe walls would rupture before reaching that pressure in most cases.

Cryogenic storage vessels should never be totally filled with liquid, and usually a part of the storage volume above the liquid surface (called ullage) is reserved for the gas. Typical ullage volume is a minimum of 10% of the total volume of the vessel. If a cryogenic storage vessel is closed off and not allowed to vent boil-off gas proportional to the heat leaked into the vessel, the storage pressure will rise and the temperature of the stored fluid will rise with it. The thermal expansion coefficients of the common cryogens are listed in Table 11-5. That they are large can be seen from the comparison with water at its normal boiling point. If the temperature of the liquid rises sufficiently,

**Table 11-5 Thermal expansion
coefficients of various fluids at the
normal boiling point $[1/V(dV/dT)_p]$**

Substance	Coefficient
Liquid helium	0.210/K
Liquid hydrogen	0.0164/K
Liquid neon	0.0144/K
Liquid nitrogen	0.0057/K
Liquid argon	0.0044/K
Liquid oxygen	0.0044/K
Water (for comparison)	0.0007/K

the liquid can completely fill the vessel, a situation that is termed "liquid full." At this point a much faster pressure rise rate can be expected, which can lead quickly to the explosion of the vessel.

Another frequently encountered mechanism for a more rapid pressure rise in a closed cryogenic system is that of thermal stratification. The heat that enters the storage volume at the bottom of the vessel will heat the entire volume of contained fluid. However, the heat that enters the sides warms the adjacent liquid, which then travels up along the wall of the vessel until it accumulates at the liquid surface. Because the pressure in the vessel is established by the temperature of the liquid surface, this unequal distribution of incoming energy will cause a pressure rise rate that can be as great as ten times the normal rise rate if all of the incoming heat were to be distributed equally within the entire volume of the liquid (see Fig. 11-3).

In cases where it is necessary to close off a storage volume, some mechanism to prevent thermal stratification is usually provided to preclude the premature venting of the fluid and maintain acceptable pressures within the vessel. Because of the vibration, a

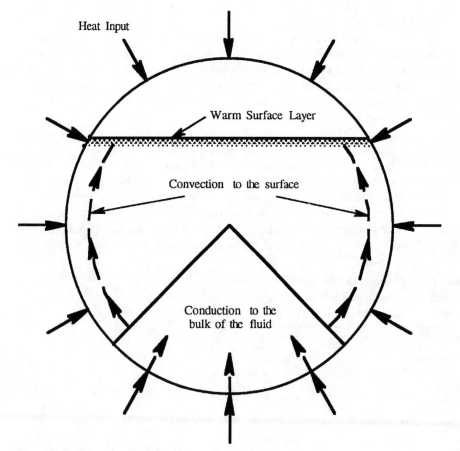

Figure 11-3 Schematic of heat flows into a cryogenic dewar.

highway transport will have a lower pressure rise rate as long as it is driven over the road. When the highway transport is stopped, the pressure rise rate can increase dramatically owing to thermal stratification [1]. Another method to prevent thermal stratification that has been proven effective is the inclusion of thermal shorts of high-thermal-conductivity material, which tend to equalize the temperature between the surface and the lower regions in the storage volume. Even the addition of a noncondensable gas stream at the bottom of the vessel to stir the fluid has been effective in preventing thermal stratification [1].

Because of the potential of unacceptable pressures arising within a cryogenic system it is necessary to provide for pressure relief in case the pressure in the system should start to rise above an acceptable level. There are several types of volumes that require pressure relief. The most obvious of these volumes is that in which the liquid is present, such as a storage volume or cryogen bath. A similar volume is found in a transfer line between two valves that can be closed. A less obvious volume is that containing a gas or condensed liquid in a volume being cooled by an external bath of cryogen or a flowing stream of refrigerant gas.

For the storage of the lower-boiling cryogenic liquids (neon, hydrogen, or helium), an evacuated insulation space is usually necessary for thermal isolation of the cold system. These three liquids are sufficiently cold that if any air were to enter the evacuated insulation system, the air will condense on the cold inner surface of the insulation space and at that temperature will exert essentially zero vapor pressure. Table 11-6 presents some approximate vapor pressures of higher-boiling substances at the temperature of liquid hydrogen and liquid helium. The condensed solid air will, therefore, give no evidence of its presence until the colder liquid being stored is removed. At that time the trapped air can evaporate and exert its full pressure, which can be sufficient to explode the outer vacuum jacket or implode the inner vessel. For this reason pressure relief must also be provided for the vacuum jackets in systems containing the lower-boiling cryogenic liquids.

A standard for pressure relief devices is given by the Compressed Gas Association [12]. In general the relief valves should be sized to allow the maximum flow of

Table 11-6 Vapor pressure of some gases at selected temperatures (Torr)

Vapor	4 K	20 K	77 K	150 K	Triple[a] point temperature
Water	b	b	b	10^{-7}	273
Carbon dioxide	b	b	10^{-8}	10	217
Argon	b	10^{-13}	160	c	84
Oxygen	b	10^{-13}	150	c	54
Nitrogen	b	10^{-11}	730	d	63
Neon	b	30	d	d	25
Hydrogen	10^{-7}	760	d	d	14

Note: Estimates; useful for comparison purposes only.
[a] Solid and vapor only at equilibrium below this temperature; no liquid.
[b] Less than 10^{-13} Torr.
[c] Greater than 1 atmosphere.
[d] Above the critical temperature, liquid does not exist.

exiting fluid that can be anticipated at the maximum allowable pressure in the storage volume. Usually a failure of the insulation system (such as a complete loss of vacuum) is considered. Also, in the case of a transport vessel, the possible upset of the vessel should be considered because it might result in the gas vent location being below the liquid surface. In this case it will be necessary to vent a liquid volume sufficient to maintain a safe pressure within the vessel. If the vessel contains a device capable of storing energy, such as a superconducting magnet, the pressure rise caused by the sudden dissipation of the stored energy into the fluid must also be considered.

Another mechanism for increasing the rate of pressure rise in a cryogenic storage volume is that of pressure oscillations. In the case of heating a flowing cryogenic liquid, the possibility and severity of these pressure oscillations depend upon the rate of heat transfer. A correlation describing the onset and severity of these oscillations is available in the literature [1]. For the colder-boiling cryogens, hydrogen and helium, oscillations can be excited by connecting the cold storage volume to ambient temperature by means, for example, of a tube to a pressure gauge. If this problem occurs, a change in the pressure measurement system might be necessary. The important parameters are the ratio of the temperatures at the ends of the tube, the tube diameter, and the temperature gradient along the tube [13].

Table 11-7 shows that the colder the normal boiling point of the cryogen, the more difficult is its handling. As seen in Table 11-7, this increased difficulty occurs because, as the normal boiling point temperature becomes lower, the heat of vaporization per unit volume of liquid also decreases. Added to this is the fact that, as the boiling temperature becomes lower, the difference in temperature (the driving force inducing heat into the cold system) is also increasing.

The storage of LNG presents a special hazard of pressure rise. This has been termed "rollover." Liquefied natural gas is not a single component fluid. Rather, it consists of several constituents, each with a different vapor pressure and a different density at a given temperature. Heat enters the tank both at the sides and the bottom. The liquid at the top can lose heat by evaporation, whereas the bottom can only lose heat by conduction to the top layer. This results in a warmer layer at the bottom, which becomes less dense as its temperature rises. At the same time the top of the liquid becomes heavier as it loses

Table 11-7 Temperature difference and heat of vaporization for various substances

Substance	Normal boiling point (K)	Heat of vaporization (J/cm^3)	Delta T^a (K)
Oxygen	90	243	210
Nitrogen	77	160	223
Neon	27	104	273
Hydrogen	20	32	280
Helium	4	2.5	296
Water^b	373	2255	–

Note: Both temperature difference and heat of vaporization affect pressure rise rate.
^{a}Temperature difference from ambient to normal boiling point.
^{b}For comparison only.

its lighter components. Eventually the difference in densities can cause a rolling over of the liquid so that the warmer liquid moves to the top, where it will evaporate more rapidly without the pressure of the hydrostatic head above it [14]. The large increase of boil-off vapors can be a hazard because they are combustible.

11-4-3 Condensation of Atmospheric Gases and Higher-Boiling Substances

All cryogens can condense water vapor and carbon dioxide and many other compounds. Table 11-6 shows how low the vapor pressure is for several substances that could be condensed. Liquid nitrogen, liquid hydrogen, and liquid helium (or even the cold vapors from the latter two) can condense oxygen or air. This is likely to occur if these fluids, or cold vapors from these fluids, are passed through an uninsulated pipeline.

In general, the condensate from atmospheric air, condensing on an exposed surface at liquid nitrogen temperature, or colder, is more hazardous than liquid air. The composition of this condensate is about 50% oxygen, and subsequent evaporation can further enrich the oxygen content. Figure 11-4 shows the composition of condensate if air with 21%

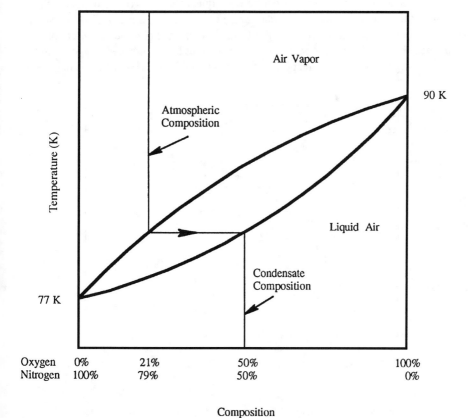

| Oxygen | 0% | 21% | 50% | 100% |
| Nitrogen | 100% | 79% | 50% | 0% |

Composition

Figure 11-4 Oxygen–nitrogen phase diagram showing ambient and condensate compositions.

oxygen is condensed on a cold surface. This condensate, liquid air, or liquid oxygen can all change the combustibility characteristics of many materials and, if falling upon combustible materials, can cause fire or explosion hazards.

The cold liquid can also cause low-temperature embrittlement if it falls upon materials that are not suitable for low-temperature service. Such an event has caused the cracking of deck plates of a barge being used to carry liquid hydrogen and has also cracked the carbon steel outer shell of a liquid hydrogen storage Dewar. In improperly purged systems, this type of condensation will take place internally. Even if there is no combustibility hazard, the presence of an inert solid can still cause safety problems by blocking the opening to relief valves or causing erosion of valve seats, for example.

11-4-4 Stresses Caused by Thermal Contraction

Dimensional changes can cause excess stresses. The thermal expansion coefficient decreases as temperature is lowered and is very small by the time 77 K is reached. Figure 11-5 shows the behavior of the thermal expansion coefficient of copper as a function of temperature. The behavior of steels is similar. Because the thermal expansion coefficient decreases so much by the time the temperature of liquid nitrogen is reached, not much further contraction occurs below this temperature. For detailed design, actual values should be used, but, as a rule of thumb, we can estimate the thermal contraction of copper and steels to be about 0.3% from room temperature down to liquid nitrogen temperature and any lower temperature. The corresponding value for aluminum is about 0.4%. In general,

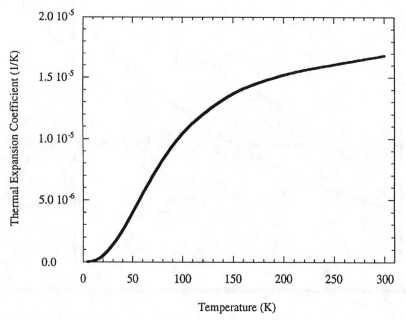

Figure 11-5   Copper thermal expansion coefficient ($1/L(DL/Dt)$).

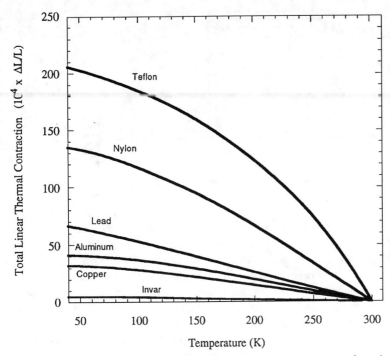

Figure 11-6   Total linear thermal contraction from 300 K to plotted temperature for various materials.

plastics have much higher thermal expansion coefficients, but they vary considerably. Figure 11-6 shows total thermal contraction of various materials as the temperature is lowered from ambient temperature to temperatures within the cryogenic range [1].

In general this contraction must be accommodated. Consider the stress that could result if steel were held fast and not allowed to contract while being cooled to a cryogenic temperature. From the rule-of-thumb for steel mentioned in the previous paragraph, the strain will be 0.3% (or 0.003). Using an elastic modulus E of 30 million pounds per square inch one can compute the resulting stress. Because E is equal to stress/strain, stress = E × strain = 90,000 psi if contraction is not allowed. This is greater than the yield stress and might be greater than the tensile strength. With Invar it might be acceptable to restrict thermal contraction because the total contraction is only about one-sixth as great, and the elastic modulus is also smaller. However, the stress on the rest of the system would have to be considered.

Dimensional changes caused by thermal contraction must be considered in transfer line design.* This can be done by using expansion bellows or by building in flexibility ("U" sections or elbows). One can analyze a piping system for thermal stresses by hand calculations for simple cases; for large systems a computer analysis is needed (a number of computer codes exist). First allow the line to contract to its new dimensions; then stretch the ends back to the anchors and compute stresses, bending moments, and

---

*Additional information on transfer line design may be found in chapter 5 of this handbook.

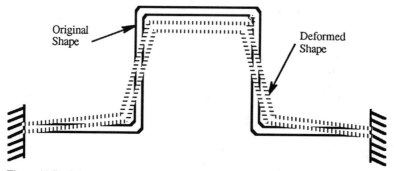

Figure 11-7 Schematic of cryogenic transfer line before and after cooling.

displacements. (Figure 11-7 shows an exaggerated view of the line after cooling to operating temperature.) If stresses are found to be too great, it is necessary to include more or larger "U" bends or elbows. If this is not desirable, flexible piping can be used if the additional pressure drop is not excessive. For vacuum-jacketed lines it may also be necessary to allow for motion of the vacuum jacket by the use of expansion bellows.

The previous considerations are for a case at thermal equilibrium. Thermal transients can give rise to thermal gradients (and stresses) during processes like cooling a piece of equipment from room temperature down to operating temperature. A thick flange can reach liquid hydrogen temperature at the inner surface while still at room temperature at the outer surface. Under these conditions it is also necessary to know something about the temperature gradient to estimate the thermal stress because the stresses can depend upon the shape of the thermal gradient as well as the total temperature difference. Therefore, cooling flow rates must not be too fast, and some maximum permissible cooling flow rates have been calculated by Novak [15].

Cooling a piece of equipment like a long, horizontal transfer line too slowly can result in another type of thermal stress. Usually a transfer line is cooled by introducing a flow of the cryogen through the line when it is initially at ambient temperature. The line is then cooled by evaporation of the cryogen. A snapshot illustration of the line at some time during the cooling process shows that several types of flow can occur within the line. When the line is partially cooled, the initial portion of the line will be filled with liquid. Downstream of this portion is a length that is still not at the temperature of the liquid and therefore is being cooled by heating the liquid and causing some two-phase flow. Even further downstream the liquid has all been evaporated, and the cold gas is precooling the line while the vapor is warming up to close to ambient temperature. If the two-phase flow is stratified flow, it is possible for the bottom of the line to cool faster than the top. This can cause the line to bow upwards and may cause unacceptable thermal stresses. A more detailed discussion of this phenomenon may be found in the literature [1].

11-5 COMBUSTION HAZARDS

Two of the commonly encountered cryogens (hydrogen and LNG) are flammable and can give rise to the hazard of unwanted combustion. In addition, oxygen is a strong promoter of combustion and can present a similar hazard. Although this latter hazard is more obvious in the case of pure oxygen, liquid air is also hazardous, and, as pointed out in section 11-4-3, air condensing from the normal atmosphere can have an oxygen concentration of up to 50% (see Fig. 11-4) and is even more hazardous than liquid air.

11-5-1 Fuels (Hydrogen and LNG)

Three ingredients are needed for combustion to occur. These are a fuel, an oxidizer, and an ignition source. Safety of operation requires that, wherever possible, the attempt should be made to eliminate two of these three at a given location. Consequently, every effort must be made to eliminate ignition sources. Ignition sources include such obvious things as open flames, smoking, and welding. Less obvious and more difficult to control ignition sources include static electricity, sparking devices, high-velocity impact of solid particles, heat of rapid compression, and friction. The elimination of these ignition sources requires precautions such as using approved electrical devices, assuring the absence of unwanted solid particles within the system, properly designing equipment, and properly operating the system [1].

Combustible mixtures must also be avoided. This effort involves complete purging of residual air from the system before introducing the combustible cryogen. In the case of hydrogen, everything other than helium can be condensed to a solid at the temperature of the liquid hydrogen. This results in another reason for complete purging because, even if not combustible, such particles can cause erosion of valve seats or can block access to relief valve ports.

Flammable substances are ignitable within a range of composition that is dependent upon temperature and pressure of the mixture. Combustion can be a reaction of fuel and oxidizer that is controlled by heat transfer from the burning substances into the adjacent combustible mixture, heating it to its ignition temperature. This combustion reaction is called "deflagration." A more vigorous reaction occurs if the combustible mixture is heated to the ignition temperature by a shock wave. This is termed "detonation." Although either of these reactions presents a definite hazard, detonation is generally much more serious. Concentration ranges of combustibility and detonability can be found in the literature [1,16,17].

11-5-2 Oxidizers

Oxygen is sufficiently reactive that almost anything that is not already completely oxidized can be made to burn if the right conditions exist. Stainless steel has been known to burn in the presence of liquid oxygen. Consequently, in the handling of oxygen, two of the three ingredients necessary for combustion (fuel and oxidizer) are almost always present. This fact makes even more important the elimination of ignition sources, including all of those mentioned above.

Liquid air (21% oxygen) and air condensed from the atmosphere are also hazardous substances, but, as the oxygen content is increased, the mixture becomes even more hazardous. Figure 11-8 illustrates the increase in reactivity of a substance as the oxygen concentration is increased. In this case an adhesive (HT-424) is used as an illustration.

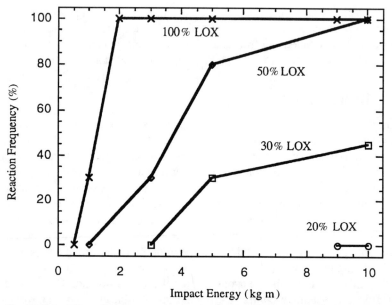

Figure 11-8 Effect of liquid oxygen (LOX) concentration on reaction of HT-424 adhesive.

However, similar behavior is obtained with many materials. The data shown are for tests in which a variable mass is dropped on a striker pin attached to the specimen, which is immersed in the liquid oxygen–nitrogen mixture. From the number of ignitions, as shown in Fig. 11-8, it can be seen that, although a 50% oxygen mixture is not as reactive as 100% oxygen, it still is much more reactive than true liquid air (21% oxygen) [18].

Safety in working with oxygen requires the proper selection of materials and scrupulous cleanliness. Materials with high ignition temperatures, high specific heats, high thermal conductivity, and low heats of reaction are desirable [1,19]. Cleanliness is important because most impurities will have lower ignition temperatures. If the impurities ignite, this combustion can subsequently ignite materials that otherwise would not have been ignited. Several cleaning methods and cleaning agents are recommended [1,20].

11-6 REGULATIONS, STANDARDS, AND GUIDELINES

There are three types of safety documents. Regulations are enacted by governmental bodies and have the force of law. Standards (also known as codes) are usually issued by associations with a wide range of members as a means of ensuring that common safety interests are met in a uniform and predictable manner. Standards are typically thought of as representing the consensus of technical experts on the subject at hand. Guidelines are developed by organizations based on their specific needs. The three types of documents are not mutually exclusive. Regulations frequently incorporate standards, either directly or by reference, thus giving them the force of law. Standards often refer to other standards or regulations to avoid repetition and to reduce inconsistencies, which can develop when differing groups cover the same subject matter. Guidelines can require members or employees of their organization to follow standards and frequently cite relevant regulations and standards to ensure they are applied when appropriate.

There are usually several levels at which governmental regulations can be established. These range from cities or counties at the local level, to states or provinces at the regional level, and to the federal or national government at the highest level. In the United States, for example, national regulations are found in the Code of Federal Regulations (CFR). The two titles most relevant to cryogenics are Title 29, Labor, which covers occupational safety and health and Title 49, Transportation, which covers the transportation of hazardous materials. In addition, groups of nations can develop consistent standards through organizations such as the International Standards Organization (ISO) and then incorporate these standards into regulations or treaties.

In addition to the ISO, many nations have their own standards organizations. It is not possible to list them all here, but representative associations in the United States include the following: American Society of Mechanical Engineers (ASME), American National Standards Institute (ANSI), American Society for Testing and Materials (ASTM), National Fire Protection Association (NFPA), Factory Mutual Engineering and Research (FM), and the Compresssed Gas Association (CGA). In addition to their safety value, many of these standards provide useful design information.

Guidelines are developed by companies, laboratories, and universities to address the specific needs of each organization. They are frequently available upon request and can provide valuable information and advice. All of the above documents can change with time, and thus one must be aware of the latest developments to ensure that current safety documents are followed.

11-7 CONCLUSIONS

At this point it should be clear that safety is a philosophy that must be integrated into all aspects of any cryogenic project. It is not an afterthought that can be adequately addressed after a system has been designed or built. Consideration of safety should begin at the conceptual design phase and continue through final design, procurement of equipment, fabrication, and assembly. Careful consideration at the conceptual design phase can often eliminate problems that will require complicated and expensive corrections if addressed later.

Safety is not finished when a project becomes operational. Operation requires planning, which includes established standard operating procedures and written checklists as well as previously thought-out responses to unexpected behavior of systems and emergencies (contingency checklists). It is important to avoid modifying any system without examining all of the possible consequences. Many accidents are caused by the unexpected consequences of quick repairs instituted without a thorough understanding of all aspects of system operation.

Finally, training of personnel should be a continuing effort and should not merely be passed from one employee to the next without some referral back to the fundamental safety requirements of the system. Without structured training of new personnel there is no way to be sure that all hazards are identified and all safety issues are adequately addressed.

REFERENCES

1. Edeskuty, F. J., and Stewart, W. F., *Safety in the Handling of Cryogenic Fluids* (New York: Plenum Press, 1996).
2. Gonzalez, F., and Walton, R. L., "Cold-Induced Tissue Injuries," Chap. 199 in *The Clinical Practice of Emergency Medicine*, A. Harwood-Nuss, C. H. Linden, R. C. Luten, G. Sternbach, and A. B. Wolfson, eds. (Philadelphia: J. B. Lippincott Co., 1991).
3. Klainer, P., "Hypothermia," Chap. 200 in *The Clinical Practice of Emergency Medicine*, A. Harwood-Nuss, C. H. Linden, R. C. Luten, G. Sternbach, and A. B. Wolfson, eds. (Philadelphia: J. B. Lippincott Co., 1991).
4. *Oxygen Deficient Atmospheres (less than 19.5%)*, Compressed Gas Association Bulletin CGA SB-2 (Arlington, Varginia: Compressed Gas Association, 1992).
5. *Carbon Dioxide*, Compressed Gas Association Bulletin CGA G-6 (Arlington, Virginia: Compressed Gas Association, 1984).
6. *Safe Handling of Liquid Carbon Monoxide*, Compressed Gas Association Bulletin CGA-P-13 (Arlington, Virginia: Compressed Gas Association, 1989).
7. American Conference of Government Industrial Hygienists Technical Information Office (Glenway Ave. Bldg. D-7, Cincinnati, OH 45211, 1993).
8. *1992–1993 Threshold Limit Values for Chemical Substances and Physical Agents and Biological Exposure Indices* (Cincinnati, Ohio: American Conference of Governmental Industrial Hygienists, 1992).
9. Gatwood, G. T., and Murphy, G. F., "Safety in the Chemical Laboratory: Ozone Hazards," *J. Chem. Ed.* 46, 1969):A103–A105.
10. Zabetakis, M. G., *Safety with Cryogenic Fluids* (New York: Plenum Press, 1967).
11. Dodge, B. F., *Chemical Engineering Thermodynamics* (New York: McGraw–Hill, 1944).
12. "Pressure Relief Device Standards, Part 2—Cargo and Portable Tanks for Compressed Gases," CGA S-1.2 (Arlington, VA: Compressed Gas Association, 1994).
13. Gu, Y., and Timmerhaus, K. D., "Experimental Verification of Stability Characteristics for Thermal Acoustic Oscillations in a Liquid Helium System," *Adv. Cryog. Eng.* 39B (1994):1733–1740.
14. Johnson, P. C., "Liquefied Natural Gas," Chap. 3 in *Liquid Cryogens*, vol. II, K. D. Williamson, Jr., and F. J. Edeskuty, eds. (Boca Raton, Florida: CRC Press, 1983).
15. Novak, J. K., "Cool-down Flow Rate Limits Imposed by Thermal Stresses in Liquid Hydrogen or Nitrogen Pipelines," *Adv. Cryog. Eng.* 15 (1970):346–353.
16. Coward, H. F., and Jones, G. W., *Limits of Flammability of Gases and Vapors*, U.S. Bureau of Mines Bulletin 503 (Washington, D.C.: U.S. Government Printing Office, 1952).
17. Zabetakis, M. G., *Flammable Characteristics of Combustible Gases and Vapors*, U.S. Bureau of Mines Bulletin 627 (Washington, D.C.: U.S. Government Printing Office, 1965).
18. Key, C. F., *Compatibility of Materials with Liquid Oxygen*, vol. 1, NASA Technical Memorandum, NASA TM X-64711 (Alabama: George C. Marshall Space Flight Center, October 1972).
19. Schmidt, H. W., and Forney, D. E., *ASRDI Oxygen Technology Survey*, vol. IX, *Oxygen Systems Engineering Review*, NASA Report SP-3090 (Springfield, Virginia: National Technical Information Service, 1975).
20. "Cleaning Equipment for Oxygen Service," CGA G-4.1 (Arlington VA: Compressed Gas Association, 1985).

INDEX*

ALLPROPS, 21, 71
aluminum alloys, 261, 485
    thermal expansion, 351T, 493F
ammonia, 7T
argon, 1, 7T, 51–60, 489T
Arrhenius equation, 127, 149
asphyxiation, 483–484

bayonet joints, 275, 276F, 367–369
Benedict–Webb–Rubin (BWR) equation, 15
Bi, Pb (2223) tapes,
    anisotropy in critical current, 108
    critical current, 104–109
    enhancement of matrix resistivity, 110
    fabrication, 103–107
    limitations on engineering critical current, 111
    reinforcement by dispersion hardening, 110
Blausius correlation, 459

CFCs, 281, 285, 284T
cable-in-conduit conductors, 330
    stability of, 344–345
carbon dioxide, 1, 7T, 484, 489T
Carnot cycle, 288–290
coefficient of performance, 288, 289
cold compressors, 393–399
    bearings, 396F
    ejectors, 394, 398–399, 400F, 401F, 402F
    performance, 399F
    range of operation, 394F
    turbocompressors, 394–398

cold end recovery, 342–343
cold seals, 263–266
combustion, 494–496
composite materials, 261, 346
    advantages of, 92
    comparisons to metals, 95–96
    design with, 96–98
    examples of use, 99–101
    fatigue in, 94, 97F
    fibers, 92–93
    laminates, 92
    nomenclature, 101–102
    properties of, 94–97
copper, 261
    thermal conductivity, 214T
    thermal expansion, 347T, 351T, 492F, 493F
critical current. *See* superconductors,
critical heat flux for helium, 181–185
cryocoolers,
    actual efficiency, 299F
    adsorption cryocoolers, 318–319
    applications, 287
    choosing, 319
    compound Gifford McMahon and
        Joule–Thomson cryocoolers, 306–307
    future trends, 311–318
    Gifford McMahon cryocooler, 113, 116,
        291–292, 302–306
    inefficiencies in, 295–298
    Joule–Thomson cryocooler, 299–301
    pulse tube cryocoolers, 314–317
    Stirling cryocooler, 292–293, 308–311

*T denotes Table
 F denotes Figure

cryocoolers, (*contd.*)
    summary of, 313T
    thermodynamics, 288–295
cryostat,
    design considerations, 259–260
    design with vapor cooled shields, 268–269
    requirements, 259
    supports, 98–100, 267–268
    useful materials for, 260–263
Curie temperature, 113, 118
current leads,
    comparison of cryogenic loads, 409F, 411T
    conduction cooled, 399, 403–404, 405F
    gas cooled, 400, 404–408
    heat sinking of, 412
    hybrid, 400, 408–413
    optimization of, 408, 410T, 410F

DC breakdown voltage. *See* dielectric strength,
density, 10
    argon, 51–60
    helium, 23–32
    nitrogen, 33–40
    oxygen, 9F, 41–50
    parahydrogen, 61–70
density wave oscillations, 378–380
Dewar. *See* cryostat,
diamagnet, 118
dielectric strength,
    helium, 347T
    polymers, 154, 156T, 347T

E-glass, 92, 101
Er_3Ni, 113, 118F, 312, 314F, 423
electrical resistivity, 410T
    rare earth elements, 116T
embrittlement, 484–486
emittance, 188–191
enthalpy,
    argon, 51–60
    helium, 23–32
    nitrogen, 33–40
    oxygen, 41–50
    parahydrogen, 61–70
entropy,
    argon, 51–60
    helium, 23–32
    nitrogen, 33–40
    oxygen, 41–50
    parahydrogen, 61–70
entropy generation, 413–414
equal area (Maddock) criterion, 342–343
Ericsson cycle, 289–290
ethane, 1, 7T
exergy, 394, 413

ferrimagnet, 118
ferromagnet, 119
flowmeters,

angular momentum, 242–243
    doppler shift, 243–244
    fluidic, 244
    He II, 475–478
    hot wire, 243
    laminar flow, 246–247
    oriface plate, 245–246
    positive displacement, 244
    suppliers of, 252–253
    temperature pulse, 244
    thermal, 243
    turbine, 244
    Venturi, 246
fluids,
    calculation of properties using scaling laws, 5–7,
        9F–20F
    computer programs for property calculation, 21,
        71
    critical properties, 7T
    impact of critical point, 15–16, 180
    state properties, 2–18
    strongly and weakly divergent parameters,
        16–18
    thermophysical properties, 1–21
    transport properties, 18–21
    See also specific fluids,
friction,
    coefficients, 75, 76
    data, 80–83
    dynamic, 74, 76–77
    experimental measurement of, 78–80
    influence on superconducting magnet design, 77,
        83–88
    lubricants, 74
    polymer aspects, 74, 88–89
    static, 74–76
    stick–slip phenomena in, 77, 81
friction factor,
    pipe, 370F
    slush hydrogen, 376F

G-10 CR, 93, 101, 261, 346
G-11 CR, 261, 346
Gadolinium Gallium Garnet (GGG), 113, 115, 117F
GASPAK, 21, 22, 71
ground loops, 210
Grüneisen parameter, 8, 141–145,

Hall effect, 248–249
Hastalloy, 262
hazards, 481–496
heat capacity. *See* specific heat,
heat exchangers,
    characteristics, 414–415
    counterflow, 415
    design of 423–429
    effectiveness, 424
    flow maldistribution, 427–429
    Hampson (coiled tube), 416, 418F

heat transfer capacity, 420T
He II, 466–470
overall heat transfer coefficient, 425
perforated plate, 419, 420F
plate fin, 416, 419
pressure drop in, 432–435
recuperative, 415–419
See also regenerators,
heat transfer coefficient correlations,
gases, 180
helium, 180
Hydrogen, 180
inside tubes, 432
liquids, 179
outside tubes, 432
plate fin surfaces, 432, 433F
regenerator surfaces, 433, 434F
supercritical fluids, 180
He II, 3
critical velocity, 453
density, 445, 447, 451
entropy, 449
expansivity, 447
film boiling heat transfer, 463
first sound, 451, 453F
flow metering, 475–478
forced flow heat transfer, 458
fountain effect, 454
heat exchangers, 466–470
isothermal compressibility, 448
Kapitza conductance, 460–462
laminar heat flow conductivity, 452T, 454
laminar mass flow, 453–455
latent heat, 449–450
peak heat flux, 457
phase diagram, 444F
phase separators, 473–475
pressure drop, 459–460
pumping, 383F, 470–473
saturation properties, 446T
second sound, 451, 453F
specific heat, 448–449
surface heat transfer, 460–463
surface tension, 449–450
transient heat transfer, 458, 459F
turbulent flow heat conductivity, 455, 456T
two fluid model, 450
viscosity, 450, 451, 452T
Helium 1, 6, 7T
Thermophysical properties of, 23–32, 490T
Helmhotz resonator, 375, 377
Hepak 21, 22, 71
high temperature superconductors. *See also* Bi, Pb
(2223), 86
hydrogen, 1, 6, 7T, 495, 489T, 490T
embrittlement, 486
ortha, 3–4
para, 3–4
slush, 374–375, 389F

thermophysical properties of, 4–5, 61–70
hypothermia, 482

ideal gas equation, 13
indium, 264
insulating materials,
electrical and thermal properties (table), 347
Invar, 262–263, 493F
ionizing radiation,
effect on polymers, 151–156
effect on temperature sensors, 221T, 222T
irreversibility distribution, 414
isenthalpic compressibility, 8
isentropic compressibility, 8
isothermal compressibility, 8

Joule–Thomson coefficient, 8, 12, 293
Joule–Thomson expansion, 293–295
gas mixtures for, 313–314
maximum inversion temperature of, 294T
Joule–Thomson refrigeration cycles, 294–296,
463–465

krypton, 1, 7T

lambda line, 3, 445T
law of corresponding states, 7
liquefied natural gas (LNG),
safety aspects, 490, 494, 495
liquid air, 495–496
liquid level sensors, 247–248, 252–253
London's equation, 454, 472
Lorentz number, 403

magnetic measurement, 248–250
magnetic refrigeration,
materials for, 112–115, 116T, 117F
nomenclature, 118–119
magnetocaloric effect, 113, 114, 119
maximum adiabatic zone (MAZ), 84–85
measurement,
AC instrumentation for, 214–215
accuracy, 205
cold electronics, 215–216
control circuits, 215
DC instrumentation for, 213–214
pulse techniques, 215
resolution, 204
system design, 203–205
uncertainty, 206–211
Meissner effect, 322–323
methane, 1, 7T
minimum propagating zone (MPZ), 84, 343–344
minimum quench energy (MQE), 84, 85, 86,
343–344
multilayer insulation systems (MLI),
description, 187
effect of vacuum pressure, 196–199
heat transfer through, 182–183, 268
ideal, parametric curves for, 193–196

multilayer insulation systems (MLI), (*contd.*)
  practical, 195–196
  testing, 188

Néel temperature, 119
neon, 1, 7T, 489T, 490T
net positive suction head (NPSH), 381
niobium aluminum, 324, 326, 328
niobium tin, 324, 326–328
  electrical insulation for, 346
  formulas for critical parameters, 327
  strand, 328
niobium titanium, 324, 325, 326
  formulas for critical parameters, 326
NIST-12, 21, 71
nitrogen, 7T, 122
  thermophysical properties, 33–40,
    489T–490T
number of transfer units (NTU), 424
Nussult number (Nu), 179,

oxidizers, 495–496
oxygen, 7T, 489T, 490T
  thermophysical properties, 9F–20F, 22, 41–
    50
oxygen deficiency, 483
  symptoms of, 483T

paramagnet, 119
polymers, 8, 74, 88–89, 346–348
  accuracy of data, 122–123
  annealing, 123
  basic properties, 125
  binding potential, 125
  bulk properties, 124T
  creep modulus, 131
  cryogenic applications of, 123–124
  damping behavior, 127–129
  deformation, 130–133
  dielectric properties, 128–129, 134, 156T
  fatigue behavior, 137–138
  fracture behavior, 135–137, 161T
  gas permeability, 147–151
  glass transitions, 127
  Grüneisen relation, 144–145
  molecular motions, 125–126
  radiation damage to, 151–156
  relaxation compliance, 131–132
  shear moduli, 133, 161T
  solubility, 149–150
  specific heat, 139–140, 155F
  stress intensity factor, 135
  tensile moduli, 130–133, 161T
  thermal conductivity, 145–146, 147T, 155F,
    160F
  thermal cycling, 123
  thermal diffusivity, 146
  thermal expansion, 141–145, 158T, 159F
  thermal vibrations, 138–139

tunneling processes, 126
  universal low temperature properties, 125
Prandtl number (Pr), 21–22, 179
pressure buildup, 486–491
pressure drop,
  bellows, 373
  bends, 372F
  coiled tubing, 373
  enlargements and contractions, 369, 373–374
  He II, 459–460
  near critical flows, 373
  plate fin surfaces, 433F
  single phase flow, 369
  tube banks, 432
  valves and fittings, 369, 371T
  woven screen, 435F
pressure oscillations. *See* thermal acoustic
    oscillations,
pressure relief valves, 489–490
pressure sensors, 236–239T
  capacitive, 241
  piezoelectric, 241–242
  piezoresistive (strain gage), 237–240
  properties of, 239T
  suppliers of, 252–253
  variable reluctance, 241
propane, 1, 7T
pumps, 380–381
  axial flow, 381
  cavitation in, 381, 386, 390F
  centrifugal, 381–390
  characteristic curves, 384, 388F–389F
  efficiency of, 381, 387
  fountain effect, 381, 472–475
  He II, 388F, 470–473
  piston, 392F
  positive displacement, 380, 392–393

quench,
  current diffusion, 350
  hot spot criterion, 351–353
  maximum current and voltage in, 350–351
  propagation, 349–350
  protection, 353–355
quench back, 353

refrigerants,
  azeotropic mixtures, 282
  classification, 279–283
  environmental impact of, 283
  properties of, 281T
  regulations concerning, 284T
  selection of, 284–285
  zeotropic, 282
Regenerators, 290, 419–423
  design of, 429–431
  magnetic materials for, 115–118, 312–313
Reynolds number (Re), 179, 459
Rutherford cable, 329

S-glass, 92, 102
sensors, 205
    calibration of, 210–211
    excitation of, 234
    self-heating in, 207–209, 231–234
    suppliers of, 252–253
    See also specific types (temperature, pressure, level, strain, magnetic),
slush hydrogen. *See* hydrogen,
sound velocity, 9, 10
specific diameter, 383, 387F
specific heat, 10
    argon, 51–60
    helium, 23–32
    nitrogen, 33–40
    oxygen, 41–50, 11, 12F, 13F
    parahydrogen, 4, 61–70
    polymers, 139–140, 155F
    rare earth elements, 116T, 314F
    regenerator materials, 118F, 314F
specific speed, 383, 387F
steel,
    nickel, 260
    stainless, 260, 268, 485
Stekly criterion, 342
Stirling cycle, 289–290
strain measurement, 234–236
superconducting magnets,
    AC losses, 334–340
    applications, 321
    conductor assembly, 329–330
    cooling, 331–332, 340–341
    coupling current losses, 337–340
    design, 330–333
    electrical insulation, 346–348
    examples of, 356–361
    friction effects on, 77, 83–88
    magnetization, 334–337
    quench protection, 332, 349–355
    stability criteria, 332, 333, 342–346
    vacuum impregnation of, 348–349
superconductors,
    critical parameters of, 322–323
    thermal behavior of, 341–342
    Type I, 323, 324T
    Type II, 323–325
    See also specific materials,
superfluid helium. *See* He II,

temperature glide, 282F
temperature sensors, 216–234
    dimensionless temperature sensitivities of, 223F
    effect of ionizing radiation, 221T, 222T
    effect of magnetic fields (magnetoresistance), 220T, 225F, 226F
    relative temperature resolutions of, 224F
    self-heating in, 231–234
    suppliers of, 252–253

thermal response time of, 219T
    types, 217T
thermal acoustic oscillations, 366, 375, 377–378
    impact on safety, 490
thermal conductivity, 9, 18–21
    argon, 51–60
    composite materials, 96, 268, 347T
    helium, 347T, 23–32
    ideal gas, 21
    multilayer insulation (MLI), 268
    nitrogen, 33–40
    oxygen, 20F, 41–50
    parahydrogen, 5, 61–70
    polymers, 96F, 145–146, 147T, 155F, 160F, 347T
    rare earth elements, 116T
    stainless steel, 268
    wires and adhesive materials, 214T
    See also thermal conductivity integrals,
thermal conductivity integrals, 163–164, 165F, 166F, 214T
thermal contact conductance, 164, 167
    effect of applied force, 167, 168, 175–177
    effect of coatings, 167, 170, 175–178
    effect of surface finish, 173–174
    experimental data, 169T, 171–178
thermal contraction (expansion),
    aluminum, 351T, 493F
    copper, 347T, 351T, 492F, 493F
    fiberglass, 347T, 351T
    Invar, 493F
    iron, 351T
    lead, 493F
    nylon, 347T
    polymers, 141–145, 158T, 159F
    stainless steel, 351T
    Teflon, 493F
thermal expansivity, 8, 10
thermal noise (Johnson), 209
thermal stratification, 488
thermocouples, 229–231, 252–253
    fits for calibration of, 230T
thermolelectric voltages, 209–210
thermoplastics, 102
thermoresins, 94, 102
thermosets, 94, 102
Thoma cavitation coefficient, 388, 390F
titanium, 262
toxicity, 484
transfer lines, 365–366
    connections in, 273, 275–277, 367–369
    design of, 269–270
    pumping out of, 275, 278
    spacers for, 270, 271–272
    thermal contraction in, 270–273, 274F, 366, 493–494
transposed critical line, 2
tribology. *See* friction,

ullage, 487

valves, 366–368, 371T
van der Waals equation, 14
vapor cooled shields, 268–269
viscosity, 9, 18–21
    argon, 51–60
    helium, 23–32
    nitrogen, 33–40
    oxygen, 19F, 41–50
    parahydrogen, 61–70

virial equation, 13, 14
Von Kármán–Nikuradse correlation, 459

Wagner equation, 15
Wiedemann–Franz law, 401, 408
wiring, 211–213
    heat sinking of, 212–213, 213T
    thermal conductivity of, 214T

xenon, 1, 7T